AF565590

Geriatric Nephrology and Urology

Edited by

EDWARD T. ZAWADA, JR.
DOMENIC A. SICA

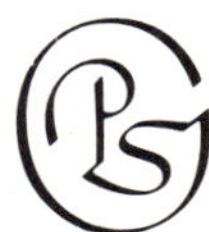

PSG PUBLISHING COMPANY, INC.
LITTLETON, MASSACHUSETTS

Library of Congress Cataloging in Publication Data
Main entry under title:

Geriatric nephrology and urology.

Includes bibliographies and index.
1. Geriatric nephrology. 2. Geriatric urology.
I. Zawada, Edward T. (Edward Thaddeus), 1947–
II. Sica, Domenic A. [DNLM: 1. Kidney Diseases–in old age. 2. Urologic Diseases–in old age.
WJ 100 G369]
RC903.G47 1985 618.97'66 84-18927
ISBN 0-88416-476-4

Published by:
PSG PUBLISHING COMPANY, INC.
545 Great Road
Littleton, Massachusetts 01460

Printed in the United States of America

International Standard Book Number: 0-88416-476-4

Library of Congress Catalog Card Number: 84-18927

Last digit is the print number: 9 8 7 6 5 4 3 2 1

CONTRIBUTORS

Ashley Bequero, MD
Transplantation Fellow
Medical College of Virginia
Richmond, Virginia

Nachman Brautbar, MD
Director of Renal Research
Associate Professor of Medicine and Pharmacology
University of Southern California
Los Angeles, California

Robert M. Centor, MD
Assistant Professor of Medicine
Medical College of Virginia
Richmond, Virginia

Kenneth L. Duchin, PhD
Associate Clinical Pharmacology Director
Squibb Institute for Medical Research
E. R. Squibb & Sons
Princeton, New Jersey

Murray Epstein, MD
Professor of Medicine
University of Miami School of Medicine
Associate Chief of Nephrology
Miami VA Medical Center
Miami, Florida

William Falls, MD
Chief, Nephrology Section
McGuire VA Medical Center
Professor of Medicine
Medical College of Virginia
Richmond, Virginia

Anthony Furlan, MD
Head, Section of Adult Clinical Neurology
Cleveland Clinic
Cleveland, Ohio

Mitchell H. Goldman, MD
Chief, Transplant Service
Associate Professor of Surgery
University of Tennessee School of Medicine
Knoxville, Tennessee

David A. Goodkin, MD
Clinical Instructor
Temple University School of Medicine
Philadelphia, Pennsylvania

Helen Gruber, PhD
Division of Nephrology
University of Southern California
Los Angeles, California

Jessie E. Hano, MD
Chief of Nephrology
Professor of Medicine
Loyola University Stritch School of Medicine
Maywood, Illinois

Antonia Harford, MD
Assistant Professor of Medicine
Medical College of Virginia
Richmond, Virginia

Frank Hinman, Jr, MD
Clinical Professor of Surgery
Department of Urology
University of California School of Medicine
San Francisco, California

Frederick A. Klein, MD
Assistant Professor of Urology/Surgery
Medical College of Virginia
Richmond, Virginia

Robert H. Lippman, MD
Assistant Professor, Pathology
Medical College of Virginia
Richmond, Virginia

Shaul G. Massry, MD
Chief, Division of Nephrology
Bernard J. Hanley Professor of Medicine and Professor of Physiology and Biophysics
University of Southern California School of Medicine
Los Angeles, California

Robert G. Narins, MD
Chief, Division of Nephrology
Professor of Medicine
Temple University School of Medicine
Philadelphia, Pennsylvania

Scott Norris, MD
Transplantation Fellow
Medical College of Virginia
Richmond, Virginia

Donald Oken, MD
Professor of Medicine
Medical College of Virginia
Richmond, Virginia

German Ramirez, MD
Chief, Nephrology Section
Tampa VA Medical Center
Associate Professor of Medicine
University of South Florida
Tampa, Florida

Sabiba R. Saba, MD
Chief, Blood Bank
Laboratory Service
Tampa VA Medical Center
Assistant Professor of Pathology
University of South Florida
School of Medicine
Tampa, Florida

Lakhi Sakhrani, MD
Assistant Professor of Medicine
University of Southern California School of Medicine
Los Angeles, California

Peter F. Schatzki, MD
Director, Clinical Pathology
McGuire VA Medical Center
Professor of Laboratory Pathology
Medical College of Virginia
Richmond, Virginia

Charles J. Schleupner, MD
Chief, Infectious Disease
Salem VA Medical Center
Associate Professor of Medicine
University of Virginia School of Medicine
Charlottesville, Virginia

Domenic A. Sica, MD
Assistant Professor of Medicine
Medical College of Virginia
Richmond, Virginia

James R. Sowers, MD
Chief, Endocrinology and Hypertension
Professor, Medicine and Physiology
Wayne State Medical School
Detroit, Michigan

William K. Stacy, MD
Chief, Dialysis Unit
Chief, End Stage Renal Disease Program
McGuire VA Medical Center
Associate Professor of Medicine
Medical College of Virginia
Richmond, Virginia

Barry M. Stults, MD
Assistant Professor of Medicine and Geriatrics
University of Utah Medical Center
Salt Lake City, Utah

Keith Van Arsdalen, MD
Assistant Professor of Urology
University of Pennsylvania School of Medicine
Philadelphia, Pennsylvania

Robert Waldman, MD
Associate Director of Hemodialysis
Ushawl Artificial Kidney Centers
Los Angeles, California

Alan J. Wein, MD
Chairman, Division of Urology
Professor of Urology
University of Pennsylvania School of Medicine
Philadelphia, Pennsylvania

Allen I. Wolfert, MD
Instructor, Department of Medicine
Medical College of Virginia
Richmond, Virginia

Edward T. Zawada, Jr, MD
Chairman, Division of Nephrology and Hypertension
Associate Professor of Medicine, Physiology and Pharmacology
University of South Dakota School of Medicine
Sioux Falls, South Dakota

CONTENTS

This volume is dedicated
to friendship and its role
in furthering scholarly activity.

FOREWORD

Geriatric Nephrology and Urology represents an important undertaking in the realm of geriatric subspecialty texts. The subject matter of this book exemplifies the nearly continuous growth that the geriatric field has experienced over the last decade. Although medical knowledge in this area has rapidly advanced, much of what we know rests on a groundwork of information acquired during the 1950s. Because of this, the goal of this geriatric textbook has been not only to address the integrally related disciplines of nephrology and urology but also to examine how current concepts in these areas might have become so commonplace.

The textbook encompasses "traditional" topics such as fluid and electrolyte abnormalities and urinary incontinence. In this respect it differs little from previously published texts in the geriatric field. Where this text substantially departs from prior efforts in this area is in the thoroughness with which nephrologic and urologic structure, function and disease are addressed in geriatric patients who represent the most rapidly expanding sector of society.

Within the nephrology section the case is made for protein excess causing hyperfiltration with resultant glomerular sclerosis and renal senescence, a concept currently undergoing intensive investigation. Diseases of the glomeruli, tubules, and lower urinary tract are systematically examined. Aspects of fluid and electrolytes including hyponatremia, acid-base disturbances and renal function testing are carefully explored.

Chapters on acute and chronic renal failure clearly point out the different ways in which these entities develop and progress in the elderly. Though management of renal failure is difficult in these patients it is surmountable. Notwithstanding this, special problems exist in the elderly if one is to utilize either dialysis or transplantation as part of a therapeutic strategy. Chapters on both of these topics carefully address these considerations. Similarly, the chapters in the area of hypertension carefully consider the uniqueness of hypertension in the elderly and examine medical and surgical considerations in this increasingly important area.

Genitourinary malignancies occupy a large section of the urology section. An extensive review of staging, surgical management and the roles of radiation and chemotherapy is offered. In this section the interdisciplinary convergence of nephrology and urology is further demonstrated by discussions of urinary tract infections, voiding disturbances, and obstructive uropathy. Finally, the growing interest in sexuality among the elderly led to the inclusion of a chapter on this important subject.

Nephrology and urology have always been closely linked disciplines but nowhere more so than in the field of geriatrics. It is hoped that this effort not only bridges the gap between these specialty areas but also that each area is considered in sufficient detail so that the reader perceives the salient features of each topic. Thus, physicians should gain a gerontologic data base of sufficient scope to facilitate diagnosis and management of our increasingly large elderly population.

Edward T. Zawada Jr, MD
Domenic A. Sica, MD

ABOUT THE EDITORS

Edward T. Zawada Jr., M.D. is Associate Professor of Internal Medicine, Physiology, and Pharmacology, and Chief of the Division of Nephrology and Hypertension for the University of South Dakota School of Medicine. Doctor Zawada graduated *summa cum laude* from Loyola University in 1969 and also *summa cum laude* as class valedictorian from Loyola University Stritch School of Medicine in 1973. All of his postgraduate training in internal medicine and nephrology was done at UCLA Hospitals and Clinics. A diplomate of the American Board of Internal Medicine in both internal medicine and the subspeciality of nephrology, he is a member of 15 scientific societies and a Fellow of the American College of Physicians, the American College of Chest Physicians, and the American College of Nutrition. Doctor Zawada is President of the Minnehaha Division of the Dakota Affiliate of the American Heart Association. He is the author of over 85 publications related to internal medicine, chest medicine and surgery, nephrology and hypertension, and urology.

Domenic A. Sica, M.D. is Assistant Professor of Internal Medicine in the Division of Nephrology at the Medical College of Virginia in Richmond. Doctor Sica graduated from Fordham University in 1971 and the Medical College of Virginia in 1975. A diplomate of the American Board of Internal Medicine in both internal medicine and the subspecialty of nephrology, he is a member of 10 scientific societies including the American and International Societies of Nephrology and the American Federation for Clinical Research. Doctor Sica is the author of over 75 publications relating to various aspects of nephrology and pharmacology.

CHAPTER 1 Renal Physiologic Changes with Age

Murray Epstein

The kidney participates in the aging process and much attention has been devoted to studying the effects of aging on the kidney. These changes are both structural and functional. This chapter will consider briefly the changes in renal anatomy with age and follow this with a more detailed discussion of the changes in renal function with senescence. Although senescence is associated with a wide range of renal functional changes, this chapter will deal only with the following aspects of renal function: (*a*) renal plasma and blood flow; (*b*) glomerular filtration rate; (*c*) renal sodium and potassium handling; and (*d*) renal concentrating and diluting ability.

Anatomy of the Aging Kidney

The alterations in renal anatomy that accompany advancing age[1–3] are considered in detail in chapter 2. It is important to highlight a few of the florid alterations. The total and cortical renal mass, the number and surface area of glomeruli, and length and volume of the proximal tubule are known to decrease with age. Consequently, the kidneys in an average 40-year-old person, which weigh 250 g, decrease to 200 g by age 80. These anatomical changes are postulated to be a consequence of specific vascular changes involving the kidneys, but nonischemic involutional processes might also be involved.

Alterations in the arterial tree and the glomerular and tubular basement membranes have also been demonstrated by histologic studies. Medial hypertrophy, intimal proliferation, and hyalinization of the renal arterial vessels are seen with increased frequency from the third to the tenth decade. These anatomical abnormalities suggest that outer cortical blood flow decreases during senescence, while inner cortical and medullary perfusion remains relatively well preserved.

The decrease with age in the length of the proximal convoluted tubule has been found to occur in a fashion that parallels the decrease in size of the glomerulus. Thus, the ratio of the glomerular surface to the proximal tubular length remains constant. This relationship could possibly explain the *parallel* decline in glomerular and tubular function observed with age.

Changes in Renal Function with Age

As noted previously, the assessment of the effects of aging on any process in man raises two major problems. The first problem involves the selection of an appropriate population, and the second problem involves the definition of normality. Shock,[4] who has had the largest experience in this field, has stressed the importance of the sampling problem in the assessment of phenomena relating to senescence. In many studies, young individuals, frequently students, have been compared with elderly subjects. Furthermore, the elderly subjects are generally selected from nursing homes and the wards of general hospitals and chronic disease facilities and are not representative of that segment of the population still residing and functioning in the community. In an attempt to obviate many of these problems, several investigators have drawn on a unique subset of active normal individuals, ie, potential kidney donors, some of whom were in their seventh decade.[5,6] In the course of assessing their suitability for major surgery and the loss of a kidney, all undergo a thorough, extensive diagnostic evaluation that excludes unsuspected, potentially relevant disease.

Another problem that confounds the interpretation of many studies is that most gerontologic investigations have utilized a cross-sectional design to demonstrate a decline of varying functional parameters with age. Despite attempts to exclude subjects with overt renal disease, subclinical renal impairment that adversely affected renal function may have gone unnoticed. Another error inherent in the design of cross-sectional studies is the concept of "selective mortality" developed by Andres.[7] In brief, in the interpretation of cross-sectional studies, it is important to remember that subjects over the age of 75 years represent a sample of biologically superior survivors from a cohort that has experienced at least a 75% mortality. If the variable under study is related to survival, either because it is a risk factor or because it has a protective effect, a cross-sectional study will seem to show age-related differences that do not exist. In order to obviate these problems, the workers at the Gerontology Research Center in Baltimore have advocated increasing reliance on longitudinal studies.

Animal Studies and Their Relevance to an Understanding of Renal Senescence in Man

In an attempt to further understand the naturally occurring long-term changes in both structure and function of the kidney, many investigators have resorted to animal studies, and most particularly studies in the rat. Since a major segment of the literature encompassing aging and the kidney tends to extrapolate from rat to man, a cautionary note is in order. Rats, indeed most other rodents studied, may be unfortunate models from which to judge long-term effects of any variable that might affect renal structure or function, since, in the absence of any known perturbation, they spontaneously develop structural and functional nephron alterations over time.[8]

Aging nephropathy in rats has been recognized for over 50 years, and varies in incidence and functional consequences among different rat strains.[9] It is accelerated by a variety of toxins, high protein feedings, and unilateral nephrectomy, and is ameliorated in severity by food restriction. This spontaneous effect of aging appears to be a primary glomerular process in rats. Importantly, however, and in contrast to the renal pathologic changes of aging in man, there is little evidence of blood vessel pathology in the rat.[10]

The spontaneous aging nephropathy in rats in associated with progressive proteinuria.[11] Fifty percent of 12-month-old Sprague-Dawley rats demonstrate significant proteinuria, which is associated with the characteristic biochemical parameters of nephrotic syndrome in heavily proteinuric old rats. Loss of protein selectivity has also been demonstrated to attend the progressive proteinuria of aging.

In contrast to the rats, the changes of age in man assume a markedly different pattern. Glomerular sclerosis is rare in man until the average human life is more than half expended. In a study of 122 victims of sudden death, acute illness, and patients without renal disease or hypertension, Kaplan et al[12] demonstrated an incidence of less than 1.1% sclerotic glomeruli through age 30, 2.1% for those between the ages of 30 and 39, and only 3.5% between the ages of 40 and 49 years.

As eloquently summarized in a recent review by Ogden[8] "extrapolation of effects observed in rats to humans, both with respect to normal and diseased human kidneys, seems difficult at best in view of the ubiquitous, spontaneous structural, and functional age-associated nephropathy in rats."

RENAL HEMODYNAMICS

The marked morphologic changes that accompany aging result in profound functional changes, including alterations in renal hemodynamics and renal tubular function. The amount of plasma or blood perfusing the kidney can be estimated by measuring para-aminohippuric acid (PAH) or iodopyracet (Diodrast) clearance. Since PAH clearance is affected by the extraction ratio for PAH, it was necessary to ascertain if this variable changed with increasing age. Davies and Shock,[13] confirming the work of Bradley,[14] demonstrated that the extraction ratio for PAH at low arterial PAH concentrations was approximately 92% in 27 subjects of *varying* age and that this extraction ratio was not affected by age. This means that 92% of the PAH entering the kidney on the arterial side was removed in one passage through the kidney or that 8% of the arterial concentration was found in the venous side.

As early as 1940, Goldring et al[15] suggested the possibility of an age-related decrease in renal plasma flow (RPF) between the third and sixth decades. Subsequent studies by Davies and Shock[13] demonstrated a decrease in clearances of both PAH and Diodrast. Wesson[16] summarized 38 renal hemodynamic studies in 634 normal subjects over a wide age range. Total renal blood flow was well maintained through approximately the fourth decade; thereafter there was a progressive decline of about 10% per decade. Despite this observation, the relationship between the reduction in renal blood flow and the concomitant decrease in renal mass remains largely unsettled. Hollenberg et al[6] addressed the relationship between the decrement of mass and flow with age. These investigators studied 207 normal human subjects ranging in age from 17 to 76 years. Since the subjects were all potential kidney donors in a renal transplant program, this cohort represented a population in which well-being had been assured. Hollenberg et al[6] pointed out that if the reduction in renal blood perfusion is secondary to parenchymal atrophy, either a proportional decrease in flow and mass or a reduction in flow less than the reduction in mass would be anticipated. Thus, flow per unit mass would be unchanged (or conceivably even increased) but certainly not reduced. Obviously, total renal blood flow and renal mass have never been measured simultaneously.

In contrast to most technics for determining renal perfusion, the inert gas washout method (xenon 133) provides an alternative approach to the assessment of the relative reduction in renal perfusion and renal mass; xenon washout measures blood flow *per unit tissue mass.*[6] Utilizing this approach, Hollenberg et al[6] demonstrated an unequivocal progressive reduction in mean blood flow per unit mass with advancing age (Figure 1-1). In addition, these investigators demonstrated a progressive reduction in rapid- component flow rate and the percent of flow into the rapid-flow (cortical) compartment. Although interpretation of such indirect studies is difficult, in contrast to direct assessments of blood flow distribution in animals, several observations have suggested that the rapid flow compartment represents perfusion to the renal cortex.

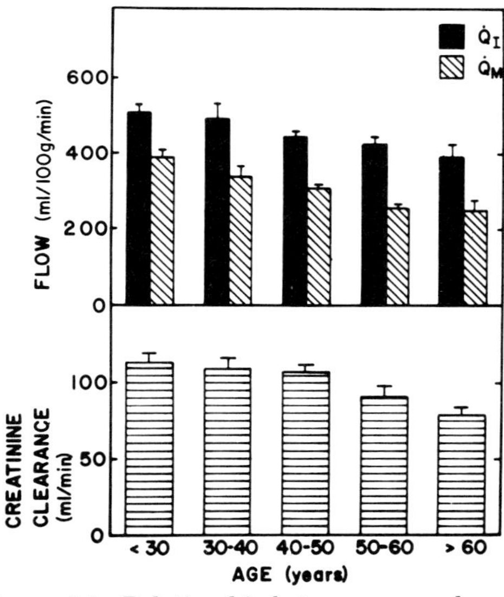

Figure 1-1 Relationship between age and renal perfusion rates in 207 normal human subjects. There is a significant reduction in mean renal blood flow (Q_M) with age ($P < .001$). A parallel reduction in the rapid-component flow rate (Q_I) also occurs with age ($P < .001$). (Reproduced with permission of Hollenberg et al and the American Heart Association.[6])

When interpreted in this context, the observations of Hollenberg et al[6] suggest that the decreased renal perfusion associated with aging is most profound in the cortex with relative sparing of flow to deeper regions. Since juxtamedullary glomeruli have a greater filtration fraction than cortical glomeruli, this redistribution of flow from cortex to medulla may account for the slight but definite increase in filtration fraction observed with advancing age.

GLOMERULAR FILTRATION RATE

The most frequently utilized and most useful measure of renal function is an estimate of the glomerular filtration rate (GFR). As early as 1938, Lewis and Alving[17] reported a decrease in urea clearance with increasing age. Subsequently, numerous investigators have corroborated, in cross-sectional studies, the progressive reduction in GFR with age. In light of the fact that the relationship of GFR to age was assessed utilizing cross-sectional studies with their attendant drawbacks,[18] and since many of the reports selected elderly subjects who were institutionalized, the problem of the effect of age on GFR was reexamined by Rowe et al.[19] These investigators employed both cross-section and serial prospective (longitudinal) analysis on a large group of active, community-dwelling men in order to establish age-adjusted normative standards. A large number of men were rigorously screened to exclude possible disease and a true creatinine method was used to assess creatinine clearance. Urine collection periods were of 24-hour duration. This study disclosed a highly significant reduction in creatinine clearance with age starting at age 34 and accelerating after age 65 years.

The decline in GFR following maturity has important implications for the management of the older patient. The dosage schedules of many drugs that are eliminated primarily by renal mechanisms are based on renal functional indexes in the young. Failure to modify the dosage schedule for these drugs to account for the 30% to 40% reduction in GFR in the elderly can lead to significant dosage errors in the administration of numerous drugs, such as digoxin or the aminoglycoside antibiotics. It is imperative that age-adjusted "normative" standards for GFR be utilized in providing dosage schedules for the elderly.

The reduction in creatinine clearance with age is attended by a parallel reduction in daily urinary creatinine excretion, reflecting decreased muscle mass.[19,20] As seen in Table 1-1, total urinary creatinine values showed a moderate decrease from the age group 20 to 29 years to the age group 50 to 59 years and thereafter a more pronounced fall was observed. The mean urinary creatinine value in milligrams per kilogram body weight per 24 hours showed a constant decrease from the youngest to the oldest age groups, and the mean values decreased from 23.8 to 9.4 mg/kg/24 h. In general all parameters for female subjects showed values lower than the corresponding values for males.

Several investigators have reported decreased urinary creatinine excretion in patients with renal failure, especially apparent when serum creatinine exceeds 6.0 mg/100 mL. These findings have not been supported by Kampmann et al.[20] The latter investigators pointed out that earlier studies failed to correct for the age of the patients. When patients with moderate azotemia (serum creatinine values ranging from 1.5 to 5.0 mg/100 mL) were compared with nonazotemic patients of corresponding age, a significant decrease in urinary creatinine was not apparent.[20]

The fall in creatinine excretion with age has a significance that has not been widely recognized in two areas. First, the relationship of serum creatinine to creatinine clearance changes with age: the net effect is constancy of serum creatinine concentration at a time when glomerular filtration rate (and creatinine clearance) declines. Thus a serum creatinine of 1 mg/100 mL may subtend a creatinine clearance of 120 mL/min at age 20, but only 60 mL/min at age 80 years. Second, since 24-hour creatinine excretion is often utilized to assess

Table 1-1
Alterations in Urinary Creatinine with Increasing Age

Age (yr)	Serum Creatinine (mg/100 mL)	Urinary Creatinine	
		(mg/24 h)	*(mg/kg/24 h)*
Males			
20–29	0.99 ± 0.16	1625 ± 137	23.8 ± 2.3
30–39	1.14 ± 0.22	1520 ± 130	21.9 ± 1.5
40–49	1.10 ± 0.20	1544 ± 421	19.7 ± 3.2
50–59	1.16 ± 0.17	1445 ± 252	19.3 ± 2.9
60–69	1.15 ± 0.14	1252 ± 364	16.9 ± 2.9
70–79	1.03 ± 0.22	919 ± 132	14.2 ± 3.0
80–89	1.06 ± 0.25	651 ± 238	11.7 ± 4.0
90–99	1.20 ± 0.16	612 ± 188	9.4 ± 3.2
Females			
20–29	0.89 ± 0.17	1135 ± 224	19.7 ± 3.9
30–39	0.91 ± 0.17	1218 ± 191	20.4 ± 3.9
40–49	1.00 ± 0.24	1056 ± 256	17.6 ± 3.9
50–59	0.99 ± 0.26	989 ± 246	14.9 ± 3.6
60–69	0.97 ± 0.17	871 ± 283	12.9 ± 2.6
70–79	1.02 ± 0.23	685 ± 184	11.8 ± 2.2
80–89	1.05 ± 0.22	578 ± 154	10.7 ± 2.5
90–99	0.91 ± 0.12	433 ± 113	8.4 ± 1.4

Data derived from Kampmann et al.[20]

the completeness of urine collections, failure to recognize the fall in creatinine excretion with age may lead to erroneous conclusions regarding the adequacy of a urine specimen.

Filtration Fraction

Changes in filtration fraction (FF) with age have been calculated from the data of Wesson, by Goldman.[21] Relatively constant values (0.20 to 0.22) were observed through the fifth decade in women and through the sixth decade in men. An increase of up to 0.28 was then observed at later decades in both sexes. Since inner cortical nephrons have larger filtration fractions than outer cortical nephrons, the preferential obliterations of the outer cortical nephrons known to occur with aging could explain this rise in FF.

Glomerular Permeability

In contrast to renal hemodynamics, relatively little information is available on the changes in glomerular permeability with age. One approach to assess permeability has entailed studies of protein excretion. Van Zonneveld,[22] in a population survey involving over 3000 persons over age 65 years, found an increasing incidence of proteinuria with age. Yet, by age 85, only 32% of his subjects had proteinuria. Lowenstein et al[23] studied glomerular clearance of free hemoglobin in 47 healthy adult males, aged 20 to 90 years, free of clinical renal disease. When free hemoglobin clearance was factored by inulin clearance, no evidence of an alteration in glomerular permeability with age was present.

Implications for Renal Transplantation

The demonstration of a reduction in renal cortical mass and GFR with advancing age suggested that the kidney of an elderly person might prove inadequate for maintaining function after transplantation. Accordingly, Darmady analyzed cumulative survival data for 6883 transplants in an attempt to assess if donor age adversely affected recipient survival.[24] Darmady has claimed that the older the donor kidney, the poorer the survival of cadaver kidney recipients. Matas et al[25] have criticized the finding of Darmady, since recipient age was not taken into account. The latter investigators compared the cumulative survival of living related transplant recipients while controlling for both donor and recipient age and failed to demonstrate a detrimental effect of donor age per se on cumulative survival. It is apparent that additional studies will be required to resolve this important issue.

Tubular Function

Proximal tubule The progressive decline in GFR with age is paralleled by a decrease in renal tubular function.[13,26] Thus, maximal reabsorption of Diodrast (Tm_D), PAH (Tm_{PAH}), and glucose (Tm_G) have been used as markers of renal tubular function. The tubular maximum of PAH or Diodrast (Tm_{PAH} or Tm_D) is a measure of the ability of the renal tubules to secrete dye when the arterial blood level is raised sufficiently to saturate the tubular transport capacity so that all of the PAH cannot be removed from the blood in one passage through the kidney.

If one assumes that kidney function at age 20 years is 100%, the GFR decreases 0.72% per year, and comparable decrements occur in Tm_D (0.68%), Tm_{PAH} (0.65%), and Tm_G (0.70%). This parallel diminution of GFR and tubular function allows constancy of the ratio between the GFR and tubular capacity over seven decades and suggests that nephron losses occur as a functional unit.

RENAL SODIUM HANDLING

Despite the critical role of the kidney in maintaining sodium homeostasis and the effect of age on a number of the determinants of renal sodium handling,[6,16,27] relatively little is known about how this important function is influenced by age. It has long been known that aged patients are capable of conserving sodium in response to an acute reduction in salt intake,[28] but the kinetics of this response had not been assessed quantitatively. Epstein and Hollenberg[5] have examined the effects of age on the capacity of the normal human kidney to respond to the restriction of sodium intake. Renal conservation of sodium and the response of dietary sodium restriction were assessed in 89 healthy subjects who were potential kidney transplant donors. All subjects were free of cardiovascular or renal disease. Following acute restriction of dietary intake to 10 mEq sodium and 100 mEq potassium per day, the daily reduction in urine sodium was determined and found to conform well to an exponential function, defined by an unweighted least-squares fit. The half-time for the reduction in renal sodium excretion in subjects under 25 years was -17.6 ± 0.7 hours, significantly faster than for subjects aged over 60 years, in whom the half-time was -30.9 ± 2.8 hours (Figure 1-2). These observations indicate that age significantly influences the kidney's capacity to conserve sodium.

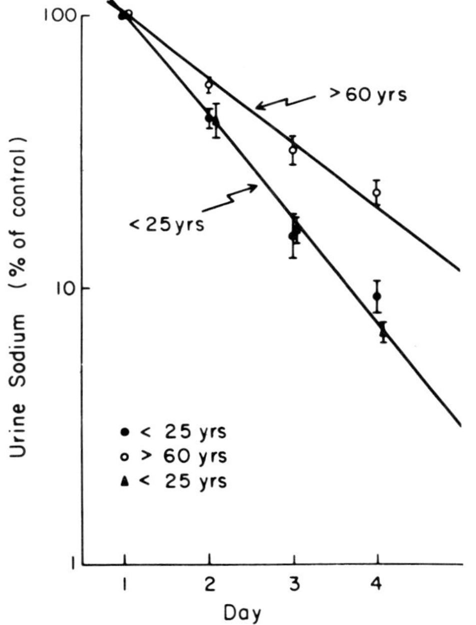

Figure 1-2 Response of urinary sodium excretion to restriction of sodium intake in normal man. The mean half-time for eight subjects over 60 years of age was -30.9 ± 2.8 hours, exceeding the mean half-time of -17.6 ± 0.7 hours for subjects under 25 years of age ($P < 0.01$). (Modified with permission from Epstein and Hollenberg.[5])

The factors responsible for the age-related changes in renal sodium handling remain incompletely defined. Glomerular filtration rate, physical factors determined by hemodynamics, and the renin-aldosterone system all are major determinants of renal sodium handling, and each has been demonstrated to vary significantly with age.[6,13,16,27]

Both renal blood flow and glomerular filtration rate decline with advancing age. Since a decrease in both renal blood flow and glomerular filtration rate per nephron would favor enhanced conservation of sodium by the kidney,[5] this mechanism clearly cannot account for the reduced capacity in the elderly. Cortical blood flow is another determinant of renal sodium handling that also falls with advancing age.[6] None of these phenomena can account for the reduced capacity of the kidney to conserve sodium. They are in the wrong direction. Indeed, one might speculate that teleologically the reduction in renal blood flow and in GFR are protective alterations in the sense that they may aid in limiting sodium loss in the elderly when intake is restricted or extrarenal losses occur.

To the extent that a reduced number of nephrons may have contributed to the decrease in glomerular filtration rate, the resultant increased solute load per nephron may have contributed to the sluggish sodium conservation in the older subjects. This concept is consistent with earlier suggestions regarding the role of increased solute load per nephron as a determinant of renal sodium conservation in patients with chronic renal failure.

The increase in the rate of aldosterone secretion in response to dietary sodium deprivation is one of the homeostatic mechanisms mediating sodium conservation. Recent studies by several investigators have demonstrated sluggish renin-aldosterone responsiveness to acute stimuli with advancing age.[27] The reduction in aldosterone levels is in a direction that could contribute to a reduced capacity for sodium retention with increasing age, but too little is known at present about the responsiveness of the renal tubule to alterations in circulating aldosterone in the elderly to permit an unequivocal assessment of the role of this possibility.

Even though the factors responsible for the age-related changes in renal sodium conservation remain incompletely defined, it is apparent that such changes must be considered in any assessment of human disease. The results of the studies of Epstein and Hollenberg[5] provide an approach for assessing changes in renal sodium handling in the elderly.

Sodium Retention

In analogy with the increased tendency of the older patient to develop volume depletion when deprived of sodium, the elderly are also more prone to develop extracellular fluid volume expansion when challenged with increased sodium intake or an intravenous (IV) sodium load. As a consequence of the progressive decrease in GFR, the senescent kidney's ability to excrete an acute salt load is impaired as compared with the younger kidney. Thus, when placed in a clinical setting where sodium access is increased, such as dietary indiscretion, the inappropriate administration of sodium-rich fluids, or after the administration of sodium-rich radiographic contrast agents, geriatric patients may develop an expanded extracellular fluid volume. Usually, in the absence of preexisting myocardial disease, the acquisition of excess salt does not result in acute precipitation of frank congestive heart failure; rather, the patient experiences modest weight gain and the appearance of mild peripheral edema. The excess sodium is generally excreted over the course of the next several days. In contrast, patients with pre-existing cardiac disease may develop pulmonary congestion necessitating aggressive emergency therapy often including the IV administration of potent loop-type diuretics, such as furosemide or ethacrynic acid.

POTASSIUM BALANCE

Hyperkalemia

Theoretical considerations suggest that several renal and hormonal events associated with aging act in concert to increase the risk of the elderly patient developing hyperkalemia. First, as noted earlier, increasing age is associated with a suppression of renin and aldosterone.[27] Through its action on the distal renal tubule, aldosterone increases sodium reabsorption and facilitates the renal excretion of potassium. Aldosterone represents one of the major protective mechanisms that prevent hyperkalemia during periods of potassium challenge. Since GFR (another major determinant of potassium excretion) is also impaired in older patients, serious elevations of plasma potassium are likely to develop.

This tendency to develop hyperkalemia is aggravated by several superimposed events. One such event is the presence of gastrointestinal (GI) bleeding (a major source of potassium) or when potassium salts are prescribed. This potential toward hyperkalemia might be further aggravated in any clinical setting associated with acidosis, since the senescent kidney is sluggish in its response to acid loading, resulting in prolonged depression of pH and concomitant potassium elevation. Similarly, diuretics such as spironolactone or triamterene, which impair renal potassium excretion, should be administered with caution to the elderly, and the concomitant administration of these agents and potassium should be avoided.

Although such considerations suggest that the older patient is at an increased risk of hyperkalemia it must be emphasized that at the time of this writing no clear-cut *clinical* studies have been reported that have addressed this important point. A recent study in rats, however, is of interest. Bengele et al[29] examined the effect of aging on acute potassium tolerance and potassium adaptation in rats. Following acute potassium chloride infusion, the fraction of the potassium load excreted was compared in young (3 to 4 months) and old (21 to 22 months) animals. They observed that aged rats have a defect in both renal and extrarenal potassium homeostasis. Of note, these defects were manifest only in those rats which had ingested a high potassium diet prior to loading; no differences in the renal or extrarenal response to potassium loading were observed between the old and young groups of animals previously maintained on a normal potassium diet.

In summary, despite the absence of clear-cut studies establishing an impairment in renal potassium handling in *man*, prudence dictates that drugs having the potential to impair potassium homeostasis (ie, potassium-sparing diuretics, β-adrenergic blocking drugs, etc) should be prescribed with circumspection in the older patient.

RENAL CONCENTRATING ABILITY

Urine concentrating ability has long been known to decline with age after maturity.[21,30] A degree of reservation has attended these findings in view of the cross-sectional design of many studies, and the proclivity of many investigators to select institutionalized patients for their elderly cohort. Rowe et al[30] have collaborated in a carefully performed longitudinal study utilizing community-residing male volunteers. They have demonstrated that elderly subjects were less able than young and middle-aged subjects to significantly alter urine flow rate, urine osmolality, or osmolar clearance following 12 hours of dehydration. No major differences in protein or salt intake were documented between groups, and similarity in total solute excretion during the initial clearance period suggested that differences in solute intake cannot explain the differences in solute excretion during water deprivation.

Several investigators have attributed the decreased concentrating ability of the aged kidney to the concomitant decline in GFR. In contrast, Rowe et al[30] failed to demonstrate a significant relationship between the decrement in creatinine clearance and either urine osmolality or flow after water deprivation. These authors concluded that although a decline in GFR may contribute to the age-related decrease in concentration ability, it cannot constitute a major determinant. Additional mechanisms postulated to account for the impaired concentrating ability of the aged include relative increases in medullary blood flow through a washout of medullary tonicity and subsequent decline in the efficacy of the countercurrent system,[30] and a possible defect in solute transport from tubular lumen to medullary interstitium.

A decline in renal concentrating ability with age has been firmly established. In contrast, the interaction of the pituitary release of vasopressin and renal responsiveness to vasopressin has only recently been elucidated.

Recently, Miller has evaluated the influence of age on the capacity of the neurohypophyseal system of the rat to secrete arginine vasopressin (AVP).[31] The secretory capacity of isolated hypothalamic-neurohypophyseal (HNP) units was assessed by an in vitro perfusion system capable of quantitating AVP release over time under base-line conditions following exposure to stimuli. It was observed that aging in the rat is accompanied by an increased capacity of the neurohypophyseal system to secrete AVP under both basal and stimulated conditions. This hypersecretory state is expressed in the intact animal as an increase in plasma AVP concentration.

Helderman et al[32] examined the effect of age on the hypothalamic-hypophyseal-renal axis in normal man by assaying plasma AVP responses to inhibitory and to secretory stimuli. These investigators demonstrated that the infusion of 3% NaCl stimulated AVP release to varying degrees in young (aged 22 to 48 years) and elderly (aged 52 to 66 years) subjects. In the younger group, the increase in serum osmolality induced by hypertonic saline resulted in an increase in plasma AVP from its basal level to 2.5 times the basal concentration by the end of the hypertonic load. Although the older group experienced a similar rise in serum osmolality, the associated increment in plasma AVP was 4.5 times the basal concentration. A plot of the slope of plasma AVP concentration on serum osmolality as an index of the sensitivity of the osmoreceptor disclosed that osmoreceptor sensitivity was greater in the older group. Thus, it would appear that the apparent sensitivity of the hypothalamic-neurohypophyseal unit increases with age in normal man. It is possible that the heightened sensitivity of the AVP response to hyperosmolality in the elderly may serve to compensate for the reduced renal ability to conserve water in the aging man.

In addition to diminished water conservation by the kidneys, it has been proposed that reduced thirst and fluid intake in the presence of physiologic need may play a role in producing hypernatremia. Reduced thirst may be particularly important in predisposing to dehydration, since a deficit in body water content can be corrected only by fluid intake. Recently, Phillips et al[33] compared thirst, fluid and electrolyte responses, and hormonal responses to 24 hours of water deprivation in seven healthy active elderly men and seven healthy young men who were matched for weight loss during water deprivation. Following water deprivation, the older men had greater increases in plasma osmolality, sodium concentration, and vasopressin levels. Nevertheless, their urinary osmolality was lower, and they were less thirsty and drank less after water deprivation so that, in contrast to the controls, their plasma and urine were not diluted to predeprivation levels.[33] Although the mechanism for this thirst deficit has not been established, central nervous system disease or a reduced physiologic sensitivity of the thirst mechanism to osmotic or volume stimuli have been proposed. Regardless, it is clear that the clinician should be alert to this abnormality. Remembering anything may be a challenge for the elderly, but remembering to drink when they are not thirsty may be more than we should expect of them. Perhaps physicians should routinely *prescribe* a glass of water every 4 hours to compensate for this derangement.

Although the decline in water-conserving capacity is not so severe as to have clinical significance under conditions of free access to water, it becomes important when fluid intake is limited. Under such conditions, geriatric patients might manifest elevations of the serum sodium concentration to levels that may impair CNS function and result in obtundation.

RENAL DILUTING ABILITY

While a decline in renal concentrating ability with age is firmly established, data regarding renal diluting ability are relatively sparse. Theoretical considerations suggest that water intoxication could constitute an equally threatening but less well-recognized electrolyte disorder in geriatric patients. If the observations of enhanced osmoreceptor sensitivity in the elderly have clinical implications, it is conceivable that diverse events such as the stress of anesthesia and surgery, or the administration of a number of drugs that enhance vasopressin action may act in concert to impair renal diluting ability and render the elderly patients susceptible to the complication of water intoxication due to excess ADH secretion. Despite such theoretical considerations, evidence supporting an alteration in renal diluting capacity is tenuous.

Two decades ago, Lindeman et al[34] reported that maximum diluting ability, as measured by minimum urine osmolality achieved, decreased with age (Table 1-2). It must be emphasized, however, that one must be careful in interpreting these data.

In older persons, total solute excretion should approximate that of younger persons if they are ingesting a similar diet. Actually, older persons do have some decrease in total solute excretion but it is much less than the decrease in GFR with age. As a consequence, each surviving nephron in the elderly person is exposed to an increased solute load. Even if all surviving nephrons were completely normal, the solute diuresis per nephron would decrease the ability of the kidney to develop maximal and minimal osmolalities when dehydrated or hydrated respectively. Thus, in order to compare concentrating and diluting abilities in young and old subjects, it is necessary to determine these functions when solute excretion per nephron is comparable.

Another way to compare concentrating and diluting abilities in young *v* old persons would be to compare negative free water clearance ($T^c_{H_2O}$) and free water clearance (C_{H_2O}), respectively, corrected for nephron mass as follows:

$$\frac{T^c_{H_2O} \times 100}{\text{Observed GFR}} = T^c_{H_2O}\ 100/\text{mL GFR}$$

$$\frac{C_{H_2O} \times 100}{\text{Observed GFR}} = C_{H_2O}/100\ \text{mL GFR}$$

Utilizing such a correction a reinterpretation of the data of Lindeman et al[34] (Table 1-2) suggests that maximal renal diluting ability is not altered by age.

Taken together, these findings suggest that the effects of aging on vasopressin release and renal water handling may predispose the elderly patient to two life-threatening but diametrically opposite complications in time of stress and intercurrent disease: hypernatremia and hyponatremia. Physicians caring for the elderly should be aware of these "normal" senescent changes and should have a high degree of suspicion of these two complications when faced with lethargic, confused, or obtunded older patients.

Table 1-2
Maximum Diluting Capacity in Young, Middle-Aged, and Elderly Male Subjects after Ingestion of a Water Load of 20 mL H_2O/kg/Body Weight

	Young	Middle-Aged	Elderly
No. of subjects	7	7	7
Mean age (yr)	31	60	84
Mean GFR (mL/min)	149 ± 9	92 ± 8	65 ± 4
Urine flow (mL/min)	19.8 ± 1.7	11.1 ± 1.5	8.5 ± 1.2
Urine osmolality (mosm/kg H_2O)	52 ± 3	74 ± 6	92 ± 11
Total solute excretion/ 100 mL GFR	690	840	1120
C_{H_2O} (mL/min)	16.2 ± 1.4	8.4 ± 1.3	5.9 ± 1.0
C_{H_2O}/100 mL GFR (mL/min)	10.9	9.1	9.1

Data derived from Lindeman et al.[34]

MECHANISMS OF THE AGING KIDNEY

One of the major unanswered questions remains: How does kidney function decline with age in the individual person? As shown in Figure 1-3, two general formulations have been advanced to explain the observed decline in renal function.[35] One invokes a progressive involutional change characterized by sequential loss of nephron units systematically through the life of the individual (dashed line in the figure). Alternatively, stable renal function may be interrupted by various pathologic processes that cause an acute decrease in renal function perhaps with decreasing ability to regenerate or replace injured or destroyed nephrons or cells. If the first were true, then renal function in individual subjects followed longitudinally would conform to the dashed line in this figure. On the other hand, diverse acute renal injuries (ie, undetected glomerulonephritis, pyelonephritis, due to bacterial or viral infections, or nephrotoxic responses to several drugs) might produce independent decreases in renal function. Many of these asymptomatic episodes might well go unrecognized since no simple diagnostic tests are available for many of them. At the time of this writing there is no readily apparent answer to this conundrum. It is hoped that ongoing longitudinal studies from a number of gerontology centers will answer this question.

ACKNOWLEDGMENT

I would like to acknowledge the critical review and suggestions of Dr. James Oster.

Portions of this chapter have been modified from reference 1 with permission.

REFERENCES

1. Epstein M: Effects of aging on the kidney. *Fed Proc* 1979;38:168–172.
2. Roessle R, Roulet F: *Nieren, in Mass und Zahl in der Pathologie.* Berlin, Julius Springer, 1932, pp 63–66.
3. Dunnill MS, Halley W: Some observations on the quantitative anatomy of the kidney. *J Pathol* 1973;110:113–121.

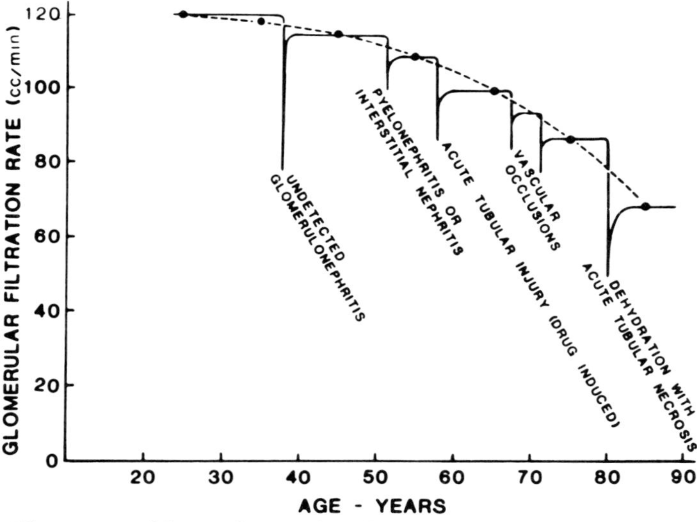

Figure 1-3 Mean glomerular GFRs as determined by cross-sectional studies plotted against age. Whether the kidney ages by a steady progressive involutional decrease in renal function (dashed line) or whether renal function remains stable until some pathologic process intervenes with incomplete recovery (solid line) remains undetermined. (Reproduced with permission from Lindeman.[35])

4. Shock NW: Current trends in research on the physiological aspects of aging. *J Am Geriatr Soc* 1967;15:995–1000.
5. Epstein M, Hollenberg NK: Age as a determinant of renal sodium conservation in normal man. *J Lab Clin Med* 1976;87: 411–417
6. Hollenberg NK, Adams DF, Solomon HS, et al: Senescence and the renal vasculature in normal man. *Circ Res* 1974;34: 309–316.
7. Andres R: Physiological factors of aging significant to the clinician (summary of remarks). *J Am Geriatr Soc* 1969;17: 274–277.
8. Ogden DA: Consequences of renal donation in man. *Am J Kid Dis* 1983;2: 501–511.
9. Elema JD, Arends A: Focal and segmental glomerular hyalinosis and sclerosis in the rat. *Lab Invest* 1975;33:554–561.
10. Gray JE, Weaver RN, Purmalis A: Ultrastructural observations of chronic progressive nephrosis in the Sprague-Dawley rat. *Vet Pathol* 1974;11:153–164.
11. Couser WG, Stilmant MM: Mesangial lesions and focal glomerular sclerosis in the aging rat. *Lab Invest* 1975;33:491–501.
12. Kaplan C, Pasternack B, Shah H, et al: Age-related incidence of sclerotic glomeruli in human kidneys. *Am J Pathol* 1975; 80:227–234.
13. Davies DF, Shock NW: Age changes in glomerular filtration rate, effective renal plasma flow, and tubular excretory capacity in adult males. *J Clin Invest* 1950;29: 496–506.
14. Bradley SE: The validity of the clearance technique in the measurement of renal blood flow in normal man and in patients with essential hypertension, in Zweifach BW, Shorr E (eds): *Transactions of the First Conference on Factors Regulating Blood Pressure.* New York, Josiah Macy Jr Foundation, 1947, pp 118–123.
15. Goldring W, Chasis H, Ranges HA, et al: Relations of effective renal blood flow and glomerular filtration to tubular excretory mass in normal man. *J Clin Invest* 1940; 19:739–750.
16. Wesson LG Jr: Renal hemodynamics in physiological states, in Wesson LG Jr (ed): *Physiology of the Human Kidney.* New York, Grune & Stratton, 1969, pp 96 –108.
17. Lewis WH Jr, Alving AS: Changes with age in the renal function in adult men. *Am J Physiol* 1938;123:500–515.
18. Rowe JW: Clinical research on aging: strategies and directions. *N Engl J Med* 1977;297:1332–1336.
19. Rowe JW, Andres R, Tobin JD, et al: The effect of age on creatinine clearance in man: A cross-sectional and longitudinal study. *J Gerontol* 1976;31:155–163.
20. Kampmann J, Siersbaek-Nielsen K, Kristensen M, et al: Rapid evaluation of creatinine clearance. *Acta Med Scand* 1974;196:517–520.
21. Goldman R: Aging of the excretory system: Kidney and bladder, in Finch CE, Hayflick L (eds): *Handbook of the Biology of Aging.* New York, Van Nostrand Reinhold, 1977, pp 409–431.
22. Van Zonneveld RJ: Some data on the genito-urinary system as found in old age surveys in the Netherlands. *Gerontol Clin* 1959;1:167–173.
23. Lowenstein J, Faulstick DA, Yiengst MJ, et al: The glomerular clearance and renal transport of hemoglobin in adult males. *J Clin Invest* 1961;40:1172–1177.
24. Darmady EM: Transplantation and the ageing kidney. *Lancet* 1974;2:1046–1047.
25. Matas AJ, Simmons RL, Kjellstrand M, et al: Transplantation of the aging kidney. *Transplantation* 1976;21:160–161.
26. Watkin DM, Shock NW: Agewise standard value for C_{In}, C_{PAH} and Tm_{PAH} in adult males. *J Clin Invest* 1955;34:969.
27. Weidman P, Demyttenaere-Bursztein S, Maxwell MH, et al: Effect of aging on plasma renin and alsosterone in normal man. *Kidney Int* 1975;8:325–333.
28. Sporn N, Lancestremere RG, Papper S: Differential diagnosis of oliguria in aged patients. *N Engl J Med* 1962;267:130–132.
29. Bengele HH, Mathias R, Perkins JH, et al: Impaired renal and extrarenal potassium adaptation in old rats. *Kidney Int* 1983; 23:684–690.
30. Rowe JW, Shock NW, DeFronzo RA: The influence of age on the renal response to water deprivation in man. *Nephron* 1976; 17:270–278.
31. Miller M: Vasopressin hypersecretion in the aging rat, in *Abstracts of the Endocrine Society,* 65th Annual Meeting, San Antonio, Texas, June 8–10, 1983, p 253.
32. Helderman JH, Vestal RE, Rowe JW, et al: The response of arginine vasopressin to intravenous ethanol and hypertonic saline in

man: The impact of aging. *J Gerontol* 1978;33:39–47.

33. Phillips PA, Rolls BJ, Ledingham JGG, et al: Reduced thirst after water deprivation in healthy elderly men. *N Engl J Med* 1984;311:753–759.
34. Lindeman RD, Lee TD Jr, Yiengst MJ, et al: Influence of age, renal disease, hypertension, diuretics, and calcium on the antidiuretic responses to suboptimal infusions of vasopressin. *J Lab Clin Med* 1966;68: 206–223.
35. Lindeman RD: Age changes in renal function, in Goldman R, Rockstein M (eds): *The Physiology and Pathology of Human Aging.* New York, Academic Press, 1975, pp 19–38.

CHAPTER 2 Renal Anatomy and Nephropathology of Aging

Robert H. Lippman
Peter F. Schatzki

ANATOMY

Embryology

To understand the age-related changes in the kidney and its function a brief description of renal embryology and anatomy is essential. The renal excretory system develops from a mesodermal derivative called the metanephros which includes the glomerulus and Bowman's capsule, the proximal tubules, Henle's loop, and the distal tubules. The collecting ducts develop from an earlier-appearing mesodermal structure, the mesonephros.

The individual units of the excretory system, the nephrons, are not fully developed at birth. Nephrons are functional in the third trimester of intrauterine life. No new nephrons are produced after birth.[1] Postnatally the glomerulus matures and enlarges. The renal tubules undergo extensive elongation postnatally, increasing in cell number and tubule length, growing down into the medulla.[2] Only after this maturation can the infant nephron produce hypertonic urine.

There is a lack of agreement regarding the ability of the kidney to hypertrophy. Postmaturity, hypertrophy is limited to the proximal tubules.[3] Darmady stated that the capability for hypertrophy decreases with advancing age.[4] Korenchevsky cited other studies which showed capacity for renal tubular hypertrophy in aged rats equal to or greater than that in younger but mature rats.[5] This remains a controversial question.

Macrostructure

The gross anatomy of the adult kidney is shown in Figure 2-1. The kidneys attain adult size by age 20 years.[2] At this age the subcapsular cortex is smooth and glistening, distorted only by varying degrees of persistent fetal lobulation. The capsule strips freely from the cortex. On cross-section the cortex has a uniform thickness. Glomeruli are grossly visible as pinpoint-sized depressions most easily seen in the outer cortex. Nephrons with glomeruli in the superficial cortex have short tubules and may be completely contained within the cortex. The longer tubules rising from glomeruli in the deep cortex extend into the medulla as the loops of Henle. The medulla also contains collecting tubules and ducts, and vascular structures. These elements are orientated perpendicular to the capsule, imparting a striated appearance to the medulla. The medulla abuts the calyceal system which drains into the renal pelvis.

Microstructure

Vascular system The renal arteries arise bilaterally from the aorta and divide into the anterior artery with segments supplying the midanterior and polar aspects of the kidney, and the posterior arteries supplying the midposterior aspect. Variant distributions are commonly found. The segmental arteries divide at the corticomedullary junction to form the arcuate arteries which give rise to the interlobular arteries. No vascular anastomoses are present and all arteries are essentially end-arteries. The afferent arterioles branch from the interlobular arteries to form the glomerular capillary tuft. One or more glomeruli arise from each afferent arteriole.[6] Each glomerular tuft is made of up to eight capillary lobules with intralobular and possibly interlobular anastomoses. Exiting glomerular capillaries reconverge as the efferent arteriole. Capillaries from the efferents supply the tubules as an intertubular plexus. The renal papillae are supplied by the vasa recta, a network of larger diameter juxtamedullary efferent arterioles and infrequent arterioles arising directly from the interlobular arteries. Oliver states that these vessels are a compensatory neovascularization and are not present at birth.[7] Branches of arteries in the adventitia of the minor calyces also supply the papillae. Capillaries drain into interlobular veins. Larger veins follow the arteries in a retrograde fashion emptying into the renal vein.

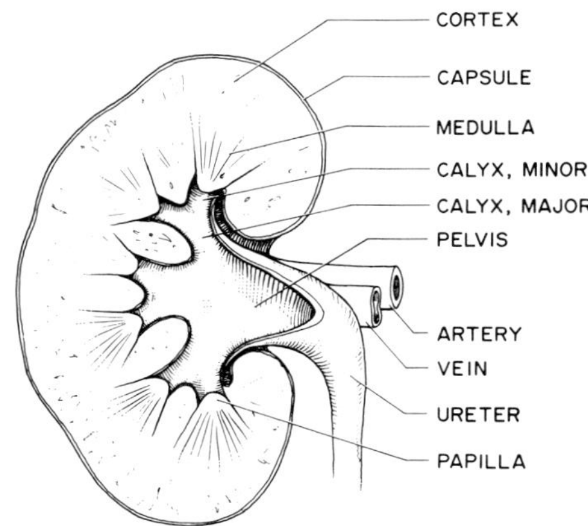

Figure 2-1 Gross anatomy of the kidney (cross sections of left kidney).

The nephron Figure 2-2 shows the structure of the kidney unit, the nephron. Each kidney contains more than 1 million nephrons which begin with the glomeruli. Each glomerulus invaginates into an epithelial pouch, Bowman's capsule. Visceral epithelial cells cover the individual glomerular capillaries; the parietal epithelium encapsulates the glomerular unit. Urinary spaces originate within the epithelial pouch. Mesangial cells, modified phagocytic smooth muscle cells with similarities to cells in arteriolar media, are present in the intercapillary tuft supporting matrix. The parietal epithelium continues as the tubular epithelium. The first tubular region is the proximal convoluted tubule (PCT). Extending towards the medulla it abruptly narrows, becoming the thin limb of the loop of Henle. It turns back upon itself as the thick ascending limb. There is an abrupt enlargement of the tubular cells forming the distal convoluted tubule (DCT). A portion of the initial aspect of the DCT contacts both the afferent and efferent arterioles at the glomerular hilus. The cells in direct contact with the arterioles are stratified and larger than the single-layered cuboidal cells of the opposite wall and the rest of the tubule. This focus is the macula densa. The specialized arteriolar and mesangial cells of the glomerular hilus combined with the macula densa form the juxtaglomerular apparatus. The tubular cells gradually transform into collecting tubules. The latter drain into an arborized system of collecting ducts which condense and empty into the calyces and the renal pelvis.

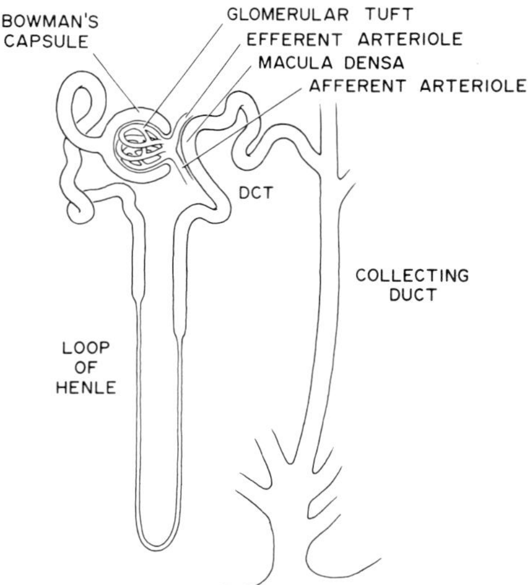

Figure 2-2 The nephron. DCT=distal convoluted tubule.

Ultrastructure

The glomerular basement membrane (GBM) lies between the glomerular endothelium and the visceral epithelium. It is continuous with the basement membrane (BM) of Bowman's capsule and the afferent and efferent arterioles and the mesangial matrix as shown in Figure 2-3. It is made of filamentous collagen and carbohydrates

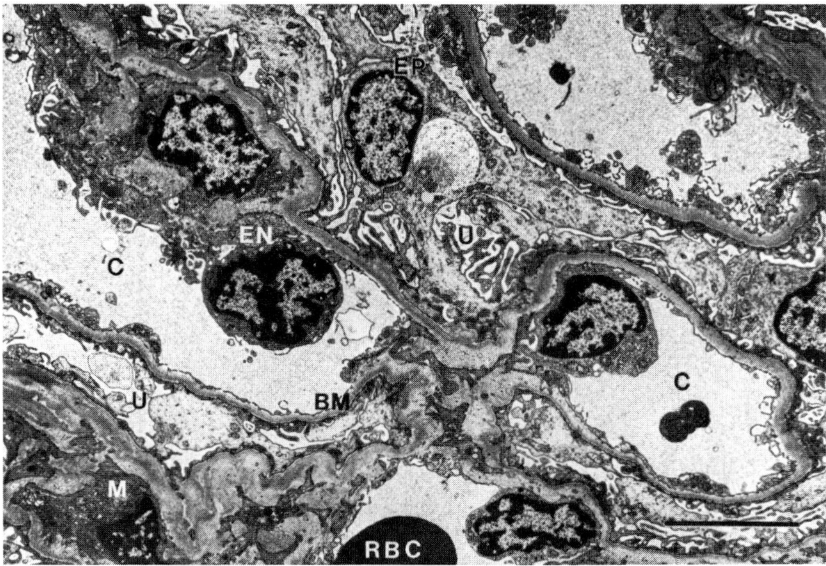

Figure 2-3 Glomerular capillary tuft: Note the uniform trilaminar basement membrane. BM=basement membrane, C=capillary lumen, EN=endothelial cell, EP=epithelial cell, M=mesangial cell and matrix, P=podocytes (epithelial), RBC=erythrocyte, U=urinary space. The patient was a 19-year-old female renal transplant donor who died from an intracerebral hemorrhage. Scale bar=5000 nm.

and is possibly secreted by epithelial cells. It functions as a molecular sieve. Its thickness varies with age and disease and will be described below. The GBM infrastructural appearance is affected by the method of fixation. Most technics suggest a trilaminar composition with a central dense layer and rarefied inner subendothelial and outer subepithelial layers. The endothelial and epithelial cells do not cover the total GBM surfaces. Fenestrations of up to 100-nm diameter punctuate the endothelium. Branched epithelial cell extensions called foot processes are embedded in the outer aspect of the GBM, 20 to 50 nm apart. Slit membranes bridge the gaps between the foot processes. Because the arborized processes of the epithelial cells interdigitate, adjacent foot processes belong to many epithelial cells as shown in Figures 2-4 and 2-5. The entire epithelial cell surface, including foot processes, is covered with acid mucosubstances rich in sialomucins. Mesangial cells have an ultrastructural appearance like that of myofibroblasts. They probably secrete the basement membrane–like mesangial matrix.

Three elements compose the juxtaglomerular apparatus. The endothelium of the terminal afferent arteriolar cells, and occasionally cells of the efferent arteriole,[1] which are in contact with the DCT, are distinctly different from the usual arteriolar endothelium. These cells contain single membrane bound granules of moderate electron density (Figure 2-6). The secretory granules contain the enzyme renin. Renin content is greater in the outer cortical glomeruli than in the juxtamedullary glomeruli. Also, a higher density of granules is found in ischemic kidneys. These findings correlate well with hemodynamic theories of glomerular sclerosis described at the end of this chapter.

The tubular cells of the macula densa are distinctly different ultrastructurally from the outer DCT cells. Compared to the usual DCT cells described below, the cells of the macula densa have fewer invaginations of the basilar plasma membrane[8] and smaller but more numerous interdigitations of the lateral plasma membrane between adjacent cells.[9] The Golgi apparatus is located on the basilar side of the

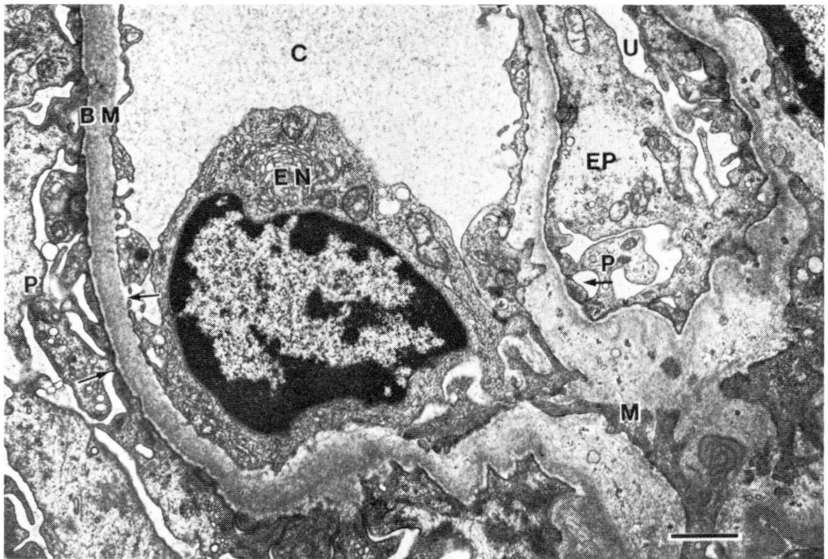

Figure 2-4 Normal glomerular basement membrane. Same patient as Figure 2-3. The GBM is contiguous with the mesangial matrix. Endothelial cell fenestrations (arrows) and podocyte slit membranes (arrowheads) are evident. Characters same as Figure 2-3. Scale bar=1000 nm.

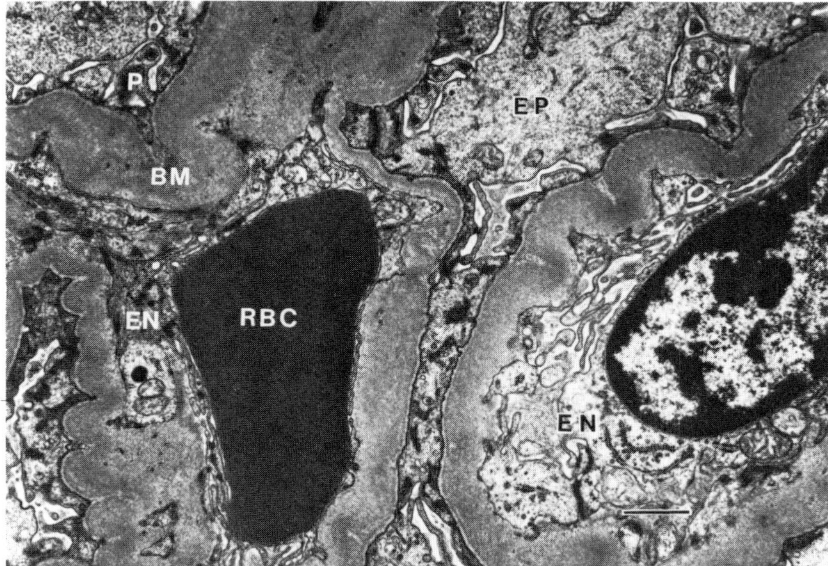

Figure 2-5 Glomerulosclerosis in a 55-year-old male with nephrosclerosis and renal cell carcinoma. Same magnifications as Figure 2-4. Note the uneven thickening of the GBM. The foot processes are within normal limits. Characters same as Figure 2-3. Scale bar=1000 nm.

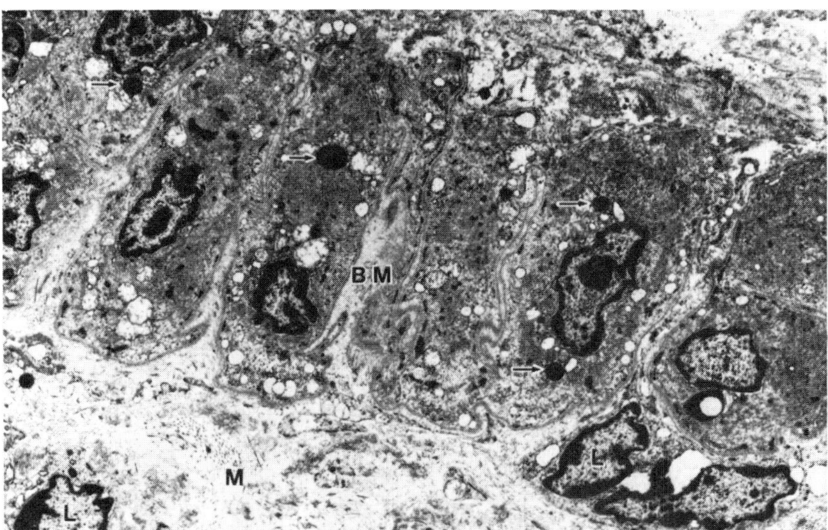

Figure 2-6 Afferent arteriole of macula densa. The endothelial cells are pseudostratified. Within the endothelial cell cytoplasm are membrane-bound electron-dense vesicles containing the enzyme renin. The polkissen matrix appears to merge into a poorly defined arteriolar basement membrane. Lacis cells are present in the matrix. The patient was a 28-year-old male with anorexia nervosa. BM= arteriolar basement membrane, L=lacis cell, M= polkissen matrix, arrows=renin granules. Scale bar=2000 nm.

nucleus, and the mitochondria are smaller than those in other cells of the DCT and are less oriented relative to the base of the cell. Between the arterioles and the macula densa is a collection of cells called the polkissen. The individual cells are known as lacis cells. The lacis cells are continuous with those of the arteriolar media and the mesangium, both of which they resemble. Usually agranular, the cells may develop granules in some human disease states. The basement membrane of the macula densa is continuous with that of the arterioles, the glomerulus, and the polkissen. It is variably described as deficient[8] or thicker[9] relative to other sites in the nephron. In Figure 2-6, for example, the BM is poorly defined.

The cells of the first portion of the PCT, the pars convoluta, are tall cuboidal cells. The basal plasma membrane has extensive infoldings, increasing the surface area at the tubular basement membrane (TBM). Elongated mitochondria pack the basal infoldings. The brush border of the apical cell membrane greatly increases the luminal surface area. Rare cilia are present along the microvilli of the brush border. Adjacent cell borders have extensive interdigitation of plasma membranes increasing the area of cell contact. Vesicles and granules are common in the apical cytoplasm and are related to active endocytotic and exocytotic activity. The cytoplasm also contains a prominent network of smooth and rough endoplasmic reticulum and a well-developed paranuclear Golgi apparatus. Cells of the distal aspect of the PCT, the pars recta, are shorter in height than the cells of the pars convoluta. They have a heavier brush border but few basal membrane invaginations, fewer and small mitochondria, few apical vesicles, a smaller Golgi apparatus, and a higher density of ribosomes relative to cells of the pars convoluta. The TBM is composed of a laminated, tightly packed fibrillar network.[8,9]

The thin limb of Henle's loop is lined by flattened epithelium with few basal invaginations, short and few microvilli, and fewer cytoplasmic organelles relative to the PCT, including mitochondria. The TBM, here and throughout the tubular system, is similar to that of the PCT with the exception of the macula densa. The thick ascending limb has columnar cells, slightly smaller than the epithelium of the PCT. Despite few apical microvilli, the thick limb has prominent basal infoldings containing abundant mitochondria oriented perpendicular to the TBM. The mitochondria are longer than those in the PCT. High levels of ATPase activity are present along the basal membrane. The rough endoplasmic reticulum and Golgi apparatus are prominent. The ultrastructure is compatible with active ion transport.[8,9]

Cells of the DCT are cuboidal and have very extensive basal infoldings packed with short mitochondria with large internal surface area. The mitochondria are not strictly oriented in relation to the TBM and may even by located apical to the nucleus. Membrane interdigitations are rare at the apices. Cellular organelles are abundant but fewer than in the PCT. Numerous membrane-active enzymes are present in the DCT.[8,9]

The collecting tubules have cuboidal cells which increase in size as the tubules approach the collecting ducts. Basal infoldings decrease until absent at the collecting ducts. A moderate number of microvilli are present at the apex. Mitochondria are irregular in shape; nuclei are large. Two cell varieties can be identified. Dark cells have more cytoplasmic organelles than light cells. Dark cells decrease in number as the collecting ducts are approached. They become more numerous in potassium depletion and may reflect higher cellular activity. Light cells have small lateral membrane interdigitations and basal infoldings with a low number of mitochondria.[8,9]

Interstitial cells are prominent in the medulla and particularly in the papilla. The cells are elongated in shape and are oriented perpendicularly to the tubules and capillaries. They contain abundant rough endoplasmic reticulum, a prominent Golgi apparatus, elongated mitochondria, microfilaments, and lipid droplets which may have vasodepressor activity.[8]

NEPHROPATHY OF AGING

Gross Appearance

The senile changes found on gross examination of the kidney have been subject to generalizations. Warren[10] was purposefully vague when citing the changes listed by Laroche and Mathe[11]: (*a*) atrophy, (*b*) renal capsular thickening with subcapsular adhesions, and (*c*) cortical surface irregularities. Warren further cites Howell and Piggott[12] who on gross examination of kidneys from 300 patients over 65 years of age found no gross lesions in 47% of patients and observed the classical senile change of coarse cortical scarring in only 14%.[10] The above generalizations are not too helpful in understanding renal aging. Careful statistical analyses provide a better basis for understanding these changes. The following sections describe more careful statistical analyses of anatomic changes in the kidneys with aging known as macroscopic and microscopic morphometric data. Micromorphometrics provides valuable explanations of gross phenomena such as the generally constant cortical thickness in adulthood up through the fourth decade and decreased thickness after age 40.

Morphometrics

Renal size Age-related decrease in renal size and weight is proportional to the decreased size and weight of all organs with aging. Tauchi et al[13] studied the macromorphometrics and micromorphometrics of 240 Japanese and 180 white male postmortem kidneys of individuals with no evidence of renal dysfunction. At all ages, kidneys of whites had significantly greater mass than Japanese kidneys ($P<.001$). Below 39 years of age the kidneys of whites had a mass of 432.1 ± 36.69 g. In the same age group, Japanese kidneys had a mean combined mass of 320.7 ± 11.38 g. These authors noted significant decreases ($P<.001$) in renal mass with advancing age in both races, perhaps slightly greater in the Japanese. In whites, renal mass decreased 10.1% between the third and fourth decades relative to the fifth decade, 5.8% between the fifth and sixth decades, 3.0% between the sixth and seventh decades, 7.9% between the seventh and eighth decades, and 9.8% between the eighth decade and beyond. Over the same intervals, Japanese renal mass decreased 4.0%, 9.4%, 10.6%, 10.2%, and 18.2%. The mean renal mass in the sixth decade was 365.8 ± 20.24 g for whites and 279.1 ± 9.96 g for Japanese. In the eighth decade the renal mass was 327.0 ± 10.89 g for whites and 224.5 ± 9.50 g for the Japanese. Age-related decreased renal mass in whites did not correlate with the degree of sclerosis of intrarenal arteries as it did in the Japanese subjects. The authors cited earlier work in which they emphasized that arterial changes and medullary fibrosis were not necessary for renal senile atrophy. They infer that their data represent pure age-related changes in whites but in the Japanese subjects the age-related changes are compounded by nutritional-induced atherosclerotic change.

Micromorphometry of the nephron and glomerulus Numerous studies have evaluated changes in components of the nephron with age. Unfortunately the parameters measured have not always been comparable and the results not always compatible. Virtually all studies have shown a decrease in the number and size of nephrons with advancing age. In hypertension, glomerular and arterial sclerosis is most prominent in the juxtaglomerular cortex with initial sparing of superficial glomeruli.[14] Schram et al emphasized that glomerulosclerosis of aging is a distinct entity independent of nonage- related glomerulopathy such as that of diabetes mellitus and hypertension.[15] However, when

Kaplan et al evaluated the percentage of sclerosed glomeruli in the subcapsular, mid-, and inner cortical zones from 122 patients without clinical evidence of renal disease or hypertension, they observed no significant differences between these zones.[16] They studied kidneys of male and female patients of ages less than 1 year old up to 89 years of age. They were able to establish a 95% confidence interval for the percent sclerotic glomeruli in a normal population spanning nine decades. These findings are shown in Figure 2-7. No sexual bias was found except for female predominance in the third decade; male in the ninth decade. Ninety-five percent of the population between 40 and 45 years old would be expected to have less than 10% glomerulosclerosis. Individuals in this age group with greater than 10% sclerosis would have a 95% probability that the etiology of glomerulosclerosis would be a disease process beyond natural aging. Morphometric studies by Kappel and Olsen[16] on transplant donor kidneys and postmortem kidneys from patients without evidence of renal disease confirmed the

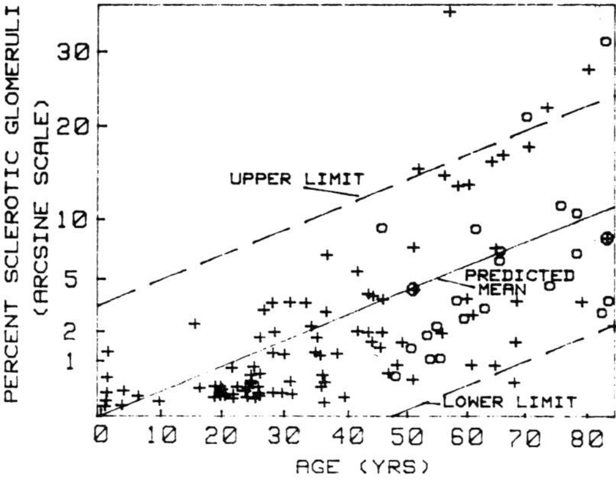

Figure 2-7 Percent sclerotic glomeruli in kidneys from 122 autopsied patients plotted against age (arcsine scale). Observed cases indicated by crosses for medical examiner cases; circles for hospital cases. The regression line for the predicted mean percent sclerotic glomeruli (Y axis) at any age (X axis) is given by the equation Y=0.0084X. Outer lines indicate 2 SD from the mean. (Reproduced with permission from Kaplan et al.[17])

studies of Kaplan et al.[17] They observed only 0% to 1% glomerulosclerosis to age 40, increasing to approximately 30% beyond age 80. Donor kidneys ranged in age from 9 to 70 years old. Autopsy kidneys ranged from 30 to almost 100 years old. The percent glomerulosclerosis significantly correlated with age in both groups ($2P<.01$ and $2P<.001$, respectively). There was no significant difference between sexes. A lower percentage of glomerulosclerosis in the donor group than in the autopsy group implied undiagnosed renal diseases in the latter group. Regression lines for percent glomerulosclerosis with aging crossed the X axis in the late third decade implying that physiologic glomerular obsolescence begins at this age.

A similar conclusion was reached by Darmady et al based on decreases in glomerular surface area and proximal tubular lengths and volume with age.[2] Changes in glomerular size with aging have been documented by several different approaches. Tauchi et al,[13] and Darmady et al,[2] measured glomerular cross-sectional area and surface areas, respectively. Tauchi et al found that in whites glomerular cross-sectional area did not vary with age (under 39 years old, 189.5 ± 1.07 μm; 50 to 59 years old, 191.9 ± 1.38 μm; above 80 years old, 185.1 ± 0.98 μm). However, they found that in the Japanese kidneys there was a significant correlation between glomerular cross-sectional area and age, $P<.001$. Under 39 years old, the mean area was 175.6 ± 0.63 μm; at 50 to 59 years old, the area was 168.8 ± 0.53 μm; over 80 years old, the area averaged 148.5 ± 0.81 μm. They also found that the number of cells in glomerular tufts significantly decreased ($P<.001$) in both races. Darmady et al, examining microdissections of nephrons, calculated glomerular surface areas. They found they steadily decline from a peak of 0.262 mm^2 at 40 to 59 years of age to 0.155 mm^2 at 80 to 101 years of age.[2]

Renal tubules Darmady et al, using microdissection, also calculated proximal tubular volume in 100 nephrons evenly divided between subcapsular, midcortical, and juxtamedullary zones from 105 postmortem kidneys (the age range was term birth to 101 years old) with no evidence of renal or hypertensive disease.[2] They found a steady, gradual decline in both PCT length and volume after age 20. In the 20- to 39-year-old age group (21 cases) the average length was 19.36 mm (the volume 0.076 mm^3). In the 80- to 101-year-old group (15 cases) the average volume was 0.052 mm^3. The ratio of glomerular surface area to PCT volume was almost constant in all age groups after maturity. Tauchi et al counted epithelial cells *per* random convoluted tubule in histologic cross-section. In whites a significant decrease ($P<.001$) was found only after age 60; in Japanese, only in the fifth decade, with no significant change thereafter.[13] Darmady et al, also compared PCT parameters for the entire cortex and the juxtamedullary zone alone. This inner zone has the longest tubules. At age 20 years the juxtamedullary nephrons constituted 8% of all nephrons and had 15% of the total PCT volume. At age 84 years the inner nephrons constituted 6% of all nephrons and had 9% of the total PCT volume. The authors felt that this apparent selective loss of nephrons possessing the longest loops of all cortical zones might be important in explaining the mechanism of reduced urine concentrating abilities in the elderly. They felt that the constancy of the ratio of glomerular surface area to PCT volume, with aging, indicated "that renal function, although reduced, is still balanced," and argued against compensatory tubular hyperplasia.[2]

An additional finding of Darmady et al and their microdissections was a linear increase in diverticula of the DCT from age 4 years onward. They postulated these tubular pouches to be related to degenerative changes in tubular elastin and basement membrane. They attached no definitive significance to the finding other than evidence of a general gradual tubular degeneration and possible relation to infection because of occasional organisms they identified within the blind pouches.[2]

Interstitial fibrous tissue In general, studies show an increased amount of interstitial fibrous tissue with aging. Darmady et al, in the process of microdissection of nephrons, and electron microscopy, noted increased fibrosis with aging, particularly after age 70 years.[2] Kappel and Olsen found the percentage of cortical interstitial fibrous tissue, including that found in TBM, to be age-dependent.[16] Statistical differences between their transplant donor and autopsy kidneys were similar to those described in their glomerular evaluations. Tauchi et al noted an increase in medullary fibrosis with age in both whites and Japanese with more marked changes in the latter.[13]

Pelvis Schramm et al described no significant age-specific changes in the renal pelvis.[15]

Vascular tree By both microscopic and micromorphometric analyses there is no evidence that vascular changes, particularly atherosclerotic vascular disease, initiate age-related nephropathy. Hypertension produces well-defined renal changes and exerts a large part of its renal effects through vascular changes. The accelerated atherosclerosis of hypertension serves as a model for the consequences of atherosclerosis. Davidson et al evaluated the angiographic changes with aging relative to those seen in kidneys of hypertensive patients.[18] Postmortem kidneys from 28 males and 23 females who in life had documented diastolic pressures below 90 torr and no evidence of age-independent renal disease on clinical history and pathologic examination were examined by in vitro angiography analogous to in vitro study. Hypertensive renovascular changes include loss of gradual tapering of the segmental arteries with increased tortuousity and luminal irregularities. The arcuate arteries show more acute angulation at the corticomedullary junction and an abrupt decrease in luminal diameter of the branches. Davidson et al[18] demonstrated senile vascular changes similar to those in hypertension but expressed only at advanced age (greater than 80 years old). Little change was seen before age 50. The earliest and predominant changes were seen in the most distal arteries visualized. There were no arcuate artery changes before age 40; essentially no segmental artery changes before age 50. Beyond age 70, all arcuate arteries showed abnormalities. Beyond age 80, all segmental arteries showed changes. When severe change was noted, it was frequently most prominent in the poles of the kidney. Kidneys with segmental arteries demonstrating the most severe changes also showed sharply circumscribed notching of those arteries immediately distal to major bifurcations. No sex differences were observed. Davidson et al (citing microangiography data of Ljungqvist[19]) noted the earliest changes evolved slowly and occurred in the small cortical vessels with secondary changes in the arcuate and segmental vessels. The earliest changes appreciable on conventional angiography were in the arcuate arteries. The authors hypothesized that the loss of functional renal tissue without loss of stroma causes the loss of the normal tapered appearance in the segmental artery. This opinion was also expressed by other authors. Tauchi et al[20] emphasized, as stated above, that arterial changes were not essential for senile renal atrophy. Tauchi et al[13] found no correlation between atherosclerotic change and decreased renal mass in whites. However, in Japanese they found that atherosclerosis, particularly in small and medium-sized vessels, appeared earlier and was more advanced than in whites. In Japanese decreased renal mass correlated with the atherosclerotic change and suggested nutritional-based disease.[13] The data of Darmady et al suggested that parenchymal and vascular changes occurred simultaneously and that vascular changes did not cause the decreased renal mass with aging.[2]

As stated above, renal changes with aging are subject to generalization. Those renal age-related changes that can be morphologically measured may be summarized in four generalized statements:

1. Age-related renal changes are not evident before the end of the fourth decade.
2. After age 40, aging produces a gradual atrophy of the components of the kidney.
3. Age-related renal changes tend to accelerate after the seventh decade.
4. These changes are independent of sex.

Morphologic Basement Membrane and Mesangial Changes With Aging

The preceding section on morphometrics described macroscopic and microscopic changes in the aging kidney and discussed little concerning the pathogenesis of these changes. Most theories of the pathogenesis of renal age-related lesions relate to basement membrane (BM) changes. Proposed mechanisms for the BM lesions include biochemical changes, senescence, immune phenomena, toxic/metabolic damage, and hemodynamic changes.

It is well established that mammalian glomerular basement membranes (GBM) show thickening with age (Figures 2-8 and 2-9).[2,14,21–29] Analogous to the onset of demonstrable human age-related renal changes at the end of the fourth decade, numerous investigators found that GBM thickening in several strains of rats was minimal before maturity.[21–23,25] The age of onset at which GBM thickening increased proportionally to advancing age differed with the strain of rat examined. Concurrent thickening of the mesangial matrix has been shown for both the rat[21,23] and guinea pig.[24] Bolton and Sturgill[23] demonstrated, in fact, an age-related thickening of all renal BM including the tubular basement membrane (TBM) as well as the GBM and mesangial matrix.[23] Darmady et al

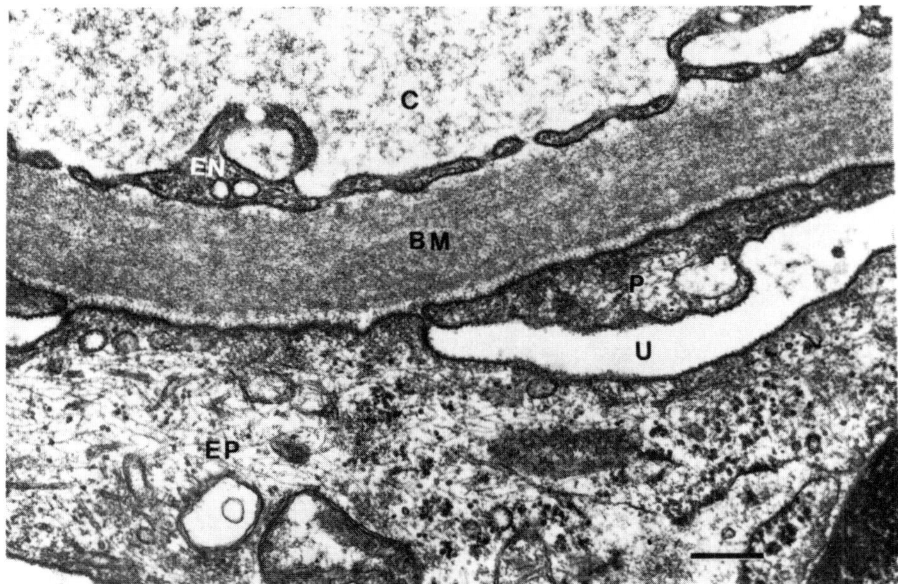

Figure 2-8 Glomerular basement membrane from the same patient as Figure 2-3. There is uniform thickening of the GBM. Foot process fusion is present. Characters same as Figure 2-3. Scale bar=250 nm.

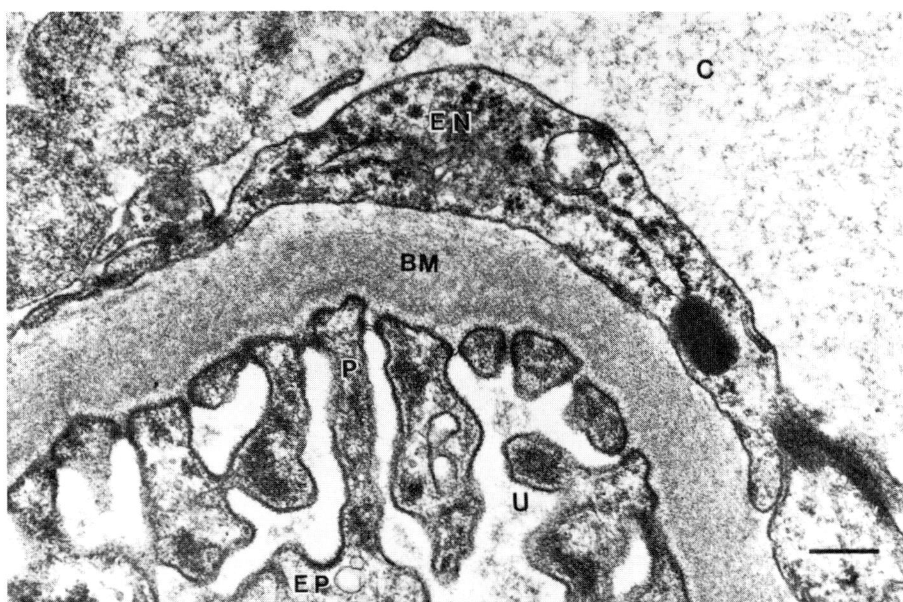

Figure 2-9 Glomerular basement membrane from the same patient as Figure 2-5. There is uneven thickening of the GBM. Foot processes are within normal limits. Characters same as Figure 2-3. The magnification is identical to Figure 2-8. Scale bar=250 nm.

confirmed age-dependent thickening of the TBM in humans. They found this change to be progressive and gradual, but focal, similar to the irregular thickening seen in older rats by Bolton and Sturgill.[2] Additional GBM-related findings included clumped eosinophilic material within the glomerulus, seen on light microscopy. Langner et al occasionally observed such material in and around the glomerular tuft in nondiabetic and, to a greater extent, in diabetic guinea pigs.[24] Couser and Stilmant observed this material in advanced glomerulosclerosis in rats; it was equivalent to subendothelial electron-dense deposits on electron microscopy.[21] Age-related increased GBM material on biochemical analysis in the rat and humans correlates with age-related GBM thickening.[30,31]

Theories on the Pathogenesis of Age-Related Nephropathy

Diabetes mellitus is but one factor known to produce increased BM thickening and glomerulosclerosis with advancing time. Diabetes mellitus and hyperglycemia may be considered to be part of a broad category of dietary effects. Other factors known to produce BM thickening and/or glomerulosclerosis include hypertension, compensatory renal growth following partial kidney ablation, and irradiation. This chapter will now be directed toward evaluating theories of pathogenesis of BM thickening and/or glomerulosclerosis and end with a unifying concept.

Diet Dietary effects are perhaps among the best known causes of glomerulosclerosis, particularly diabetes mellitus. Kimmelstiel and Wilson described the nodular glomerulosclerosis pathognomonic of diabetes mellitus in 1936.[32] This diabetic lesion is a focal proliferation of capillary tuft BM and contiguous BM-like material of the mesangial matrix. It appears to be an exaggerated focal BM thickening reminiscent of the focal BM thickening with age described above. Basement membrane thickening in both aging and diabetes is not restricted to the kidney. Age-related BM thickening and diabetes-related BM thickening have been described in the capillaries of other organ systems including muscle.[26] Further similarities between aging and diabetes will be discussed below under biochemical changes in BM.

Over-nutrition independent of diabetes is also associated with BM thickening and glomerulosclerosis. Kennedy found that hypothalamic-induced hyperphagia produced renal lesions in rats identical to those which occur spontaneously with aging.[27] These changes were independent of and preceded vascular changes. Kennedy also observed renal tubule cell proliferation in the hyperphagic rats. In addition, the same changes occurred in non-hyperphagic rats subjected to uninephrectomy. Further significance of this finding is discussed below. Langner et al found that hyperglycemia enhanced the glomerulopathy of aging.[24] Johnson and Barrow found that GBM thickening in the mouse was induced by aging and to a greater extent by a high protein diet.[28] Everitt et al found that both high caloric and high protein diets accelerated the BM thickening and glomerulosclerosis of aging in the rat without affecting blood pressure or serum protein concentration.[29] Though high protein diet does not induce accelerated renal lesions in normal aging individuals, the effect may be significant in patients with decreased renal mass. Low calorie and low protein diets have been suggested for renal compromised patients.[29,33,34]

Toxins Many nephrotoxins are known in the pharmacopoeia and in the environment. Unidentified toxins have been suggested as one cause for the age-related renal changes.[21,23] Because of the similarities of renal lesions related to protein intake and that of aging, amino acids have been questioned as a possible toxin.[23] Inorganic phosphate has been implicated as well, and there have been recent recommendations to reduce its content in the diet of patients with compromised renal function.[29,33] Bolton and Sturgill interpreted ultrastructural findings to indicate that senescence, possibly enhanced by toxins, produces glomerulosclerosis.[23]

Immune mechanisms Immunologic mechanisms are known to play active roles in many glomerulopathies. Humoral immune mechanisms have been suggested as a component of age-related nephropathy by many authors.[2,21-23,35] However, some of these same authors have excluded immune mechanisms as the sole cause. Bolton et al[22] found no correlation between glomerular immunoglobulin and complement deposition with age. Couser and Stilmant felt that mesangial IgM deposits in the aging rats were the result of nonspecific trapping of proteins reaching mesangium because of increased glomerular permeability with aging.[21] Bolton and colleagues, however, could not exclude a cell-mediated immune factor.[22,23]

Mesangial overwork As the BM of glomerular capillaries is intimately connected to the BM-like mesangial matrix, and the mesangial cells are believed to secrete the matrix, the mesangial cells are suspect in the pathogenesis of the thickening of the matrix if not also of the GBM. Increased mesangial matrix in glomerulosclerosis of any etiology must be the result of overproduction or decreased catabolism. Mesangial cells have phagocytic activity which decreases with age.[21] They also maintain the mesangial matrix integrity. Accumulation of substances which stimulate production of the mesangial matrix could produce a thickened matrix.[34] Accumulation of cellular toxins might decrease the ability of the mesangial cells to maintain the matrix.[21,35] Simple overload of mesangial cells by macromolecules filtered through the GBM and phagocytosed by mesangial cells could have a similar effect.[21,25] Couser and Stilmant stated that increasing glomerular BM permeability precedes proteinuria and the subsequent development of mesangial lesions which produce glomerulosclerosis.[21] Romen felt that thickening of the mesangial matrix and GBM results from the inability of mesangial cells to degrade accumulating BM due to senescence or decreased digestibility of the modified BM.[35]

Biochemical changes in basement membrane Romen's suggestion of decreased digestibility of modified aging BM leads directly to the discussion of the biochemical changes in BM with aging. On a general level, Korenchevsky felt that hypertrophy and atrophy are both components of aging in the kidney.[5] At a molecular level, Bolton and Sturgill favored the failure to degrade and repair BM ("abiotrophy") as the mechanism of senescent changes in the rat kidney.[23] Taylor and Price found that with aging the chemical composition of rat glomerular BM becomes more similar to type IV collagen, suggesting an increase in type IV collagen.[30] They based this conclusion on an increased proportion of hydroxylated proline and lysine (collagen-specific amino acids) to the total amino acid (proline, hydroxyproline, lysine, hydroxylsine) content. They also found an age-related increase in the collagenous and disaccharide components of rat GBM, and an age-related decrease in the solubility of GBM. Analyses of human GBM and TBM by Langeveld et al showed an increased hydroxylation of proline and lysine with maturation and aging up to age 65, but decreased hydroxylation beyond age 65.[36] Smalley also noted decreased hydroxylation; all but four of his 23 patients were of advanced age.[31] All these authors also, however, observed an increased saccharide binding in aged BM, particularly to hydroxylysine and hydroxyproline residues. DeBats et al found increased hydroxylation and increased content of hexose and hexosamine in the GBM of humans of advanced age relative to young normal patients.[26] They found identical but greater changes in the GBM of diabetics of advanced age relative to young normal patients.

Morphologic and biochemical similarities between GBM and TBM have already been described. Biochemical differences between the two types of BM have also been found.

Langeveld et al found that human GBM contains more 3-hydroxyproline and heterosaccharides than human TBM.[36] They also found that hydroxylation of TBM occurs later in life and continues for a longer duration than in GBM. They found these differences in numerous mammalian species as well as humans. They believed the differences between GBM and TBM may be related to the different cells producing the BM in the different sites. Langeveld et al[36] and Taylor and Price[30] theorized that BM hydroxylation, positively correlating with the age-related modification of BM composition, reflects increased collagen cross-linking. The resultant increased stability and decreased enzymatic-digestibility would decrease BM collagen catabolism producing thickened BM.[30,36] Smalley speculated that the age-related incorporation of saccharide moieties might impart resistance to enzymatic digestion.[37] DeBats et al suggested that the biochemical BM changes might result from increased hydroxylase and glycosyl transferase activity or spontaneous chemical changes from increased autooxidative processes.[26] Functionally, changes in the chemical constituents and ionic charges of the BM could affect mechanical support, hydraulic conductivity, molecular sieving, and charge-selective properties.[34,36]

Renovascular and hemodynamic theories A heterogeneous assortment of theories related to the pathogenesis of age-related nephropathy are based on renovascular and hemodynamic changes. Known causes of renovascular disease have been evaluated as models of age-related nephropathy. Hypertension has been discussed above. Radiation nephropathy is another possible model. Renal changes following irradiation do not become clinically evident until weeks to months after the insult. The lesions which evolve resemble spontaneous nephrosclerosis and involve the vascular, nephronal, and interstitial compartments. The earliest changes seen are degeneration of arterioles and capillaries with vasodilation and fluid transudation into the interstitium. Subsequent fibrinoid necrosis occasionally evolves. Later changes include independent glomerulosclerosis, tubular atrophy, interstitial edema, and mild chronic inflammatory infiltrates. The later changes seem closely related to capillary lesions. The latest events are renal fibrosis and scarring.[8,38] Radiation, however, induces changes that are more reminiscent of those of malignant hypertension than aging. It may also induce hypertension, a finding not found with aging.[14,29]

Ischemia has also been suggested as the etiology of age-related nephropathy. Oliver, noting that renal degeneration and atrophy were accompanied by renovascular atherosclerosis, suggested that atherosclerotic-induced ischemia was the primary effect in the nephropathy of aging. He stated further that aging of the kidneys is a special case of aging of the vascular system.[7] Darmady et al refuted this theory. Citing a quote from Oliver acknowledging arteriosclerosis itself as a disease, Darmady et al considered atherosclerosis distinct from aging. They supported this concept with their data which showed that vascular changes are concurrent with, rather than precedent to, the progressive renal changes in aging.[2] Romen[35] invoked ischemia as one possible contributing factor to decreased collagen catabolism with subsequent collagen accumulation within the thickening BM. He cited Chvapil who found normal dermal collagen synthesis but decreased dermal collagen degradation during partial anoxia.

Hydraulic theories bridge the domains of morphology and hemodynamics. Shock[3] felt that age-induced vascular changes at the nephron level are the primary factor in decreased renal function with age. He observed a steady decline in effective renal plasma flow per unit of tubular excretory capacity after the fourth decade not attributable to decreased cardiac output or hypotension. The age-induced reduction in renal blood flow was partially reversible during the course of a pyrogen reaction (killed typhoid, intravenous). Shock felt therefore that age-induced vascular changes are not the result solely of structural changes in the renal vessels. Schurek et al[25] documented age-related elevation in the blood pressure in male rats in a strain without spontaneous hypertension. Blood pressure elevation was concurrent with increasing GBM width. They postulated that the blood pressure elevation was compensatory for the decreased hydraulic conductance imparted by the thickening GBM. Blood pressure fell in rats of advanced age. The glomerular filtration rate remained relatively constant until advanced age. In contrast, Feld et al[14] found no variation in blood pressure in male rats from a strain without spontaneous hypertension. They observed the rats through middle age. Everitt et al[29] studied male rats of the same strain as Schurek et al but found no age-related change in blood pressure through advanced age, even with caloric and protein diet modifications.

Micropuncture arteriolar and glomerular capillary pressure and resistance studies by Azar et al[39] in spontaneously hypertensive rats without renal damage showed an increase in afferent and efferent arteriolar resistance at the single nephron level. They regarded the increased afferent arterial resistance in the presence of hypertension as an autoregulatory function. They performed similar studies on aging normotensive rats without renal disease. Up until maturity there was a progressive increase in body weight, renal mass, and single nephron glomerular filtration rate (SNGFR). From maturity (7.5 months of age) to 10 months of age, body and renal mass did not change. However, the SNGFR continued to rise.

Renal ablation has been used as a model of reduced renal mass as would occur at a slow progressive rate with aging. Kennedy found that the changes induced in the remaining kidney following uninephrectomy were equivalent to those found in hypothalamic hyperphagia, and in both experimental conditions the discriminating factor was the duration after the insult.[27] Azar et al[39] measured renal hemodynamics in the rat via micropuncture technics. They also used unilateral nephrectomy as the means of reducing renal mass. Renal ablation produced increased glomerular plasma flow and a lesser magnitude increase in transcapillary hydraulic pressure. There was no significant change in total kidney GFR relative to renal mass, but SNGFR increased significantly to about 150% of normal ($P<.01$). No hypertension developed and the single nephron filtration fraction was unchanged. Uninephrectomy in rats made hypertensive by a high salt intake postweaning produced a large increase in transcapillary hydraulic pressure and a large decrease in arteriolar resistances with resultant greatly increased glomerular plasma flow relative to normals ($P_5.001$) and uninephric normotensives ($P<.005$). The SNGFR of uninephric hypertensive rats exceeded that of normals by 200%. With advancing age the single nephron filtration rate fell significantly ($P<.001$). The GFR relative to renal mass in the hypertensives fell to about 60% of normal ($P<.025$).[39] Hostetter et al, using micropuncture and 11/12ths renal ablation in normotensive rats, found identical pathologic changes to those found by Azar et al including a greater significance and magnitude of rise in glomerular plasma flow ($P<.005$) than in capillary hydraulic pressure ($p<.025$).[40] Furthermore, they found a low protein diet negated any changes in the ablated rat relative to sham-operated normals. They felt their data suggested that single nephron hyperfiltration damaged remnant glomeruli.[40] Azar et al[39] and Hostetter et al[40] described the microscopic changes produced by their experiments. Azar et al found that by light microscopy in hypertensive ablated rats, glomerular capillary lesions—complete or partial glomerulosclerosis, GBM thickening, focal mesangial hypercellularity, epithelial proliferation, and capsular adhesions—were prominent, whereas arteriolar changes were minimal even in the arterioles of sclerosed glomeruli. They suggested that the degeneration was purely glomerular and was attributable to increased capillary pressure.[39] Hostetter et al[40] examined their animals by light, scanning electron, and transmission electron microscopy. The ablated normal diet animals showed protein-filled lysosomes in glomerular and tubular epithelial cells, glomerular epithelial cytoplasmic blebs, foot process fusion, and mesangial expansion. No vascular changes were found. All lesions were more frequent in the outer cortex. No lesions were present in the sham group, few in the low protein ablated group; with no podocyte change, no protein droplets, and no mesangial change. The physiologic data suggest that (1) renal ablation produces a compensatory increase in glomerular plasma flow; (2) the "post-salt" hypertension model produces a decreased arteriolar resistance and increased hydraulic pressure; (3) these forces are additive to increase SNGFR; (4) hyperfiltration causes glomerulosclerosis; and (5) autoregulation can be returned (physiologic effects of ablation or hypertension mollified) by a low protein diet. The constant total kidney GFR in the face of a rise in SNGFR implies continued nephron loss. If in advanced age the nephrons can no longer undergo anatomic and functional hypertrophy, total kidney GFR will decrease as found by Schurek et al.[25]

Unifying concept Brenner et al[34] have proposed an integrated hypothesis to explain the interrelation of the various pathophysiologic conditions discussed above which result in glomerulosclerosis. Their hypothesis is based on a centralizing feature of hyperfiltration. Figure 2-10 is a modification of their diagrammed hypothesis. Aging and the changes it induces have been integrated into the overall scheme. The age-related changes can be followed along the outside of the diagram from aging through BM and mesangial matrix alteration to glomerulosclerosis. A direct path from age-induced BM changes to increase mesangial matrix is not drawn to avoid clutter. Hyperfiltration effects become important as a compensatory response to the decreased glomerular plasma flow secondary to age-related BM changes and the decreased renal mass caused by glomerular sclerosis. Other initiating con-

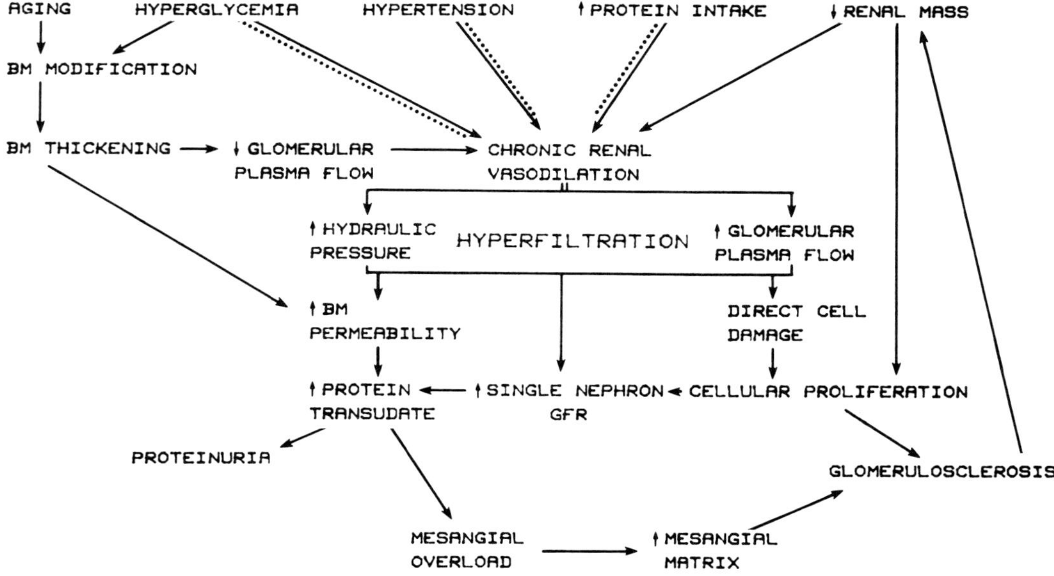

Figure 2-10 Pathogenesis of glomerulosclerosis integrating various etiologies including aging. Composite lines indicate unequal effects of elevated hydraulic pressure and increased glomerular plasma flow in producing hyperfiltration via some etiologies. Solid lines indicate which side of the flow chart predominates. (Modified with permission from Brenner et al.[34])

ditions such as hyperphagia, hyperglycemia, hypertension, and high protein intake enter the pathway via chronic vasodilation. Chronic vasodilation produces hyperfiltration through the synergistic effects of increased hydraulic pressure and increased glomerular plasma flow rates. Diabetes mellitus exerts its effect by way of both BM alteration and chronic renal vasodilation. Renal ablation equates with decreased renal mass. It enters the pathway by two routes. Decreased renal mass causes chronic renal vasodilation and compensatory cellular proliferation (hypertrophy/hyperplasia). The latter leads directly to glomerular sclerosis or indirectly via mesangial matrix expansion. Many other initiating factors are not integrated into the diagram. Radiation injury and other sources of direct cellular damage including toxins and complement-mediated immune complex disease will adversely affect the maintenance of BM and mesangial matrix, accelerating BM and matrix degeneration. It is important to understand that aging and other initiating factors in the pathogenesis of glomerulosclerosis are part of a self-perpetuating process. Because of built-in renal reserve, aging and other factors usually do not result in overt renal insufficiency.

REFERENCES

1. Moore RA: The total number of glomeruli in the normal human kidney. *Anat Rec* 1931;48:153–168.
2. Darmady EM, Offer J, Woodhouse MA: The parameters of the aging kidney. *J Pathol* 1973;109:195–209.
3. Shock NW: Age changes in renal function, in Lansing AI (ed): *Cowdry's Problems of Aging. Biological and Medical Aspects.* Baltimore, Williams & Wilkins, 1942, pp 614–630.
4. Darmady EM: Growth, ageing, and hypertrophy, in Darmady EM, MacIver AG (eds): *Renal Pathology.* London, Butterworths, 1980 pp 43–66.
5. Korenchevsky V: Chapter 21, in Bourne GH (ed): *Physiological and Pathological Aging.* New York, Hafner Publishing Co, 1961, pp 432–441.
6. Allen AC: Anatomy, in Allen AC: *The Kidney. Medical and Surgical Diseases,* ed 2. New York, Grune & Stratton, 1962, pp 19–63.
7. Oliver JR: Urinary system, in Lansing AI (ed): *Cowdry's Problems of Aging, Biological and Medical Aspects.* Baltimore, Williams & Wilkins, 1952, pp 631–650.
8. Heptinstall RH: Anatomy, in Heptinstall RH (ed): *Pathology of the Kidney.* Boston, Little Brown & Co, 1974, pp 1–50.
9. Trump BF, Bulger RE: Morphology of the kidney, in Becker EL (ed): *Structural Basis of Renal Disease.* New York, Hoeber Medical Division, Harper & Row Publishers, 1968, pp 1–92.
10. Warren A: The urinary system, in Warren A (ed): *The Anatomy of Aging in Man and Animals.* New York, Grune & Stratton, 1971, pp 172–182.
11. Laroche CL, Mathe G: Le rein senile, in Benit L, Bourliere FR (eds): *Trecis de Gerontologie.* Paris, Masson et Cie, 1955, pp 329–347.
12. Howell TH, Piggot AP: The kidney in old age; a preliminary communication. *J Gerontol* 1948:2–3;124–128.
13. Tauchi H, Tsuboi K, Okutoni J: Age changes in the human kidney of the different races. *Gerontology* 1971;17:87–97.
14. Feld LG, Vanliew JB, Galaske RJ, et al: Selectivity of renal injury and proteinuria in the spontaneously hypertensive rat. *Kidney Int* 1977;12:332–343.
15. Schramm A, Genett M, Gerhart KH: Veräendernde Nierenfunktion und Morphologie im Alter. *Z Gerontol* 1981;15:354–369.
16. Kappel B, Olsen S: Cortical interstitial tissue and sclerosed glomeruli in the normal human kidney, related to age and sex. *Virchows Arch [Pathol Anat]* 1980;387: 271–277.
17. Kaplan C, Pasternack B, Shah H, et al: Age-related incidence of sclerotic glomeruli in human kidneys. *Am J Pathol* 1975; 80:227–234.
18. Davidson AJ, Talner LB, Downes WM III: A study of the angiographic appearance of the kidney in an aging normotensive population. *Radiology* 1969;92:975–983.
19. Ljungqvist A: The intrarenal arterial pattern in the normal and diseased human

kidney. A micro-angiographic and histologic study. *Acta Med Scand* 1963;174(suppl 1401):1–38.
20. Tauchi H, Tsuboi K, Sato K: Histology and experimental pathology of senile atrophy of the kidney. *Nagoya Med J* 1958;4:71–97.
21. Couser WG, Stilmant NM: Mesangial lesions and focal glomerular sclerosis in the aging rat. *Lab Invest* 1975;33(5):491–501.
22. Bolton WK, Benton FR, Maclay JG, et al: Spontaneous glomerular sclerosis in aging Sprague-Dawley rats, 1. Lesions associated with mesangial IgM deposits. *Am J Pathol* 1976;85:277–302.
23. Bolton WK, Sturgill BC: Spontaneous glomerular sclerosis in aging Sprague-Dawley rats, 2. Ultrastructural studies. *Am J Pathol* 1980;98:339–356.
24. Langner PH, Lang CM, Singh SB, et al: Glomerular basement membrane changes in aging non-diabetic and diabetic guinea pigs. *Exp Aging Res* 1981;7(2):93–105.
25. Schurek HJ, Panzer J, Weimeyer A, et al: Effects of ageing on glomerular capillaries, blood pressure, and renal function in rats. *Contrib Nephrol* 1982;30:157– 162.
26. DeBats A, Rhodes EL, Gordon AH, et al: Biochemical differences in human glomerular basement membrane related to diabetes and age. *Ann Clin Biochem* 1982;19: 17–21.
27. Kennedy GS: Effects of old age on overnutrition on the kidney. *Brit Med Bull* 1957;13:67–70.
28. Johnson JE Jr, Barrow CH Jr: Effects of age and dietary restriction on the kidney glomeruli of mice: Observations by scanning electron microscopy. *Anat Rec* 1980; 196:145–151.
29. Everitt AV, Porter BD, Wyndham JR: Effects of caloric intake and dietary composition on the development of Proteinuria-associated renal disease and longevity in the male rat. *Gerontology* 1982;28:168–175.
30. Taylor SA, Price RG: Age-related changes in rat glomerular basement membrane. *Int J Biochem* 1982;14:201–206.
31. Smalley JW: Age-related changes in the amino acid composition of human glomerular basement membrane. *Exp Gerontol* 1980;15:43–52.
32. Kimmelstein P, Wilson C: Intercapillary lesions in glomeruli of kidney. *Am J Pathol* 1936;12:83–98.
33. Hostetter TH, Rennke HG, Brenner BM: Compensatory renal hemodynamic injury: A final common pathway of residual nephron destruction. *Am J Kidney Dis* 1982;1(5): 310–314.
34. Brenner BM, Meyer GW, Hostetter TH: Dietary protein intake and the progressive nature of kidney disease: The role of hemodynamically mediated glomerular injury in the pathogenesis of progressive glomerular sclerosis in aging, renal ablation, and intrinsic renal disease. *N Engl J Med* 1982; 307(11):652–659.
35. Romen W: Licht und Elektronenmikroskopische Untersuchungen zur Pathogenese der altersbedingten Glomerulosklerose. *Verh Dtsch Ges Pathol* 1975;59:370–375.
36. Langeveld JPM, Veerkamp JH, Duyf CMP, et al: Chemical characterization of glomerular and tubular basement membranes of men of different ages. *Kidney Int* 1981;20: 104–114.
37. Smalley JW: Age-related changes in hydroxylysylglycosides of human glomerular basement membrane collagen. *Exp Gerontol* 1980;15:65–66.
38. Anderson RE. Radiation injury, in Anderson WAD, Kissane JM (eds): *Pathology.* St. Louis, CV Mosby Co, 1977, pp 326–368.
39. Azar S, Johnson MA, Hertel B, et al: Single-nephron pressures, flows, and resistances in hypertensive kidneys with nephrosclerosis. *Kidney Int* 1977;12:28–40.
40. Hostetter TH, Olson JL, Rennke HG, et al: Hyperfiltration in remnant nephrons: A potentially adverse response to renal ablation. *Am J Physiol* 1981;241:F85–F93.

CHAPTER 3 Tests of Glomerular and Tubular Function in the Elderly

Domenic A. Sica
Robert M. Centor

Anatomical changes occur in the senescent kidney affecting glomeruli,[1] tubules,[2] and the interstitial compartment of the kidney.[2,3] The extent of histologic alterations and their physiologic consequences is more fully discussed in earlier chapters. Certain of these anatomical changes need to be considered in detail in order to reach a fuller understanding of the clinically observed functional changes that occur with aging. Most studies have demonstrated a greater decline in renal cortical mass than that of the medulla.[4,5] Distinctive intrarenal vascular changes accompany this alteration in mass. Hyalinization and collapse of the glomerular tuft with obliteration of the preglomerular arteriole characterizes one type of vascular change. Anatomical continuity between afferent and efferent arterioles localized primarily to the juxtamedullary area, occurs in the other type.[6] Despite a poor correlation between age and the number of glomeruli present, glomeruli generally decrease in number with age.[7] Furthermore, an increasing percentage of the glomeruli remaining become sclerotic and obsolescent.[3] Since new glomeruli are not formed after birth,[7] maintenance of adequate renal function requires that elements of the remaining functioning glomeruli[1] undergo hypertrophy. The condition of the renal vasculature affects this hypertrophy and may, in part, lead to the gradual decline in function of residual nephrons by a hyperfiltration phenomenon[8] in those functioning glomerular tufts that remain. The absence of a linear age-related decline in filtration supports this hypothesis (filtration has an increased rate of decline after the fifth decade).[9,10]

The ratio of glomerular surface area to proximal tubule length remains constant with age since proximal tubule length changes proportionally with glomerular size.[2] This anatomical observation may, in part, explain the parallel decline in glomerular and proximal tubule function that occurs with age.[9] This parallel decline may have several etiologies in that the pathologic changes in the proximal tubule include reduplication as well as thickening of the basement membrane,[2] and these changes may, in part, contribute to the observed functional disturbances.

Distal tubular sites control concentration, dilution, and acidification, and these functions are all disturbed to a varying extent in the senescent kidney. In spite of this, anatomical correlates of distal tubular functional changes are limited to the development of diverticula which clearly increase in number with age.[2,11] Finally, there have been a limited number of observations as regards interstitial changes with age.[2,3,12] Interstitial fibrosis becomes much more evident in the medullary portion of the kidney than in the cortex[3] and may relate to decreases in the acid mucopolysaccharide content of the medullary region.[13] This finding may explain, in part, the observed difference between the gradual rate of decline of creatinine clearance with age as compared to the more precipitous drop in urinary concentrating ability.[14]

A number of renal function tests deviate from the normal range in the face of senescence in the kidney. Table 3-1 lists these by the anatomical site in the nephron where control of the functional process is primarily exercised.

Table 3-1
Alterations in Renal Function Testing in the Elderly

Proximal Tubule
Tubular reabsorption of phosphate[19]
Maximal excretion of:
Diodrast (Tm_D)[54]
PAH (Tm_{PAH})[9,54]
Glucose (Tm_G)[15,16]
Distal Nephron
Ability to excrete an acid load[23,24,26–28]
Diluting ability[33–35]
Concentrating ability[14,37–40]
Sodium conservation[47–49]
Glomerulus
Inulin clearance[9,50,54]
Creatinine clearance[50,51,58,61,74,77]

PROXIMAL TUBULE

As mentioned above, previous anatomical work has described a constancy in the ratio between glomerular size and proximal tubular length with both declining with age.[2] Functional observations parallel this histologic finding in that glomerular filtration rate (GFR) and renal tubular function both decline with age. In this respect, proximal tubular functions studied include the maximal excretion of para-aminohippurate (PAH),[9] Diodrast (Tm_D),[9] and glucose (Tm_G).[15] If one assumes that maximal rates of glomerular filtration are attained by age 20 years, then, as an individual ages, there is a loss of renal function of, approximately, 0.72% per year. This is closely matched by the yearly loss of tubular transport capacity for glucose Tm_G (0.7%), Tm_D (0.68%), and Tm_{PAH} (0.65%). Figure 3-1 illustrates the constancy of the Tm_{PAH}/inulin clearance ratio with age. These observations suggest the existence of a relationship between the rate of decline of glomerular and tubular function and that this decrement represents a loss of nephron function as a unit.[9]

The close correlation between the decline in Tm_G and in that of the clearance of inulin can be seen in Figure 3-2. This lowering of the glucose threshold is not borne out by clinical observation since elderly patients fail to manifest glycosuria

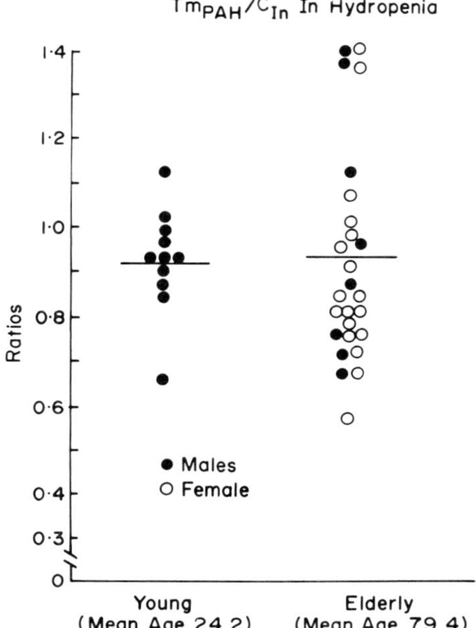

Figure 3-1 Ratio of Tm_{PAH}/C_{In} in a group of young and elderly subjects. Despite the ratios being comparable there is a wide scatter in the elderly group. (Reproduced with permission from Dontas et al.[32])

as readily as their younger counterparts. Butterfield et al have suggested that the renal threshold for glycosuria increases with age, particularly among women[16] with a similar but less evident phenomenon present in males. Close inspection of these data reveals that there seldom existed an absence of glycosuria when serum values exceeded 210 mg/dL for males and 220 mg/dL for females. In their patient population a number of elderly patients manifested glycosuria despite blood sugar values well below an expected threshold value. Considering this analysis[15,16] it is evident that considerable interpatient variability exists as regards the onset of glycosuria and that urine glucose determinations are difficult to interpret in the elderly.

The decline in most proximal tubular functions is predicated on a decrease in function based on involutional changes following ischemia. Certain alterations in proximal tubular function ensue from adaptational changes to a declining nephron mass. One such change is the rise in immunoreactive parathyroid hormone (PTH) that occurs with age,[17,18] which, in turn, is linked to the decline in renal function.[10,19] This causes a decrease in serum phosphate resulting from a decrease in the tubular reabsorption of phosphate and in the ratio of Tm_{PO_4} to GFR,[19] both of these measures being proximal tubular functions. Though a rise in immunoreactive PTH occurs with age, it is not always closely correlated with the level of renal function and may alternatively reflect alterations in calcium homeostasis that result in hypocalcemia.[10,17,18] Such alterations include decreases in hepatic-25-hydroxylation[20] and in 1-hydroxylation by the kidney.[21]

DISTAL TUBULE

Nephron functions such as acidification, concentration and dilution, and sodium excretion are controlled beyond the proximal tubule and abnormalities in each of these functions have been demonstrated in the elderly. In the senescent kidney there is little problem under basal conditions in attaining urinary pH values below 6.0.[22,23]

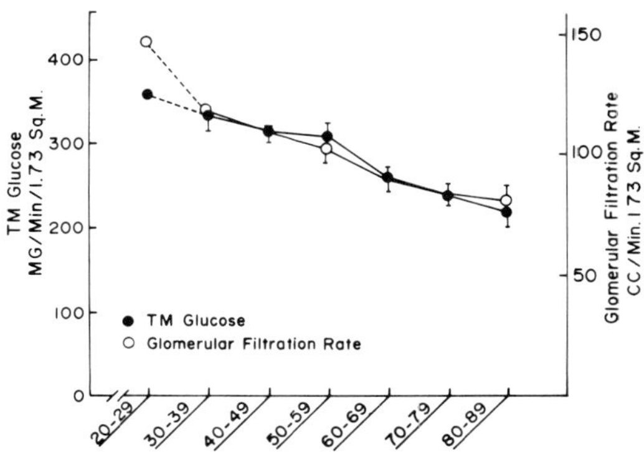

Figure 3-2 Comparison of the maximum rate of renal tubular reabsorption of glucose (Tm_G) with glomerular filtration rate as determined by inulin clearance. The mean values are connected for each decade with the vertical lines representing ± 1 SEM. (Reproduced with permission from Miller et al.[15])

This ability to acidify urine normally permits the maintenance of both a normal blood pH and bicarbonate concentration in the elderly.[24,25] However, when the senescent kidney is stressed with an acid load, its response is sluggish.[22,23] Defects exist in both the minimum urinary pH attained and the time course of net acid excretion following ammonium chloride loading.[22,23] If prolonged ammonium chloride administration is utilized as a testing maneuver, the elderly person remains uncompensated, in a state of metabolic acidosis, much longer than a younger control.[26] Figures 3-3A and 3-3B illustrate the percentage of an administered ammonium chloride acid load excreted in the subsequent eight hours. The reduction in net acid excretion appears to be the result of defects in ammonium excretion rather than in titratable acid excretion and reflect the decline in functioning renal mass that occurs in the elderly.[22,23] When ammonium excretion is factored by the decline in GFR, there appears to be no additional defect in its excretion.[22]

At variance with this work has been a subsequent study[23] that demonstrates a persistent defect in ammonium excretion independent of any correction for a lowered GFR. This observation has been suggested as evidence for a specific defect within the collecting duct of the senescent kidney, a site where urinary acidification and ammonium excretion occurs. The major determinants of ammonium excretion include acid-base status, plasma potassium, urinary pH, and urine flow rate.[27,28] In the two published studies[22,23] values in the young and elderly subjects are similar for all of these determinants *except* for urine flow rate. Until further studies are performed in the elderly, controlling for all variables affecting a change in ammonium excretion, a specific tubular defect in ammonium excretion should remain speculative.

The ability to adequately dilute the urine serves a critical role in preventing the development of dilutional hyponatremia. Urinary diluting ability is clinically

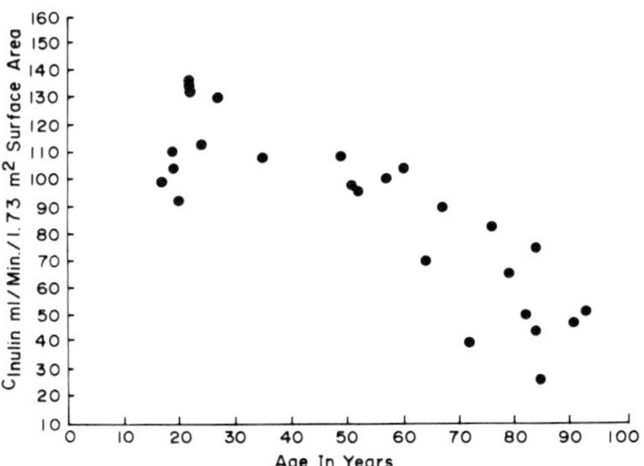

Figure 3-3A Clearance of inulin (mL/min/1.73 m^2 surface area) in relationship to age in 26 subjects. The elderly subjects were housed on the National Institutes of Health gerontology ward and were screened for renal disease. (Reproduced with permission from Adler et al.[22])

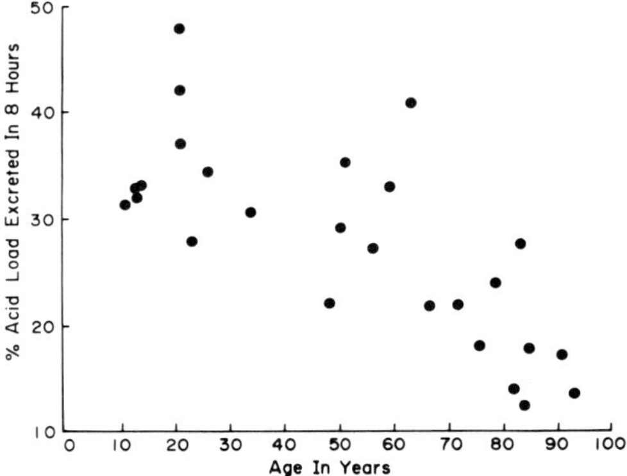

Figure 3-3B Effect of age on the percentage of ingested acid excreted in urine over a subsequent eight-hour period. Subjects were fasted overnight and then given 10 mL/kg body weight of water in the morning followed by an ammonium chloride load (0.1 g/kg body weight). (Reproduced with permission from Adler et al.[22])

assessed by the response to an ingested water load. This test is performed by having the patient ingest 20 mL/kg water over 30 minutes. A normal result requires an adequate *quantitative* excretion of water (80% ingested load/4 h) as well as a *qualitatively* normal urine (osmolality $<$ 100 mosm/kg). Urinary dilutional abnormalities may then result either from inadequate excretion of the ingested water load or from an inability to attain an appropriate diminution in urinary osmolality. As one views the normal dilution process, there are three mechanisms that impair the ability to dilute urine. These are (1) inadequate delivery of tubular fluid (sodium and water) to the diluting region (ascending limb); (2) reduced reabsorption of sodium and water in the ascending limb; and (3) increased permeability of the collecting tubule to water. Any assessment of diluting ability in the elderly must be careful to assess the *healthy* aged individual who is not ingesting medications such as diuretics[29,30] (thiazides and furosemide) or oral hypoglycemic agents[31] (chlorpropamide), both of which are capable of altering maximal water diuresis and are not infrequently utilized in the aged.

There have been few studies that have carefully addressed the intrinsic ability of the senescent kidney to attain maximum degrees of free water clearance (C_{H_2O}) as well as to reach minimum urinary osmolality.[32,33] Those studies performed have demonstrated the existence of a major defect in C_{H_2O} for relatively similar levels of free water volume expansion when comparing young to aged study subjects.[32,33] In addition, in a carefully performed study by Lindeman et al, following ingestion of a standard water load (20 mL/kg) the minimum osmolality attained in a young group of subjects (mean age 31) was 52 ± 3 mosm/kg H_2O compared to an elderly group (mean age 84) who only attained minimum urinary osmolalities of 74 ± 6 mosm/kg/H_2O.[33] Both of these observations (↓C_{H_2O} and ↓ minimum urinary osmolality) may be explained by phenomena associated with the decline in glomerular filtration rate that occurs with aging. This means that the concept of free water clearance must be assessed in light of the fact that a decrease in glomerular filtration rate impairs the ability to excrete water in a quantitative manner. Therefore, any assessment of C_{H_2O} must be factored by measured GFR (C_{H_2O}/100 mL GFR). Figure 3-4 illustrates C_{H_2O} measurements factored per 100 mL GFR from the study of Lindeman et al.[33] Reinterpreting their data in this way suggests that maximal C_{H_2O} is not truly defective but reflects the diminished GFR in the elderly. This correction of C_{H_2O} for diminished GFR has not always led to a normalization of C_{H_2O}. Studies by Dontas et al[32] and Nunez et al[34] suggest that a persistent defect exists in C_{H_2O}/GFR in *elderly females* but not in elderly males.

A final consideration is that of the minimum urinary osmolality that can be attained in the elderly. As total nephron mass declines the remaining nephron population must assume an increasing share of the workload. This increased solute load in residual nephrons initiates an osmotic diuresis and thereby impairs the ability to attain minimum urinary osmolality values.[35] Such a postulate can be proved correct by demonstrating that a further diminution in urinary osmolality occurs following water loading if solute load per nephron is decreased. Limiting salt intake (solute) in individuals with varying degrees of azotemia does, in fact, result in an improvement in the minimum urinary osmolality that can be attained;[36] this finding is consistent with the aforementioned solute load postulate and probably explains the observed values for minimum urinary osmolality in the elderly.[32,33]

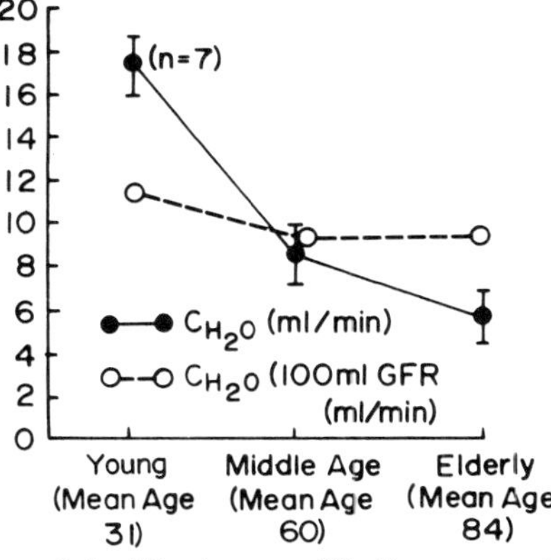

Figure 3-4 Maximum diluting capacity in young, middle aged, and elderly male subjects following ingestion of 20 mL H_2O/kg body weight. Data for C_{H_2O} are ±SEM. (Adapted with permission from Lindenan et al.[33])

An inability of the aged kidney to concentrate urine has been observed since the studies of Lewis and Alving.[37] There have been numerous confirmatory studies of this phenomenon in man[32,38,39] as well as in the rat.[40] Most of these studies have employed a cross-sectional[32,37,39] rather than a longitudinal study design[14] and have employed small numbers of patients often representing a chronically debilitated population. A longitudinal study conducted by Rowe et al utilized male volunteers who had been carefully screened for concurrent medical illness.[14] This study demonstrated that following 12 hours of dehydration, elderly subjects were less able than young or middle-aged subjects to alter urinary volume, urinary osmolality, or osmolar clearance. Since dietary intake was similar in all groups studied, it was not apparent why there existed differences in total solute excretion among the study groups.

It is unclear as to what the actual defect in concentrating ability is due to though a number of possibilities exist (Table 3-2). These possibilities can be listed under the categories of glomerular abnormalities, alteration in antidiuretic hormone levels or its degree of activity, or as intrarenal factors. Several authors have attributed the decline in concentrating ability to the concomitant decline in GFR.[32,39] Despite this, Rowe et al, in their study of elderly subjects, could not demonstrate a relationship between the observed level of creatinine clearance and either urinary flow rate or osmolality (U_{osm}) following 12 hours of fluid deprivation. In their older age group (60 to 79 years), maximum U_{osm} attained was 882 ± 49 mosm/kg compared to a younger group (20 to 39 years) in whom maximum U_{osm} reached was 1109 ± 22 mosm/kg. Though a decline in GFR is undoubtedly contributory to the concentrating defect, it probably is not the sole determinant.

It is possible that with age there occurs a defect in the release of antidiuretic hormone (ADH) thereby limiting the extent to which urine is concentrated. In fact, insensitivity of ADH release to baroreceptor stimuli has been demonstrated in an elderly group of subjects (68 to 81 years old). This group did not increase plasma ADH levels appropriately when the nonosmotic stimulus (supine to upright) of positional change was employed.[41] Despite this observation, all remaining evidence pertaining to ADH release in the elderly points to a limited suppressibility of its release. Miller[42] employed an in vitro system of isolated hypothalamic-neurohypophyseal units obtained from aged rats. In this system ADH release was clearly greater, in both the basal and stimulated states, in units obtained from aged rats. Posterior pituitary content of ADH was also consistently greater in older animals

Table 3-2
Factors Influencing Urinary Concentrating Ability in the Elderly

Glomerular
Decrease in GFR[14]

Antidiuretic Hormone
Increased levels in response to a hyperosmolar stimulus[43]
Decreased suppressibility with ethanol[43]
Baroreceptor insensitivity to positional change[41]
Increased capacity for release of ADH in isolated neurohypophyseal systems[42]
Normal response to submaximal ADH infusion[33]
Decreased maximal urinary osmolality to high-dose vasopressin[38]

Intrarenal
Increased solute load per remaining nephron[44]
Relative increase in medullary blood flow[46]
Defect in generation of medullary interstitial gradient[34,40]

than in their younger counterparts. Also, when the percentage of release was compared between young and old animals it was consistently greater in the latter. In the intact animal, this hypersecretory state was expressed as an increase in plasma ADH concentration. Analogous results have been obtained from the work of Helderman et al.[43] In these studies, stimuli known to inhibit ADH release (ethanol) and to stimulate its release (3% NaCl) were utilized in elderly test subjects (52 to 66 years) and in younger (22 to 48 years) subjects. Despite similar alterations in serum osmolality by an administered 3% NaCl load, the older aged group increased plasma ADH by 450% whereas the younger controls only developed a 250% increment in ADH levels. Osmoreceptor sensitivity, as obtained by plotting the slope of plasma ADH concentration *v* serum osmolality, was demonstrably greater in the older age group. In these same subjects, following the administration of intravenous (IV) ethanol, the suppressibility of ADH was much less in the older age group. These observations suggest that a deficiency in ADH is not present in the elderly.

Since ADH levels would appear not to be decreased in this group, we might, in fact, be dealing with a form of nephrogenic diabetes insipidus, that is, an abnormal response to adequate circulating levels of ADH. Lindeman et al[33] examined the urinary osmolality response to submaximal doses of ADH (8 mU/h during water diuresis). He observed no age-related decline in renal responsiveness to the submaximal dose of vasopressin (Pitressin) administered. However, maximum urinary osmolality that can be attained with high-dose vasopressin is significantly diminished in elderly subjects undergoing a water diuresis. In the studies of Miller and Shock[38] mean values for the urine/plasma (U/P) inulin ratio were determined in each of three age groups (Figure 3-5) undergoing a water diuresis and receiving IV vasopressin (0.5 mU/kg body weight). There clearly existed a negative correlation between the maximum U/P inulin ratio obtained and age; this finding then suggests a defect in the distal nephron's ability to perform maximal osmotic work when supplied with ADH in a standardized amount. It is unclear if this defect represents diminished medullary tonicity or occurs due to an alteration in the renal receptor for vasopressin.

Most likely there exists an intrarenal mechanism that causes the concentrating defect in the elderly. It is possible that an increased solute load in remaining intact nephrons results in an osmotic diuresis.[44] This would then limit the generation of a maximal interstitial medullary gradient and thereby lower the upper limit of urinary osmolality that can be attained in the elderly.

Clearance technics in subjects undergoing water diuresis have been employed to demonstrate the extent of solute transport in the thick ascending limb of the

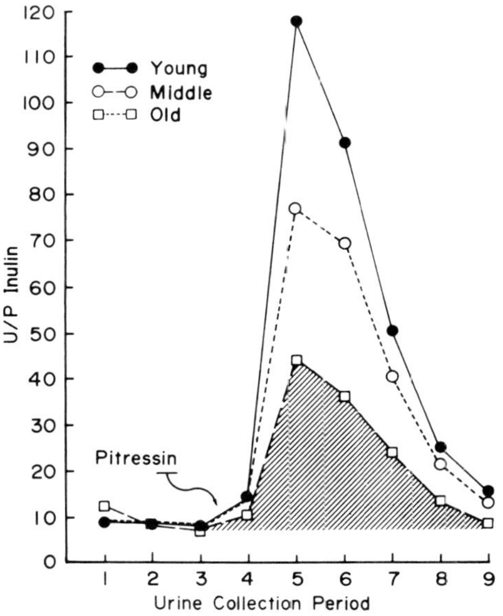

Figure 3-5 Maximum U/P inulin ratio obtained following administration of vasopressin 0.5 mU/kg body weight in subjects undergoing water diuresis. Each urine collection period was 12 minutes in duration. Cross-hatching illustrates maximum U/P inulin ratio attained in elderly subjects. (Reproduced with permission from Miller and Shock.[38])

loop of Henle. Free water clearance/glomerular filtration rate may be employed as a measure of loop salt transport which in turn is affected by rates of distal solute delivery with distal delivery terms being V/GFR or $(C_{H_2O} + C_{Na})$/GFR.[45] In studies done by Nunez et al[34] solute free water generation (C_{H_2O}/100 mL GFR) was always lower in elderly patients for equivalent amounts of sodium delivery to the distal tubule ($C_{H_2O} + C_{Na}$/100 mL GFR). This defect in solute transport might then help explain the defect in urinary concentration based on the theory of diminished medullary hypertonicity. This observation may be species specific since in the aged rat[40] the relationship between C_{H_2O} and $(C_{H_2O} + C_{Na})$ was not found to be different from that in young rats.

A final consideration in the genesis of the concentrating defect in the elderly is the role of medullary blood flow in controlling the removal of solute from the medullary interstitium. Studies by Takazakura et al[6] in the aging kidney have shown that the medullary vascular supply is better maintained than that of the cortex. Studies by Hollenberg et al[46] have provided physiologic support for this observation. They studied 207 prospective kidney donors (17 to 76 years old) assessing their renal hemodynamics by xenon washout studies. These studies showed an inverse relationship between age and cortical blood flow. A *relative* increase in medullary blood flow was suggested which might then enhance removal of solute from the medullary interstitium.

A synthesis of the data on urinary concentrating ability in the elderly is difficult. It would seem that any defect present is multifactorial having a relationship to the age-related decrease in GFR as well as to mechanisms limiting the extent to which the medullary gradient can be generated. Fortunately, this defect in water conservation in the *healthy* elderly subject is not sufficient to contribute significantly to the development of hypertonic volume depletion.

The final urinary sodium concentration is typically thought of as a tubular function. Despite this, a number of additional determinants of renal handling of sodium exist. Several of these are affected by aging including a decrease in renal blood flow,[9] a relative increase in medullary blood flow,[46] and a certain degree of sluggishness of the renin-aldosterone system when acutely stimulated.[47]

Until recently it was not clear as to how the aged kidney would respond to the extremes of sodium intake. It had been known for several years that the aged kidney was capable of conserving sodium in response to an acute diminution in intake.[48] The rapidity with which this sodium conservation occurred was debated until the definitive studies of Epstein and Hollenberg were reported.[49] In these studies the half-time for renal sodium excretion was determined in 89 potential transplant donors of various ages who were placed on controlled sodium intake. In those subjects under 30 years of age the half-time for renal sodium excretion was 17.6 ± 0.7 hours whereas in subjects over 60 years of age, the half-time was prolonged to 30.9 ± 2.8 hours. This observation remains unexplained as to its physiologic basis and to its clinical significance. The diminished conservation of sodium could relate to the increased solute load occurring in remaining functioning nephrons in the older subjects, thereby simply reflecting the sequel to an osmotic diuresis,[44] or it may be a manifestation of the limitations in the secretory rate of aldosterone observed in the elderly.[47] The clinical significance of these observations lies in the fact that net renal sodium conservation in the elderly, though somewhat slower, is certainly more than adequate for maintenance of sodium and water balance. In fact, in studies by Weidmann et al[47] following dietary sodium restriction for six days, the weight loss in elderly subjects (60 to 70 years) of 1.65 ± 0.85/kg body weight was quite comparable to that seen in younger study subjects (20 to 30 years) 1.62 ± 0.85/kg body weight. In both groups studied, 2.5% of body weight was lost as they came into sodium balance.

GLOMERULUS

Glomerular filtration rate (GFR) remains the most frequently employed measure of renal function. The GFR can be measured by a number of technics. Regardless of which technic is utilized it must be reproducible and capable of reflecting the known age related decline in GFR.[9,37,50,51]

For a substance to be an effective measure of GFR, it should be metabolically inert and freely filterable through the glomerulus. Once filtered, it should neither be reabsorbed nor secreted by the renal tubules. Finally, it should be easily measurable with consistent accuracy in both plasma and urine.[52]

The only substance meeting all of these criteria is the fructose polysaccharide inulin (molecular weight 5000) and its clearance is generally accepted as the reference standard for GFR.[53] Early studies in elderly patients clearly demonstrated an age-related decline in inulin clearance.[9,54] Studies employing inulin clearance have the greatest accuracy, but inulin is not an endogenous substance and requires an IV infusion. Additionally, analysis of inulin requires laboratory sophistication. For these reasons the utilization of inulin clearance as a measure of GFR has not been employed to a major extent in clinical medicine.

A number of other substances have been examined as substitutes for inulin. The substance that has attained the widest application in clinical practice has been the concentration of endogenous creatinine in serum and, therefore, the endogenous creatinine clearance.

Several variables determine the serum creatinine concentration including the rate of production, the volume of distribution, the rate of excretion, and the noncreatinine chromogen contribution to the serum measurement.[55] Creatinine is formed in muscles as an end product of the metabolism of creatine and phosphocreatine. Creatine is primarily formed in the liver, and when released it is taken up against a concentration gradient by muscle and other tissues. Creatine and phosphocreatine are interconverted in muscle by the enzyme creatine kinase.[56] In muscle, both creatine and phosphocreatine are nonenzymatically dehydrated to a cyclic anhydride, creatinine, at a rate of 1% to 2% of the body stores of phosphocreatine-creatine[57] (Figure 3-6). The rate of creatinine production is closely related to the weight, age, and sex of the patient. The age-related decline in creatinine production is explained by the decrease in lean body mass.[58–60] A similar explanation applies to the lesser rate of creatinine production in females which averages about 90% of that in males of the same age and weight.[58,61] A reasonable approximation of the expected daily creatinine excretion can be obtained by application of the following formula: 28−(0.2 age) mg/kg body weight in males and the same formula multiplied by 0.85 in females.[61] Very little is known as regards regulation of the rate of creatinine production in man. There is some evidence that production is diminished in individuals with dystrophic muscle diseases,[62,63] or in individuals with advanced renal failure.[64] An increase in the nonrenal elimination of creatinine in chronic renal failure has been proposed as an explanation for this declining urinary excretion.[65]

The apparent volume of distribution of creatinine is equivalent to total body water irrespective of the level of renal function. Most textbooks quote total body water as 60% of total body weight but there is in reality considerable interindividual variability in this measurement as well as a gradual decline with age.[66] It is of interest to note that the rate of decline of total body water with age parallels the decrease in creatinine excretion as well as the decrease in lean body mass.[67] It would then appear that the best measure of total

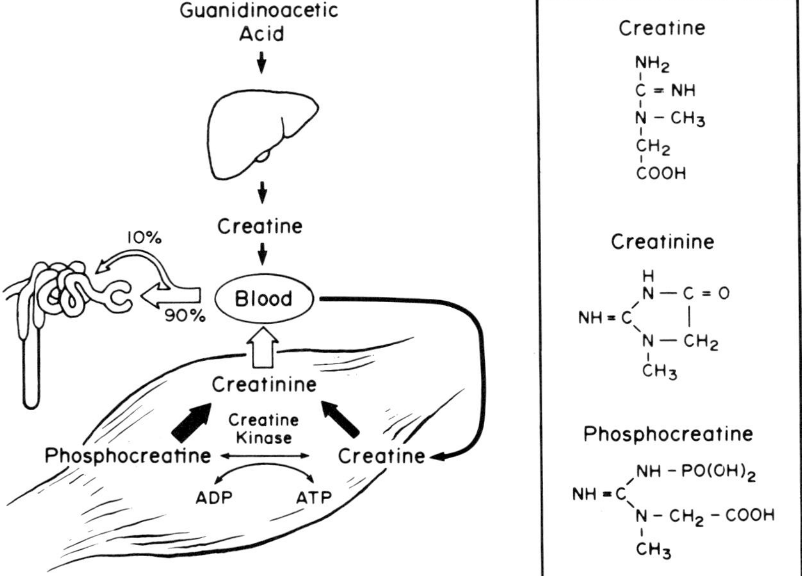

Figure 3-6 Schematic representation of creatinine metabolism in man. Guaninidoacetic acid is a precursor of creatine which, primarily in the liver, is methylated in an irreversible manner to form creatine. Creatine is then taken up by active uptake into muscle, where it exists in two forms: phosphocreatine and creatine. Both substances dehydrate to creatinine at a fixed daily rate (phosphocreatine > creatine) of about 2%. The creatinine so formed diffuses from the cell appearing in the urine as a function of its filtration and secretion.

body water and creatinine production might be lean body mass.

A number of variables affect day-to-day creatinine excretion. Exercise can increase creatinine excretion by 10%.[62] Creatinine excretion can also be raised by the ingestion of preformed creatine or creatinine or the amino acid precursors of creatine.[56] Creatinine excretion also declines with age (Figure 3-7). This most likely represents the age-related decline in muscle mass but dietary factors may contribute to the decrease in urinary creatinine since the elderly tend to ingest less meat. As GFR decreases, urinary creatinine excretion declines, becoming particularly noteworthy when the serum creatinine exceeds 6 mg/dL. Studies by Mitch and colleagues have demonstrated two alternative catabolic pathways for creatinine in renal failure. They include a recycling of creatinine to creatine and an increased intestinal degradation of creatinine to non-creatine byproducts.[65,68] Finally, there exists a considerable day-to-day intrasubject variability in creatinine excretion that has a demonstrated coefficient of variation of from 10.5% to 14.4%.[69]

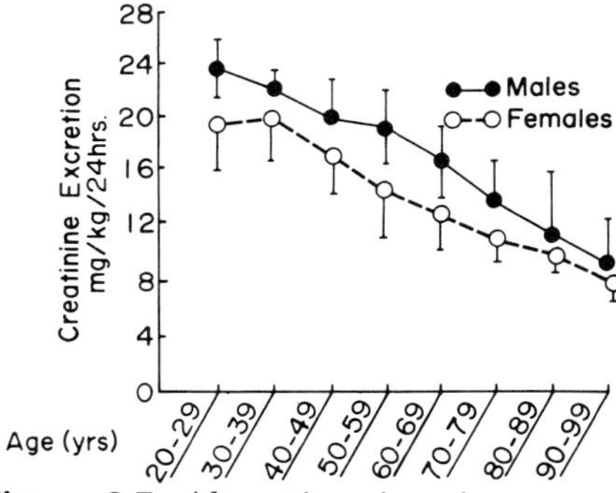

Figure 3-7 Alterations in urinary creatinine excretion with age. Patients were divided into 10-year age groups. Urinary creatinine was determined in three separate 24-hour collections and the mean obtained. Points are ± SEM and represent the means for all patients in that age group. (Adapted with permission from Kampmann et al.[58])

The serum creatinine value is measured by the alkaline picrate method of Jaffe. This method may overestimate the concentration of creatinine in blood since it also reads noncreatinine chromogens.[70] This overestimation may be up to 20%.[62] It has been argued that the overestimation of true serum creatinine by the inclusion of noncreatinine chromogens (denominator) is counterbalanced by the secretory component of urinary creatinine excretion (numerator) thereby leaving the creatinine clearance unchanged. This argument is spurious, since there is no true correlation between these two variables. The best approximation of creatinine clearance to inulin clearance is obtained when a true serum creatinine is obtained.[62,71] An intriguing phenomenon that affects the serum creatinine value is the ability of certain drugs to block the secretory component of creatinine. The resultant rise in serum creatinine invalidates its use in the clearance formula necessitating use of an alternative method such as chromium 51 ethylenediaminetetraacetate. Two such drugs in common use in the elderly are cimetidine[72] and trimethoprim-sulfamethoxazole.[73]

Data on GFR changes with aging have been criticized since the studies relied upon were cross-sectional studies in institutionalized patients. In the study of Rowe et al[50] mentioned above, a true creatinine methodology was employed and there was comparison of simultaneously obtained 24-hour creatinine clearances and inulin clearances. This study demonstrated a highly significant reduction in creatinine clearance beginning at age 34 and accelerating once the age of 65 was reached. These data then permitted the development of a nomogram which facilitates determination of an individual's age-adjusted percentile rank for creatinine clearance (Figure 3-8).[74] A number of studies have demonstrated that the clearance of true creatinine exceeds that of inulin[62,71] by a variable degree, depending on the state of renal function.[75] In the study by Rowe et al,[50] where simultaneous inulin and creatinine clearances were performed, it was shown that the renal handling of creatinine relative to inulin did not change. Therefore, a decline in renal tubular creatinine secretion is not a sufficient explanation for the age-related decline in creatinine clearance.[50,76]

The difficulty in obtaining accurate 24-hour collections is readily apparent. For this reason several authors have suggested the use of formulas based on age, weight, and serum creatinine to determine creatinine clearance thereby obviating the need for urine collection. Several of these "urine-free" formulas are listed in Table 3-3. In a study by Gral and Young[77] a comparison was made between endogenous

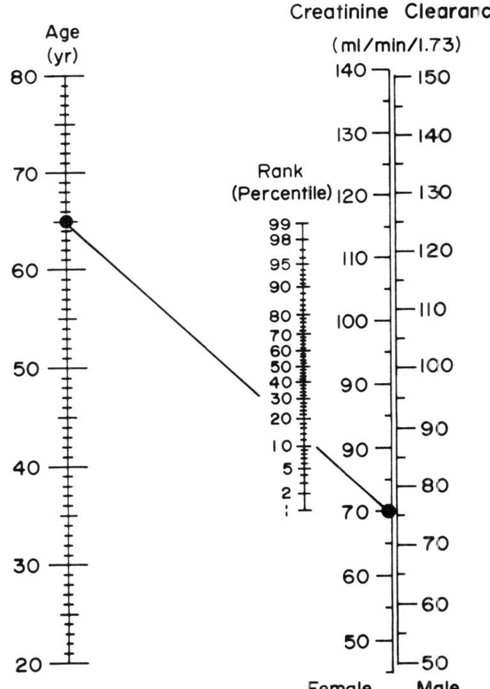

Figure 3-8 Nomogram for determining age-adjusted percentile rank in creatinine clearance. This nomogram is constructed to utilize creatinine values as determined by the "total chromogen" method. A line through the patient's age (70 years) and creatinine clearance (75 cc) intersects the percentile rank line, which in this instance is 20%. (Reproduced with permission from Rowe et al.[74])

Table 3-3
Commonly Used Urine-Free Formulas for Estimation of Creatinine Clearance

Formula	Reference
$\dfrac{(140 - \text{age})\ \text{body weight(kg)}}{72 \times \text{S creatinine}}\ (\text{mL/min})$	(1) 61
$\dfrac{(140 - \text{age}) \times \text{lean body weight.}}{72 \times \text{S creatinine}}$	(2) 78
$\dfrac{100}{\text{S creatinine}} - 12\ (\text{mL/min/1.73 m}^2)$	(3) 79
$\dfrac{98 - 16\dfrac{(\text{age} - 20)}{20}(\text{mL/min/1.73 m}^2)}{\text{S creatinine}}$	(4) 80
$\dfrac{94.3}{\text{S creatinine}}$	(5) 81

creatinine clearance and formulas (1) and (2) (see Table 3-3): Of the 26 patients studied, 23 had what might be considered a normal serum creatinine (0.7 to 1.5 mg/dL) though measured creatinine clearance was reduced in all patients. The measured clearance correlated well with the formula of Cockcroft and Gault[61] (r=.80) and that of Lott and Hayton[78] (r=.85). Despite certain inherent drawbacks in the use of formulas which do not require urine measurements, this study suggests that in the elderly a good correlation exists between these formulas and measured clearance. The merit of the use of such formulas in the elderly is obvious and the rough approximation of GFR obtained with a urine-free formula is more than sufficient to make clinical judgments.

The preceding discussion has indicated that the elderly manifest distinct changes in serum and urine creatinine which may affect their clinical management. Unless adjustments are made for the decreased creatinine excretion occurring with aging, erroneous conclusions may be reached about the adequacy of a 24-hour urine collection. Second, the same serum creatinine concentration may reflect markedly different levels of renal function. With age there is a parallel reduction in both creatinine production and renal function with the result being little, if any, change in serum creatinine. Unless this fact is ppreciated, dosage adjustments for potentially nephrotoxic drugs may not be properly made in the elderly.

REFERENCES

1. Goyal VK: Changes with age in the human kidney. *Exp Gerontol* 1982;17:321–331.
2. Darmady EM, Offer J, Woodhouse MA: The parameters of the aging kidney. *J Pathol* 1973;109:195–207.
3. Kappel B, Olsen S: Cortical interstitial tissue and sclerosed glomeruli in the normal human kidney, related to age and sex. *Virchows Arch [Pathol Anat]* 1980;387: 271–277.
4. Dunmill MS, Holley W: Some observations on the quantitative anatomy of the kidney. *J Pathol* 1973;110:113–121.
5. Griffiths GJ, Robinson KB, Cartwright GO, et al: Loss of renal tissue in the elderly. *Br J Radiol* 1976;49:111–117.
6. Takazakura E, Sawabu N, Handa A, et al: Intrarenal vascular changes with age and disease. *Kidney Int* 1972;2:224–230.
7. McLachlan MS, Guthrie JC, Anderson CU, et al: Vascular and glomerular changes in the aging kidney. *J Pathol* 1977;121:67–78.

8. Brenner BM, Meyer TW, Hostetter TH: Dietary protein intake and the progressive nature of kidney disease: the role of hemodynamically mediated glomerular injury in the pathogenesis of progressive glomerular sclerosis in aging, renal ablation, and intrinsic renal disease. *N Engl J Med* 1982;307:652–659.
9. Davies DF, Shock NW: Age changes in glomerular filtration rate, effective renal plasma flow, and tubular excretory capacity in adult males. *J Clin Invest* 1950;29: 496–507.
10. Marcus R, Madvig P, Young G: Age related changes in parathyroid hormone and parathyroid hormone action in normal humans. *J Clin Endocrinol Metab* 1984; 58:223–230.
11. Boert L, Steg A: Is the diverticulum of the distal and collecting tubules a preliminary state of the simple cyst in the adult? *J Urol* 1977;118:707–710.
12. Inove G, Sawada T, Fukunaga Y, et al: Levels of acid mucopolysaccharides in aging human kidneys. *Gerontologia* 1970; 16:261–265.
13. Keresztury S, Megyeri L: Histology of renal pyramides with special regard to changes due to aging. *Acta Morphol Acad Sci Hung* 1962;11:205–215.
14. Rowe JW, Shock NW, DeFronzo RA: The influence of age on the renal response to water deprivation in man. *Nephron* 1976; 17:270–278.
15. Miller JH, McDonald RK, Shock NW: Age changes in the maximal rate of renal tubular reabsorption of glucose. *J Gerontol* 1952;7:196–200.
16. Butterfield WJ, Keen H, Whichelow MJ: Renal glucose threshold variations with age. *Br Med J* 1967;4:505–507.
17. Gallagher JC, Riggs BL, Jerpbak CM, et al: The effect of age on serum immunoreactive parathyroid hormone in normal and osteoporotic women. *J Lab Clin Med* 1980;95:373–385.
18. Wiske P, Epstein S, Bell NH, et al: Increases in immunoreactive parathyroid hormone with age. *N Engl J Med* 1979; 300:1419–1421.
19. Berlyne GM, Ben-Ari J, Kushelevsky A, et al: The aetiology of senile osteoporosis: secondary hyperparathyroidism due to renal failure. *Q J Med* 1975;44:505–521.
20. Rushton C: Vitamin D hydroxylation in youth and old age. *Age Ageing* 1978;7: 91–95.
21. Gallagher JC, Riggs BL, DeLuca HF: Effect of age on calcium absorption and serum 1,25$(OH)_2$D. *Clin Res* 1978;26: 680A.
22. Adler S, Lindeman RC, Yeingst MJ, et al: Effect of acute acid loading on urinary acid excretion by the aging human kidney. *J Lab Clin Med* 1968;72:278–289.
23. Agorwal BN, Cabebe FG: Renal acidification in elderly subjects. *Nephron* 1980;26: 291–295.
24. Shock NW, Yiengst MJ: Age changes in the acid-base equilibrium of the blood of males. *J Gerontol* 1950;5:1–4.
25. Leask RG, Andrews GR, Caird FI: Normal values of sixteen blood constituents in the elderly. *Age Ageing* 1973;2:14–23.
26. Hilton JG, Goodbody MF, Krusi OR: The effect of prolonged administration of ammonium chloride on the blood acid-base equilibrium of geriatric subjects. *J Am Geriatr Soc* 1955;3:697–703.
27. Tizianello A, Deferrari G, Garibette, G, et al: Renal ammoniagenesis in an early state of metabolic acidosis in man. *J Clin Invest* 1982;69:240–250.
28. Tannen RB: The relationship between urine pH and acid excretion—the influence of urine flow rate. *J Lab Clin Med* 1969; 74:757–769.
29. Ashraf N, Locksley R, Arieff A: Thiazide induced hyponatremia associated with death or neurologic damage in outpatients. *Am J Med* 1981;70:1163–1168.
30. Sunderam SG, Mannikar GO: Hyponatremia in the elderly. *Age Ageing* 1983;12: 77–80.
31. Weissman PN, Shrenkman L, Gregerman R: Chlorpropamide hyponatremia: drug-induced inappropriate antidiuretic hormone activity. *N Engl J Med* 1971;234: 65–71.
32. Dontas AS, Marketos SG, Papanayiotou P: Mechanisms of renal tubular defects in old age. *Postgrad Med J* 1972;48:295–303.
34. Nunez JFM, Iglesias CG, Roman AB, et al: Renal handling of sodium in old people: A functional study. *Age Ageing* 1978;7: 178–181.
35. Kleeman CR, Adams DA, Maxwell MN: An evaluation of maximal water diuresis in chronic renal disease. I. Normal solute

intake. *J Lab Clin Med* 1961;58:169–184.
36. Adams DA, Kleeman CR, Bernstein LH, et al: An evaluation of maximal water diuresis in chronic renal disease. II. Effect of variations in sodium intake and excretion. *J Lab Clin Med* 1961;58:185–196.
37. Lewis WH, Alving AS: Changes with age in the renal function of adult men. Clearance of urea, amount of urea nitrogen in blood, concentrating ability of kidneys. *Am J Physiol* 1938;123:505–515.
38. Miller JH, Shock NW: Age differences in the renal tubular response to antidiuretic hormone. *J Gerontol* 1953;8:446–450.
39. Lindeman RD, Van Buren HC, Raisz L: Osmolar renal concentrating ability in healthy young men and hospitalized patients without renal disease. *N Engl J Med* 1960;262:1306–1309.
40. Bengele HH, Mathias RS, Perkins JH, et al: Urinary concentrating defect in the aged rat. *Am J Physiol* 1981;240:F147–150.
41. Rowe JW, Minaker KL, Sparrow D, et al: Age-related failure of volume-pressure-mediated vasopressin release. *J Clin Endocrinol Metab* 1982;54:661–664.
42. Miller M: Vasopressin secretion in the aging rat, in *Abstracts of the Endocrine Society*, 65th Annual Meeting, San Antonio, Texas, June 8–10, 1983, p 253.
43. Helderman JH, Vestal RE, Rowe JL, et al: The response of arginine vasopressin to intravenous ethanol and hypertonic saline in man: the impact of aging. *J Gerontol* 1978;33:39–47.
44. Coburn JW, Gonick HC, Rubini ME, et al: Studies of experimental renal failure in dogs. I. Effect of 5/6 nephrectomy on concentrating and diluting capacity of residual nephrons. *J Clin Invest* 1965;44:603–614.
45. Eknoyan G, Martinez-Maldonado M, Suki WN: The use of clearance methods for the determination of sites of action of diuretics in the kidney, in Martinez-Maldonado M (ed): *Methods in Pharmacology. Renal Pharmacology.* New York, Plenum Press, 1976, pp 99–120.
46. Hollenberg NK, Adams DF, Solomon HS, et al: Senescence and the renal vasculature in normal man. *Circ Res* 1974;34:309–316.
47. Weidmann P, DeMyttenaere-Bursztein S, Maxwell MH, et al: Effect of aging on plasma renin and aldosterone in normal man. *Kidney Int* 1975;8:325–333.
48. Sporn N, Lancestremere RG, Papper S: Differential diagnosis of oliguria in aged patients. *N Engl J Med* 1962;267:130–132.
49. Epstein M, Hollenberg NK: Age as a determinant of renal sodium conservation in normal man. *J Lab Clin Med* 1976;87: 411–417.
50. Rowe JW, Andres R, Tobin JD, et al: The effect of age on creatinine clearance in men. A cross-sectional and longitudinal study. *J Gerontol* 1976;31:155–163.
51. Gault MH, Cockcroft DW: Creatinine clearance and age. *Lancet* 1975;2:612–613.
52. Kampmann JP, Hansen JM: Glomerular filtration rate and creatinine clearance. *Br J Clin Pharmacol* 1981;12:7–14.
53. Shannon JA, Smith HW: The excretion of inulin, xylose, and urea by normal and phlorizinized man. *J Clin Invest* 1935;14: 393–401.
54. Watkin DM, Shock NW: Agewise standard value for C_{IN}, C_{PAH}, and TM_{PAH} in adult males. *J Clin Invest* 1955;34:969.
55. Bjornsson TD: Use of serum creatinine concentration to determine renal function. *Clin Pharmacokinet* 1979;4:200–222.
56. Heymsfield SB, Arteaga C, McManus C, et al: Measurement of muscle mass in humans: Validity of the 24-hour urinary creatinine method. *Am J Clin Nutr* 1983;37:478–494.
57. Walker JB: Creatine: biosynthesis, regulation, and function. *Adv Enzymol* 1979; 50:177–242.
58. Kampmann J, Siersbak-Nielsen K, Kristensen M, et al: Rapid evaluation of creatinine clearance. *Acta Med Scand* 1974; 196:517–520.
59. Bulusu L, Hodgkinson A, Nordin BE, et al: Urinary excretion of calcium and creatinine in relation to age and body weight in normal subjects and patients with renal calculus. *Clin Sci* 1970;38:601–612.
60. Forbes GB, Reina JC: Adult lean body mass declines with age: some longitudinal observations. *Metabolism* 1970;19:653–663.
61. Cockcroft DW, Gault MN: Prediction of creatinine clearance from serum creatinine. *Nephron* 1976;16:31–41.
62. Doolan PD, Alpen EL, Theil GM: A clinical appraisal of the plasma concentrations and endogenous clearance of creatinine: *Am J Med* 1962;32:65–79.
63. Fitch CD, Sinton DW: A study of creatine

metabolism in diseases causing muscle wasting: *J Clin Invest* 1964;43:444–452.
64. Effersoe P: Relationship between endogenous 24-hour creatinine clearance and serum creatinine concentration in patients with chronic renal disease. *Acta Med Scand* 1957;156:429–434.
65. Mitch WE, Walser M: A proposed mechanism for reduced creatinine excretion in severe chronic renal failure. *Nephron* 1978;21:248–254.
66. Edelman IS, Leibman J: Anatomy of body water and electrolytes. *Am J Med* 1959; 27:256–277.
67. Forbes GB: The adult decline in lean body mass. *Hum Biol* 1976;48:161–173.
68. Mitch WE, Collier VU, Walser M: Creatinine metabolism in chronic renal failure. *Clin Sci* 1980;58:327–335.
69. Greenblatt DJ, Ransil BJ, Harmatz JS, et al: Variability of 24-hour urinary creatinine excretion by normal subjects. *J Clin Pharmacol* 1976;16:231–238.
70. Narayanan S, Appleton HD: Creatinine: a review. *Clin Chem* 1980;11:1119–1126.
71. Healey JK, Graeme GR: Clinical assessment of glomerular filtration rate by different forms. *Am J Med* 1968;44:343–358.
72. Dubb JW, State RM, Familiar RG, et al: Effect of cimetidine on renal function in normal man. *Clin Pharmacol Ther* 1978; 24:76–83.
73. Berglund F, Killander J, Pompeius R: Effect of trimethoprim-sulfamethoxazole on the renal excretion of creatinine in man. *J Urol* 1975;114:802–808.
74. Rowe JW, Andres R, Tobin JD, et al: Age adjusted standards for creatinine clearance. *Ann Intern Med* 1976;84:567–569.
75. Bauer JH, Brooks CS, Burch RN: Clinical appraisal of creatinine clearance as a measurement of glomerular filtration rate. *Am J Kidney Dis* 1982;2:337–346.
76. Sawyer WT, Canady BR, Poe TE, et al: A multicenter evaluation of variables affecting the predictability of creatinine clearance. *Am J Clin Pathol* 1982;78: 832–838.
77. Gral T, Young M: Measured versus estimated creatinine clearance in the elderly as an index of renal function. *J Am Geriatr Soc* 1980;28:492–496.
78. Lott RS, Hayton WL: Estimation of creatinine clearance from serum creatinine concentration—A review. *Drug Intell Clin Pharm* 1978;12:140–150.
79. Jelliffe RW: Estimation of creatinine clearance when urine cannot be collected. *Lancet* 1971;1:975–976.
80. Jelliffe RW: Creatinine clearance. Bedside estimate. *Ann Intern Med* 1973;79:604–605.
81. Edwards KD, Whyte HM: Plasma creatinine level and creatinine clearance as tests of renal function. *Aust Ann Med* 1959;8:218–233.

CHAPTER 4 Primary Glomerulonephritis in the Elderly

German Ramirez
Sabiba R. Saba

Abnormalities of renal function in the elderly are attributable to a variety of causes, the most common of which include nephrosclerosis, hypertension, and malignancy.[1] However, with the widespread use of nonsteroidal anti-inflammatory drugs, nephrotoxicity due to this group of medications as well as a variety of additional drugs is now becoming an increasingly more common problem in the geriatric population.[2–5] Finally, urinary tract infections and obstructive uropathy constitute an important part of those renal diseases capable of affecting the elderly.[6–8]

There are four major categories of medical renal disease: (1) primary glomerular diseases, (2) secondary glomerular diseases, (3) pyelonephritis and obstructive uropathy, and (4) tubulointerstitial disease. This chapter will be limited to a review of the glomerulopathies only.

Primary glomerular diseases constitute a heterogenous collection of disorders in which the glomeruli are the sole or predominant tissue involved by the disease process. In the majority of cases, the primary glomerular diseases are of unknown etiology, or idiopathic. However, the majority of so-called primary glomerular diseases are associated with immune complex deposition in the glomeruli and may or may not have circulating immune complexes. Secondary glomerular diseases are clinicopathologic entities in which glomerular involvement is a result of a systemic disease rather than the main pathologic process. An example of secondary glomerular disease is the renal involvement present in either systemic lupus erythematosus or diabetes mellitus.

The clinical manifestations of glomerular diseases are variable, but can present as: (1) an acute process, with rapid deterioration of renal function; (2) chronic, with slow, progressive deterioration of renal function which takes years in association with persistent urinary sediment abnormalities; or (3) a nephrotic syndrome in which the main problem is a massive leakage of protein by the glomeruli with all of its attendant consequences.

Primary glomerular diseases are classified according to either their histologic pattern or their clinical characteristics and include: (1) acute glomerulonephritis, (2) rapidly progressive glomerulonephritis, (3) IgA nephropathy or Berger's disease, (4) mesangioproliferative glomerulonephritis, (5) minimal change disease, (6) focal sclerosing glomerulonephritis, (7) membranous glomerulonephritis, and (8) membranoproliferative glomerulonephritis.

We will describe the main histologic and clinical characteristics of each of the abovementioned diseases, as well as their frequency and clinical presentation in reference to the elderly population. (Elderly or aged population is here defined as persons aged over 60 years.)

ACUTE GLOMERULONEPHRITIS

Acute glomerulonephritis is synonymous with postinfectious glomerulonephritis and is characterized by the appearance of blood, protein, red cell casts, white cells, and granular casts (nephritic sediment) in the urine. In the majority of cases, it is accompanied by a rapid deterioration in renal function. Usually the renal manifestations are preceded by an acute infectious event which may have occurred from 1 to 2 weeks prior to the renal symptomatology. By light microscopy, the glomeruli appear enlarged and hypercellular. The capillary lumina are occluded by a proliferation of both mesangial and endothelial cells. This is accompanied by variable degrees of infiltration with polymorphonuclear leukocytes, monocytes, and eosinophils within capillary lumina and the mesangium. By electron microscopy, the most characteristic finding is the presence of electron-dense, dome-shaped deposits projected outward from the epithelial side of the basement membrane. Immunofluorescence studies show immunoglobulin IgG, and less often IgM and IgA, in an irregular, usually granular pattern along the capillary walls and mesangium. C_3 is usually present in the same pattern as IgG. Immune complexes containing IgG and C_3 are often present in the circulation.[9] Early in the course of the disease, the serum levels of total hemolytic complement activity (CH_{50}) and C_3 will generally be reduced.[10,11] Acute glomerulonephritis in the elderly occurs with less frequency than in the young,[12–16] but the exact incidence is unknown. The prognosis and course of acute glomerulonephritis appears to be generally benign in the young population.[17,18] In the older population, the course following acute glomerulonephritis may not be quite as favorable.[19,20] Limitations in renal functional reserve as well as the presence of extrarenal diseases frequently lead to early and sustained symptomatology. The ultimate prognosis in this particular segment of the population is variable but probably is not as benign as in the younger population.[21–23]

RAPIDLY PROGRESSIVE GLOMERULONEPHRITIS

Rapidly progressive glomerulonephritis (RPGN) is a clinical syndrome manifested by a progressive decline in renal function occurring over days to months (usually no longer than 6 months). The glomerular disease is characterized by an extensive and exuberant proliferation of cells within Bowman's space, forming what are characteristically termed crescents.

Rapidly progressive glomerulonephritis is a clinical and histologic diagnosis that can follow from the onset of a variety of systemic disorders. These include systemic lupus erythematosus, polyarteritis nodosa, Wegener's granulomatosis, Henoch-Schönlein purpura, cryoglobulinemia, and subacute bacterial endocarditis, among others. Therefore, one should be careful in any analysis of published reports dealing with this entity as a primary occurrence. Furthermore, the histologic findings of RPGN can be seen in a number of other primary renal diseases such as acute glomerulonephritis, membranoproliferative glomerulonephritis, and Goodpasture's syndrome.[23-25] For a rational analysis of the literature, it should be understood that when no etiologic factors are known, and histopathologic findings indicate the presence of extensive glomerular crescents arising within Bowman's capsule, we are dealing with a case of so-called idiopathic RPGN. In the case of idiopathic RPGN, immunofluorescence studies do not show linear deposition of immunoglobulins in capillary loops of the glomerulus. When linear basement membrane fluorescence occurs, the diagnostic term becomes RPGN of the antiglomerular basement variety. When concomitant clinical and/or histologic involvement of the lungs is present, the defining term becomes Goodpasture's syndrome.

Reports[21,22,26-28] indicate that RPGN is the most common type of glomerulonephritis leading to acute renal failure in the elderly. Two recent studies[22,26] have stressed the fact that when RPGN appears in the elderly, the majority of cases prove to be idiopathic. This is proved to be the case since immunofluorescence patterns did not reveal linear deposition of immunoglobulins, circulating antibodies against glomerular basement membrane were not detected, and immune deposits were absent from the glomeruli.

RPGN, if left untreated, carries a grave prognosis. A number of therapeutic modalities have been tried including corticosteroids, anticoagulants, immunosuppressive agents, and more recently, plasmapheresis. Oral corticosteroids, administered alone or in conjunction with other immunosuppressive drugs, have rarely modified the course of the disease.[29,30] Anticoagulants, either alone or with other agents, offer a better therapeutic alternative in that their use may on occasion stabilize or even improve renal function.[31,32] A drawback to any interpretation of the results of therapy in RPGN remains the fact that corticosteroids are concurrently utilized with any additional treatment that is employed.[31-33] In addition, therapeutic success is also difficult to assess accurately because rapidly progressive glomerulonephritis is a clinical-pathologic syndrome which includes several different diseases.[34] Most reports have included all forms of RPGN as a single group regardless of the underlying cause.[34] When the results of therapy for idiopathic RPGN are analyzed,[34-36] it appears that high doses of intravenous (IV) steroids, when given early in the evolution of the disease, can be moderately successful in both arresting the progression of the disease and in some instances actually improving renal function. A further characteristic of those responding to high-dose IV steroids is that they are generally normotensive and have sustained a shorter disease interval. Biopsies of these patients have shown that crescents are predominantly cellular in nature, with minimal interstitial fibrosis, and few sclerotic glomeruli.[34] Any such histologic characterization must be cautiously interpreted in the aged since there is a progressive loss of renal mass with age,[37] which occurs predominantly in the renal cortex with relatively little loss occurring from the medulla. The number of glomeruli decrease and mesangial expansion occurs.[38,39] Both glomerular and tubular basement membranes increase in thickness,[40] and sclerotic changes occur in the walls of the large renal vessels, even in the absence of hypertension.[41] With all these changes related to aging alone, the histologic interpretation of a renal biopsy becomes particularly difficult in the elderly. Perhaps the normal renal dysfunction which follows from the aging process contributes to the poor prognosis that is seen in this population. Despite the histologic abnormalities that follow aging, three studies that specifically reported the results of therapy for idiopathic RPGN[34–36] demonstrated that some of the patients that responded were above the age of 60 years. This observation suggests that the prognosis for idiopathic RPGN may depend more on its early diagnosis than on the age of the affected individual.

IgA NEPHROPATHY OR BERGER'S DISEASE

IgA nephropathy is characterized clinically by the finding of hematuria with or without proteinuria in the absence of any identifiable systemic illness. By light microscopy, the glomeruli may show minimal alterations, including focal or segmental proliferative changes, as well as mesangial expansion and segmental hypercellularity. Berger and Hinglais, in the late 1960s, reported the localization of both IgA, and to a lesser extent of IgG, within the mesangium of numerous glomeruli. The pattern of deposition was granular. These findings were in a group of children where the clinical presentation was that of hematuria and variable degrees of proteinuria.[42,43] Since that time, patients with hematuria and renal histology characterized by IgA deposition in the glomeruli are said to suffer from IgA nephropathy or Berger's disease. Furthermore, although IgA has proved to be the predominant immunoglobulin deposited in the glomeruli, C_3 is present and with a frequency similar to that of IgA. The absence of C_{1q} or C_4[42,44] on immunofluorescence suggests that any activation of the complement cascade is mainly through an alternate pathway mechanism.

The frequency of this disease in the general population has been reported to be as high as 20% to 25% of all cases of primary glomerulonephritis,[45,46] although some authors dispute this figure.[47,48] The disease is usually diagnosed in the young adult, although it can be present in the elderly as well, and its occurrence is predominantly in males.[49] The most common clinical presentation is that of recurring episodes of gross hematuria,[50–52] although a number of other symptoms, including loin pain, may be present as well.[53,54]

It has also been reported that the concentration of IgA in the serum of patients with this type of glomerulonephritis is elevated.[55,56] However, this has been found to be of little diagnostic value because serum IgA is increased in only half of the patients with IgA nephritis.[57] Although the role of IgA in the pathogenesis of the renal lesion is presently unknown, several pieces of evidence suggest that circulating immune complexes may play a role in the deposition of IgA, despite uniformly unsuccessful attempts to detect circulating immune complexes in serum.[58,59] In a recent report, Hall et al[60] were able to detect IgA-containing immune complexes in the serum of 50% of patients with IgA nephritis. In addition, this same IgA was the predominant immunoglobulin localized to the mesangium of the glomeruli in these patients. Whatever the pathogenesis of IgA nephritis, the course of the disease tends to be chronic and renal failure may develop in up to 25% of patients.[61,62]

The frequency of IgA nephritis in the elderly population is unknown at the present time. Hematuria in the elderly is more commonly attributed to problems of the lower urinary tract and prostate than to glomerulonephritis. This, as well as a general reluctance to biopsy elderly individuals for hematuria alone, has limited our assessment of this disease in the aged. So, although this disease has been reported in the elderly,[26] its course and prognosis in this group awaits a more careful characterization.

MINIMAL CHANGE DISEASE

Minimal change disease, additionally termed either nil disease or lipoid nephrosis, is a common cause of nephrotic syndrome in children.[63] It appears also that when idiopathic nephrotic syndrome occurs in the adult population, from 10% to 30% of cases may be due to lipoid nephrosis, although the incidence declines with age.[64-69] This disease has also been reported to occur in the elderly population.[64-66] If the nephrotic syndrome occurs in the aged as the result of a primary glomerular lesion, about 25% of cases will be due to minimal change nephropathy.[70]

The therapy of minimal change disease consists of the administration of steroids for a short period of time. It is encouraging to know that this glomerulopathy responds well to corticosteroids in the geriatric population,[64,68] a therapeutic response not dissimilar to that observed in children with nil disease.

MESANGIOPROLIFERATIVE GLOMERULONEPHRITIS

Mesangioproliferative glomerulonephritis is characterized clinically by the presence of hematuria[71,72] and is usually associated with proteinuria.[73,74] The glomerular changes in the biopsy specimen consist of diffuse mesangial proliferation as the sole or predominant abnormality with the presence of three or more nuclei per mesangial area constituting mesangial proliferation.[75] The presence of multiple nuclei is considered the most reliable clue in estimating the extent of mesangial proliferation. The histopathologic finding of mesangial proliferation can also be found in IgA nephritis, or other diseases such as systemic lupus erythematosus, resolving postinfectious glomerulonephritides, or Henoch-Schönlein purpura.[76] Therefore, care should be taken to exclude these diseases before settling on a diagnosis of mesangioproliferative glomerulonephritis.

The course is variable and the nephrotic syndrome may or may not be responsive to the administration of steroids. A frequent finding is the deposition of IgM in the mesangium,[77,78] but the significance of this finding is still not fully understood. In the evolution of this disease, it is possible to observe focal segmental sclerosing lesions in the glomeruli,[71] and to see the gradual development histologically of a focal sclerosing glomerulonephritis.[79] Some authors have also observed the evolution of minimal change disease into focal sclerosing glomerulonephritis with the transitional stage being that of mesangial proliferation.[79,80] In trying to assess the varied evolutionary stages of this lesion, it becomes apparent that there exist inherent difficulties in interpretation of the renal biopsies of elderly individuals, a population in whom sclerosed glomeruli and widening of the mesangium are ordinary findings. Therefore, it is difficult to assess the frequency of this type of glomerulonephritis in the aged. We still do not know if mesangioproliferative glomerulonephritis should be considered a separate entity from focal sclerosing glomerulonephritis or an early form of this latter entity.

In our own experience, we have followed five patients over a period of 5 years whose histologic diagnosis was that of mesangioproliferative glomerulonephritis. In each instance, the original biopsy lesion evolved from mesangioproliferative to focal sclerosing glomerulonephritis.

FOCAL SCLEROSING GLOMERULONEPHRITIS

Focal sclerosing glomerulonephritis is characterized clinically by the presence of nephrotic syndrome and hematuria. It is the cause of nephrotic syndrome in some 10% to 20% of cases that occur in adults and children. Kidney involvement is localized (focal), with variable numbers of glomeruli showing segmental sclerosing lesions. This has been described by Spargo et al[81] as "a solidified area within the glomerular tuft, which is adherent to Bowman's capsule and has a hard glossy character in hematoxylin and eosin and PAS stained sections." The unaffected glomeruli appear normal by light microscopy, though on occasion they reveal diffuse mesangial proliferation. Tubular changes are common and consist of focal thickening of the basement membrane and tubular atrophy. By electron microscopy, the glomeruli show diffuse or segmental foot process alterations and diffuse mesangial cell hyperplasia. Immunoglobulin M, C_{1q}, and C_3 may be deposited in an irregular, granular, or nodular distribution pattern in the area of sclerosis within the glomerulus. The glomeruli without sclerosing lesions do not demonstrate immune deposits.[82,83] These histologic characteristics, as seen by light microscopy, can be found in a variety of circumstances or as late complications of other diseases. These may include such diverse diseases as sarcoidosis,[84] massive obesity,[85] or heroin abuse,[86] and care should be taken to rule out such entities prior to establishing the diagnosis of focal sclerosing glomerulonephritis as an idiopathic entity.

Focal sclerosing glomerulonephritis (FSG) can present as two separate clinicopathologic patterns.[79] The first is characterized by the presence of nephrotic syndrome associated with the typical histopathologic findings of FSG. These histologic changes are present at or near the time of onset of the nephrotic syndrome. This group of patients fare poorly, eventually developing renal failure and resistance to medical therapy.[82,87,88] The second group of patients are initially steroid-responsive patients whose biopsies have shown less prominent sclerotic changes in the glomeruli. Many of them are classified initially as suffering from minimal change disease. These patients appear to have a more benign prognosis[79] and need not progress inevitably to renal insufficiency.

Kincaid-Smith and Young[89] have added more subtleties to the diagnosis of focal sclerosing glomerulonephritis based on its histologic appearance on light microscopy:

1. Focal sclerosing. In this group of patients, the focal lesion involves some, but not all of the glomeruli. The glomeruli involved show increased fibrillar material due to both collapse and condensation of the basement membrane (silver-positive).
2. Focal and segmental hyalinosis. In this group again, some, but not all of the glomeruli are involved, and those involved contain cellular structural material composed of glycoproteins (silver-negative) in the glomerular tuft.
3. Focal and segmental proliferation. Again, some of the glomeruli are involved with proliferating cells; the majority of these cells are extracapillary, resulting in segmental crescent formation, with or without associated fibrin deposition.

Of these groups of patients, the ones with proliferation had the worst prognosis. Over a 10-year period, 37% of males with extracapillary proliferation either died or required dialysis, while only 11% of females died or developed renal failure. Individuals with focal and segmental hyalinosis fared better, with 75% of males and 93% of females surviving over a 10-year period. The patients with a focal sclerosing lesion have the best prognosis, with none of them developing any evidence of renal failure during a 10-year follow-up. The histology of focal sclerosis is often predictable based on the response to steroids when utilized for the therapy of the nephrotic syndrome. Those initially responsive to therapy, with improvement or resolution of the nephrotic syndrome, usually have a better prognosis. Frequently they demonstrate a focal sclerosing lesion with an absence of extracapillary proliferation.

It is clear that the term focal sclerosing glomerulonephritis represents a confusing array of histologic pictures which manifest variable levels of renal disease. An additional concern in the interpretation of the renal biopsy is that ischemic changes can simulate this entity. Seeking early renal biopsy in the nephrotic syndrome will improve our understanding of this disease, and by repeating biopsies, when indicated, our knowledge will increase. Although focal sclerosing glomerulonephritis has been reported in persons above the age of 60 years,[90] its frequency in the elderly is unknown. In addition, little is known about either the prognosis or the course of this disease when it occurs in the aged.

MEMBRANOUS GLOMERULONEPHRITIS

Membranous glomerulonephritis is usually associated with the nephrotic syndrome. This disease, when present in the absence of systemic diseases, is termed idiopathic membranous glomerulonephritis. Despite its occurrence as an idiopathic entity, it can also be associated with a variety of diseases, including infections,[90-93] multisystem collagen vascular diseases, such as systemic lupus erythematosus,[94-96] and neoplasias.[97-99] A number of other diseases, such as Guillain-Barré syndrome, sickle cell disease,[100-102] as well as medication ingestion[103-105] have also been associated with membranous nephropathy.

Membranous glomerulonephritis is characterized histologically by a diffuse and uniform thickening of the capillary wall of the glomerulus, usually without significant proliferation of endothelial, mesangial, or epithelial cells.[106] By immunofluorescence, immunoglobulin G is almost always present in a uniform granular distribution outlining many of the capillary loops. By electron microscopy, electron-dense deposits are usually found in the subepithelial region of the basement membrane

Membranous glomerulonephritis is a common cause of the nephrotic syndrome in the adult[107,108] as well as in the elderly.[26,70] However, when membranous glomerulonephritis is diagnosed in the elderly, up to 22% of cases may be associated with a concurrent malignancy,[70] though an association of this magnitude has not been observed in other studies.[26] Nevertheless, a careful search for malignancy should be initiated in the aged if membranous or membranoproliferative glomerulonephritis is found on biopsy. Therapy directed toward remission of the nephrotic syndrome in the elderly is not as successful as in young adults,[26,70] and specific data on whether declining renal function can be stabilized are currently lacking. The therapy in the aged is fraught with complications, since prednisone is commonly included. The complications that follow from steroid therapy are of particular concern in the selection of therapy since it has yet to be convincingly demonstrated that steroid therapy is better than no therapy at all in these patients.

MEMBRANOPROLIFERATIVE GLOMERULONEPHRITIS

Membranoproliferative glomerulonephritis (MPGN) appears to exist in two histologic forms, each quite different from the other in its immunofluorescence pattern, electron microscopic appearance, and in the clinical evolution. In general, the disease is characterized by a light microscopic appearance that combines capillary wall thickening with endocapillary proliferation of cells. The thickening of the glomerular capillary wall may occur by different pathophysiologic mechanisms and is what separates this disease into its component entities: membranoproliferative glomerulonephritis types I and II.

In the type I variant of MPGN, there is a subendothelial extension or interposition of mesangial cytoplasm and matrix that produces an apparent splitting of the basement membrane.[109,110] This mesangial interposition is usually associated with subendothelial immune deposits.[111] In the type II variant of MPGN the capillary wall of the glomerulus is thickened by a peculiar dense transformation of the basement membrane.[112] These patterns can be readily separated by electron microscopy. Immunofluorescence studies of renal tissue in type I MPGN shows that C_3 is almost always present in the capillary loops and, on some occasions, in the mesangial area.[113] These immune deposits can be visualized by electron microscopy as electron-dense deposits along the endothelial side of the basement membrane. The deposits are separated from the endothelial cells by mesangial interposition. Electron-dense deposits can on occasion be found in the mesangial areas as well. In MPGN type II, the immunofluorescence appearance is characterized by homogeneous deposits of C_3 in the mesangial area and along the glomerular basement membrane.

The clinical picture of MPGN-I is usually that of hematuria and heavy proteinuria. Despite a variable clinical course up to 50% of patients will eventually develop renal failure.[113] The MPGN-II is similar to type I, but the latter occurs predominantly in children and young adults. In our experience, this type of glomerulonephritis seldom occurs in patients older than 50 years.

Membranoproliferative glomerulonephritis, without distinction between types I and II, has been classically associated with low levels of C_3 in the blood.[114] Type I-MPGN may have persistently low levels of C_3, but in the majority of cases, the level fluctuates and may remain relatively normal. In our experience with adults, rarely has a low C_3 been found in blood, despite multiple determinations. Furthermore, it appears that in type I-MPGN complement activation occurs by way of the classic pathway,[115] suggesting a possible role for immune complexes in the pathogenesis. In type II-MPGN, C_3 levels in blood remain persistently low while C_{1q} and C_4 levels remain in the normal range.[114] C_3 nephritic factor activity is almost always present in type II-MPGN. All these findings indicate that, in type II-MPGN, complement is activated almost exclusively through the alternative pathway and probably as the result of the presence of C_3 nephritic factor. Whatever the pathophysiologic mechanisms that produce the changes in the basement membrane of the glomeruli, it appears that any damage occurring is initiated by way of immune mechanisms with resultant activation of either the classical or alternative complement pathways and eventual consumption of components of the complement cascade.

Membranoproliferative glomerulonephritis is not an uncommon disease in adults, and it has been reported in the aged as well.[26] However, its frequency, as well as which type predominates, is not known.

CONCLUSIONS

In the previous review of primary glomerulonephritis, it is obvious that little is known about the frequency of these diseases or their prognosis in the elderly. Perhaps this segment of the population behaves differently from their younger counterparts, and it is possible that some primary glomerular diseases can be seen with higher frequency than in the younger population.

The literature suggests that if an elderly patient has a rapid deterioration of renal function in the presence of a nephritic sediment, the most likely diagnosis would be rapidly progressive glomerulonephritis. This disease carries an ominous prognosis if not diagnosed or treated early, especially in the aged. We can say, however, that if the nephrotic syndrome is encountered in the aged, we might expect that the patient suffers from membranous glomerulonephritis, a potentially treatable disease. Any therapy of glomerulonephritis in the elderly should be carefully considered. Steroids can be harmful and their use in the absence of any deterioration of renal function should be questioned.[70] What is not clear is, if membranous nephropathy in the elderly implies the possibility of a hidden malignancy, should, as some authors have suggested,[71] an aggressive workup seeking malignancy be done in all patients?

To widen our understanding of primary

glomerulonephritis in the elderly population, we have reviewed the renal biopsy material from the Tampa Veterans Administration Medical Center from the years 1974 to 1982. This medical facility maintains the unusual position of being one of the few centers in the western part of Florida capable of processing renal biopsy material for light, immunofluorescence, and electron microscopy. Particularly germane to this discussion, also, is the very high proportion of geriatric patients in our sampling population.

In that period of time (1974–1982), 970 renal biopsies were processed at the Tampa VA Medical Center and, of these biopsies, 277 were performed in patients above the age of 60 years (28.6% of the total renal biopsies performed in the community). Of these 277 biopsies, 166 were performed in male patients and 111 in females. The age of patients biopsied in this group of 277 ranged from 60 to 84 years. Table 4-1 lists the frequency of primary glomerular disease as diagnosed by these 277 biopsies. The most frequent primary glomerular disease diagnosed was membranous glomerulonephritis, which represented 20.5% of the total biopsies. The second most frequent diagnosis was rapidly progressive glomerulonephritis thereby confirming previous reports[21,22,26–28] attesting to its frequency. However, in contradistinction to what is described in the literature, very few of the RPGNs in our series were idiopathic (1.4%). In the majority of cases (13/17) linear deposition of IgG was demonstrated in addition to the classical subepithelial crescent formation (Figures 4-1A and B.) In two cases (0.7%), in addition to the kidney involvement, the patients had lung involvement, which allowed for the probable diagnosis of Goodpasture's syndrome. Unfortunately, we do not know if circulating antibodies against the glomerular basement membrane (GBM) were present, since that information was not made available to us. So in our series, when RPGN histology was found by light microscopic examination, the chances were that in 65% of the cases the disease was most likely the result of antiglomerular basement membrane antibodies. We must be aware, however, that in our series this diagnosis was made by finding linear deposition of IgG in the absence of other diseases capable of affecting basement membrane deposition of antibodies, such as lupus erythematosus or diabetes mellitus. In addition, we lacked any information concerning the presence of circulating GBM antibodies.

The third most common diagnosis of primary glomerulonephritis in the elderly pa-

Table 4-1
Frequency of Primary Glomerular Disease in 277 Biopsies Performed in Patients Above Age 60 Years

Diagnosis	No.	% of Total
Acute glomerulonephritis	5	1.8
Rapidly progressive glomerulonephritis	17	6.1
Idiopathic RPGN	4	1.4
Antiglomerular basement disease (without lung involvement)	11	4.0
Goodpasture's syndrome	2	0.7
IgA nephritis	14	5.1
Minimal change disease	16	5.8
Mesangioproliferative glomerulonephritis	5	1.8
Focal glomerular sclerosis	12	4.3
Membranous glomerulonephritis	57	20.5
MPGN type I	12	4.3
MPGN type II	1	0.4
Total	139	50.1

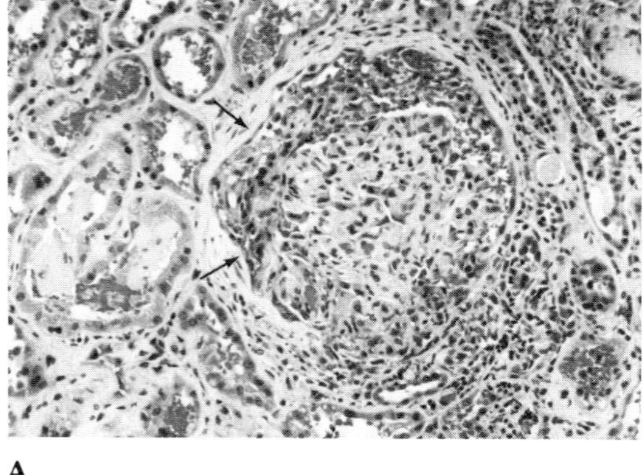

A

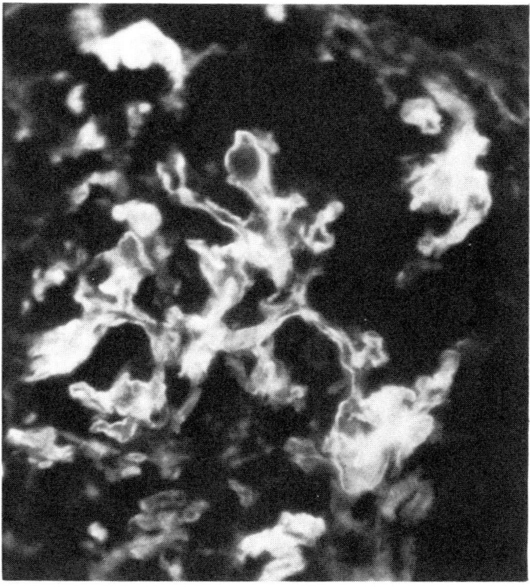

B

Figures 4-1A and B Rapidly progressive glomerulonephritis. **A** Representative glomerulus of a renal biopsy performed in a 67-year-old white male with rapid deterioration of renal function and nephritic urinary sediment. The glomerular tuft is surrounded by a cellular epithelial crescent (arrows). Tubular atrophy is notorious and an inflammatory infiltrate is present in the interstitium (H & E × 480). **B** Immunofluorescence microscopy showed linear deposits of IgG along the glomerular capillary wall. No pulmonary symptomatology was present and the patient did not have circulating anti-GBM antibodies (×1200).

tients was minimal change disease (5.8%), although this diagnosis is not readily reached histologically, since age-related abnormalities make biopsy interpretation difficult (Figures 4-2A and B). IgA nephritis follows minimal change disease as the fourth most common diagnosis (5.1%), followed by all the other primary glomerulopathies, such as MPGN type I, and FGS. It is interesting to note that mesangioproliferative glomerulonephritis was diagnosed in only 1.8% of renal biopsies, reflecting the considerations previously mentioned and the changes illustrated in Figures 4-3A and B. One case of MPGN type II was diagnosed in a 66-year-old woman (Figures 4-4A–E), but this proved to be an unusual finding.

Therefore, from our series it is evident that if an elderly patient develops nephrotic syndrome the most likely diagnosis will be membranous glomerulonephritis. In two patients in our series, membranous nephropathy followed the use of gold and was felt to be the result of therapy with this agent. Thus far, we have not resolved the specific issue of the association of membranous glomerulonephritis with malignancy, since sufficient information to make this determination was lacking. Therefore, it remains open to question to what extent a malignancy search should be initiated when membranous nephropathy is found on renal biopsy.

If acute nephritic syndrome occurs in the elderly population, its etiology, in the majority of cases, is likely to be due to a rapidly progressive glomerulonephritis.

IgA nephritis was the fourth most common diagnosis in our series. We presume that this diagnosis could be made with more frequency if all cases of unexplained hematuria in the elderly population were more vigorously evaluated.

Approximately 50% of renal biopsies performed in elderly individuals resulted in a diagnosis of primary glomerulopathy. However, there were other diagnoses made as the result of the renal biopsies that were performed and their findings are displayed

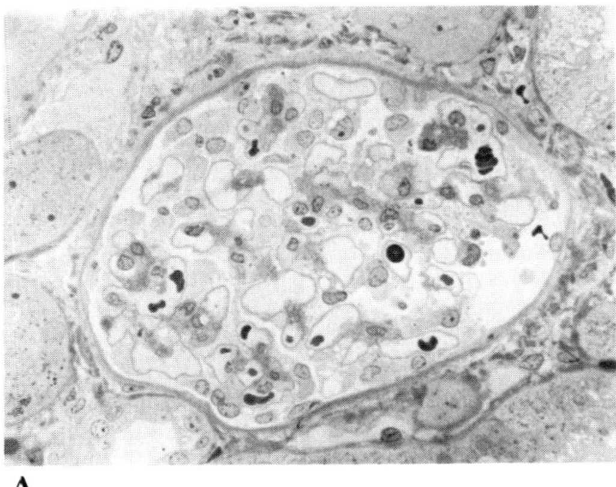

A

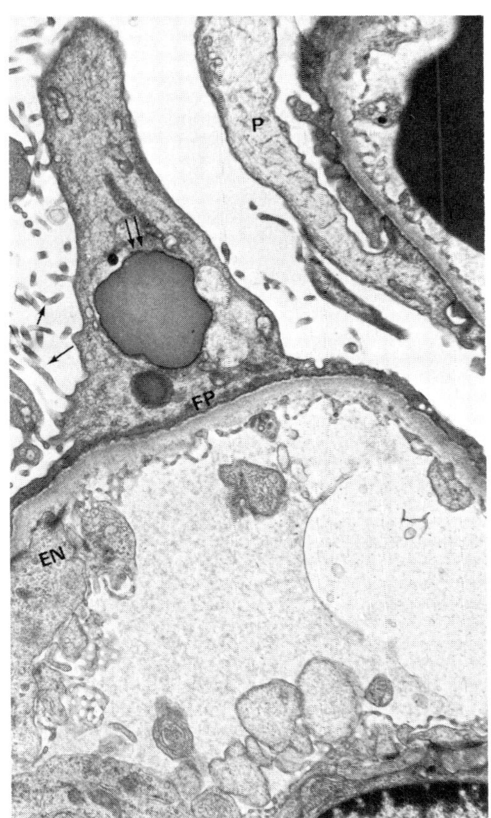

B

Figures 4-2A and **B** Minimal change disease. **A** A 1-μm-thick section of an essentially normal glomerulus. However, mild mesangial sclerosis and periglomerular fibrosis are present, in addition to moderate interstitial fibrosis (H & E × 1200). **B** Electron microscopy demonstrates effacement of the epithelial foot processes (FP). Fat droplets are present in the epithelial cytoplasm (double arrow) and marked edema is present in the endothelial cells (EN) and podocytes (P) (× 13050).

in Table 4-2. Diabetic glomerulopathy was diagnosed in 5.1% of renal biopsies. However, this diagnosis was seldom a solitary finding and was usually associated with a concurrent primary glomerulonephritis or some other form of renal involvement. This is the reason why the combined percentage of Tables 4-1 and 4-2 exceeds 100% and probably reflects the reluctance to biopsy individuals to whom diabetes is an evident cause of the nephrotic syndrome.

Interestingly, acute interstitial nephritis was the most common diagnosis in the nonprimary glomerulonephritis category. The majority of these cases were secondary to the administration of antibiotics or nonsteroidal anti-inflammatory agents. However, with the available information, we were often unable to ascertain the immediate reason for the acute interstitial nephritis in a number of cases. This interesting finding must be pursued in the

Table 4-2
Other Diseases Found in 277 Renal Biopsies Done in Patients Above Age 60 Years

Diagnosis	No.	% of Total
Acute interstitial nephritis	23	8.3
Renal amyloidosis	19	6.9
Arteriolar nephrosclerosis	18	6.5
Diabetic glomerulopathy	14	5.1
Lupus erythematosus	12	4.3
Myeloma kidney	9	3.2
Chronic interstitial nephritis	9	3.2
Acute tubular necrosis	6	2.2
Wegener's granulomatosis	4	1.4
Secondary renal amyloidosis	3	1.1
Cholesterol emboli	3	1.1
Cancer of the bladder	3	1.1
Scleroderma	2	0.7
Henoch-Schönlein purpura	2	0.7
Acute pyelonephritis	1	0.4
Hemolytic uremic syndrome	1	0.4
Microangiopathic polyarteritis	1	0.4
Unknown	19	6.91
Total	149	55.0

future since drug usage is a common accompaniment to therapy in the elderly population and, at least in our series, served as an important proximate cause of renal dysfunction. Primary renal amyloidosis is another common cause of the nephrotic syndrome in the aged within the nonglomerulonephritis category.

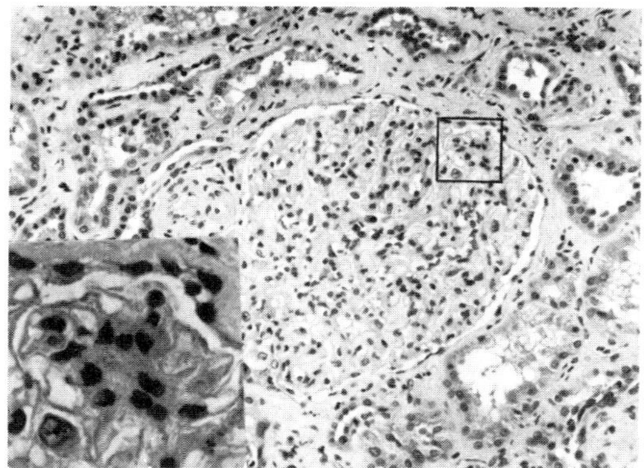

Figure 4-3A Mesangioproliferative glomerulonephritis. **A** A 63-year-old female patient with nephrotic syndrome. The glomerulus demonstrates increased cellularity and mesangial widening (H & E × 480). The insert in the lower left (× 1200) clearly demonstrates increased mesangial cells and mesangial matrix. Noticeable in this biopsy is the presence of interstitial fibrosis and tubular atrophy.

It is clear from our data and that of other authors that glomerulonephritis of a primary or secondary nature does occur in the elderly. The presenting signs and symptoms of this entity may be masked by symptomatology peculiar to extrarenal organ system dysfunction. This requires maintenance of a high degree of suspicion by the clinician who might then by judicious use of renal biopsy find a lesion that is potentially treatable. This approach to the elderly subserves a dictate that not all of that which occurs in the elderly should be attributed to the inexorable effect of aging on the reference organ system.

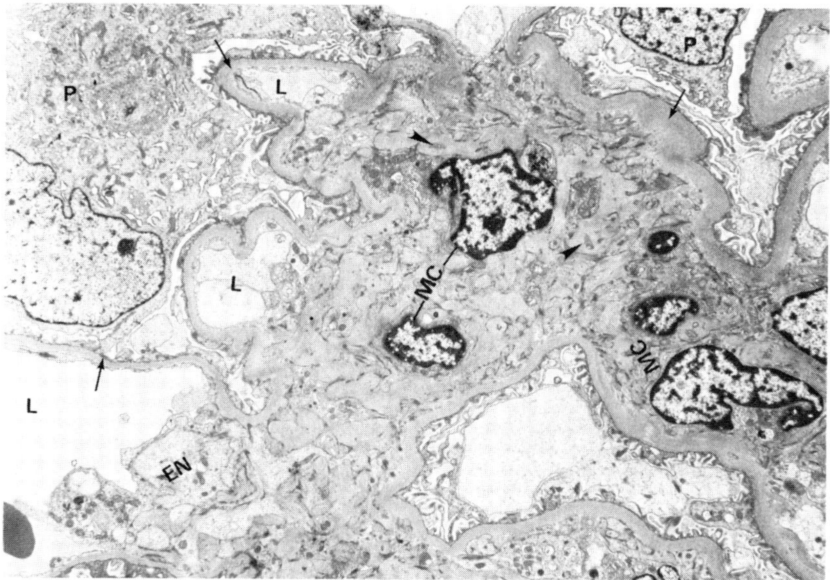

Figure 4-3B Electron microscopy demonstrates mesangial widening produced by increased number of mesangial cells and mesangial matrix. Some electron-dense deposits are present in the mesangium (arrow head) (× 3610). Arrows indicate basement membrane, P = epithelial cell, MC = mesangial cell, L = capillary lumen, EN = endothelial cell.

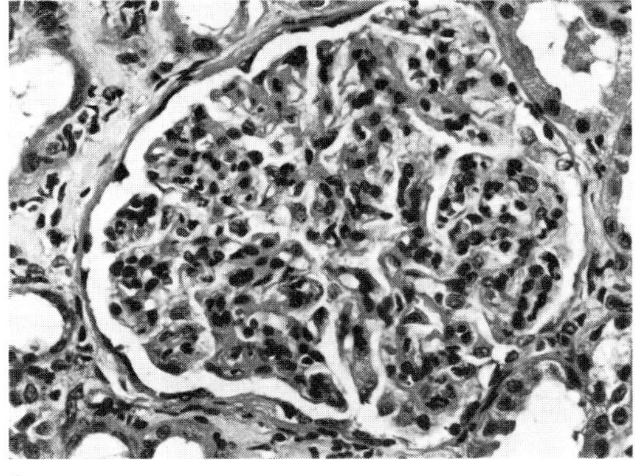

A

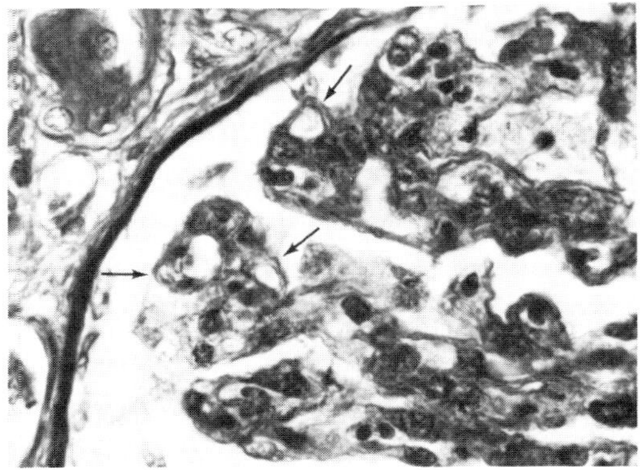

B

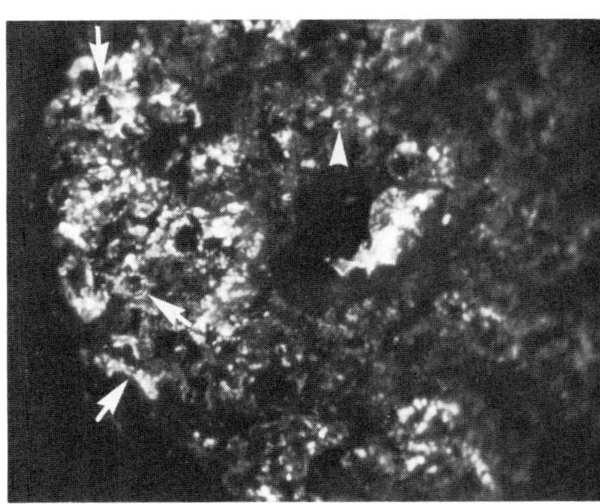

C

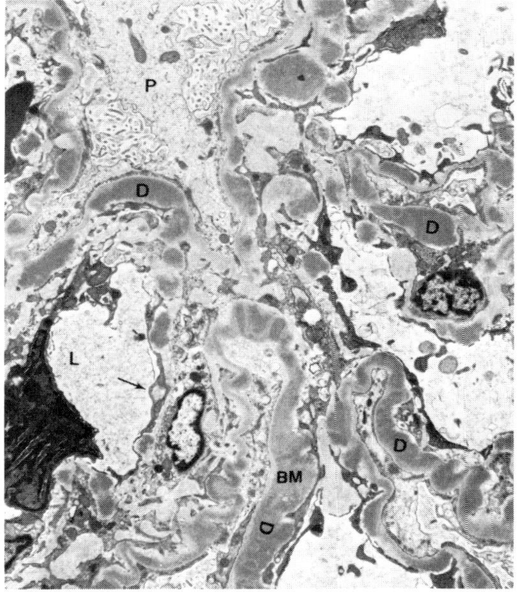

D

Figures 4-4A–E Membranoproliferative glomerulonephritis. **A** A 66-year-old white female with nephrotic nephritic urinary sediment. Renal biopsy by light microscopy showed increased cellularity and mesangial matrix in the glomerulus with some lobular accentuation of the capillary loop. Focal tubular atrophy and interstitial inflammatory infiltrate was also present (H & E × 1200). **B** Under higher magnification (PAS × 3000) a double contour (arrows) is present in some of the capillary loops. **C** The immunofluorescent study demonstrates extensive C_3 deposits in the mesangial area and peripheral capillary loops. The immune deposition is not homogeneous and appears to be present in both sides of the basement membrane (arrow). Bright granular deposits are present in the mesangium and a few of them have a ring-like appearance (arrowhead) (×3000). **D** Electron microscopy showed very dark deposits (D) following the outline of the capillary basement membrane (BM). In some areas the electron-dense deposits are discontinuous and inside the basement membrane, producing expansion of this stricture (× 5510).

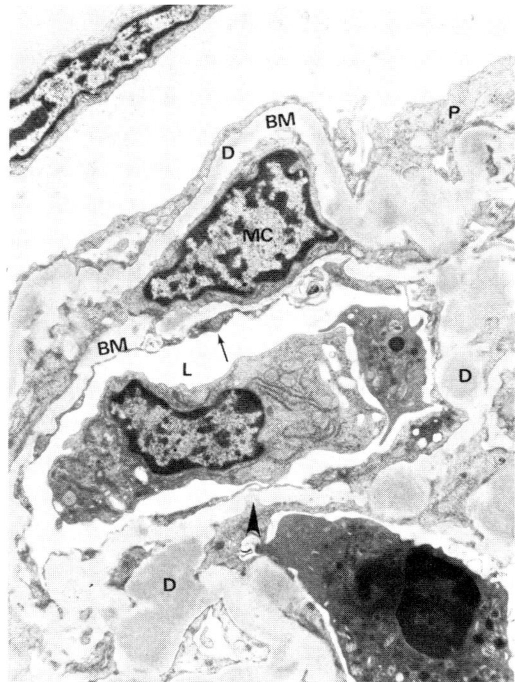

E In other areas the basement membrane is split (BM) with mesangial cell (MC) interposition and reduplication of the basement membrane (arrow). Some disruption of the basement membrane is also present (arrowhead) (× 8550). L = capillary lumen, P = epithelial cell.

ACKNOWLEDGMENTS

This work was supported by the Veterans Administration Research Funds and the Renal Research and Education Funds of the Tampa VA Medical Center. The authors are grateful to Mrs Virginia Shrader for secretarial help, Ms Diane E. Heckerman for technical assistance, Dr Charley Gutch and Ms Vera Rhodes for review of the manuscript and valuable suggestions.

REFERENCES

1. Rosen E: Renal disease in the elderly. *Med Clin North Am* 1976;60:1105–1119.
2. Stewart RB, Hale WE, Mark RG: Effects of nonsteroidal anti-inflammatory drugs on renal function in the elderly. *South Med J* 1982;75:824–826.
3. Katz SM, Capaldo R, Everts EA, et al: Tolmetin association with reversible renal failure and acute interstitial nephritis. *JAMA* 1981;246:243–245.
4. Kimberly RP, Bowden RE, Keiser HR, et al: Reduction of renal function by newer nonsteroidal anti-inflammatory drugs. *Am J Med* 1978;64:804.
5. Marketos S, Papayiotou P, Dontas AS: Glomerular filtration rate in elderly men and women under the influence of a new anabolic steroid. *Nephron* 1969;6:478–483.
6. Perlman CV, Kennedy BW, Hayner NS: Primary and secondary renal failure in a total community (Tecumseh, Michigan): Preponderance in the elderly and possible antecedent factors. *J Am Geriatr Soc* 1974;22:25–32.
7. Carter CB, Olichney MJ, Westlervelt FB: Renal failure in the elderly. *South Med J* 1970;63:805–808.
8. Riehle RA, Darracott-Vaughan E: Genitourinary disease in the elderly. *Med Clin North Am* 1983;67:445–461.
9. Mohammed I, Ansell BM, Holborow EJ, et al: Circulating immune complexes in subacute infective endocarditis and post streptococcal glomerulonephritis. *J Clin Pathol* 1977;30:308–311.
10. Lange K, Craig F, Oberman J, et al: Changes in serum complement during the course and treatment of glomerulonephritis. *Arch Intern Med* 1951;88:433–445.
11. Lewis EJ, Carpenter CB, Schur PH: Serum complement levels in human glomerulonephritis. *Ann Intern Med* 1971;75:555–560.
12. Boswell D, Eknoyan G: Acute glomerulonephritis in the aged. *Geriatrics* 1968;23:73–80.
13. Lee HA, Stirling G, Sharpstone P: Acute glomerulonephritis in the middle aged and elderly patient. *Br Med J* 1966;2:1361–1363.
14. Samiy AH, Fields RA, Merrill JP: Acute glomerulonephritis in elderly patients. *Ann Intern Med* 1961;54:603–609.
15. Nesson HR, Robbins SL: Glomerulonephritis in older age group. *Arch Intern Med* 1960;105:47–56.
16. Arieff AI, Anderson RJ, Massry SG: Acute glomerulonephritis in the elderly. *Geriatrics* 1971;26:74–84.
17. Dodge WF, Spargo BH, Travis LB, et al:

Poststreptococcal glomerulonephritis, a prospective study in children. *N Engl J Med* 1972;286:273–278.
18. Mota-Hernandez F, Briseno-Mondragon E, Gordillo-Paniagua G: Glomerular lesions and final outcome in children with glomerulonephritis of acute onset. *Nephron* 1976;16:272–281.
19. Jennings RB, Earle DP: Poststreptococcal glomerulonephritis: histopathologic and clinical studies of the acute, subsiding acute and early chronic latent phases. *J Clin Invest* 1961;40:1525–1557.
20. Baldwin DS, Gluck MC, Schacht RG, et al: The long-term course of poststreptococcal glomerulonephritis. *Ann Intern Med* 1974;80:342–358.
21. Potvliege PR, Deroy G, Dupuis F: Necropsy study on glomerulonephritis in the elderly. *J Clin Pathol* 1975;28:891–898.
22. Montoliu J, Darhell A, Torras A, et al: Acute and rapidly progressive forms of glomerulonephritis in the elderly. *J Am Geriatr Soc* 1981;29:108–116.
23. Heptinstall RH: Rapidly progressive glomerulonephritis, in Heptinstall RH (ed): *Pathology of the Kidney.* Boston, Little, Brown & Co, 1974, pp 371–391.
24. Spargo BH, Ordonez MG, Ringus JC: The differential diagnosis of crescentic glomerulonephritis: The pathology of specific lesions with prognostic implications. *Hum Pathol* 1977;8:187–204.
25. Forland M, Jones RE, Easterling RE, et al: Clinical and renal biopsy observations in oliguric glomerulonephritis. *J Chronic Dis* 1966;19:163–177.
26. Moorthy AV, Zimmerman SW: Renal disease in the elderly: Clinicopathologic analyses of renal disease in 115 elderly patients. *Clin Nephrol* 1980;14:223–229.
27. Beirne GJ, Wagnild JP, Zimmerman SW, et al: Idiopathic crescentic glomerulonephritis. *Medicine* 1977;56:349–381.
28. Morrin PAF, Hinglais N, Nabarra B, et al: Rapidly progressive glomerulonephritis: A clinical and pathologic study. *Am J Med* 1978;65:446–460.
29. Brown CB, Turner D, Ogg CS, et al: Combined immunosuppression and anticoagulation in rapidly progressive glomerulonephritis. *Lancet* 1974;2: 1166–1172.
30. Camerson JS, Gill D, Turner DR, et al: Combined immunosuppression and anticoagulation in rapidly progressive glomerulonephritis, letter. *Lancet* 1975; 2:923–925.
31. Kincaid-Smith P, Saker BM, Fairley KF: Anticoagulants in "irreversible" acute renal failure. *Lancet* 1968;2:1360–1363.
32. Arief AT, Pinggera WF: Rapidly progressive glomerulonephritis treated with anticoagulants. *Arch Intern Med* 1972; 129:77–84.
33. Lockwood CM, Pinching AJ, Sweny P, et al: Plasma exchange and immunosuppression in the treatment of fulminating immune-complex crescentic nephritis. *Lancet* 1977;1:63–67.
34. O'Neill WM, Etheridge WB, Bloomer HA: High dose corticosteroids. Their use in treating idiopathic rapidly progressive glomerulonephritis. *Arch Intern Med* 1979;139:514–518.
35. Bolton WK, Couser WG: Intravenous pulse methylprednisolone therapy of acute crescentic progressive glomerulonephritis. *Am J Med* 1979;66:495–502.
36. Oredugba O, Mazumdar DC, Meyer JS, et al: Pulse methylprednisolone therapy in idiopathic, rapidly progressive glomerulonephritis. *Ann Intern Med* 1980; 92:504–506.
37. Rower JW: Aging and renal function. *Annu Rev Gerontol Geriatrics* 1980;1: 161–179.
38. Sorensen FH: Quantitative studies of the renal corpuscle. *Acta Pathol Microbiol Scand* [A] 1977;85:356–366.
39. Tauchi H, Tsuboi K, Okutomi J: Age changes in the human kidney of the different races. *Gerontology* 1971;17:87–97.
40. Ashworth CT, Erdmann RR, Arnold BS: Age changes in the renal basement membrane in rats. *Am J Pathol* 1960;36: 165–179.
41. Darmady EM, Offer J, Woodhouse MA: The parameters of the aging kidneys. *J Pathol* 1973;109:195–207.
42. Berger J, Hinglais N: Les dépôts intercapillaries d'IgA-IgG. *J Urol Nephrol* 1968;74:694–695.
43. Berger J: IgA glomerular deposits in renal disease. *Transplant Proc* 1969;1:939–944.
44. Morel-Maroger L, Leathem A, Richet G: Glomerular abnormalities in nonsystemic diseases. Relationship between findings

by light microscopy and immunofluorescence in 433 biopsy specimens. *Am J Med* 1972;53:170–184.

45. Barbiana Di Belgiojoso G, Tarantino A, Civati G, et al: Glomerulonefrite a depositi intercapillari di IgA-IgG: studio clinico e morfologico di 63 casi. *Clin Lab* 1973;3(suppl 1):30–42.
46. Druet P, Bariety J, Bernard D, et al: Les glomerulonéphrites primitives a dépôts mesangiaux d'IgA et d'IgG. Étude clinique et morphologique de 52 cas. *Presse Med* 1970;78:583–587.
47. McCoy RC, Abromowsky CR, Tisher CC: IgA nephropathy. *Am J Pathol* 1974;76: 123–144.
48. Lowance DC, Mullins JD, McPhaul JJ: Immunoglobulin A (IgA) associated glomerulonephritis. *Kidney Int* 1973;3: 167–176.
49. Clarkson AP, Seymour AE, Chan YL, et al: Clinical pathological and therapeutic aspects of IgA nephropathy, in Kincaid-Smith P, d'Apice AJF, Atkins RC (eds): *Progress in Glomerulonephritis.* New York, Wiley Medical Publications, 1979, pp 247–259.
50. Sissons JGP, Woodrow DF, Curtis JR, et al: Isolated glomerulonephritis with IgA deposits. *Br Med J* 1975;3:611–614.
51. Zimmerman SW, Burkholder PM: Immunoglobulin-A nephropathy. *Arch Intern Med* 1975;135:1217–1223.
52. Alexander F, Barabas AZ, Jack RGJ: IgA nephropathy. *Hum Pathol* 1977;8:173–185.
53. MacDonald I, Fairley KF, Hobbs JB, et al: Loin pain as a presenting symptom in idiopathic glomerulonephritis. *Clin Nephrol* 1975;3:129–133.
54. Clarkson AR, Seymour AE, Thompson AJ, et al: IgA nephropathy: a syndrome of uniform morphology, diverse clinical features and uncertain prognosis. *Clin Nephrol* 1977;8:459–471.
55. Cordonnier D, Vialtel P, Chenais F, et al: Augmentation due taux des IgA serques dors les glomerulonéphrites avec d'IgA dans le mesangium. *Nouv Presse Med* 1974;3:2264–2265.
56. Lagrue G, Hirbec G, Fournel M, et al: Glomerulonéphrite mesanguiale à dépôts d'IgA. Étude des immunoglobulines sergues. *J Urol Nephrol* 1974;80:385–387.
57. Berger J: Idiopathic mesangial deposition of IgA, in Hamburger J, Crosneir J, Grunfeld JP (eds): *Nephrology.* Paris, John Wiley & Sons, 1974, pp 535,541.
58. Pussell BA, Lockwood CM, Scott DM, et al: Value of immune complex assays in diagnosis and management. *Lancet* 1978;2:359–363.
59. Tung KSH, Woodroffe AJ, Ahlin TD, et al: Application on the solid phase C_{1q} and Raji cell radioimmunoassays for the detection of circulating immune complexes in glomerulonephritis. *J Clin Invest* 1978; 62:61–72.
60. Hall RP, Stachura I, Cason J, et al: IgA containing circulating immune complexes in patients with IgA nephropathy. *Am J Med* 1983;74:56–63.
61. Van Der Peet J, Arisz L, Brentjens JRH, et al: The clinical course of IgA nephropathy in adults. *Clin Nephrol* 1977;8: 335–340.
62. D'Amico G, Ferrario F, Colasanti G, et al: IgA mesangial nephropathy (Berger's disease) with rapid decline in renal function. *Clin Nephrol* 1981;16:251–257.
63. Habib R, Kleinknecht C: The primary nephrotic syndrome of childhood. Classification and clinicopathologic study of 406 cases. *Pathol Annu* 1971;6:417–474.
64. Morthy AV: Minimal change nephrotic syndrome–a benign cause of proteinuria in the elderly. *Am J Med Sci* 1978;275: 65–73.
65. Facet IW, Hilton PJ, Jones HF, et al: Nephrotic syndrome in the elderly. *Br Med J* 1971;2:387–388.
66. Khokhar N, Akavaram HR, Qunones EM: Lipoid nephrosis in the elderly. *South Med J* 1980;73:790–791.
67. Hooper J, Ryan P, Lee JC, et al: Lipoid nephrosis in 31 adult patients: renal biopsy study by light, electron and fluorescence microscopy with experience in treatment. *Medicine* 1970;49:321–341.
68. Cameron JS, Turner DR, Oggs CS, et al: The nephrotic syndrome in adults with "minimal change" glomerular lesions. *Am J Med* 1974;43:461–488.
69. Hayslett JP, Kashgarian M, Bensch KG, et al: Clinicopathological correlations in the nephrotic syndrome due to primary renal disease. *Medicine* 1973;52:93–120.
70. Zech P, Colon S, Pointet PH, et al: The

nephrotic syndrome in adults aged over 60: Etiology, evolution, and treatment of 76 cases. *Clin Nephrol* 1982;18:232–236.
71. Waldherr R, Gubler MC, Levy M, et al: The significance of pure mesangial proliferation in idiopathic nephrotic syndrome. *Clin Nephrol* 1978;10:171–179.
72. Brown EA, Upadhyaya K, Hayslett JP, et al: The clinical course of mesangial proliferative glomerulonephritis. *Medicine* 1979;58:295–303.
73. Murphy WM, Jukkola AF, Roy S: Nephrotic syndrome with mesangial cell proliferation in children. A distinct entity. *Am J Clin Pathol* 1979;72:42–47.
74. Schoeneman MJ, Bennett B, Griefer I: The natural history of focal segmental glomerulosclerosis with and without mesangial hypercellularity in children. *Clin Nephrol* 1978;9:45–54.
75. Sinniah R, Pwee HS, Lim CH: Glomerular lesions in asymptomatic microscopic hematuria discovered on routine medical examination. *Clin Nephrol* 1976;5: 216–228.
76. White RHR: Mesangial proliferative glomerulonephritis, in Kincaid-Smith P, Mathew TH, Becker EL (eds): *Glomerulonephritis: Morphology, Natural History and Treatment.* New York, John Wiley & Sons, 1976, pp 383–396.
77. Cohen AH, Border WA, Glassock RJ: Nephrotic syndrome with glomerular mesangial IgM deposits. *Lab Invest* 1978;38:610–619.
78. Rhasin HK, Abuelo JG, Nayak R, et al: Mesangial proliferative glomerulonephritis. *Lab Invest* 1978;39:21–29.
79. Cameron JS: The problem of focal segmental glomerulosclerosis, in Kincaid-Smith P, d'Apice AJF, Atkins RC (eds): *Progress in Glomerulonephritis.* New York, Wiley Medical Publications, 1979, pp 209–228.
80. Kashgarian M, Hayslett JP, Siegel NJ: Lipoid nephrosis and focal sclerosis: distinct entities or spectrum of disease? *Nephron* 1974;13:105–108.
81. Spargo BH, Seymour AE, Ordonez NG: Focal glomerulosclerosis, in Spargo BH, Seymour AE, Ordonez NG (eds): *Renal Biopsy Pathology with Diagnostic and Therapeutic Implications.* New York, John Wiley & Sons, 1980, pp 45–63.
82. Hyman LR, Burkholder PM: Focal sclerosing glomerulonephropathy with segmental hyalinosis. *Lab Invest* 1973;28: 533–544.
83. Rumpelt HJ, Thoenes W: Intraglomerular (immune) deposits in focal and segmental sclerosing glomerulopathy (nephritis). *Clin Nephrol* 1973;1:367–369.
84. Lee SM, Michael AF: Focal glomerular sclerosis and sarcoidosis. *Arch Pathol Lab Med* 1978;102:572–575.
85. Weisinger JR, Kempson RL, Eldrige FL, et al: The nephrotic syndrome: A complication of massive obesity. *Ann Intern Med* 1974;81:440–447.
86. Friedman EA, Sreepada Rao TK, Nicastri AD: Heroin associated nephropathy. *Nephron* 1974;13:421–426.
87. Hyman LR, Burkholder PM: Focal sclerosing glomerulopathy with hyalinosis: A clinical and pathologic analysis of the disease in children. *J Pediatr* 1974; 84:217–225.
88. Camerson JS, Ogg CS, Chantler C, et al: The long-term prognosis of patients with focal segmental glomerulosclerosis. *Clin Nephrol* 1978;10:213–218.
89. Kincaid-Smith P, Young CK: Focal and segmental proliferative glomerulonephritis, focal and segmental hyalinosis and sclerosis, and focal sclerosis in the adult, in Kincaid-Smith P, d'Apice AJF, Atkins RC (eds): *Progress in Glomerulonephritis.* New York, Wiley Medical Publications, 1979, pp 231–259.
90. Glassock RJ: The nephrotic syndrome. *Hosp Pract* 1979;14:105–129.
91. Brzosko WJ, Krawczynski K, Nazarewicz T, et al: Glomerulonephritis associated with hepatitis B-surface antigen immune complexes in children. *Lancet* 1974;2: 477–481.
92. Ramanujam K, Ramu G, Balakrishnan S, et al: Nephrotic syndrome complicating lepromatous leprosy. *Indian J Med Res* 1973;61:548–556.
93. Braunstein GD, Lewis EJ, Galvanek EG, et al: The nephrotic syndrome associated with secondary syphilis: An immune deposit disease. *Am J Med* 1970;48: 643–648.
94. Libit SA, Burke B, Michael AF, et al: Extramembranous glomerulonephritis in childhood. Relationship to systemic lupus

erythematosus. *J Pediatr* 1976;88:294–402.
95. Baldwin DS, Lowenstein J, Rothfield NF, et al: The clinical course of the proliferative and membranous forms of lupus nephritis. *Ann Intern Med* 1970;73: 929–942.
96. Comerford FR, Cohen AS: The nephropathy of systemic lupus erythematosus: An assessment by clinical, light and electron microscopic criteria. *Medicine* 1967; 46:425–473.
97. Eagen J, Lewis EJ: Glomerulopathies of neoplasia. *Kidney Int* 1977;11:297–306.
98. Row PG, Cameron JS, Turner DR, et al: Membranous nephropathy. Long-term follow-up and association with neoplasia. *Am J Med* 1975;44:207–239.
99. Hopper J: Tumor related renal lesions. *Ann Intern Med* 1974;81:550–551.
100. Rosen S: Membranous glomerulonephritis: Current status. *Hum Pathol* 1971; 2:209–231.
101. Ducret F, Berthous FC, Colon S, et al: Glomerulonephritis with extramembranous lesions in a patient with sickle cell disease. Confirmation of the deposits by immunofluorescence. *Presse Med* 1977;6:1395.
102. Ehrenreich T, Churg J: Pathology of membranous nephropathy. *Pathol Annu* 1968;3:145–186.
103. Silverberg DS, Kidd EG, Shnitka TK, et al: Gold nephropathy: A clinical and pathologic study. *Arthritis Rheum* 1970; 13:812–825.
104. Jaffe IA, Treser G, Suzuki Y, et al: Nephropathy induced by D-penicillamine. *Ann Intern Med* 1969;69:549–556.
105. Tait GB: Nephropathy during phenindione therapy. *Lancet* 1960;2:1198–1199.
106. Cameron JS: Pathogenesis and treatment of membranous nephropathy. *Kidney Int* 1979;15:88–103.
107. Rastogi SD, Hart-Mercer J, Kerr DMS: Idiopathic membranous glomerulonephritis in adults. Remissions following steroid therapy. *Q J Med* 1968;38: 335–350.
108. Pollak VE, Rosen S, Pirani CL, et al: Natural history of membranous glomerulonephritis. *Ann Intern Med* 1969;69: 1171–1196.
109. Jones DB: The nature of scar tissue in glomerulonephritis. *Am J Pathol* 1963; 42:185–199.
110. Arakawa M, Kimmelstiel P: Circumferential mesangial interposition. *Lab Invest* 1969;21:276–284.
111. Habib R, Kleinknecht C, Gubler MC, et al: Idiopathic membranoproliferative glomerulonephritis in children. *Clin Nephrol* 1973;1:194–214.
112. Habib R, Gubler MC, Loirat C, et al: Dense deposit disease: A variant of membranoproliferative glomerulonephritis. *Kidney Int* 1975;7:204–215.
113. Levy M, Gubler MC, Habib R: New concepts on membranoproliferative glomerulonephritis, in Kincaid-Smith P, d'Apice AJF, Atkins RC (eds): *Progress in Glomerulonephritis.* New York, Wiley Medical Publications, 1979, pp 177–205.
114. West CD, McAdams AJ, McConville JM, et al: Hypocomplementemic and normocomplementemic persistent (chronic) glomerulonephritis: Clinical and pathological characteristics. *J Pediatr* 1965;67: 1089–1109.
115. Ooi YM, Vallotta EH, West CD: Classical complement pathway activation in membranoproliferative glomerulonephritis. *Kidney Int* 1976;9:46–53.

CHAPTER 5

Tubulo-Interstitial Nephritis in the Elderly

William F. Falls

Tubulo-interstitial nephritis (TIN) spans a broad etiologic and pathogenetic spectrum. This chapter will be devoted to a discussion of this renal disease category as it occurs in the aged but will exclude two disorders which may have a major tubulo-interstitial component: acute tubular necrosis (vasomotor nephropathy) and bacterial pyelonephritis. These disturbances in the elderly are covered in other chapters in this book. As will be elaborated subsequently, TIN may be either acute or chronic. Such a classification may be somewhat arbitrary but has both a clinical and pathologic basis.

Tubulo-interstitial nephritis is seen in all age groups. There is probably nothing unique about its occurrence in the elderly; however, attainment of old age, per se, diminishes the likelihood of new onset disease being caused by a congenital or hereditary disorder. Although most patients with congenital or hereditary renal disease will have reached end-stage by age 65 years, some with adult polycystic disease[1] or females with Alport's syndrome[2] may survive into the later decades. Both these disorders will usually have been recognized earlier in life and will not be considered in this chapter.

The clinical and pathologic picture of TIN in the elderly may be subtly tinted by the aging process itself. As noted in chapter 2, an indolent, atrophic process occurs in the kidneys of all persons after the fifth decade.[3] This process involves all histologic elements of the kidney. Medial hypertrophy, intimal proliferation, and hyalinization are seen in small arteries. Mild, focal glomerular basement membrane thickening and sclerosis are frequent. Tubular atrophy, tubular basement membrane thickening, interstitial infiltration with mononuclear cells, and interstitial fibrosis are commonly noted. The latter may be particularly notable in the medullary area after the seventh decade. The functional correlates of these anatomical changes are a decreased glomerular filtration rate (GFR)[4] and diminished ability to modulate sodium,[5] water,[6] and acid-base metabolism.[7] Even in the absence of any specific renal disease the older patient is unable to maximally concentrate his urine, severely limit sodium excretion, or rapidly excrete an acid load. The tubular systems for maximal transport of glucose, iodopyracet (Diodrast), para-aminohippurate (PAH), and probably other reabsorbed and secreted substances are impaired.[8] In addition, the renin-angiotensin-aldosterone system seems to be operative at a lower level than in younger persons.[9] Thus, the elderly patient suffers a loss of renal reserve. As a consequence, any new insult will be superimposed on a histologically altered kidney and the resultant functional changes may be disproportionately severe.

A particularly important aspect of tubulo-interstitial renal disease in the elderly is its relation to drug administration. The elderly have a higher incidence of both drug exposure and adverse reactions than younger persons.[10] The incidence of adverse reactions relates to alterations in both pharmacokinetics and pharmacodynamics.[11] The most important pharmacokinetic change is the delayed clearance of many drugs secondary to decreased glomerular filtration.[12] Toxic serum concentrations of drugs primarily excreted by the kidney may develop at usual dosages. Much of this toxicity is renal tubulo-interstitial damage. In the aged patient a vicious cycle of renal damage and rising serum drug concentrations may be encountered when potentially nephrotoxic agents cleared by the kidneys are administered. Although less well studied, alterations in drug pharmacodynamics may also predispose older patients to adverse effects above and beyond those related to specific toxic serum concentrations.

The serum creatinine determination is an inadequate marker of GFR in older patients.[13] This is true because the total quantity of creatinine produced as a byproduct of muscle metabolism diminishes with aging. This loss of muscle mass essentially parallels the age-related reduction in GFR. Thus, the serum creatinine may remain relatively normal with aging despite a significant fall in GFR.

ACUTE TUBULO-INTERSTITIAL NEPHRITIS

General Overview

Pathology The subject of acute TIN has been extensively reviewed.[14-20] The finding of acute TIN on routine pathologic examination is not specific for any particular etiologic process. Gross, postmortem examination reveals large, edematous kidneys. On light microscopic examination, the cortical interstitium is edematous with a cellular infiltrate composed of varying proportions of lymphocytes, plasma cells, and eosinophils. The infiltrates may be either patchy or diffuse (Figure 5-1). Early on, some polymorphonuclear cells may be seen but their presence is usually suggestive of a superimposed bacterial infection. Tubular lesions are variable and include flattening and swelling of the epithelial cells with occasional exfoliation and necrosis. Lymphocytes may either abut the outer tubular surface or be found within the tubular basement membrane interposed between tubular cells. Severe tubular damage with rupture of the tubular basement membrane has been described. The tubular lumen may be filled with amorphous debris

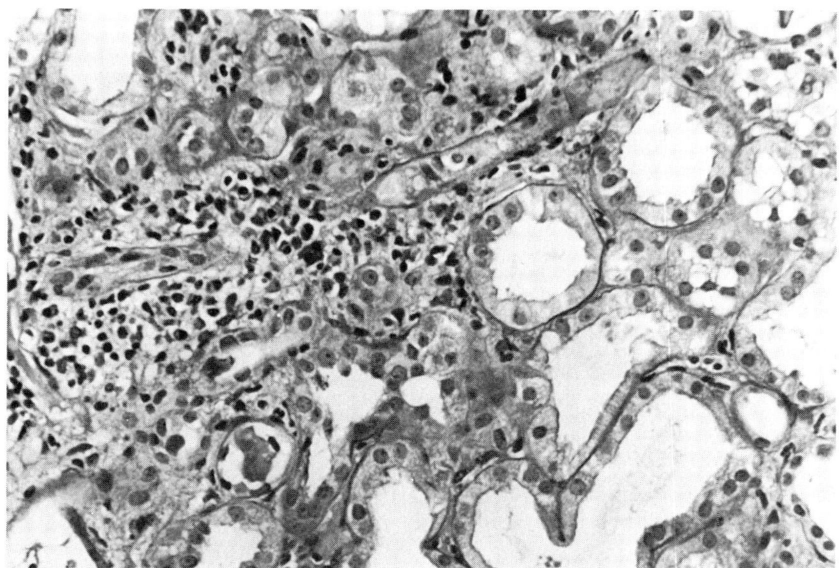

Figure 5-1 Acute interstitial nephritis. Note the focal infiltration of inflammatory cells interspersed between the tubules. Tubular compression is noted (×160).

and necrotic tubular cells. Glomerular changes are usually minimal but segmental mesangial proliferation may be seen. Vascular changes are usually not impressive and when present would suggest a concomitant vasculitis. Notably, there is usually no evidence of fibrosis or other chronic change; however, in the elderly patient, underlying atrophic alterations may alter the histologic picture. In the circumstances where an underlying immunologic insult is attacking both the interstitium and the glomeruli (see below), typical patterns of primary glomerular involvement may accompany the interstitial change. The immunofluorescent picture may be more specific in pinpointing a given etiology and will be defined in greater detail with the discussion of individual diseases which follows. Electron microscopy has generally been less helpful in defining tubulo-interstitial as compared to glomerular pathology.

Clinical picture The clinical picture of acute TIN is characterized by the abrupt onset of renal insufficiency. Urinary output is usually not greatly diminished, but acute oliguric renal failure and fluid overload have been described. Hypertension is not part of the typical picture. Heavy proteinuria (greater than 2.5 g/24 h) is rare and its presence suggests an accompanying glomerular abnormality. The urine sediment may contain red cells, white cells, and casts with white cell and granular inclusions. Red cell casts are seldom seen. Eosinophils may be noted if the urine is stained with Wright's stain, particularly in those patients with a drug-induced nephropathy. Other laboratory studies are usually not very helpful diagnostically, but the kidneys may appear to be enlarged by urography or sonography. It has been suggested recently that gallium uptake may be increased in kidneys with an acute TIN and that a gallium scan may assist in diagnosis.[21]

The course of acute TIN is highly variable and depends on the underlying disease process. Specific management is usually directed at recognition and correction of the basic disease and will be discussed with each separate entity. Supportive care including the use of peritoneal or hemodialysis is used in the same fashion as in patients with acute renal failure of any cause.

Specific Causes

Infectious diseases Acute TIN was originally described in association with such infectious diseases as diphtheria, scarlet fever, and septicemic states.[22] In this setting the renal disease was frequently overshadowed by other clinical manifestations and resolution depended on improvement in the overall disease process. In current medical practice, acute TIN is recognized more frequently as a complication of several specific infectious processes listed in Table 5-1.

Acute TIN is the renal lesion most frequently seen in patients with leptospirosis.[23] Its etiology is uncertain. Because of the onset of infiltration early in the course of disease and the frequent presence of a major element of tubular necrosis, some have suggested a toxic mechanism.[24] However, a recent case demonstrated glomerulonephritis with positive glomerular immunofluorescence accompanying the acute TIN lesion.[25] These findings were interpreted as suggesting the possibility of an immunologic mechanism for both the glomerular and interstitial involvement. In most patients the renal insufficiency disappears with resolution of the infection; however, progression to chronic disease has been described and dialysis has been necessary to tide others over the acute insult. It has been suggested that the disease may be more severe in the elderly.

Legionnaires' disease secondary to infection with the gram-negative bacillus, *Legionella pneumophilia*, is frequently complicated by the development of renal failure.[26] The renal failure may be severe and occurs in the setting of unexplained pulmonary infection and fever. Renal pathologic findings are variable and have included both acute tubular necrosis and acute TIN. This infection appears to have a particular propensity to attack elderly and immunosuppressed individuals. Clearing of the renal insufficiency usually occurs with recovery from the infection after therapy with erythromycin. Dialysis has been required in some cases, however.[27]

An occasional patient with infectious mononucleosis may have evidence of renal involvement.[28] This is usually recognized only as an abnormality of the urine sediment and overt renal insufficiency is rare. Renal biopsies have shown both TIN alone and in association with glomerular involvement.

Infection with *Brucella* organisms may be accompanied by an acute TIN with focal glomerular abnormalities.[29] Resolution may be incomplete despite antibiotic therapy and progression on to chronic TIN with renal insufficiency has been described.

Other infectious diseases in which a predominant acute TIN pattern has been described include toxoplasmosis, measles, syphilis, *Mycoplasma* pneumonia infection, and Rocky Mountain spotted fever.[30] The pathogenesis of tubulo-interstitial involvement is poorly understood but an immunologic response to either the infectious agent or an antigenic component which has lodged in the interstitium seems to be a likely explanation for the disease.

Drug-related acute tubulo-interstitial disease

Hypersensitivity There is great contemporary interest in drug-related acute TIN. A large number of agents have been incriminated as causes (Table 5-2) and several interesting pathologic mechanisms have been suggested by the study of biopsy material. Although most cases have not been in the elderly, one might expect an increasing incidence in patients of this age group because of their frequency of drug exposure. Indeed, this now seems to be the case for instances of reactions to non-steroidal anti-inflammatory agents.[31]

Acute TIN induced by methicillin or other penicillins is the prototype of drug-induced disease and has been the most thoroughly studied.[32-35] The classic clinical picture is characterized by the onset of fever, erythematous skin eruption, and renal insufficiency 1 to 3 weeks after institution of drug therapy. Nausea, vomiting, and flank pain are also frequent complaints. The magnitude of renal insufficiency is variable. Anuria and a picture of acute renal failure may be seen. Red and white blood cells are usually noted in the urine sediment. Eosinophils in the urine are seen more frequently with methicillin-induced disease than with other causes of TIN.[34] An elevation of blood eosinophils and serum IgE concentration may be noted in some patients.[14] Occasionally all manifestations of hypersensitivity may be absent and the urine sediment may be free of eosinophils. In such situations the disease must be suspected by the presence of recent drug exposure and an abnormal urinary sediment containing red cells, white cells, or granular casts. A presumptive diagnosis can be made by observing the response to discontinuation of the suspected offending drug. Confirmation may be obtained by performing a renal biopsy or by rechallenging the patient with a specific drug. Recrudescence of fever and a rise in serum creatinine concentration in a patient being treated for an infectious disease with antibiotics may be the first indication of incipient acute TIN. All too frequently, patients with presumed TIN have

Table 5-1
Infectious Diseases Associated with Acute Tubulo-Interstitial Nephritis

- *a.* Diphtheria
- *b.* Streptococcal scarlet fever
- *c.* Leptospirosis
- *d.* Legionnaires' disease
- *e.* Brucellosis
- *f.* Syphilis

2. Mycoplasma
   Mycoplasma pneumonia
3. Rickettsia
   Rocky Mountain spotted fever
4. Viruses
   - *a.* Infectious mononucleosis
   - *b.* Measles
5. Protozoa
   Toxoplasmosis

Table 5-2
Drugs Associated with Acute Tubulo-Interstitial Nephritis

I. Antibiotics
- *a.* Penicillins
  1. Methicillin
  2. Penicillin G
  3. Ampicillin
  4. Amoxicillin
  5. Nafcillin
  6. Oxacillin
  7. Carbenicillin
- *b.* Cephalosporins
  1. Cephalothin
  2. Cefoxitin
  3. Cephalexin
  4. Cephradine
  5. Cefotaxime
- *c.* Aminoglycosides
- *d.* Tetracyclines
- *e.* Rifampin
- *f.* Sulfonamides
- *g.* Trimethoprim
- *h.* Vancomycin

II. Antituberculous agents

III. Nonsteroidal anti-inflammatory agents
- *a.* Ibuprofen
- *b.* Fenoprofen
- *c.* Mefenamic acid
- *d.* Zomepirac
- *e.* Tolmetin
- *f.* Indomethacin
- *g.* Phenylbutazone
- *h.* Naproxen
- *i.* Antipyrine
- *j.* Diflunisal

IV. Amphotericin B

V. Diuretics
- *a.* Hydrochlorothiazide
- *b.* Furosemide
- *c.* Triamterene
- *d.* Tienilic acid
- *e.* Chlorthalidone

VI. Miscellaneous drugs
- *a.* Phenytoin
- *b.* Barbiturates
- *c.* Lithium
- *d.* Clofibrate
- *e.* Sulfinpyrazone
- *f.* Cimetidine
- *g.* Propranolol
- *h.* Allopurinol
- *i.* Phenindione
- *j.* Glafenin
- *k.* Aspirin
- *l.* Carbamazepine
- *m.* Azathioprine
- *n.* Phenylpropanolamine
- *o.* Methyldopa

an infectious illness and are receiving more than one drug that could cause acute TIN. This makes identification of the specific offending agent difficult. There is no evidence of dose dependence in the induction of acute TIN. Cross-reactivity between the penicillin and cephalosporin groups of antibiotics appears to occur with acute TIN just as it does with other types of hypersensitivity responses. The actual incidence of acute TIN as a complication of therapy with penicillin-related drugs is unclear but probably is quite low.

Certain unique features have been noted with the disease caused by other agents. Rifampin-associated disease almost always seems to occur following a hiatus in therapy.[36] When therapy has been reinstituted in some patients an acute illness characterized by fever, arthralgia, myalgia, nausea, vomiting, hypertension, and rapidly progressive renal insufficiency has developed. The renal failure has usually lasted for a week or so and ultimately been reversible, although permanent damage has been described. Lithium may produce a functional state of nephrogenic diabetes insipidus as well as both acute and chronic TIN.[37] Recognition of acute TIN secondary to diuretic agents may be particularly difficult because they may have been prescribed to a patient with edema and an underlying glomerulopathy.[38] Suspicion of a superimposed interstitial process may be raised by a suddendeterioration in function in a previously stable patient.

The nonsteroidal anti-inflammatory agents[39] may produce functional renal changes as well as induce TIN. They may acutely lower GFR, reduce sodium excretion, and cause potassium retention without producing any anatomical change. These functional changes are rapidly reversible with discontinuation of the drug and are particularly likely to occur when the drug is administered to the elderly. These changes probably relate to inhibition of prostaglandin synthesis by the offending agent. The induction of acute TIN by these drugs, on the other hand, is usually associated with the onset of nonoliguric acute renal failure without systemic manifestations of hypersensitivity or eosinophilia. In addition, several patients have been described with the simultaneous development of acute TIN and minimal change glomerulopathy.[40] These patients have had a nephrotic syndrome as well as a urine sediment suggestive of TIN. Both the heavy proteinuria and the acute TIN have resolved when the drug has been discontinued.

Several different pathogenetic mechanisms have been proposed to explain drug-induced acute TIN. Evidence for both an antitubular basement membrane antibody[41] and an immune complex[42] mediated pathogenesis has been presented. The original studies of methicillin nephritis showed linear deposition of antisera to IgG and dimethoxyphenyl penicilloyl hapten along the tubular basement membranes.[43] These findings suggested that an antibody which cross-reacted with a portion of the methicillin molecule and a component of the tubular basement membrane was induced by drug administration. The inflammatory reaction itself was thought to be mediated by activation of the complement cascade following combination of the antigen and antibody. Similar lesions have been noted in patients with Goodpasture's syndrome who display both circulating antiglomerular and antitubular basement membrane antibodies.[44]

Immune complex–mediated disease has been suggested by observation of granular deposits of immunofluorescent material in and around tubular basement membranes.[42] The complexes could form either in the circulation or in situ. Such a mechanism is less well established than the antibasement membrane mechanism, but clear evidence for a complex–mediated pathogenesis has been noted in patients with lupus renal disease[42] and in IgA nephropathy.[45] Most of these patients have had glomerular involvement overshadowing that of the tubules. Animal models of concomitant glomerular and peritubular immune complex–mediated inflammation have also been developed.[46]

One problem with the acceptance of either an antibasement membrane antibody or an immune complex–mediated mechanism as a total explanation for the development of acute TIN is the observation that the infiltrate in acute TIN is characteristically composed of lymphocytes, plasma cells, and eosinophils. Such a finding would be atypical for a complement-mediated inflammatory process where polymorphonuclear leukocytes usually predominate. The observed cell pattern suggests that cellular immunity must play a role in at least some cases of acute TIN. This concept is further strengthened by the frequent inability to identify immunoglobulin or complement components in human biopsy material despite the presence of an extensive interstitial reaction. Recent studies in both animals[47] and man[48,49] suggest that cellular immunity plays a major role in the pathogenesis of at least some cases of acute TIN. Cellular mechanisms could be involved by a classic delayed type hypersensitivity reaction in which the inflammation is triggered by contact of a few sensitized lymphocytes with antigen residing in tubular or peritubular areas (perhaps presented on the surface of macrophages) followed by the release of lymphokines causing the influx of effecter cells. Acute TIN could also be mediated by direct T-cell-mediated cytolysis. This mechanism might be particularly likely to occur in association with viral infections. Antibody-dependent, cell-mediated cytotoxicity also may play a role.

Actual identification of T-cell subsets in human pathologic material has been limited but recently Husby et al[48] have identified a predominance of suppressor cells in the infiltrate in TIN. Watson et al[49] have studied the make-up of the lymphocyte population in a patient with cimetidine-induced disease and also found a predominance of cytotoxic/suppressor T-cells. They have suggested that there may be some similarity of this reaction to that seen with acute transplant rejection where similar cells seem to be the effectors. Stachura et al also found disproportionate numbers of cytotoxic/suppressor T-cells in two patients with acute TIN secondary to fenoprofen toxicity.[50] The ratio of these cells to helper cells was corrected following resolution of the disease after steroid therapy in one patient. Obviously, one can anticipate rapid advances in our understanding of the pathogenesis of acute TIN as newer immunologic tools are applied to the problem. The course of acute drug-induced TIN is variable, but generally is one of rapid improvement when the offending agent is withdrawn. In some cases improvement has seemed to occur more rapidly after steroid administration.[34] Aggressive management with hemodialysis is indicated for those patients who manifest renal failure and an impending uremic syndrome.

Intratubular obstruction Methotrexate is an antineoplastic agent that may be associated with acute nephrotoxicity when given in high doses (> 1 g/m^2).[51] The agent is highly insoluble in an acid urine and produces an acute intratubular obstructive process with the formation of methotrexate-containing casts. The disease can be avoided by urinary alkalinization and adequate hydration at the time the drug is given.

Metabolic causes of acute tubulointerstitial disease Several metabolic disturbances may lead to an acute TIN. The most notable of these are hypercalcemia,[52] hyperuricemia,[53] and hypokalemia.[54] With marked acute elevation in the serum calcium concentration, a series of events including reduction in GFR, blood pressure elevation, inhibition of urinary concentrating ability, and precipitation of calcium in and about tubules may occur (Figure 5-2). Marked hypercalcemia of any cause may induce this process and lead to relatively rapid deterioration in renal function culminating in a uremic syndrome. The process is usually reversible with lowering of the serum calcium concentration by any feasible means. The administration of oral sodium phosphate, volume expansion with saline solutions while inducing a saline diuresis with furosemide, steroid administration, calcitonin administration, mithramycin administration, and the use of dialysis against a calcium-free dialysate are accepted therapeutic measures. Acute hypercalcemic nephropathy may be expected with increasing frequency in the elderly because of the high incidence of neoplasia and associated hypercalcemia in older individuals.

Acute hyperuricemic nephropathy is usually characterized by the formation of uric acid microlithiasis in the collecting ducts. The clinical presentation is one of renal failure, frequently with oliguria.[53] Usually the disorder is seen in the setting of abrupt tumor lysis and a general catabolic state. Although hyperuricemic nephropathy may occur spontaneously with very rapidly proliferating tumors, it is usually seen during the treatment of multiple myeloma or leukemia with chemotherapy or during radiation of very sensitive, large solid tumors. A rapidly developing uremic syndrome may be noted. The disorder is preventable by pretreatment with allopurinol to suppress uric acid formation. Once established, treatment consists of alkalinization of the urine, induction of an osmotic diuresis, administration of allopurinol, and dialysis if necessary.[55] Survival is usually dependent on the activity of the underlying neoplasm and not on renal failure per se.

Although both functional and structural changes have been noted in hypokalemic animals,[56] the entity of hypokalemic nephropathy is poorly defined in humans. Nevertheless, instances of defective urinary concentrating ability and mild renal insufficiency have been described in patients with profound hypokalemia secondary to laxative or diuretic abuse.[54] The syndrome appears to be totally reversible with potassium replacement.

CHRONIC TUBULO-INTERSTITIAL NEPHRITIS

General Overview

Pathology The pathologic picture of chronic TIN is characterized by the presence of interstitial fibrosis, mononuclear cell infiltrates, tubular atrophy, glomerular sclerosis, vascular hyalinization, and periglomerular fibrosis[57] (Figure 5-3). Ischemic changes may be marked and culminate in areas of infarction, particularly in the papillae. The location of the most marked alteration will vary depending on etiology.

The above-mentioned histologic picture may be difficult to distinguish from the alterations associated with the aging process itself. This is particularly true of vascular changes (hyaline alterations and thickening of the arterial walls). An interstitial infiltration of mononuclear cells may also be noted with aging but this is usually modest in comparison to that seen with chronic TIN.[3]

Clinical picture There is some overlap between acute and chronic TIN and occasionally acute cases progress on to chronicity. Nevertheless, the clinical picture of the two is usually distinct. The onset is abrupt in acute disease, and much more indolent in chronic. On occasion signs and symptoms of renal insufficiency may be overshadowed by those related to the involvement of other organ systems. In chronic disease, the patient may present with severe anemia, dehydration, or metabolic acidosis as the first manifestation of renal disease. The presence or absence of hypertension will be variable. Patients may display significant azotemia or a full-blown uremic syndrome when first seen. Urinalysis usually shows minimal proteinuria and a sediment that is either relatively benign or characterized by modest numbers of white cells, red cells, and granular casts. Renal glycosuria may occur as a manifestation of the predominantly tubulo-interstitial involvement.[58]

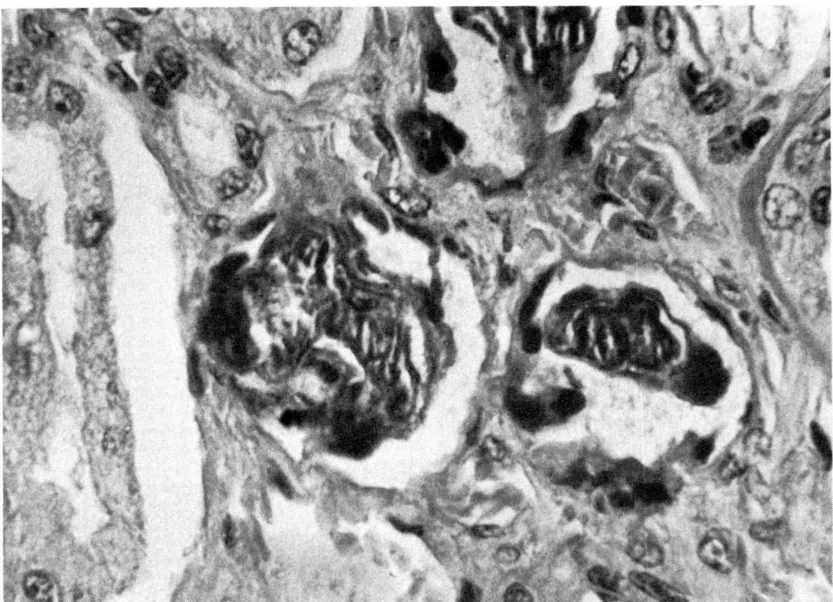

Figure 5-2 Acute hypercalcemic nephropathy. Note the intraluminal precipitation of dark, calcium-containing casts (×320).

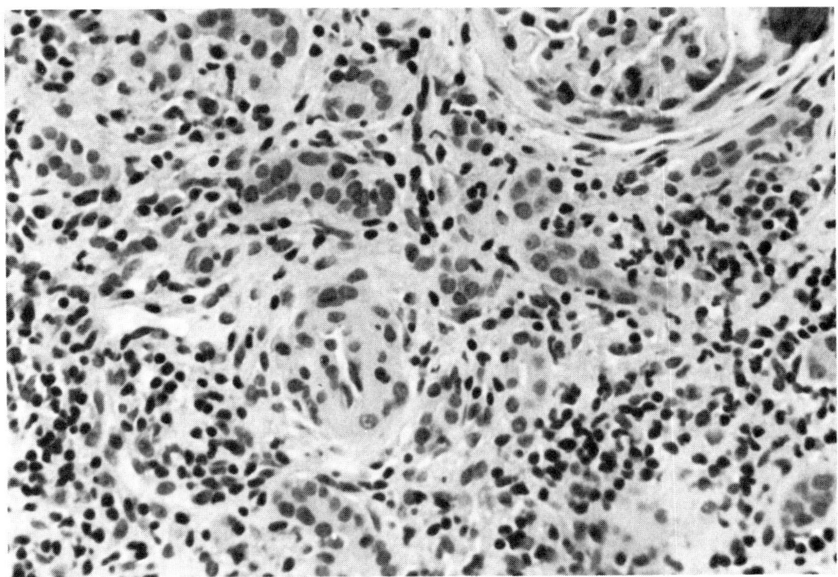

Figure 5-3 Chronic interstitial nephritis. Note the diffuse interstitial infiltration of inflammatory cells and periglomerular fibrosis suggesting chronicity of disease (×160).

Not infrequently secondary bacterial infection will be superimposed upon the underlying process. The causes of chronic TIN are listed in Table 5-3.

Table 5-3
Diseases Associated with Chronic Tubulo-Interstitial Nephritis

1. Infectious disease
   a. Tuberculosis
   b. Leprosy
2. Drug-related
   a. Lithium
   b. Analgesic abuse
3. Antineoplastic agents
   a. Cisplatin
   b. Nitrosourea compounds
   c. Streptozocin
4. Heavy metals
   a. Lead
   b. Cadmium
5. Immunologically mediated
   a. Lupus erythematosus
   b. IgA Nephropathy
   c. Sjögren's syndrome
6. Radiation injury
7. Metabolic causes
   a. Hypercalcemia
   b. Hyperuricemia
   c. Oxalate nephropathy
8. Neoplastic disease
   a. Tumor cell invasion
   b. Myeloma kidney
9. Miscellaneous disorders
   a. Sarcoidosis
   b. Balkan nephropathy
10. Tubulo-interstitial disease with unusual manifestations
   a. Megalocytic interstitial nephritis
   b. Xanthogranulomatous pyelonephritis
   c. Malakoplakia
11. Noncellular tubulo-interstitial diseases
   a. Amyloidosis
   b. Light chain disease

Specific Causes

Infectious disease Tuberculosis may affect the kidney unassociated with obvious clinical involvement of other areas and remain relatively quiescent for many years.[59] This may be particularly notable in the elderly with reactivation of a latent focus. Renal tuberculosis usually is associated with characteristic alterations in the collecting system by urography but on occasion such changes may be absent and the disease recognized only as an interstitial nephritis by biopsy.[60] Suspicion of renal tuberculosis should be raised in a patient with unexplained pyuria or hematuria. Adequate therapy requires initiation of treatment with three antituberculous drugs followed by a prolonged course with two drugs after the organism's sensitivities have been determined.[61]

Several different patterns of histologic involvement may be seen in the kidneys of patients with leprosy.[62] These include membranous and membranoproliferative glomerulopathy, amyloidosis, and lepromatous interstitial nephritis. The latter is quite rare, but a nonspecific interstitial reaction, possibly secondary to drugs, may be seen in as many as 20% of patients.

Drug-related chronic tubulo-interstitial disease

Lithium Some controversy exists as to the frequency of TIN with the therapeutic use of lithium.[37] Evidence of distal tubular dysfunction with impaired urine concentrating ability is seen frequently and a disturbance in distal acidification mechanisms has also been described.[37] In some patients renal biopsies have demonstrated alterations in distal tubular and collecting duct morphology as well as an interstitial cellular infiltrate.[63] Severe renal insufficiency has been noted very rarely, however. In those patients with a concentrating defect and tubulo-interstitial changes, sterile pyuria may be noted. It is of interest that an equal incidence of interstitial change has been observed in the renal biopsies of psychiatric patients with or without lithium therapy when compared to normal controls.[64] This suggests an unexplained susceptibility of psychiatric patients to chronic TIN. Appropriate therapy of lithium nephropathy is discontinuation of the drug.

Analgesic abuse nephropathy Analgesic nephropathy is an intriguing cause of TIN and a public health problem of worldwide scope.[65] A particularly high prevalence has been noted in Switzerland, the Scandinavian countries,[66] and Australia.[67] In the latter country it may account for 20% of patients in dialysis programs. Although probably not as prevalent in the United States, it is being recognized with increasing frequency and may be the cause of renal failure in as many as 20% of patients with tubulo-interstitial disease.[68] Although usually diagnosed before age 65, the fact that the incidence of analgesic use increases with advancing age places the elderly in jeopardy.

The disorder is recognized most frequently in females of middle age and is characterized by the insidious onset of renal insufficiency in association with dyspepsia, polyuria, skin hyperpigmentation, and anemia.[65,67] There is usually a 10- to 20-year history of analgesic mixture abuse in kilogram quantities; however, such a history may be elicited only with difficulty in many patients. The analgesics have usually been purchased over the counter and have been taken for nonspecific headache and arthritic complaints. Not infrequently, other substance abuse, particularly alcohol, may also have been a problem.

The diagnosis of analgesic abuse nephropathy is virtually certain if papillary necrosis is recognized in the clinical setting mentioned above.[67] Necrotic papillae may be passed in the urine as dark "fleshy" stones or they may be identified as classic filling defects on intravenous or retrograde urography.[69] Gross hematuria may accompany the papillary necrosis or microscopic hematuria, and sterile pyuria may be noted during periods of relative disease quiescence. Secondary infections with the usual urinary pathogens and hypertension frequently complicate the clinical picture.

Kidneys from patients with uncomplicated analgesic abuse nephropathy initially show predominant changes in the medulla.[70] There is marked ischemic damage to the medullary structures. The interstitium is infiltrated with mononuclear cells unless secondary bacterial infection has supervened in which case polymorphonuclear cells are encountered. Collecting ducts in the involved area are necrotic. With overt papillary necrosis there is demarcation between viable and necrotic tissue with sloughing of entire papillae into the caliceal lumen. Histologic examination of papilla passed in the urine is quite characteristic and shows an acellular, necrotic tissue, with only the ghosts of necrotic collecting ducts remaining (Figure 5-4). This fact makes histologic examination of any material passed by a patient with suspected papillary necrosis mandatory.

Determination of the pathogenesis of analgesic abuse nephropathy has remained elusive. Initial studies suggested a strong correlation of disease incidence with the use of phenacetin-containing preparations,[71] and in some countries where phenacetin has been removed from analgesic mixtures the incidence has declined.[66] However, the disease has by no means been totally eradicated. Current thinking would suggest that toxic metabolites produce oxidative injury to the metabolic machinery of collecting duct cells and result in tubular necrosis as the first pathogenetic event.[65,72] It is likely that these drug metabolites are concentrated in the papillary area by the same countercurrent mechanism that is responsible for producing a high papillary urea concentration. It has also been suggested that inhibition of medullary prostaglandin synthesis may be of importance in pathogenesis and contribute to ischemic vascular change.[65] Prostaglandins are vasodilators. Most of the components of analgesic mixtures are prostaglandin synthetase inhibitors; consequently reduction in medullary prostaglandins by analgesic administration may lead to an imbalance of pressor influences on the medullary vessels with consequent ischemic change. The two proposed mechanisms are not mutually exclusive and both may play a role.

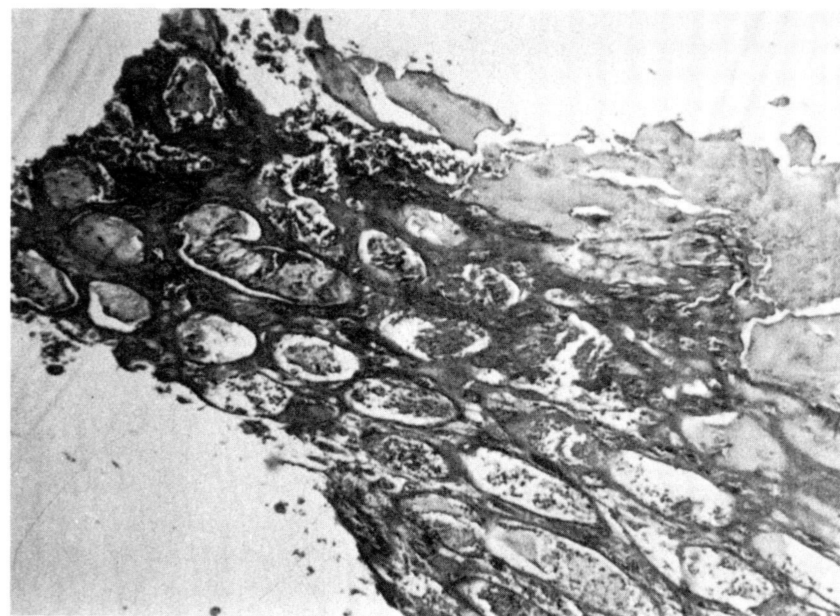

Figure 5-4 Papillary necrosis. Note the total necrosis of the papillary tip which was passed in the urine by an analgesic abuser. Only the ghosts of tubules remain (×80).

Treatment of analgesic nephropathy requires discontinuation of the analgesic mixture. In many patients, if the drugs are discontinued, progression of renal insufficiency will be inhibited and in some cases functional improvement may occur. Secondary pyelonephritis and hypertension also must be treated appropriately. Recently it has been recognized that carcinomas of the uroepithelium have an increased incidence in patients with analgesic abuse nephropathy and this may prove to be a common complication of the disorder.[73]

Antineoplastic agents Both cisplatin[74] and nitrosourea compounds[75] have been reported as causes of chronic TIN. The former is usually associated with an episode of acute tubular necrosis followed by residual TIN. Instances of insidiously progressive TIN have been described, however. Renal magnesium wasting has also been noted as a complication of therapy. The acute effects of cisplatin are dose-related and can be mitigated to at least some degree by a forced saline diuresis and the administration of mannitol during the period of drug administration.[74]

The disease associated with nitrosourea compounds is characterized by progressive loss of renal function after the administration of 1200 to 2000 mg/m^2.[75] Renal biopsies have demonstrated tubular atrophy, interstitial fibrosis, and glomerular sclerosis. No glomerular proliferative changes or immunoglobulin deposition have been noted.

Streptozocin is a chemotherapeutic agent that has been used in the treatment of islet cell carcinomas of the pancreas and hepatic carcinoma. Most frequently its renal toxicity has been indicated by the development of renal phosphate wasting and renal tubular acidosis.[76] On occasion the development of a chronic TIN-like picture has been noted, however.[77]

Antibiotics The initial manifestation of renal disease caused by antimicrobial agents is usually seen in the form of acute TIN or acute tubular necrosis. However, some patients with aminoglycoside toxicity have displayed a rather insidious course and shown predominant chronic TIN changes as described by Kowrilsky et al.[78] Some of these patients may progress to end-stage disease.

Heavy metal toxicity Lead[79,80] and cadmium[81] have been incriminated as causes of chronic TIN. Of these the former is the more frequent and has been described in three settings: after industrial exposure,[80] as a residual of childhood pica,[79] or as the result of ingestion of illicit whiskey distilled in a lead-containing apparatus.[82] Early on, the renal involvement may be heralded by tubular dysfunction as manifest by glycosuria and aminoaciduria. These changes correlate with characteristic acid-fast intranuclear inclusion bodies which may be seen in proximal tubular cells on renal biopsy.[83] Later, progressive renal insufficiency and hypertension develop, frequently in association with clinical gout and a normochromic, normocytic anemia. Pathologic examination in more advanced cases is characterized by prominent interstitial inflammation and arterial vascular changes. In many patients with advanced disease, the serum lead concentration and free erythrocyte protoporphyrin measurements will be normal and the body's increased lead burden can only be identified by examination of the urine after mobilization from bone and tissue by calcium ethylenediaminetetraacetate chelation.[80,82] Whether or not protracted chelation therapy is helpful in reversing well-established renal disease is uncertain, but improvement in GFR after this type of treatment has been noted. Patients with associated gout and hypertension may require long-term therapy with allopurinol and antihypertensive medications.

Cadmium toxicity usually occurs in association with environmental rather than industrial exposure.[81] Initially there is proximal tubular damage followed later by the development of chronic TIN. The proximal tubular damage may be manifest by glycosuria, aminoaciduria, phosphaturia, proximal renal tubular acidosis, increased β-2-microglobulin excretion, and urinary calcium wasting. The latter may be reflected by both the development of renal stones and metabolic bone disease.

Immunologic mechanisms Immunologic mechanisms are much less well characterized in the mediation of chronic TIN as compared to the acute process. Some patients with active lupus nephritis have been shown to have an element of interstitial inflammation in biopsy specimens.[84] Immunofluorescent studies in such patients have been interpreted as being consistent with an antigen-antibody complex–mediated pathogenesis.[42] Such lupus patients have also tended to have disturbances in distal tubular function including a diminished ability to acidify the urine and an insensitivity to aldosterone with consequent hyperkalemia.[85] Cellular immune mechanisms may play an even more important role but are poorly characterized in most situations.

Sjögren's syndrome is a disorder in which disturbed immune mechanisms are postulated to play a role in chronic TIN.[86] Sjögren's syndrome is clearly not a homogeneous disease entity. The syndrome may appear in idiopathic form or in association with a connective tissue disease such as rheumatoid arthritis or systemic lupus erythematosus. In either case the renal involvement is characterized clinically by a picture of distal tubular dysfunction. An acidification defect leading to systemic hyperchloremic acidosis, defective urinary concentration with concomitant polyuria, and a tendency to dehydration may be noted.[87] These findings are seen in conjunction with the typical keratoconjunctivitis sicca, dry mucous membranes, and, on occasion, purpura of the distal extremities. Most of the patients are women above age 40. Abnormalities of both the humoral and cellular arms of the immune system have been postulated as playing a role in pathogenesis. Antisalivary gland antibody is found with a high incidence in patients with rheumatoid arthritis–associated disease but less frequently in the idiopathic form. Nonorgan-specific antinuclear antibodies of three different types, as well as circulating immune complexes, are seen frequently. A cellular infiltrate of the same type of lymphocytes found invading the salivary glands is seen extensively involving the renal interstitium.[88] Whether or not this infiltration represents a primary cell-mediated hypersensitivity reaction is not clear, but peripheral lymphocytes cytotoxic for renal tubular cells have been identified in some patients. Therapy of the renal manifestations of Sjögren's syndrome includes treatment of the underlying disorder and the administration of sodium bicarbonate if acidosis is present. Adequate administration of water must be assured if a concentrating defect exists. Rarely is therapy with hydrochlorothiazide indicated for the nephrogenic diabetes insipidus-like picture.

Radiation injury For years loss of renal function has been noted as a manifestation of renal damage secondary to ionizing radiation.[89] Clinically the picture either may be one of acute or chronic injury. In the former there is loss of renal function in association with hypertension beginning 6 to 12 months after radiation exposure. An indolent loss of renal function and modest hypertension beginning years after exposure is seen in the latter. The pathologic picture is characterized by marked vascular change including fibrinoid necrosis and hyalinization of glomeruli, interstitial scarring, and interstitial infiltration with mononuclear cells in the more rapidly progressive illness. The chronic process is marked to a greater degree by fibrosis and scarring. Such injury is likely to occur at any time the renal tissue has received a dose greater than 2300 rad. The primary radiation toxicity is probably vascular and the interstitial changes are secondary to ischemia. Once established there is no definite therapy except for control of blood pressure to avoid further damage to the kidney and other organ systems from the pressure alone. Rare cases of unilateral radiation nephritis and poorly controlled hypertension have been described in which nephrectomy cured the hypertension.[90]

Metabolic causes The major metabolic disturbances leading to chronic TIN include hypercalcemia,[52] hyperuricemia,[91] and oxalate nephropathy.[92] Chronic hypercalcemia of any cause may lead to varying combinations of stone disease with obstructive uropathy and TIN. The latter is induced by calcium microlithiasis in the collecting ducts, and peritubular deposition of calcium salts. The course may be quite indolent with slowly progressive renal failure and polyuria because of abnormal urinary concentrating ability. Episodes of dehydration may be encountered. On pathologic examination all of the features of a chronic, nonspecific TIN may be noted but in addition careful evaluation may reveal calcium deposition in and about the collecting ducts. Appropriate therapy involves treatment of the underlying disease with concomitant normalization of the serum calcium concentration. When such a goal is achieved, improvement in renal function frequently occurs.

Debate exists as to the incidence of chronic renal disease secondary to sustained hyperuricemia. The work of Yü and Berger[93] has clearly shown that mild elevations of uric acid are seldom related to the development of renal insufficiency in the absence of hypertension, renal vascular disease, or overt tophaceous change. Although chronic TIN can be clearly the result of long-standing tophaceous gout[91] (Figure 5-5), this is rarely a problem today because most patients with clinical gout are treated with allopurinol or uricosuric agents long before renal involvement ensues.[94] As noted previously the occurrence of chronic TIN and gout may reflect underlying lead intoxication.[79,80,82] Very few patients are encountered in dialysis or transplant programs with gout as the predominant cause of renal failure.

Oxalate-related renal disease may be associated with the formation of calcium

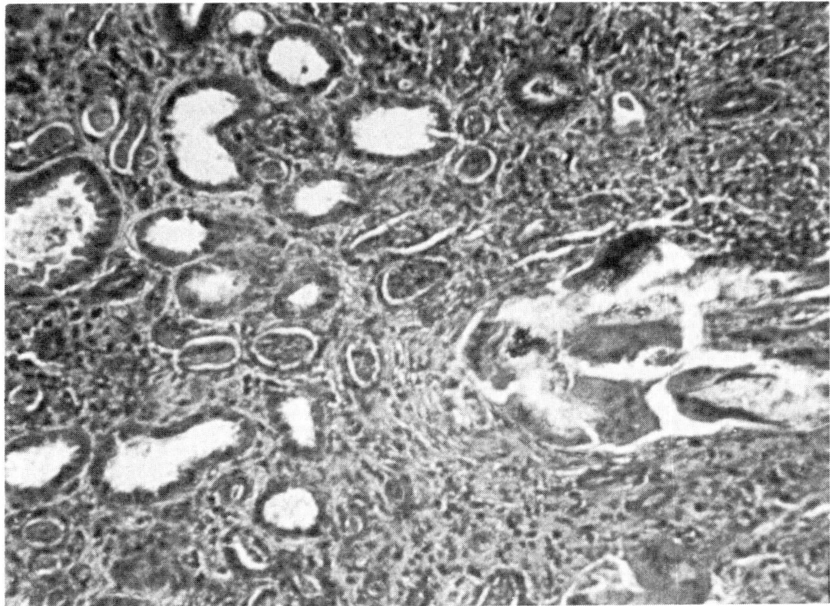

Figure 5-5 Gouty nephropathy. Note the extensive chronic interstitial inflammatory reaction and the large tophaceous deposit from a patient with long-standing untreated tophaceous gout (×160).

oxalate stones or intrarenal deposits of calcium oxalate crystals.[92] The latter usually occurs in the form of microlithiasis of the collecting tubules. This may occur acutely following the ingestion of ethylene glycol[95] or the administration of methoxyflurane anesthesia.[96] The acute episode may be followed by the development of chronic TIN with progressive scarring and fibrosis of the kidney.

Recently it has been recognized that chronic, insidious deposition of oxalate crystals, nephrocalcinosis, and an associated TIN may occur because of gastrointestinal (GI) disturbances involving the small bowel.[92] This has been particularly noted following ileal bypass surgery for morbid obesity, but may also be seen in other types of diseases which interfere with ileal absorptive function. It is thought that oxalate absorption is increased in these disorders because of increased binding of calcium to malabsorbed bile acids. This malabsorption of bile acids results from damage to mucosal surfaces or from shortening of available absorptive surface area (bypass) in the gut. Insufficient free calcium is then available in the ileum to bind oxalate. Free oxalate is then readily absorbed within the colon.

Treatment of oxalate nephropathy must be directed at correction of the underlying bowel disease as well as the maintenance of a steady urine output to lower the concentration of oxalate within the urine, since the solubility of oxalate in urine is little influenced by other variables such as manipulation of the urinary pH.

Neoplastic disease

Tumor cell invasion Renal insufficiency from diffuse infiltration of the renal interstitium with neoplastic cells has been described on occasion with leukemia, lymphoma, and sarcoma.[97] This type of infiltration is usually accompanied by extensive involvement of the bone marrow and other organs. There may be deterioration of renal function and radiographic evidence of enlarged kidneys with a thickened cortex and stretching of the calyces. Frequently there is concomitant hydronephrosis because of extrinsic compression of the ureters by neoplastic invasion of perirenal tissue or lymph nodes. Renal function usually improves if the neoplasm is one that is responsive to radiation or chemotherapy. Renal failure in and of itself seldom is the cause of death. The patient's prognosis frequently rests on the responsivity of the underlying malignancy to therapeutic measures.

Myeloma kidney Renal involvement may take several different forms in multiple myeloma.[98] Hypercalcemic nephropathy, urate nephropathy, and amyloid involvement may be noted and are discussed in other sections. The classic histologic type of myeloma involvement is that produced by the deposition of globulin light chains in the renal tissue. Both lambda and kappa light chains are easily filtered by the glomerulus. Occasionally they may be reabsorbed and crystalize in proximal tubular cells where they may interfere with transport processes and produce a Fanconi syndrome.[99] Kappa chains are usually associated with this type of involvement. More frequently light chains have been noted to precipitate as casts in the collecting ducts causing intratubular obstruction. With progression of disease the tubular cells may be disrupted, inflammatory cells may appear, and a chronic TIN may be induced. Certain clinical events such as the development of dehydration and the administration of x-ray contrast media may hasten the development of this type of disease. Immunofluorescent studies may clearly identify the type of light chain precipitated in the intratubular casts.[100]

Multiple myeloma is a frequent disease in the elderly and as such must be considered in any patient with bone pain, anemia, and renal insufficiency. Its presence can be suspected by finding an abnormal paraprotein on electrophoresis of the serum. Myeloma renal disease is suggested by the findings of an excessive concentration of light chains in the urine either by electrophoresis or by the conventional Bence Jones protein determination. A routine dipstick determination for urine protein will not identify light chains.

The first order of treatment of myeloma kidney is to reduce the light chain burden by shrinking the overall neoplastic mass with chemotherapy using prednisone and cyclophosphamide or phenylalanine mustard.[101] Remarkable improvement in renal function has been described with this type of therapy. Provision of a water diuresis and alkalinization of the urine may also be helpful by inhibiting light chain precipitation within the collecting ducts.

Miscellaneous disorders

Sarcoidosis Most frequently the renal disease of sarcoidosis is secondary to hypercalcemia or immune complex–mediated glomerular disease; however, on occasion progressive renal insufficiency may develop as a result of extensive interstitial involvement by the sarcoid inflammatory process.[102] An interstitial infiltrate with mononuclear cells and eosinophils may be seen in conjunction with formation of noncaseating granulomata (Figure 5-6). Usually, but not always, there is extensive evidence of sarcoid involvement elsewhere. Dramatic improvement in renal function may be seen when steroids are administered.[103]

Balkan nephropathy There is a high incidence of slowly progressive renal disease in the inhabitants of a small area of the Balkans along the Danube.[104] The etiology of this disease is unknown. The disorder does not appear to be inherited and no specific nephrotoxic etiology has been identified despite extensive research. Patients with Balkan nephropathy demonstrate the clinical picture of progressive renal failure, relatively scant proteinuria, and a sediment that is most consistent with tubulo-interstitial damage. Renal biopsies have shown minor glomerular change and extensive chronic TIN. Hypertension is infrequent or modest. It is a disease of young adults and the middle-aged. No therapy is available for this disorder and most patients will have either died with uremia or

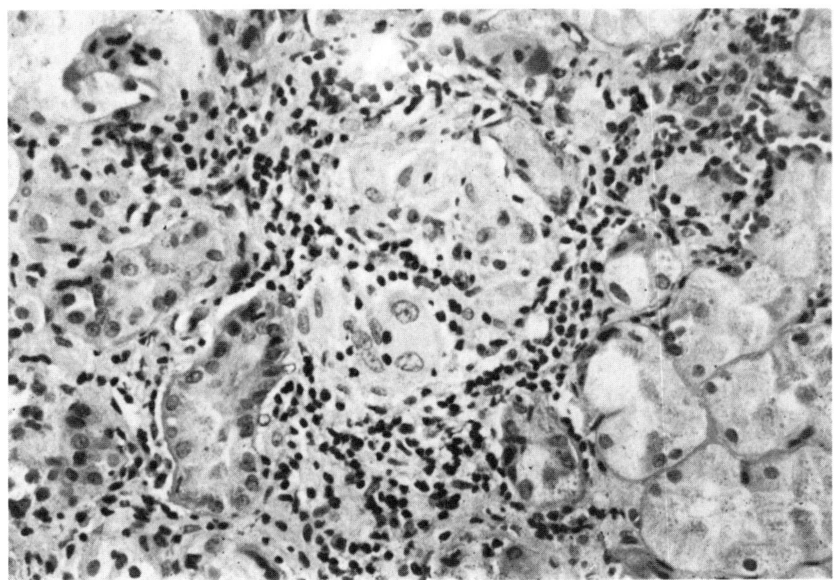

Figure 5-6 Sarcoid nephropathy. Extensive interstitial inflammatory reaction with a small sarcoid granuloma in the center of the field from a patient with nonhypercalcemic sarcoid nephropathy (×160).

require chronic dialysis prior to reaching old age.

Tubulo-interstitial disease with unusual manifestations Megalocytic interstitial nephritis, xanthogranulomatous pyelonephritis, and malakoplakia are three rare pathologic processes which involve the renal interstitium and are of unknown etiology.[105] In each of these processes PAS-positive, diastase-resistant material is noted within the cytoplasm of histiocytes in the renal interstitium. Megalocytic interstitial nephritis usually is manifest by one or more nodular lesions of the renal cortex that by routine radiographic studies are suggestive of neoplasia.[106] Presenting symptoms may include gross hematuria or pyuria and the diagnosis is made on histologic evaluation of the renal mass. The lesions may be single or multiple. Xanthogranulomatous pyelonephritis also usually presents as a mass lesion which involves both the cortex and medulla. Nonfunction of the involved kidney, renal calculi, and urinary tract infection accompany the pathologic process.[107] Malakoplakia tends to occur in immunosuppressed individuals and primarily involves the renal pelvis with secondary extension into the parenchyma. Characteristic Michaelis-Gutman bodies are seen in the inflammatory process and are helpful in making the diagnosis.[108] Urinary tract infection is a commonly associated finding. The etiology of these disorders is unknown, but it has been suggested that each represents an unusual host response to inflammation and that bacterial antigens may be of importance in disease induction.[104,107]

Noncellular tubulo-interstitial disease In a certain sense infiltration of the renal interstitium with amyloid[109] or light chain fragments[110] may be considered a type of tubulo-interstitial disease. Most frequently renal amyloidosis is associated with extensive glomerular involvement and the nephrotic syndrome; however, rarely the involvement may be primarily of the tubulo–and peritubulo-interstitial tissue with consequent manifestations of tubular dysfunction.[109] The same holds for light chain disease. Nephrogenic diabetes insipidus and defective urinary acidification have been described as a consequence of such distal tubular involvement.[109]

Special Functional Disturbances with Chronic Tubulo-Interstitial Nephritis

Renal salt wasting Although the elderly cannot conserve sodium as readily as younger persons, this alteration is relatively minor and can only be identified with severe dietary restriction.[5] Sodium balance is, thus, usually easily maintained in older individuals with normal cardiovascular function. Severe sodium wasting on an ordinary diet may be encountered, however, in some patients with chronic and, rarely, acute TIN. This functional change is particularly likely if there is damage to the collecting ducts or papillae.[111] The mechanism for this sodium-wasting tendency is not entirely clear but probably relates to loss of the deep cortical nephrons which are so important for maximal sodium reabsorption. Aldosterone deficiency or tubular unresponsiveness to aldosterone is not an important factor in the development of sodium wasting. Management requires the administration of large quantities of sodium. This is usually given as sodium chloride, but if there is concomitant metabolic acidosis supplemental sodium bicarbonate may also be necessary.

Nephrogenic diabetes insipidus As noted earlier the ability to produce a maximally concentrated urine is lost by the aging kidney.[6] This seldom causes a problem stricted in his access to water by cerebral or neuromuscular disease. Even the elderly can usually concentrate above isosthenuria. With damage to the collecting ducts and medullary interstitium as seen with lithium administration,[37] hypercalcemic nephropathy,[52] analgesic nephropathy,[65,66] medullary amyloidosis,[109] and Sjögren's syndrome,[87] hypotonic urine with a true nephrogenic diabetes insipidus may be seen. Treatment consists of maintenance of adequate hydration and, on occasion, the administration of hydrochlorothiazide. This agent reduces urine volume by enhancing proximal tubular reabsorption after causing mild extracellular fluid volume depletion. Its effect can be sustained only if dietary sodium is restricted during the therapeutic period.

Defective acidification An impairment in maximal urinary acidification and ammonium excretion has been recognized in normal elderly individuals.[7] This defect is mild and not associated with a persistent metabolic acidosis. Hyperchloremic acidosis may be associated with chronic TIN. It may be of the type 1 or distal variety in which there is an abnormal pH gradient across the collecting duct.[112] This is encountered most frequently in Sjögren's syndrome. Rarely there may be a true bicarbonate leak suggesting proximal tubular dysfunction as may be seen in some cases of multiple myeloma.[99] Most frequently, the ability to lower the urine pH is well maintained and the acidosis is classified as a type 4 renal tubular acidosis (RTA).[113] This usually accompanies hyperkalemia in the setting of selective hypoaldosteronism as will be discussed below. Therapy in all cases involves the judicious use of sodium bicarbonate.

Hyperkalemia Recently in some patients with chronic renal disease there has been considerable interest in a syndrome of hyperkalemia disproportionate to the degree of renal insufficiency. These patients have been heterogeneous in regard to the cause of their renal disease, but the underlying etiology has usually been diabetes, TIN, or nephrosclerosis.[114] The majority of the patients have either been middle-aged or elderly. Because both renal patients and animal models of renal failure display potent adaptive mechanisms for maintaining normokalemia until end-stage renal disease has been reached,[115] it is likely that these patients have a defect in some component of the adaptive response.

Schambelan et al demonstrated in the

largest series of patients with moderate renal insufficiency and hyperkalemia published to date significant abnormalities in the aldosterone axis. Of 31 patients, 23 (75%) had hypoaldosteronism when compared to normals.[114] Of those with hypoaldosteronism all but four also displayed reduced plasma renin activity (19/31); thus, 67% of the hyperkalemic patients had hyporeninemic hypoaldosteronism. Tan and Burton obtained similar results in a survey of 100 hyperkalemic patients: 19% of these patients had unexplained hyperkalemia and of these about 50% had hyporeninemic hypoaldosteronism.[116] These findings suggest that hyporeninemic hypoaldosteronism is the major cause of disproportionate hyperkalemia for the level of renal insufficiency, but that other abnormalities of the complex group of factors controlling the serum potassium concentration may be of importance in a substantial minority of patients.

Studies in individuals of this minority group have revealed production of an inactive big renin,[117] enzymatic defects along the chain of aldosterone biosynthesis,[118] and end-organ unresponsiveness to aldosterone[85] as additional causes of the syndrome. With the exception of those with end-organ unresponsiveness hypoaldosteronism seems to be the common denominator of the syndrome. Berl et al have suggested that high levels of aldosterone secretion represent an important component of the adaptive mechanism for potassium regulation as renal function deteriorates in man.[115] Both renin activity and aldosterone secretion decline in aging,[9] and it is likely that expression of the syndrome may occur with greater frequency in the elderly for this reason.

The clinical significance of the syndrome is uncertain. Clearly, a few patients, like the classic case described by Hudson et al,[119] may have problems with potentially life-threatening cardiac conduction disturbances. On the other hand, follow-up of a large number of patients in our center has revealed remarkably few clinical events that definitely could be attributed to hyperkalemia per se. Optimal therapy is also uncertain. Although large doses of mineralocorticoids such as fludrocortisone may stimulate potassium secretion and consequently lower the serum potassium concentration, these agents also may accentuate sodium retention, exacerbate hypertension, and reduce glucose tolerance, particularly in the diabetic patient. As a consequence, it is probably wise to be very cautious in their use. It may be preferable to attempt to manage the hyperkalemia with a combination of dietary potassium restriction and supplemental diuretics where practical. Because many of the patients have a mild hyperchloremic acidosis (type 4 RTA), administration of sodium bicarbonate may also be helpful.

SUMMARY

Several general conclusions follow from the preceding review. Tubulo-interstitial nephritis may be categorized roughly into acute and chronic processes on the basis of the clinical presentation and histopathologic picture. A heterogeneous group of disorders may be associated with either the acute or chronic type. With a few exceptions such as hypercalcemic nephropathy and myeloma kidney the histologic picture is nonspecific in both the acute and chronic forms. Disturbances in tubular function such as sodium wasting, defective urine concentration, renal tubular acidosis, and disproportionate hyperkalemia may provide a clue that TIN, particularly of the chronic type, is present. Subtle histologic and functional changes mimicking those seen in chronic TIN may occur in the aging kidney. There is loss of renal reserve in the elderly. As a consequence, the development of TIN in an elderly patient may be particularly devastating. Acute TIN is likely to occur in the elderly secondary to immunologically mediated drug hypersensitivity, in association with the complications of neoplasms or their treatment, and secondary to infections such as legionnaires' disease. Chronic TIN in older persons may be a manifestation of chronic infection such as tuberculosis, or of direct drug nephrotoxicity from analgesic mixtures or antineoplastic agents. It may also represent a metabolic complication of an underlying disease, such as the hypercalcemic nephropathy of metastatic bone malignancy or the light chain–induced myeloma kidney. The threads of immune hypersensitivity and direct drug nephrotoxicity run throughout the pathogenesis of both acute and chronic TIN but in most instances the mechanisms of renal damage are incompletely understood.

REFERENCES

1. Grantham JJ: Polycystic renal disease, in Earley LE, Gottschalk CW (eds): *Strauss and Welt's Diseases of the Kidney,* ed 3. Boston, Little Brown & Co, 1979, pp 1123–1146.
2. Suki WN, Caskey CT: Hereditary chronic nephropathies, in Earley LE, Gottschalk CW (eds): *Strauss and Welt's Disease of the Kidney,* ed 3. Boston, Little, Brown & Co, 1979, pp 1167–1195.
3. McLachlan MSF: The aging kidney. *Lancet* 1978;2:143–146.
4. Rowe JW, Reubin A, Tobin JD, et al: The effect of age on creatinine clearance in men: A cross-sectional and longitudinal study. *J Gerontol* 1976;31:155–163.
5. Epstein M, Hollenberg NK: Age as a determinant of renal sodium conservation in normal man. *J Lab Clin Med* 1976; 87:411–417.
6. Rowe JW, Shock NW, DeFronzo RA: The influence of age on the renal response to water deprivation in man. *Nephron* 1976;17:270–278.
7. Adler S, Lindeman RD, Yiengst MJ, et al: Effect of acute acid loading on urinary acid excretion by the aging human kidney. *J Lab Clin Med* 1968;72:278–289.
8. Miller JH, McDonald RK, Shock NW: Age changes in the maximal rate of renal tubular reabsorption of glucose. *J Gerontol* 1952;7:196–200.
9. Weidman P, Myttenaere-Bursztein SD, Maxwell MH, et al: Effect of aging on plasma renin and aldosterone in normal man. *Kidney Int* 1975;8:325–333.
10. Vestal RE: Drug use in the elderly: A review of problems and special considerations. *Drugs* 1978;16:358–382.
11. Crooks J, Stevenson IH: Drug response in the elderly–sensitivity and pharmacokinetic considerations. *Age Ageing* 1981; 10:73–80.
12. Crooks J, O'Malley K, Stevenson IH: Pharmacokinetics in the elderly. *Clin Pharmacokinet* 1976;1:280–296.
13. Rowe JW: Clinical research on aging: Strategies and directions. *N Engl J Med* 1977;297:1332–1336.
14. Ooi BS, Wellington J, First MR, et al: Acute interstitial nephritis. A clinical and pathologic study based on renal biopsies. *Am J Med* 1975;59:614–629.
15. Martin DW, Naughton JL, Smith LH: Tubulo-interstitial nephropathies–a pathophysiologic approach. *West J Med* 1980;132:134–140.
16. Laberke HG: Drug-associated nephropathy. Part II: Tubulo-interstitial lesions. A: Acute interstitial nephritis, nephrotoxic lesions, analgesic nephropathy. *Curr Top Pathol* 1980;69:184–215.
17. Papper S: Interstitial nephritis. *Contrib Nephrol* 1980;23:204–291.
18. Lespier-Dexter LE: Tubulo-interstitial disease. *Contrib Nephrol* 1981;27:12–19.
19. Dixon AJ, Winearls CG, Dunnill MS: Interstitial nephritis. *J Clin Pathol* 1981; 34:616–624.
20. Cotran RS, Brenner BM, Stein JH (eds): *Tubulo-Interstitial Nephropathies.* New York, Churchill Livingston, 1983.
21. Linton AL, Clark WF, Driedger AA, et al: Acute interstitial nephritis due to drugs. *Ann Intern Med* 1980;93:735–741.
22. Councilmann WT: Acute interstitial nephritis. *J Exp Med* 1898;3:393–420.
23. Sitprija V, Evans H: The kidney in human leptospirosis. *Am J Med* 1970;49:780–788.
24. Ooi BS, Chen BTM, Tan KK, et al: Human renal leptospirosis. *Am J Trop Med Hyg* 1972;21:336–341.
25. Lai KN, Aarons I, Woodroffe AJ, et al: Renal lesions in leptospirosis. *Aust N Z J Med* 1982;12:276–279.
26. Friedman HM: Legionnaires' disease in non-legionnaires. A report of five cases. *Ann Intern Med* 1978;88:294–302.
27. Poulter N, Gabriel R, Porter KA, et al:

Acute interstitial nephritis complicating legionnaires' disease. *Clin Nephrol* 1981;15:216–220.
28. Woodroffe AJ, Row PG, Meadows R, et al: Nephritis in infectious mononucleosis. *Q J Med* 1974;43:451–460.
29. Dunea G, Kark RM, Lannigan R, et al: Brucella nephritis. *Ann Intern Med* 1969;70:783–790.
30. Appel GB, Kunis CL: Acute tubulo-interstitial nephritis, in Cotran RS, Brenner BM, Stein JH (eds): *Tubulo-interstitial Nephropathies*. New York, Churchill Livingstone, 1983, pp 175–176.
31. Appel GB, Kunis CL: Acute tubulo-interstitial nephritis, in Cotran RS, Brenner BM, Stein JH (eds): *Tubulo-interstitial Nephropathies*. New York, Churchill Livingstone, 1983, pp 69–171.
32. Schrier RW, Bulger RJ, VanArsdel PP Jr: Nephropathy associated with penicillin and homologues. *Ann Intern Med* 1966; 4:116–127.
33. Ditlove J, Weidmann P, Bernstein M, et al: Methicillin nephritis. *Medicine* 1977; 56:483–491.
34. Galpin JE, Shinaberger JH, Stanley TM, et al: Acute interstitial nephritis due to methicillin. *Am J Med* 1978;65:756–765.
35. Appel GB: A decade of penicillin related acute interstitial nephritis–more questions than answers. *Clin Nephrol* 1980; 13:151–154.
36. Kleinknecht D, Adememar JP: Les insuffisances rénales aiguës dues a la rifampicine. *Med Mal Infect* 1977;7:117–121.
37. Ramsey TA, Cox M: Lithium and the kidney: A review. *Am J Psychiatry* 1982; 139:443–449.
38. Lyons H, Pinn VW, Cortell S, et al: Allergic interstitial nephritis causing reversible renal failure in four patients with idiopathic nephrotic syndrome. *N Engl J Med* 1973;288:124–128.
39. Koch-Weser J: Nonsteroidal antiinflammatory drugs. *N Engl J Med* 1980;302: 1179–1185, 1237–1243.
40. Finkelstein A, Fraley DS, Stachura I, et al: Fenoprofen nephropathy: Lipoid nephrosis and interstitial nephritis. *Am J Med* 1982;72:81–87.
41. McCluskey RT: Anti-tubular basement membrane (TBM) nephritis. *N Engl J Med* 1975;292:914–915.
42. Lehman DH, Wilson CB, Dixon FJ: Extraglomerular immunoglobulin deposits in human nephritis. *Am J Med* 1975;58: 765–786.
43. Baldwin DS, Levine BB, McCluskey RT, et al: Renal failure and interstitial nephritis due to penicillin and methicillin. *N Engl J Med* 1968;279:1245–1252.
44. Andres G, Brentjens J, Kohli R, et al: Histology of human tubulo-interstitial nephritis associated with antibodies to renal basement membranes. *Kidney Int* 1978;13:480–491.
45. Fransca GM, Vangelista A, Biagini G, et al: Immunological tubulo-interstitial deposits in IgA nephropathy. *Kidney Int* 1982;22:184–191.
46. Klassen J, Milgrom FM, McCluskey RT: Studies of the antigens involved in an immunologic renal tubular lesion in rabbits. *Am J Pathol* 1977;88:135–141.
47. McCluskey RT, Bahn AK: Cell-mediated mechanisms in renal diseases. *Kidney Int* 1982;21:S6–S12.
48. Husby G, Tung KSK, Williams RC Jr: Characterization of renal tissue lymphocytes in patients with interstitial nephritis. *Am J Med* 1981;70:31–38.
49. Watson AJS, Dalbow MH, Stachura I, et al: Immunologic studies in cimetidine-induced nephropathy and polymyositis. *N Engl J Med* 1983;308:142–145.
50. Strachura I, Jayakumar S, Bourke E: T and B lymphocyte subsets in fenoprofen nephropathy. *Am J Med* 1983;75:9–16.
51. Pittman SW, Frei E; Weekly methotrexate-calcium leucovorin rescue: Effect of alkalinization on nephrotoxicity; Pharmacokinetics in the CNS; and use in CNS non-Hodgkin's lymphoma. *Cancer Treat Rep* 1977;695–701.
52. Lins LE: Reversible renal failure caused by hypercalcemia. *Acta Med Scand* 1978;203:309–314.
53. Conger JD: Acute uric acid nephropathy. *Semin Nephrol* 1981;1:69–74.
54. Relman AS, Schwartz WB: The kidney in potassium depletion. *Am J Med* 1958; 24:764–773.
55. Maher JF, Rath CE, Schreiner GE: Hyperuricemia complicating leukemia. *Arch Intern Med* 1969;123:198–200.
56. Hollander W Jr, Blythe WB: Nephropathy of potassium depletion, in Strauss MB,

Welt LG (eds): *Diseases of the Kidney*, ed 2. Boston, Little Brown & Co, 1971, Vol 2, pp 933-972.

57. Heptinstall RH: Interstitial nephritis, in Heptinstall RH: *Pathology of the Kidney*, ed 2. Boston, Little Brown & Co, 1974, Vol 2, pp 829-831.
58. Cogan MG: Classification and patterns of renal dysfunction, in Cotran RS, Brenner BM, Stein JH (eds): *Tubulo-interstitial Nephropathies*. New York, Churchill Livingstone, 1983, p 41.
59. Christensen WI: Genitourinary tuberculosis: Review of 102 cases. *Medicine* 1974;53:377–390.
60. Mallinson WJW, Fuller RW, Levison DA, et al: Diffuse interstitial renal tuberculosis–an unusual cause of renal failure. *Q J Med* 1981;198:137–148.
61. Narayana AS: Overview of renal tuberculosis. *Urology* 1982;19:231–237.
62. Phadnis MC, Menta MC, Bharaswadker MS, et al: Study of renal changes in leprosy. *Int J Lepr* 1982;50:143–147.
63. Hestbech J, Hansen HE, Amdisen A, et al: Chronic renal lesions following long-term treatment with lithium. *Kidney Int* 1977;12:205–213.
64. Walker RG, Bennett WM, Davies BM, et al: Structural and functional effects of long-term lithium therapy. *Kidney Int* 1982;21:S13–S19.
65. Schreiner GE, McAnally JF, Winchester JF: Clinical analgesic nephropathy. *Arch Intern Med* 1981;141:349–357.
66. Gloor FJ: Changing concepts in pathogenesis and morphology of analgesic nephropathy as seen in Europe. *Kidney Int* 1978;13:27–33.
67. Nanra RS, Stuart-Taylor J, De Leon AH, et al: Analgesic nephropathy: Etiology, clinical syndrome, and clinicopathologic correlations in Australia. *Kidney Int* 1978;13:79–92.
68. Murray T, Goldberg M: Chronic interstitial nephritis: Etiologic factors. *Ann Intern Med* 1975;82:453–459.
69. Arger PH, Bluth EI, Murray T, et al: Analgesic abuse nephropathy. *Urology* 1976;7:123–128.
70. Burry A: Pathology of analgesic nephropathy: Australian experience. *Kidney Int* 1978;13:34–40.
71. Fiffield MM: Renal disease associated with prolonged use of acetophenetidin-containing compounds. *N Engl J Med* 1963;269:722–726.
72. Mitchell JR, McMurtry RJ, Statham CN, et al: Molecular basis of several drug-induced nephropathies. *Am J Med* 1977;62:518–526.
73. Bengtsson U: Phenacetin and renal pelvic carcinoma. *Clin Nephrol* 1974;2:124–126.
74. Blachley JD, Hill HB: Renal and electrolyte disturbances associated with cisplatin. *Ann Intern Med* 1981;95:628–632.
75. Harmon WE, Cohen HJ, Schneeberger EE, et al: Chronic renal failure in children treated with methyl CCNU. *N Engl J Med* 1979;300:1200–1203.
76. Loftus L, Cuppage FE, Hoogstraten B: Clinical and pathological effects of streptozotocin. *J Lab Clin Med* 1974;84: 408–413.
77. Myerowitz IM, Saftizno CP, Cavallo T: Nephrotoxic and cytoproliferative effects of streptozotocin. *Cancer* 1976;38:1550–1555.
78. Kourilsky O, Solez K, Morel-Maroger L, et al: The pathology of acute renal failure due to interstitial nephritis in man with comments on the role of interstitial inflammation and sex in gentamicin nephrotoxicity. *Medicine* 1982;61:258–268.
79. Emmerson BT: Chronic lead nephropathy. *Kidney Int* 1973;4:1–5.
80. Wedeen RP, Maesaka JK, Weiner B, et al: Occupational lead nephropathy. *Am J Med* 1975;59:630–641.
81. Friberg L, Piscztor M, Nordenberg GF, et al: *Cadmium in the Environment*, ed 2. Boca Raton, Fla, CRC Press, Inc 1974, pp 101–114, 137–161, 192–195.
82. Morgan JM: Chelation therapy in lead nephropathy. *South Med J* 1975;68: 1001–1006.
83. Heptinstall RH: Sundry conditions affecting the renal tubules, in Heptinstall RH: *Pathology of the Kidney*, ed 2. Boston, Little Brown & Co. 1974, vol 2, pp 1063–1064.
84. Tu WH, Shearn MA: Systemic lupus erythematosus and latent renal tubular dysfunction. *Ann Intern Med* 1967;67: 100–109.
85. DeFronzo RA, Cooke CR, Goldberg M, et al: Impaired renal tubular potassium secretion in systemic lupus erythema-

tosus. *Ann Intern Med* 1977;86:268–271.
86. Kassan SS, Gardy M: Sjögren's syndrome: An update and overview. *Am J Med* 1978;64:1037–1046.
87. Shioji R, Furuyama T, Onodera S, et al: Sjögren's syndrome and renal tubular acidosis. *Am J Med* 1970;48:456–463.
88. Tu WH, Shearn MA, Lee JC, et al: Interstitial nephritis in Sjögren's syndrome. *Ann Intern Med* 1968;69:1163–1170.
89. Arruda JAL: Radiation nephritis, in Cotran RS, Brenner BM, Stein JH (eds): *Tubulo-interstitial Nephropathies.* New York, Churchill Livingstone, 1983, pp 275–285.
90. Shapiro AP, Cavallo T, Cooper W, et al: Hypertension in radiation nephritis. *Arch Intern Med* 1977;137:848–851.
91. Boss GR, Seegmiller JE: Hyperuricemia and gout. Classification, complications and management. *N Engl J Med* 1979; 300:1459–1468.
92. Miller MJ: Nephrocalcinosis in intestinal bypass patients. *Arch Intern Med* 1977; 137:1743–1744.
93. Yü TFA, Berger L: Impaired renal function in gout. Its association with hypertensive vascular disease and intrinsic renal disease. *Am J Med* 1982;72:95–100.
94. Fessel WJ: Renal outcomes of gout and hyperuricemia. *Am J Med* 1979;67: 74–82.
95. Smith DE: Morphologic lesions due to acute and subacute poisoning with antifreeze (ethylene glycol). *Arch Pathol* 1951;51:423–433.
96. Franscino JA, Vanamee P, Rosen PP: Renal oxalosis and azotemia after methoxyflurane anesthesia. *N Engl J Med* 1970;283:676–679.
97. Pirani CL, Silva FG, Appel GB: Tubulointerstitial disease in multiple myeloma and other nonrenal neoplasias, in Cotran RS, Brenner BM, Stein JH (eds): *Tubulo-interstitial Nephropathies.* New York, Churchill Livingstone, 1983, pp 314–317.
98. Pirani CL, Silva FG, Appel GB: Tubulointerstitial disease in multiple myeloma and other nonrenal neoplasias, in Cotran RS, Brenner BM, Stein JH (eds): *Tubulo-interstitial Nephropathies.* New York, Churchill Livingstone, 1983, pp 288–305.
99. Maldonado JE, Velosa JA, Kyle RA, et al: Fanconi syndrome in adults. A manifestation of a latent form of myeloma. *Am J Med* 1975;58:354–364.
100. Levi DF, Williams RC Jr, Lindstrom FD: Immunofluorescent studies of the myeloma kidney with special reference to light chain disease. *Am J Med* 1968;44: 922–933.
101. Durie BGM, Salmon SE: The current status and future prospects of treatment for multiple myeloma. *Clin Haematol* 1982;1:181–210.
102. Muther RS, McCarron DA, Bennett WM: Granulomatous sarcoid nephritis: a cause of multiple renal tubular abnormalities. *Clin Nephrol* 1980;14:190–197.
103. Falls WF Jr, Randall RE Jr, Sommers SC, et al: Nonhypercalcemic sarcoid nephropathy. *Arch Intern Med* 1972; 130:285–291.
104. Cracium EC, Rosculescu I: On Danubian endemic familial nephropathy (Balkan nephropathy). Some problems. *Am J Med* 1970;49:774–779.
105. Kelly DR, Murad TM: Megalocytic interstitial nephritis, xanthogranulomatous pyelonephritis, and malakoplakia. An ultrastructural comparison. *Am J Clin Pathol* 1981;75:333–344.
106. Shinkawa T, Osada Y, Ishisawa N, et al: Chronic cortical nodular interstitial nephritis. *Urology* 1982;19:325–327.
107. Malek RS, Eara S, Elder JS: Xanthogranulomatous pyelonephritis: a critical analysis of 26 cases and of the literature. *J Urol* 1978;119:589–593.
108. Garrett IR, McClure J: Renal malakoplakia. Experimental production and evidence of a link with interstitial megalocytic nephritis. *J Pathol* 1982;126:111–122.
109. Luke RG, Allison MEM, Davidson JF, et al: Hyperkalemia and renal tubular acidosis. *Ann Intern Med* 1969;70:1211–1217.
110. Smithline N, Kassirer JR, Cohen JJ: Light-chain nephropathy. Renal tubular dysfunction association with light-chain proteinuria. *N Engl J Med* 1976;294:71–74.
111. Anderson RJ, Linas SL: Sodium depletion states, in Brenner BM, Stein JH (eds): *Contemporary Issues in Nephrology.* New York, Churchill Livingstone, 1978, vol 1: *Sodium and Water Homeostasis,* pp 166–167.

112. Cogan MG, Rector FC, Seldin DW: Acid-Base Disorders, in Brenner BM, Rector FC (eds): *The Kidney*, ed 2. Philadelphia, WB Saunders, 1981, vol 1, pp 841–937.
113. Sebastian A, Hulter HN, Schambelan M: Renal hyperchlorenic acidosis with hyperkalemia type 4 renal tubular acidosis (RTA), in Barecelo R, Bergeron M, Carriere S, et al (eds): *Proceedings of the Seventh International Congress of Nephrology*. Montreal, Les Presses de L'Université de Montreal, 1978, pp 351–360.
114. Schambelan M, Stockigt JR, Biglieri EG: Isolated hypoaldosteronism in adults. A renin-deficiency syndrome. *N Engl J Med* 1972;287:573–612.
115. Berl T, Katz FH, Henrich WL, et al: Role of aldosterone in the control of sodium excretion in patients with advanced renal failure. *Kidney Int* 1978;14:228–235.
116. Tan SY, Burton M: Hyporeninemic hypoaldosteronism. An overlooked cause of hyperkalemia. *Arch Intern Med* 1981; 141:30–33.
117. Deleiva A, Christlieb AR, Melby JC, et al: Big renin and biosynthetic defect of aldosterone in diabetes mellitus. *N Engl J Med* 1976;295:639–643.
118. Tuck ML, Mayes DM: Mineralocorticoid biosynthesis in patients with hyporeninemic hypoaldosteronism. *J Clin Endocrinol Metab* 1980;50:341–347.
119. Hudson JB, Chobanian AV, Relman AS: Hypoaldosteronism. A clinical study of a patient with an isolated adrenal mineralocorticoid deficiency, resulting in hyperkalemia and Stokes-Adams attacks. *N Engl J Med* 1957;275:529–536.

CHAPTER 6 Acute Renal Failure in the Elderly

Donald E. Oken
Allen I. Wolfert
Domenic A. Sica

DEFINITIONS

Although the term "acute renal failure" has been applied in recent years to en compass decreases in renal function that cause the serum creatinine concentration to rise by as little as 1 mg/dL, we shall reserve that name here to represent a fall in glomerular filtration rate (GFR) which is so marked as to lead to serious clinical consequences unless it is reversed or substitution therapy is introduced. Such severe manifestations in adults usually are seen only at a GFR below 10 mL/min. Less marked aberrations of glomerular function that do not pose a direct threat to the patient's proximate welfare will be referred to as "renal insufficiency." An abrupt deterioration of renal function is called acute, while the condition is considered chronic if it has been present for months or years and, therefore, is very slowly progressive. We shall use the word "reversible" to indicate the potential for renal function to return to or close to its base-line level, either spontaneously or as the result of definitive therapy. The definition of irreversible renal failure is self-evident. "Oliguria" in adults is defined by common consent as a urine volume below 400 mL/24 h, and "anuria" is interpreted to mean a urine volume below 50 mL/24 h; one thus must resort to the term "total anuria" to describe a state in which urine output is unmeasurably small. An increase in blood urea nitrogen (BUN) or serum creatinine concentration that produces no major clinical or biochemical alteration here is termed "azotemia." We shall refer to "uremia" as a state in which serious biochemical and physical consequences of decreased glomerular filtration are either present or imminent. Distinction between these two entities is of some importance from the point of view of the patient's well-being, likely diagnosis, and the need for immediate dialytic therapy.

IMPORTANT CAUSES OF ACUTE RENAL FAILURE IN THE ELDERLY PATIENT

Virtually all the diseases that cause acute renal failure in the general population (obstetrical and comparable special causes excluded) may do so in the elderly as well. It is often stated that older patients are more prone to develop vasomotor nephropathy (VMN, "acute tubular necrosis") than others, but we have not been able to find reasonable documentation for such a belief either in the literature or in our own practices. Extensive surgical procedures, often performed on an emergency basis, are indeed commonplace in older patients and this same population is placed at particular risk of renal failure due to the hemodynamic consequences of sepsis, intestinal hemorrhage, myocardial infarction, mesenteric ischemia, aortic dissection, and dissecting aneurysm. Despite this, only 38 of 113 patients reported by Brown et al[1] to have developed acute renal failure following surgical operations were over age 60. In a large series of 760 patients with acute renal failure of various types reported by Kleinknecht and Ganeval,[2] fewer than one third were 60 years of age or older. This age group is, however, particularly at risk of other types of acute renal failure that are relatively uncommon in the younger age groups, most notably multiple myeloma, occlusive disease of the large renal vessels and aorta, renal atheroembolism, and urinary outflow obstruction due to carcinoma. For reasons to be discussed below, older patients also are particularly susceptible to functional renal failure and are prone to develop aminoglycoside nephrotoxicity when treated with dosage regimens that may be relatively innocuous in younger individuals.[3] In this chapter, therefore, while paying particular attention to vasomotor nephropathy, we shall also place some emphasis upon other causes of renal functional impairment that are particularly germane in the aged population.

ACUTE VERSUS CHRONIC RENAL DISEASE

In considering the cause of renal failure, the first task is to determine whether the process is acute in onset, is a chronic condition which has progressed covertly, or if it is a reflection of an acute deterioration of renal function superimposed upon chronic renal disease. The patient's history may be of great help in differentiating between acute and chronic processes. Acute renal failure is diagnosed when renal function is known to have been essentially normal or, if initially normal, to have been changing quite slowly before an episode of rapid deterioration is noted. Chronic renal failure may be suspected if there is a previous history of any degree of glomerular functional impairment, of proteinuria and/or an abnormal urinary sediment. Even when the patient has not received medical care in the recent past, he may have been told of such abnormalities years earlier in the course of pre-employment, military, insurance or other routine physical examinations. A prior history of glomerulonephritis, the nephrotic syndrome, nephrolithiasis, abdominal irradiation, severe and/or long-term hypertension, gout, diabetes, myelomatosis, pyelonephritis, lupus or other systemic diseases that might affect the kidneys, excessive ingestion of milk and calcium carbonate antacids, or lengthy exposure to cadmium, lead, mercury, or other nephrotoxins all raise the possibility of established chronic renal disease. Chronic nocturia or edema in the absence of congestive heart failure and long-standing abnormalities of micturition may be very significant in differential diagnosis. A history of excessive intake of phenacetin-containing compounds suggests the existence of chronic interstitial renal disease or papillary necrosis, and treatment with methysergide[4] for migraine headaches may have caused retroperitoneal fibrosis with chronic urinary tract obstruction. Recurrent hypertension or renal abnormalities in pregnancy (particularly early in pregnancy) may progress to renal failure decades later.[5] A family history of renal disease, particularly polycystic kidney disease, is noteworthy even in the elderly, a marked variability in expressivity of this disorder often providing the first evidence of renal disease quite late in life.[6]

Various physical findings suggest the chronicity of renal disease. It is difficult, for example, to fail to recognize classical chronic uremic skin pigmentation, that peculiar lemon-tan coloration which is not seen with acute renal failure. The finding of excoriations on the skin, particularly a mixture of healed and fresh scratch marks, indicates the presence of (possibly uremic) pruritus for some significant period of time. Grade III retinal changes on fundoscopic examination bespeak a chronic process, as would evidence of peripheral neuropathy. The radiographic changes of osteitis fibrosa cystica or severe osteomalacia in bone and the pecular gait associated with severe renal osteodystrophy are obvious signs of very protracted renal disease. Small kidneys, particularly when they are irregular in outline, staghorn calculi, or nephrocalcinosis found on a plain film of the abdomen are indicative of renal disease which is not of acute origin; notably large renal outlines may be indicative of polycystic disease, hydronephrosis, or tumor. In routine laboratory workup, severe normochromic, normocytic anemia suggests chronicity as does normochloremic (rather than hyperchloremic) acidosis, since a significant length of time is required to accumulate the required concentrations of sulfate, phosphate, organic acids, and other anions that account for the presence of normochloremia. Unfortunately, abnormalities of other serum electrolytes (including calcium and phosphate), while important in their own right, are of little help in distinguishing between acute and chronic processes.

One cannot always judge either the severity or the acuteness of renal functional impairment of a patient when he first presents to a hospital, however. Thus, a previously normal individual with fully established acute renal failure and a creatinine clearance of perhaps 2 to 3 mL/min is expected to exhibit a serum creatinine concentration of some 3 mg/dL 24 to 48 hours after the onset of the disorder. Another individual with long- standing renal insufficiency and a stable GFR of 30 mL/min would have essentially the same serum creatinine concentration. Thus, to ascertain both the severity and the acuteness of renal functional impairment of these two patients, it becomes necessary to perform serial measurements of serum creatinine which should provide stable values in the first patient and a progressive rise in serum creatinine in the second, or, perhaps preferably, to measure the creatinine clearance at the outset. Indeed, the four-hour creatinine clearance is very useful in this regard so long as the patient is not too oliguric for reasonably accurate measurement of urine volume. The creatinine clearance and serum creatinine concentration in steady state are inversely related, a stable serum creatinine concentration of 3 mg/dL roughly corresponding to a creatinine clearance that is one third of normal while a concentration of 5 mg/dL reflects a clearance that is about one fifth of normal (some 25 mL/min). The serum creatinine concentration is a reasonable indicator of the GFR only in steady state, however. If, therefore, a previously unknown patient presenting with a serum creatinine concentration of, eg, 3 mg/dL, has a measured creatinine clearance of perhaps 10 mL/min, one can: (*a*) recognize the severity of renal impairment at once, and (*b*) be assured that the process is acute because of the marked discrepancy between the serum creatinine and clearance values.

THE CONTROL OF GLOMERULAR FILTRATION

A major decrease in glomerular filtration is the hallmark of all forms of acute renal failure. It thus seems appropriate to briefly review the dynamics of glomerular filtration in normal man to promote a firmer understanding of the events that might lead to filtration failure.

As the term glomerular filtration implies, the process reflects the bulk flow of fluid from the glomerular capillary into Bowman's space. Filtration is promoted by the hydrostatic pressure within the glomerular capillary and is opposed by both the hydrostatic pressure in Bowman's space and the mean colloid osmotic pressure in glomerular capillary blood. Glomerular capillary hydrostatic pressure in turn is a function of the mean arterial blood pressure and the values at which the pre- and postglomerular vascular resistances and glomerular capillary resistance are set. An isolated increase in preglomerular resistance decreases glomerular capillary pressure as does relaxation of postglomerular resistance; an opposite change in each resistance has the inverse effect on filtration pressure and thus on filtration. The rate at which filtrate is formed at any given net transcapillary pressure is determined by the ultrafiltration coefficient (Kf) of the capillary membrane.

Current views on the control of glomerular filtration are largely based on information obtained in renal micropuncture studies performed on rats and dogs.[7,8] Comparable studies obviously cannot be performed in man, yet one can obtain a great deal of information on human glomerular dynamics without having access to the micropuncture approach. Assuming a complement of 1 million nephrons in each kidney,[9] a single kidney GFR of 60 to 65 mL/min,[10] a blood hematocrit of 45 mL/dL blood, and a filtration fraction of 0.2[11] in normal human subjects, the mean single nephron GFR can be estimated to be 60 to 65 nanoliters per minute (nL/min) while glomerular blood flow is approximately 550 nL/min. With mean arterial and renal venous pressures of 92 mmHg and 6 mmHg respectively, the total vascular resistance per nephron is calculated to be approximately 1.2×10^{10} dyne seconds cm^{-5}, a value one fourth to one fifth of that commonly reported for the rat[7] and approximately one half that reported for the dog.[8]

In theory, at least, failure of glomerular filtration might be induced by increasing preglomerular resistance, reducing postglomerular resistance, decreasing glomerular capillary hydraulic conductivity, or raising the pressure in the proximal tubule, and two or more such abnormalities might coexist. We have previously employed network thermodynamic modeling[12] to determine the degree of change in each of these parameters that, as an isolated change, would be required to produce acute renal failure in the rat and dog.[13] In view of the major interspecies differences in normal glomerular dynamic parameters found in a previous analysis,[14] however, one cannot extrapolate findings in the rat and dog directly to man. Hence the need to perform a separate analysis for human acute renal failure.

We do not know the relative values of the pre- and postglomerular vascular resistances in normal man, but one can derive maximal and minimal values for each since the total nephron resistance is known with some confidence (see above). There is a unique value for the ultrafiltration coefficient that provides the requisite normal single nephron GFR of 65 nL/min at any assigned pre- to postglomerular resistance ratio. Within these limitations, we find that the preglomerular resistance in man cannot be higher than the postglomerular resistance and it is, in all likelihood, no more than one half as high. Renal venous wedge pressure, reportedly an excellent indicator of proximal tubule pressure, is in the vicinity of 15 mmHg[15] to 25 mmHg,[16] the latter being found in more recent reports. With this information and working between the possible limiting values for pre- and postglomerular resistances, we have employed network modeling to determine the approximate degree of change in individual resistances, proximal tubule pressure, or ultrafiltration coefficient needed to reduce GFR to or below 10% of control, as expected in human acute renal failure. According to this analysis, proximal tubule pressure must rise by some 12 to 22 mmHg if tubular obstruction alone is to cause renal failure. A decrease in the glomerular ultrafiltration coefficient will depress filtration, but not in any simple fashion. Normally, ongoing filtration causes the serum protein concentration (and hence the plasma oncotic pressure) to rise progressively along the capillary's length. Net filtration pressure thus falls as blood flows along the capillary and is much lower at its distal end than at the origin. If we were to decrease the ultrafiltration coefficient below its normal value, GFR would fall early in the capillary but, because the normal rise in capillary blood oncotic pressure would then be blunted, the fall in Kf would be partially offset by the maintenance of a higher net filtration pressure more distally. The observed fall in GFR, therefore, would be much smaller than might otherwise be anticipated. A 50% reduction in ultrafiltration coefficient, for example, is estimated to lower GFR by only some 30% in man, and a 90% fall in Kf still leaves GFR at about 20% of control. Moreover, just as in the rat, a fall in ultrafiltration coefficient of this magnitude has less and less absolute effect on GFR when filtration pressure is already reduced by either preglomerular vasoconstriction or tubular obstruction. Thus, it is found that the glomerular capillary membrane would have to become virtually impermeable before acute renal failure could be attributed to that mechanism alone.

The theory of "plasma flow dependence" suggests that net filtration pressure becomes totally dissipated at some point proximal to the terminus of the glomerular capillaries,[17] leaving a state of "filtration pressure equilibrium" (FPE) where further filtration is impossible. According to this concept, any decrease in glomerular blood flow is supposed to decrease GFR simply by providing filtration equilibrium more proximally in the capillary, and such a mechanism has been invoked in one study of experimental murine acute renal failure.[18] Whether FPE exists in the normal rat is debatable, various authors finding a significant net filtration pressure remaining at the end of the capillary even in this species.[19–21] Filtration pressure equilibrium is clearly not present in the dog,[5] however, and unless one accepts the most extreme (high) value for the afferent/efferent arteriolar resistance ratio, a very substantial residual net filtration pressure must remain at the end of the glomerulus in man as well.[13] Thus, there is no reason to propose that human VMN is an extreme manifestation of the plasma flow dependence phenomenon.

Our model shows that a sufficiently large increase in preglomerular vascular resistance causes a precipitous fall in GFR, as would be expected intuitively. If preglomerular resistance (R_A) in normal man is assumed to be one third as large as postglomerular resistance (ie, 0.3×10^{10} dyne seconds cm^{-5}), and tubular hydrostatic pressure is 25 mmHg, a filtration rate of some 5% of normal will be obtained when R_A rises to $\sim 1 \times 10^{10}$ dyne seconds cm^{-5}. This degree of resistance change, our analysis shows, would decrease renal blood flow by some 40%. Assigning R_A to its maximum possible normal value of $\sim 0.5 \times 10^{10}$ dyne seconds cm^{-5}, filtration failure would be expected if that resistance were raised to only 0.9×10^{10} dyne seconds cm^{-5}, an increase that should depress renal blood flow by approximately 30%. Thus, regardless of the basal value of R_A chosen for normal man, failed filtration does not need to be accompanied by extreme renal ischemia. Put differently, a fall in cortical blood flow of 30% to 40% is quite sufficient to account for filtration failure if due to preglomerular vasoconstriction alone. An isolated decrease in postglomerular resistance (R_E) would likewise depress filtration, GFR falling almost linearly as R_E falls, but blood flow would be expected to rise markedly if R_E were lowered to a value that itself provides filtration failure. That clearly is not the case in either human or experimental VMN. Even small degrees of postglomerular vascular relaxation, coupled with preglomerular vasoconstriction, would contribute significantly to impaired filtration produced by any other means, however. Concomitant equal increases in both pre- and postglomerular resistance leave GFR remarkably well maintained while adversely affecting blood flow, a tripling of total renovascular resistances that reduces blood flow by two thirds leaves GFR at some 55% of its normal value.[13]

A change in glomerular capillary resistance has been proposed as the cause of failed filtration both in VMN[22,23] and in glomerular diseases. Indeed, the histologic changes seen in the more severe instances of glomerulonephritis are entirely compatible with that possibility, especially if accompanied by a concomitant change in capillary wall permeability. We estimate that GFR can be reduced to 10% of its normal value by increasing capillary resistance alone, but that this requires a capillary resistance that is almost twice the total vascular resistance of the normal human nephron. Blood flow would then be depressed by 60% or more.

VASOMOTOR NEPHROPATHY (VMN, "ACUTE TUBULAR NECROSIS," "ACUTE RENAL FAILURE")

Vasomotor nephropathy is a syndrome manifested by an abrupt and severe depression of renal function, most commonly following trauma, shock, sepsis, obstetrical accidents, rhabdomyolysis, poisoning, and hemolytic reactions. Each of these same conditions may produce functional renal failure which is reversed when the underlying cause is adequately treated. In vasomotor nephropathy, however, glomerular filtration remains severely depressed long after the cardiac output and blood pressure have been returned to normal. Previously called "lower nephron nephrosis," and now usually termed "acute tubular necrosis" or "acute renal failure," none of those terms is entirely appropriate inasmuch as frank tubular necrosis is found uncommonly; such injury as is found is most prominent in the proximal, and not the distal, tubule; and acute renal failure may be a manifestation of such diverse entities as glomerulonephritis, renal arterial occlusion, and allergic interstitial nephritis. The term vasomotor nephropathy has been suggested, therefore, since the syndrome is generally initiated in a substrate of hemodynamic instability and is typified by marked and persistent renal cortical ischemia throughout its course (see below).

Pathology

Initially normal in size, the kidneys become large, firm, and edematous one or two days after the onset of renal failure. Swelling of the kidney is predominantly due to interstitial edema, a finding which seems best explained by altered capillary permeability.[24] The cortical parenchyma is pale and shiny, a reflection of both interstitial edema and cortical ischemia. The medulla, by contrast, may show engorgement of the vasa recta and is then deep burgundy in color. Small patches of leukocytic infiltrate may be present in the cortical interstitium, lymphocytes being the predominant cells but with occasional plasma cells and polymorphonuclear or eosinophilic leukocytes often intermixed. Although usually sparse and patchy, such areas of infiltration may be more abundant in the occasional patient.[25]

Tubular injury is highly variable in its degree and severity. As pointed out by

Finckh et al,[26] Sevitt,[27] and others, one often sees little or no change in cellular architecture on light microscopy. Even in such cases, however, electron microscopic examination has revealed degeneration of cellular nuclei, swelling of mitochondria with distortion of their cristae, and disintegration of outer mitochondrial membranes in individual tubular cells.[28] Such changes may explain the grossly depressed transport capacity of the nephron in this syndrome. At the other extreme, frank tubular necrosis with nuclear pyknosis, cellular disruption, and shedding of masses of epithelium into tubular lumens are seen occasionally. There is, however, little correlation between the severity of the histologic lesions and the clinical status of the patient.[27,29] Whether tubular injury is severe or essentially nonexistent on postmortem examination, Bohle[30] has pointed out that tubular lumens typically are not collapsed as in other autopsy material. Luminal casts containing proteinaceous material, heme pigments, or cellular debris are found in varying degree from patient to patient. Some authorities have assumed that such material obstructs the tubules and hence serves as an important factor in the genesis of acute renal failure; others, however, point to the many instances where luminal casts cannot be found at all[27,30,31] and suggest that the intraluminal deposition of debris may be the result, rather than the cause, of filtration failure.[32]

The glomeruli and blood vessels of the kidney with vasomotor nephropathy are histologically normal on both light and electron microscopic examination.[33] Specifically, the glomerular endothelial and epithelial cells, mesangium, and basement membranes show no characteristic lesions.

With the passage of time, kidneys displaying more severe degrees of injury display increasing numbers of mitoses indicative of tissue repair, and these antedate recovery of glomerular function. Interstitial edema persists into the recovery phase, resolving slowly thereafter. With time, full healing of the renal lesions is expected, although islands of tubular atrophy and interstitial fibrosis may persist indefinitely. Very rarely, the healing process is associated with progressive parenchymal atrophy.[34]

The Cause of Filtration Failure in Human Vasomotor Nephropathy

Although the relative importance of hemodynamic factors, tubular leakage of filtrate, and tubular obstruction in the pathogenesis of experimental acute renal failure in the rat is still debated,[35-37] every study of the renal circulation in man performed to date has shown renal cortical blood flow to be reduced by 50% to 70% or more.[38-41] It has been suggested that such a degree of renal ischemia cannot account for renal failure since blood flow may be equally reduced in some patients with chronic renal insufficiency who maintain a much higher filtration rate. This frequently cited objection to a hemodynamic basis for vasomotor nephropathy does not take into account the widely different histologic and functional changes in the two conditions, however. Acute renal failure is characterized by diffuse vasoconstriction of the entire renal cortex (see Figure 6-1). Chronic renal failure, by contrast, is typified by islands of well-perfused, functioning tissue surrounded by large areas of scarring where blood flow is presumably vanishingly small. Filtrate thus is derived from those few nephrons that are still functioning, and Bricker has called particular attention to this characteristic of chronic renal failure which serves as the basis for his "intact nephron" hypothesis.[42] As shown earlier, glomerular filtration in man is expected to be totally suppressed when preglomerular resistance is raised to a degree that causes cortical blood flow to fall by only 30% to 40%. The far greater degree of cortical ischemia usually found in this syndrome is thus quite sufficient to explain failed filtration so long as the increase in

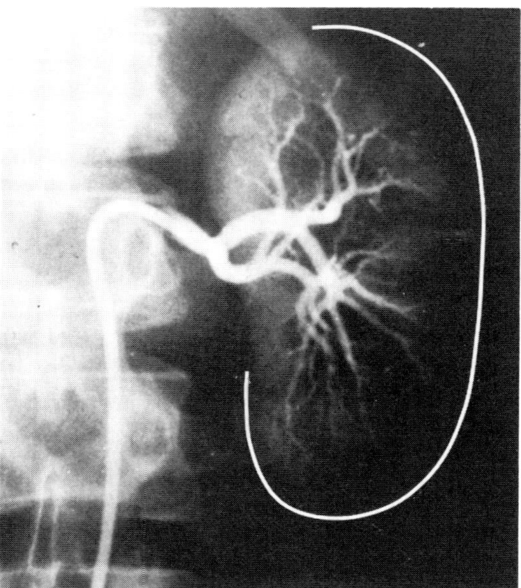

Figure 6-1 Left renal angiogram of a patient with vasomotor nephropathy. The renal outline is delineated in white. Note the characteristic absence of filling of the outer cortical vasculature attendant on the marked increase in resistance and severe cortical ischemia that characterizes this syndrome in man.

renal cortical resistance can be shown to largely involve the preglomerular circuit. Figure 6-1 shows the appearance of the intrarenal vasculature during the vascular phase of a selective renal angiogram performed on a patient with vasomotor nephropathy. It is typical of findings reported by various authors,[41,43] all of whom have shown some degree of attenuation of the larger arteries within the kidney and such marked attenuation of the arcuate and interlobular arteries that there is almost no filling of the outer cortical vasculature with opaque media. Such an ischemic appearance correlates well with the scant bleeding of the renal cortex found on open renal biopsy[38] and is fully consonant with the marked decrease in both blood flow and glomerular filtration found in human VMN. This conclusion has been questioned since cortical blood flow of subjects with this syndrome can be increased substantially during intra-arterial infusions of acetylcholine[44] or dihydralazine[45] without providing any detectable improvement in GFR. It seems, however, that the renal vasodilators exert their effect primarily on the postglomerular, rather than the preglomerular, vasculature,[46] an effect which would be expected to further decrease glomerular filtration rather than raise it.

As judged from measurements of renal venous wedged pressures performed by Munck[11] and Brun et al,[15] proximal tubule pressure is not elevated in human acute renal failure. It is thus unnecessary to suggest that tubular obstruction is superimposed upon the hemodynamic abnormalities. Nor, with such marked cortical ischemia and attenuation of the cortical vasculature, is there any cogent reason to suppose that filtration is well-maintained but that nonselective passive absorption of the filtrate formed is the true cause of vasomotor nephropathy. It cannot be disproved that *some* of the filtrate formed might be absorbed as suggested in the "passive backflow theory" of VMN, and Myers et al have produced data that suggest the possibility that some of the filtrate formed (perhaps as much as 15%) may be absorbed by such a mechanism.[47] With a true filtration rate of, eg, 5 mL/min, then, the apparent GFR would be 4.3 mL/min, a difference that is too small to measure and one which is not really of any practical concern to the patient's treatment and welfare.

Clinical Presentation

Except for the development of oliguria, the early symptoms associated with vasomotor nephropathy relate exclusively to the underlying cause. There is no flank pain attributable to the process and the kidneys are not palpable. Gross hematuria is a relatively uncommon finding and, since so many of the patients at risk of this syndrome have had indwelling bladder catheters inserted during the incipient phase of VMN, any hematuria that is observed is apt to be attributed to catheter-related bladder injury. Oliguria thus is the sole clinical hallmark of vasomotor nephropathy. It has become increasingly evident, however, that a large proportion of patients with vasomotor nephropathy are not oliguric at all,[48,49] although it is not certain that all patients included in such reports have had a sufficiently severe degree of renal impairment to merit the diagnosis of acute renal failure as defined earlier.

Vasomotor nephropathy occurs uncommonly without an obvious antecedent cause, and it is not difficult to recognize the subjects at risk. Only a very small percentage of the latter group of patients develop fixed renal failure, however. In one series, only five of some 204 patients subjected to cardiac surgery developed VMN.[50] Powers et al[51] have estimated that the syndrome occurs in some 0.1% of patients undergoing major surgery and, in reviewing 1659 cases of lower aortic surgery performed in ten centers, Kountz et al[52] found an overall incidence of VMN of only 3.8%. Although up to 36.5% of patients treated with aminoglycosides were reported to experience some degree of renal dysfunction in one report,[53] only a very small minority of those given gentamicin develop significant renal failure if the agent is used appropriately. On the other hand, these antibiotics are so widely used in seriously ill patients that approximately one half of all cases of nonoliguric acute renal failure were found by Anderson et al to be caused by aminoglycoside nephrotoxicity.[48] The role of nephrotoxic medications in the genesis of renal failure is discussed in more detail later in the chapter.

Whether oliguric or nonoliguric, vasomotor nephropathy presents with certain distinct clinical features. First, the GFR is usually less than 5 mL/min, and, most often, is only 1 to 2 mL/min. The tubule's capacity to transport salt and water is grossly impaired despite the small volume of filtrate provided, presumably as the result of tubular injury, and the ability to significantly concentrate and dilute the urine generally is lost. Since the GFR does not change greatly from day to day prior to the onset of recovery and since the ability of the tubule to transport sodium and to concentrate the urine is so severely impaired, it is not surprising that the urine volume and sodium excretion remain fairly constant from day to day and that there usually is little response to diuretic therapy. Refractoriness to furosemide's diuretic effect is further attributable to the fact that this agent must be secreted by the proximal tubule prior to its reaching the luminal surface where it then depresses ion transport in Henle's loop.[54] Tubular secretion of furosemide in renal failure is presumably as severely impaired as that of para-aminohippurate and other weak acids.[55] The serum creatinine concentration typically rises by at least 0.6 mg/dL daily, most commonly by 1 to 2 mg/dL/24 h; in patients with rhabdomyolysis[56] and in severely hypercatabolic patients, the serum creatinine concentration may rise by as much as 4 to 5 mg/dL per day.

With a markedly depressed GFR and little flexibility to adjust urine output, peripheral edema and frank congestive heart failure are apt to develop if salt and water intake is not controlled and renal failure is long-lasting. Hyponatremia was a common complication before water restriction became standard procedure in these patients. Metabolic acidosis is an expected part of acute renal failure of any etiology, but it is apt to be particularly severe in vasomotor nephropathy related to sepsis, severe trauma, or burns where an extreme degree of hypercatabolism may coexist. In less severely ill patients, however, the serum bicarbonate usually falls by only 0.5 to 1.5 mEq/L/day so that acidosis may present no major clinical challenge to the patient's welfare until late in the course, even if dialysis is withheld.

Hyperkalemia is among the most serious of all the potentially lethal complications to which the patient with acute renal failure is subject. Even when dietary potassium is eliminated and other sources of potassium (eg, blood transfusions, medications given as potassium salts) are carefully avoided, release of this ion from necrotic tissue, sequestered blood, ongoing hemolysis, and hypercatabolism of whatever cause may result in severe hyperkalemia soon after the onset of renal failure unless steps are taken to prevent such an occurrence. Hyperkalemia seems to be particularly severe in myoglobinuric VMN[56] and is apt to be enhanced in any patient with severe metabolic acidosis. Far less acute increases in serum K are found in the majority of patients, however. Hypocalcemia is an expected concomitant of any form of protracted acute renal failure, the serum concentration often falling to 6 or 7 mg/dL, an effect presumably related in part to the attendant hyperphosphatemia and possibly in part to unresponsiveness to parathyroid hormone.[57] Even when the serum calcium concentration falls to very low levels, however, tetany is rarely found. Hypermagnesemia of some degree is expected, but again usually is of no clinical concern.

Even in the absence of overt intestinal bleeding or evident hemolysis, most patients will display a slow and progressive fall in blood hematocrit, presumably the result of depressed erythropoiesis. How much of this effect is due to a specific defect in erythropoietin production and how much relates to covert hemolysis and the attendant illness of the patient is unclear. Frequent venipuncture and the removal of large volumes of blood for daily or twice daily laboratory testing can contribute significantly to the development of anemia, particularly in this setting. It is thus not unusual for a patient's hematocrit to fall by almost one half within ten to 12 days. Rapid and abrupt decreases in hematocrit, however, are usually indicative of blood loss into the intestinal tract. Leukocytosis is commonly present but generally mild in the absence of infection. It can, nonetheless, be disquieting to the physician ever alert to the risk of septic death in the immunocompromised[58] patient with acute renal failure. Thrombocytopenia per se usually is of far less significance than the intrinsic defect in platelet function as a cause of disturbed hemostasis.[59]

Anorexia, nausea, and vomiting are common concomitants of acute renal failure. Early in the course, these symptoms are most often the result of the attendant acute illness that caused renal failure in the first place. Later, however, they may be harbingers of impending uremia. Stomatitis and parotitis may be found, particularly in severely ill patients, and monilial glossitis is not uncommon. These complications can largely be avoided by good nursing practices. Gastrointestinal (GI) bleeding due to stress ulcers, nonspecific gastritis, bleeding diatheses, or enterocolitis is a common and dreaded complication, only the two latter entities being largely preventable by dialysis. Hemodialysis, in turn, may initiate intestinal bleeding because of the use of heparin during the procedure.

Infection is a leading cause of death in both the oliguric and recovery phase of vasomotor nephropathy.[60] Impaired mentation, immobilization, trauma, tissue necrosis, burns, and surgical violation of the various body cavities all contribute to the frequency with which infection is found. Central venous catheters inserted for continuous pressure measurement or for hyperalimentation, and Swan-Ganz catheters may provide easy portals of entry for invading bacteria and fungi.[61] Infection introduced by an indwelling bladder catheter is indeed unfortunate, since such catheters are rarely necessary for the care of oliguric patients. Infected arteriovenous shunts may provide a portal for systemic infection and there is always the risk of peritonitis attendant upon peritoneal dialysis. Most centers now utilize early and vigorous regimens of dialysis in hopes of improving the patient's overall clinical status, alertness, and resistance to infection, although proof of the efficacy of this approach is still somewhat weak. The awareness of the hospital staff of potential causes for sepsis in a given patient and the institution of prompt and vigorous therapy of any established infection may be of equal importance in reducing the death rate from infection in any form of acute renal failure. Delaying the onset of dialysis until severe biochemical and physical complications are present has no justification, nonetheless.

Heart failure usually is an entirely preventable complication of injudicious volume administration, but it may be seen in the absence of overhydration following open-heart surgery, myocardial infarction or contusion, cardiac tamponade, or pulmonary embolization despite careful and conservative fluid management. Hypertension, except when due to gross volume overload, is an unusual complication of vasomotor nephropathy. Arrhythmias, formerly a very common occurrence, are now far less frequently seen in uncomplicated VMN since hyperkalemia is more successfully managed and the patient's susceptibility to digitalis toxicity is widely recognized. Indeed, digitalis toxicity is expected in prolonged VMN if the dosage of digoxin is not adjusted to provide 10% to 25% of the normal dose. Digitoxin, by contrast, is largely excreted by the liver, and while the dose should be reduced by 25% to 50%, it is less likely to cause cardiotoxicity. On the other hand, the slower elimination of digitoxin makes for far more prolonged toxicity once it develops, and many authorities avoid its use in patients with renal failure for that reason. Digitalis glycosides are not significantly dialyzable if toxicity does develop. Uremic pericarditis, typically a manifestation of severe uremia, has occurred far less frequently since it has become customary to undertake early and frequent dialysis. Life-threatening pericardial effusion is relatively uncommon, despite occasional reports of hemopericardium and cardiac tamponade.[62]

Uremia is typified by severe nausea and vomiting, often with intestinal ileus. Pruritis is customary and typically severe, and hiccoughs occur commonly. Serious electrolyte disorders and acidosis are usually present, and a variety of neurologic aberrations appear preterminally. Abnormalities of affect, attitude, and mentation are the earliest CNS signs of uremia. The concentration span is short, and the patient may be restless or sullen, withdrawn and dull. Asterixis of the outstretched hand, muscular twitching, myoclonic movements, and hyperreflexia are common manifestations portending the development of convulsions or coma, and the EEG may show diffuse slowing or intermittent paroxysms of slow activity.[63] Uremic pericarditis and hemorrhagic membranous enterocolitis may supervene prior to death. Untreated, the patients usually die of volume or electrolyte disorders, arrhythmias, infection, GI bleeding, convulsions, or coma. Only with deliberate withholding of dialysis (eg, in patients with terminal cancer) is the fully established uremic syndrome likely to be found in hospitalized patients.

Despite all forms of modern therapy and the ready availability of dialysis, the overall mortality rate of patients with VMN is some 50%,[1,2,64] over half this number dying a septic death.[60] Severe posttraumatic VMN and renal failure occurring after ruptured aortic aneurysm carry a mortality rate in most centers of 80% to 90%.[65,66] A somewhat better outlook for postaneurysmectomy patients seems to have been achieved in certain centers, however.[67] There appears to be a significant excess mortality among the aged and, as might be expected, particularly those patients with more severe trauma or systemic illnesses.

FUNCTIONAL RENAL FAILURE

Acute renal failure that is not due to renal parenchymal disease, occlusion of the major vessels, urinary outflow obstruction, or urinary extravasation is generally called "prerenal" or, as we prefer, "functional" renal failure.[68] That name underscores the fact that there is no intrinsic abnormality of the kidney, the impairment of glomerular filtration being hemodynamic in origin and usually readily reversed if the immediate abnormality is removed. Importantly, however, this form of renal insufficiency is attributable to many of the same causes that produce vasomotor nephropathy and, if its treatment is delayed or inadequate, the latter may supervene ("incipient renal failure"[69]). Thus, the early recognition and prompt therapy of functional renal failure is considered important.

The healthy young kidney responds to volume depletion, hemorrhage, or any other factor that causes a reduction in cardiac output by avidly conserving sodium, concentrating the urine and ultimately, if the stimulus is sufficiently great, by significantly decreasing renal blood flow and glomerular filtration.[70] Very marked decreases in cardiac output or frank shock virtually abolish filtration, the serum creatinine concentration then rising as if vasomotor nephropathy were present when in fact it is not. Aged patients and patients with pre-existing renal disease are particularly sensitive to changes in cardiac output and may experience total (functional) renal shutdown in response to a stimulus that would cause only moderate renal insufficiency in a younger individual.

The existence of heart failure or severe hypotension is immediately evident on physical examination, but it must be recalled that the nephrosclerotic kidney may respond poorly to quite modest changes in cardiac output and blood pressure, as mentioned above. Even seriously hypovolemic patients are apt to have a normal blood pressure while lying in bed. On standing, however, they cannot tolerate the additional shrinkage of effective intravascular volume caused by pooling of blood in the capacitance vessels of the lower extremities. They thus develop a significant fall in blood pressure (orthostatic hypotension) together with tachycardia as soon as they assume the upright position. If not attributable to drug therapy, neuropathy or prolonged immobilization, such blood pressure change is a key physical indicator of serious volume depletion. The appearance of this physical finding, however, requires approximately a 10% decrease in total body water, and the function of the nephrosclerotic kidney may be seriously depressed with a far smaller degree of volume depletion. Thus, while orthostatic hypotension usually is an accurate reflection of a severe fluid deficit, its absence in no way offers assurance that the GFR of an elderly patient has *not* become severely compromised purely on the basis of hypovolemia. The other physical findings of volume depletion that are commonly cited—dry mouth and skin, loss of skin turgor, and soft ocular globes—have not proved very useful, especially in the aged. The appearance of the buccal mucosa reflects the adequacy of mouth care by the nursing staff, recent intake of fluids and, perhaps most importantly, whether the patient breathes through his mouth. A well-hydrated "mouth breather" who does not lick his lips and swallow will probably have a very dry appearing mouth, while a seriously dehydrated patient who sips fluids or has continued to eat is apt to have a more normal appearing mucosa. The loss of skin turgor with age is expected regardless of the adequacy of hydration and thus is of little help in clinical evaluation; the wide individual variation in perspiration and the response to change in body temperature, ambient temperature, and humidity all combine to make volume assessment on the basis of skin moisture very difficult.

Perhaps the most useful indicator of severe volume depletion is found in comparing the patient's recent and present weights if these are available. Knowing those values, one may discover a 2, 3, or even a 5 L fluid deficit or, on the other hand, document the existence of a significant weight gain that largely rules out volume-related functional renal failure. It should not be forgotten, however, that extracellular fluids may be distributed abnormally despite the fact that body weight may be unchanged or may even be increased. Large amounts of fluid can be sequestered as ascites or pleural effusions, within the bowel in cases of intestinal ileus, or as concealed hemorrhage, leaving plasma volume greatly depressed. While significant peripheral edema serves as prima facie evidence of plasma volume expansion in the absence of hypoalbuminemia, burns, and venous/lymphatic obstruction, the presence and degree of edema in these latter conditions show no correlation with overall fluid balance. Indeed, vigorous attempts to mobilize such hypoalbuminuric or "mechanical" edema with diuretics may result in severe plasma volume depletion while leaving the patient as edematous as ever. History too can be persuasive in diagnosis. A diabetic entering with marked hyperglycemia may be presumed to have experienced an osmotic diuresis and to have lost a large volume of fluid as urine; a history of protracted vomiting and diarrhea or documented hypodypsia[71] is notable. Lastly, except for the rare patient with essential hypernatremia,[72] a markedly elevated serum sodium concentration that is not the result of injudicious salt loading of a patient already in renal failure provides presumptive evidence for severe water depletion since there is no other way of developing such a state.

The urinary sodium and creatinine concentrations and the urine osmolality are very important parameters in differentiating between functional and organic causes of renal failure (see below). At times, however, doubt persists concerning the volume status of a given patient despite all available information. Measurement of the central venous pressure (CVP) or pulmonary capillary wedged pressure can then be extremely helpful not only diagnostically but also as a vehicle with which to monitor the replacement of fluids more safely in those patients whose cardiovascular reserve is questionable. It is generally considered that a CVP above 15 cm H_2O is indicative of either fluid overload or primary myocardial failure. Such a concept has been shown to be valid in circumstances where simple abnormalities in cardiac function or blood volume exist[73]; the question is rather more complex, however, when these aberrations intersect with abnormalities in vascular tone such as might be induced by the neural response to trauma or hemorrhage. Baek et al[73] have shown that a supernormal CVP of 18 cm H_2O not only may coexist with a decidedly low blood volume in critically ill postoperative patients but it may well fall (to an average of less than 9 cm H_2O in their case) following the infusion of 500 mL of 5% albumin solution. Cardiac output increased in parallel by some 75% in the succeeding 30 minutes. Thus, it is difficult to be sure that critically ill patients with normal to high CVP values are necessarily euvolemic unless their blood volume is actually shown to be normal by careful measurement. If left with a contracted blood volume, they may remain in functional renal failure which, at times, may be wrongly diagnosed as VMN. The response to judicious fluid administration may thus be the final key in determining the role of volume depletion as the prime cause of acute renal failure in elderly or critically ill patients.

By definition, functional renal failure is reversed when the initiating cause is removed. Thus, the restoration of blood volume, cardiac output, and blood pressure, or the treatment of sepsis not only is appropriate in care of the whole patient, but it also serves as a yardstick proving that the renal problem is indeed functional. Hypovolemic hypotension is treated by the administration of the appropriate fluids. Prolonged volume depletion may be accompanied by an increase in capacitance vessel tone, however. Thus, even when fluids initially are administered to a severely volume depleted patient at a rate of 150–200 mL/h, occasional patients will exhibit a rapid, early rise in CVP long before adequate replacement is complete. If, then, the venous catheter is removed and further fluids are withheld to "prevent" the development of heart failure, the patient remains volume-depleted, renal function may not improve, and the cause of impaired filtration may remain enigmatic. If, instead, the catheter is left in place while the infusion is slowed or stopped, the CVP will be seen to fall over a period of perhaps ten to 30 minutes–often to the preinfusion level. The cycle can then be repeated with the CVP value ultimately reflecting the true intravascular volume with some fidelity after the capacitance vessels reattain their normal tone.

At times, one may be disappointed to find that a patient with presumably functional renal failure remains oliguric despite the attainment of what appears to be adequate volume replacement. Such is not an infrequent occurrence, oliguria sometimes persisting for up to 12 hours or even longer after full fluid repletion.[74,75] The reason for this delay in restoration of urine output is unclear, but such patients often will respond promptly to furosemide administration or the infusion of 12.5 to 25 g of mannitol and maintain an appropriate urine volume and GFR thereafter. This phenomenon may account in part for some cases in which furosemide and mannitol have been thought to prevent the development of VMN in its incipient phase when, with a little more time, recovery would have occurred spontaneously.

Examination of the properties of the urine plays a very important role in differentiating between functional renal failure and VMN, as will be discussed below.

MALIGNANCIES AND THE KIDNEY

The markedly increased incidence of carcinoma in patients after age 60 contributes importantly to the development of both acute and chronic renal failure. Bladder outflow obstruction secondary to carcinoma of the bladder, colon, cervix, and prostate is found commonly in this age group. Involvement of the retroperitoneum with a variety of tumors or tumor-related retroperitoneal fibrosis is a distinct, but relatively uncommon, cause of both ureteral obstruction and of extrinsic entrapment of the major vessels.[76] Ureteral metastases from breast[77] and other[78] tumors–at times bilateral–may cause acute outflow obstruction and varying degrees of renal failure. Although infiltration of the kidney is a common finding in leukemia, myeloma, and lymphoma, renal failure rarely results from replacement of renal tissue by direct invasion of these malignancies.[79] Metastases from solid tumors to the kidney are common and often bilateral, but they rarely lead to renal failure other than by obstructing urinary outflow.

Gastrointestinal, biliary, pancreatic, hepatic, and other tumors may cause functional acute renal failure through fluid loss as vomitus or diarrhea, through relative nephrogenic diabetes insipidus induced by hypercalcemia or hypokalemia,[80] and through the rapid development of tumorous ascites or uncontrolled hemorrhage. The severe vomiting and other GI symptoms complicating therapy with a variety of chemotherapeutic agents also may lead to functional renal insufficiency and a greater susceptibility to the nephrotoxic effects of both the antineoplastic agents themselves and other toxic drugs being used concomitantly.

Chemotherapeutic agents employed in the treatment of cancer–especially cisplatin,[81] streptozocin,[82] and methotrexate given alone or combined with leucovorin[83] ("citrovorum rescue")–cause dose-related acute renal failure either by their direct nephrotoxic effects on tubular epithelial cells or by intratubular obstruction (methotrexate). Occasional instances of toxic acute renal failure have been encountered following the use of other antimetabolites in cancer therapy.

Hyperuricemia is a frequent complication of malignancies. Although the serum uric acid concentration is often elevated to 12 to 14 mg/dL,[84] such a degree of hyperuricemia is not itself apt to seriously compromise kidney function.[85] Far higher uric acid concentrations may be seen, however, if renal insufficiency has supervened for other reasons.[86] Unless preventive measures are employed, plasma urate concentrations of 20 to 30 mg/dL or higher may follow treatment of the leukemias, lymphomas, and other tumors with antineoplastic agents, and such concentrations are sufficient to cause renal failure due to either intrarenal or extrarenal crystallization of uric acid or, uncommonly, to "acute gouty nephropathy."[87] This phenomenon is largely preventable by assuring adequate hydration and minimization of uric acid synthesis by administering allopurinol before chemotherapy or radiotherapy is begun. Urine alkalinization with sodium bicarbonate and maintenance of urine output with mannitol infusion have been widely employed.

Renal failure, a common occurrence in multiple myeloma[88] may be functional and related to hypercalcemic volume depletion or volume losses from any other cause. It is then largely reversible with fluid replacement. The coprecipitation of immunoglobulin light chains with Tamm-Horsfall and other proteins within renal tubules[89] is an ominous and usually irreversible cause of acute renal failure. Indeed, several cases have been reported in which renal failure was the first clinical presentation of multiple myeloma,[90] and various biopsy studies of patients with acute renal failure of obscure origin have revealed otherwise unsuspected myelomatosis as the cause.[91] Mild or moderate renal insufficiency is present in over one half of all patients at initial diagnosis,[88] a state which makes such patients particularly prone to the complications of aminoglycoside therapy. The susceptibility of persons with multiple myeloma to develop frank renal failure after radiologic procedures that require injection of contrast media is legendary.[92]

DRUG-INDUCED RENAL FAILURE

Few patients escape treatment with drugs in hospital, and polypharmacy is commonplace. Certain agents clearly are potential nephrotoxins and others are known mediators of acute allergic interstitial nephritis in a small minority of patients exposed to them. Drugs with this reputation should become suspect whenever a patient to whom they are given exhibits an otherwise unexplained abrupt decrease in renal function. The aminoglycoside antibiotics[93] and certain antineoplastic agents[81–83] are the most notorious of the nephrotoxic drugs.

The widely used β-lactam antibiotics (the penicillins and cephalosporins) are clearly the most commonly cited causes of allergic interstitial nephritis in all age groups,[94] methicillin being the archtypical example.[95] The sulfonamides,[96] trimethoprim-sulfamethoxazole,[93] and rifampin[97] are well-recognized offenders as are most (if not all) of the nonsteroidal anti-inflammatory drugs presently in use.[98–100] A large number of other medications (eg, cimetidine,[101] phenytoin,[102] allopurinol,[103] diuretics, and phenylpropanolamine hydrochloride[104] have also been reported to cause interstitial nephritis, although not at all commonly. Intriguingly, some of the drugs listed as causes of acute interstitial nephritis (especially the penicillins and sulfonamides) may initiate allergic vasculitis as well.[105]

The elderly patient seems particularly at risk of renal failure due to the renal accumulation of nephrotoxic antibiotics.[106] In part, such susceptibility is attributable to the decrease in GFR that occurs as part of the normal aging process but is effectively masked by a concomitant decrease in creatinine production.[107] A normal serum creatinine concentration of 1 mg/dL in an octagenarian may in fact reflect a creatinine clearance that is well below 50 mL/min.[107] The seemingly exaggerated decrease in GFR displayed by the senescent kidney in response to volume depletion or congestive heart failure and the need for prolonged antibiotic therapy in many severely ill older patients also probably contribute significantly to the frequency with which aminoglycoside-induced renal failure or renal insufficiency is found in the elderly population. Thus, it is important to adjust the dosage of gentamicin sulfate, tobramycin sulfate, netilmicin sulfate, and amikacin sulfate (and, presumably, new aminoglycosides not yet released for general use) with due regard to age if nephrotoxicity is to be avoided. An empirical formula relating predicted creatinine clearance to serum creatinine concentration and age is widely used[108] such that $C_{cr} = (140 - \text{age})/(72 \times P_{creat}) \times \text{NBW}$ for males, where NBW is normal, nonedematous body weight. The formula is modified to $C_{cr} = (140 - \text{age})/(72 \times P_{creat}) \times 0.85$ NBW for females whose production of creatinine and percent water content are, on average, rather lower than those of males.[107] It is evident that a further volume correction is needed for the body weight term in markedly obese subjects. As mentioned above, moreover, the serum creatinine concentration can be extrapolated to an estimated creatinine clearance only when it is constant. A single measurement of serum creatinine, when applied to the formulas above, may give an erroneous clearance estimate. If there is any reason to suspect a degree of functional renal impairment to be present in a given patient, therefore, the creatinine measurement should be repeated 24 hours after aminoglycoside therapy is started. Preferably a four-hour creatinine clearance measurement can be obtained at the initiation of treatment to give an immediate and quite good approximation of C_{cr} free from the assumption of steady-state conditions. Renal function and serum drug levels should be followed particularly closely in any patient whose body volume, cardiac output, or GFR is subject to question.

There are no specific findings associated with nephrotoxic renal damage that clearly separate this etiology from other causes of depressed renal function. The diagnosis typically is made by inference when impaired filtration is noted to have developed in patients who are receiving potentially nephrotoxic drugs and who have no other evident reason to develop renal failure (see below). The majority of patients with nephrotoxic responses to aminoglycosides actually show only mild to moderate degrees of renal insufficiency that is usually reversible, and even those with serious renal failure may not be oliguric.[48] Patients with classical allergic interstitial nephritis caused by members of the β-lactam group of antibiotics often present with fever, a present with fever, a morbilliform rash, loin or abdominal pain, and arthralgias.[93] Hematuria, varying degrees of proteinuria, pyuria, and eosinophiliuria are commonly associated,[109] and lymphadenopathy may or may not be present.[109] Nonetheless, as demonstrated by the finding of seemingly "silent" interstitial nephritis in various biopsy series,[110,111] these agents may initiate renal failure in certain individuals without such obvious signs. It has also become increasingly apparent that interstitial nephritis due to the nonsteroidal anti-inflammatory drugs most often provides a somewhat different clinical presentation.[99] Here, the findings that typify an allergic reaction (rash, fever, and eosinophilia) generally have been lacking, and neither eosinophiliuria nor hematuria is considered the rule. Marked proteinuria has been a relatively common finding of intolerance to these agents on the other hand, and, indeed, several patients have developed the nephrotic syndrome with or without acute renal failure following the use of nonsteroidal anti-inflammatory agents.[99,112] Older individuals seem to have a particular predilection for allergic interstitial nephritis caused by nonsteroidal anti-inflammatory drugs,[99] perhaps because of the particularly widespread use of such agents in this age group for arthritic symptoms.

Captopril has been considered responsible

for the development of renal dysfunction due to nephrotoxic and idiosyncratic reactions.[113,114] Such cases have been rare, but there is now an increasing literature that incriminates this agent as a cause of frank acute renal failure in patients with either bilateral renal arterial stenosis or renal arterial stenosis of a solitary kidney.[115,116] For the most part, impairment of renal function has been reversed when the agent was withdrawn. The fact that severe renal dysfunction follows the use of captopril far more commonly than other antihypertensive agents argues that it is not the decreased blood pressure per se that impairs the GFR.[115] Rather, angiotensin has been found to exert its intrarenal vasoconstrictor effect preferentially at the efferent arteriole, relaxation of which in a kidney already displaying maximal autoregulatory dilation of the preglomerular vasculature might well reduce effective filtration pressure to a degree that seriously impairs glomerular function.

OBSTRUCTIVE UROPATHY

Obstruction to urinary outflow is a frequent cause of acute renal failure in the hospitalized population. Since lower urinary tract obstruction is readily diagnosable and, once diagnosed, is usually easily treatable, this diagnosis should be pursued promptly in any patient who presents with acute renal failure of unknown etiology. Patients with increased resistance to urinary outflow but who are otherwise compensated may experience full obstruction when ill and put to bed. Others may decompensate after receiving narcotics, sedatives, tricyclic antidepressants, or other anticholinergic medications. On history, the patient may complain of low abdominal discomfort or express an urgent but futile need to void. Total anuria for 24 hours or more, an uncommon finding in vasomotor nephropathy, should raise the possibility of urinary outflow obstruction, as should marked fluctuation in the urine output of patients who are not anuric. A history of prostatic disease, problems with micturition, or carcinoma of the prostate, bladder, cervix, or rectum increases the probability of acute renal failure due to obstruction of the bladder or the ureters. On physical examination, careful percussion and palpation of the abdomen may reveal an enlarged bladder, and a rectal or pelvic examination may reveal the cause of this abnormality. When bladder outflow obstruction is present, the careful insertion of a catheter will not only prove the diagnosis but also serve to relieve that disorder. Drainage may be achieved by suprapubic puncture where catheter insertion is not possible per urethram, but this procedure should be employed in adults only if the bladder is known to be enlarged above the pubic symphysis. While, formerly, it was deemed essential to drain an acutely distended bladder slowly and stepwise to prevent the development of "bladder shock" or bladder hemorrhage, more recent studies have shown that intracystic pressure falls abruptly very soon after the onset of drainage, thus removing the rationale for stepwise decompression.[117] Caution in drainage is to be observed nonetheless.

Ureteral obstruction must either be bilateral or present in a solitary functioning kidney if it is to produce acute renal failure. Ureteral obstruction is not an uncommon sequel to abdominal, and particularly to gynecologic surgery where the ureters might have been traumatized, cut, or inadvertently tied. Ureteral scarring or occlusion with blood clot, fungal bezoars, dislodged papillae, and papillary tumors or peripelvic cysts may present as ureteral obstruction. Stone disease is the predominant cause of ureteral obstruction in young adults. The frequency with which tumor infiltrates the retroperitoneum and its nodes and the occurrence of retroperitoneal fibrosis that may be idiopathic,[118] drug-related,[4] or secondary to an aortic aneurysm,[119] however, change the spectrum considerably in the older age group. One of the few causes of bilateral ureteral occlusion, retroperitoneal disease, produces few symptoms suggestive of urinary outflow obstruction. Renal colic comparable to that seen with renal stones, blood clots, or sloughed papillae is decidedly uncommon,[4] and such pain as is present might be referred to the back or be felt diffusely through the abdomen.[4] Thus, the diagnosis may be missed unless specifically sought with the possibility of covert obstruction in mind.

A plain film of the abdomen may provide a great deal of information in patients with acute renal failure of obscure origin. Acutely hydronephrotic kidneys are apt to be large in size and, if obstruction is due to a radiopaque calculus, that stone can be seen, its size assessed, and the need for surgical intervention determined. Intravenous pyelography may reveal dilated calyces and dilatation of the ureter proximal to the site of obstruction. Renal sonography has proven very useful in the diagnosis of ureteral and pelvoureteral obstruction without subjecting the patient to the risk of the more invasive procedures.[120,121]

ACUTE RENAL FAILURE DUE TO RENAL ARTERIAL OCCLUSION AND ATHEROEMBOLIZATION

Acute renal failure due to primary occlusion of atherosclerotic renal arteries or to embolization from aortic atherosclerotic plaques, is a well-described but infrequently recognized cause of renal failure antemortem.[122] Embolization of atrial or mural thrombi may occur as well. Such embolization of thrombi from the heart occurs particularly during the onset of conversion of atrial fibrillation[123] and in patients with cardiomyopathy or bacterial endocarditis. The possibility of such an event should be entertained particularly if concomitant embolic phenomena involving the brain, viscera, or peripheral arteries are detected in a patient whose renal function deteriorates suddenly. As shown in autopsy studies,[123] the vast majority of cases of renal arterial embolization go unrecognized during life, the diagnosis often being made by serendipity when one or both kidneys that were known to be functioning in the recent past fail to visualize on pyelography, arteriography, or renography.[122] Classically, the diagnosis of acute renal infarction is suggested by the sudden onset of flank or abdominal pain, nausea, vomiting, microscopic or gross hematuria, fever, leukocytosis, and an increase in serum lactate dehydrogenase or transaminase concentrations.[124] Unfortunately, these classical signs are by no means always found. In one large series of patients with acute renal arterial embolism, for example, pain was totally lacking in almost 25% of patients and half of those experiencing any pain at all lacked flank pain. Proteinuria was uniformly present in this series and 15 of the 17 patients had microscopic hematuria.[122] Pain was recorded in only one half of patients in the report of Goldsmith et al.[125] In yet another series, even proteinuria was found in only one third of cases in which arterial embolism was recognized clinically.[125] Thus, this entity may well account for a significant number of cases of acute renal failure in the elderly whose cause is obscure.

Formerly considered universally fatal, cholesterol or atheromatous embolization affects the kidney more often than any other organ.[126,127] The frequency with which renal failure results from atheroembolic disease is unknown, but the marked difference between the clinical incidence and that found at autopsy suggests that this is yet another important cause of "undiagnosed" acute renal failure in the elderly. In the first postmortem study relating atheromatous embolization to acute renal failure, Thurlbeck and Castleman[128] found severe atheromatous embolization to the kidneys of four of 22 patients dying after aortic surgery. Various smaller series of cases were reported subsequently. More in keeping with today's clinical practice, Ramirez et al found significant renal cholesterol embolization in over one fourth of a large group of patients who had died after aortic or coronary arteriography, an incidence far higher than the 4% rate found in a control group matched for age and atheromatous disease.[129] Contrary to older belief, it is now apparent that this disorder is not universally fatal[130,131] and we have seen three patients who have survived renal functional impairment with episodes which fit classically with a diagnosis of atheromatous embolization; the diagnosis was confirmed histologically in two of the three cases (unpublished observation).

Cholesterol emboli released from atheromatous areas of the aorta lodge in any and all more distal tissues, presenting with multiorgan system abnormalities, hypertension, and a clinical picture which has been misdiagnosed as vasculitis or periarteritis nodosa.[132] As in these disorders, moreover, the ESR may be elevated and eosinophilia may be marked.[130] Depending upon the site from which the emboli are discharged, they may provide prominent symptomatology relating to the brain, myocardium, pancreas, intestine, the limbs, digits, or any other tissue. Alternately, occlusion of small vessels in the skin may produce livedo reticularis (a peculiar reddish-blue netlike mottling of the skin of the extremities) or petechial hemorrhages; digital ulcerations or retinal cholesterol deposits lodged at the bifurcations of retinal arterioles ("Hollenhorst plaques") may be the only externally visible evidence for this disorder. Thus, whenever faced with unexplained acute renal failure in the elderly, and particularly if cardioaortic surgery or angiographic procedures have been performed in the recent past, a careful examination of the retina and skin should always be performed. Ultimately, the diagnosis depends upon microscopic examination of tissue, an area of livedo reticularis being particularly likely to provide results as would areas surrounding ulcers of the fingers and toes. Blind biopsy of muscle has at times provided evidence of the needle-shaped cholesterol clefts in small vessels that typify this entity.[130]

URINALYSIS IN THE DIFFERENTIAL DIAGNOSIS OF ACUTE RENAL FAILURE

The urinary characteristics found in functional renal failure, vasomotor nephropathy, glomerular-microvascular diseases and urinary outflow obstruction, tubulo-interstitial diseases and urinary outflow obstruction have proved very valuable as aids in differential diagnosis. Abnormalities of the urinary sediment and significant proteinuria are the hallmarks of acute renal failure due to the microvascular and glomerular groups of diseases, especially when they are so severe as to cause acute renal failure. Red blood cells and RBC casts usually can be found, although casts may be found only after a diligent search in adults with these disorders. It is noteworthy that atheromatous embolic disease typically presents with proteinuria but usually lacks the sedimentary change expected in other forms of microvascular disease involving the kidney.[130] Leukocyturia and WBC casts, often with significant numbers of eosinophils found on Wright staining of the urine sediment, typify allergic interstitial nephritis related to the β-lactam antibiotics, but such a sedimentary change is seen far less commonly in patients with interstitial nephritis due to the nonsteriodal antiinflammatory agents (see above). Proteinuria is usually moderate in degree in classical interstitial nephritis but may be far more prominent and even produce the nephrotic syndrome when interstitial nephritis follows the use of the anti-inflammatory drugs.[99] Unless superimposed on pre-existing chronic renal disease, functional renal failure presents no distinctive urinary sedimentary change and produces scant proteinuria except in subjects with congestive heart failure or a high fever. Obstructive uropathy may or may not be attended by hematuria depending upon the rate at which bladder or renal calyceal distention develops. Red blood cell casts are not an expected finding, however, and, in contrast with the hematuria of glomerular-microvascular disease, the morphology of most of the erythrocytes excreted is not abnormal.[133] Leukocytes and leukocyte casts may be present if obstruction is complicated by secondary infection or if the obstruction is inflammatory in origin. Obstruction due to retroperitoneal fibrosis usually provides no distinctive abnormality of the urinary sediment[4] although a moderate degree of proteinuria may be found.

Examination of the urinary concentrations of sodium, urea, and creatinine relative to those in plasma and the urine/plasma osmolality (U/P_{osm}) ratio has proved extremely useful in differentiating between vasomotor nephropathy and functional renal failure. Thus, with tubular injury, the kidney of patients with vasomotor nephropathy usually can neither maximally conserve sodium nor form a concentrated urine regardless of the volume status.[134] As a result, the urinary sodium concentration usually is between 30 and 90 mEq/L and the U/P_{osm} ratio is very close to 1.0. As a further indication of impaired concentrating capacity, the U/P creatinine ration (U/P_{creat}) is predictably below 15 (usually <10.0).[135] By contrast, the healthy young kidney with functional renal insufficiency will concentrate the urine to provide a U/P_{osm} ratio significantly greater than 2.0, will maximally retain sodium to provide a urinary concentration far below 10 mEq/L, and exhibit a U/P_{creat} ratio considerably higher than 20. Unfortunately, the urinary features separating functional renal failure from vasomotor nephropathy may become blurred in elderly patients and in younger patients with underlying chronic parenchymal renal disease who, although volume-depleted, may not be able to maximally conserve sodium or adequately concentrate their urine. Accordingly, more definitive diagnostic indicators have been sought in recent years. Handa and Morrin[136] proposed the renal failure index (RFI) as a superior diagnostic indicator separating functional renal failure from VMN. This index is calculated as: $RFI = [U_{Na}/(U/P_{creat})] \times 100$. The fractional excretion of sodium (FE_{Na}) is a modification of the renal failure index in which the U/P sodium concentration ratio (U/P_{Na}), is substituted for the urinary sodium concentration value, so that: FE_{Na} equals $[U/P_{Na}/(U/P_{creat})] \times 100$. With the degree of variation in serum sodium concentration generally encountered, the two indicators give results that are little different in their diagnostic significance. A fractional excretion of sodium below 1% effectively rules out the possibility of vasomotor nephropathy, reflecting a well-retained capacity to conserve sodium and concentrate the urine. Such a value also is found in many patients with vascular, glomerular and microvascular diseases of the kidney, however, so that it is not an absolute indicator of functional renal failure per se.[135] FE_{Na} values between 1% and 3% are considered indeterminate by Miller et al[137] but indicative of vasomotor nephropathy by Espinel and Gregory[138] if alternate causes of renal failure are not obviously present. In our experience, most patients with a clinical presentation that is typical of VMN in every way have had a fractional excretion of sodium of 5% or higher, although many have exhibited an FE_{Na} between 3% and 5%. A small minority have shown values between 1% and 2%, but these lowest figures have most often been obtained in cases where, on the basis of the overall clinical presentation, the diagnosis of vasomotor nephropathy has been less than certain. Very notably, some renal failure patients who clearly did not have VMN have shown marked random fluctuations in FE_{Na} within the same day or on succeeding days while not receiving diuretics or major changes in fluid therapy, some values being below 1% and others greater than 3%. Furthermore, many individuals with acute interstitial nephritis, obstructive uropathy, functional renal failure superimposed on chronic renal insufficiency or nephrosclerosis, or glomerular diseases with a prominent component of tubular injury may present with the same U_{Na}, U/P_{creat}, U/P_{osm}, and FE_{Na} found in vasomotor nephropathy; some others have values intermediate between those of functional renal failure and VMN. Thus, while the urinary characteristics may be a very useful adjunct to ruling out VMN, they cannot be used to "prove" that diagnosis. Rather, accurate diagnosis requires an integrated approach utilizing all the available information on history, physical examination, laboratory values, urinalysis, and clinical course.

Certain sources of error must be avoided when using the fractional excretion of sodium or the U_{Na} and U/P_{creat} in differential diagnosis. First, it is important to be sure that the patient has not received diuretics in the 12 hours preceding urine collection since these agents would be expected to inappropriately increase urinary sodium concentration and decrease the urinary osmolality even in subjects with marked volume depletion. The same reservation applies if the patient is experiencing a brisk osmotic diuresis because of either glycosuria or the prior administration of mannitol or radiographic contrast media. In addition, the urine obtained immediately after the admission of a severely oliguric patient to a hospital may have been formed 12, 24, or even 48 hours earlier and at a time before VMN became superimposed on functional renal failure. Thus, while the sedimentary findings of a first voided sample may be very revealing, the remainder of the examination should be accepted only with reservations. Lastly, if the patient has an indwelling catheter, it is important to ensure that the bladder has not been rinsed with saline or distilled water, the presence of either of which could greatly distort the characteristics of the urine obtained subsequently.

REFERENCES

1. Brown BB, Cameron JS, Ogg CS, et al: Established acute renal failure following surgical operations, in Friedman EA, Eliahou HE (eds): *Proc Conf on Acute Renal Failure.* US Dept of Health, Education, and Welfare publication no. (NIH) 74–608, 1973, pp 187–201.
2. Kleinknecht D, Ganeval D: Preventive hemodialysis in acute renal failure. Its effect on mortality and morbidity, in Friedman EA, Eliahou HE (eds): *Proc Conf on Acute Renal Failure.* US Dept of Health, Education, and Welfare publication no. (NIH) 74–608, 1973, pp 165–184.
3. Lane AZ, Wright GE, Blair DC: Ototoxicity and nephrotoxicity of amikacin. *Am J Med* 1977;62:911–918.
4. Graham JR, Suby HI, LeCompte PR, et al: Fibrotic disorders associated with methysergide therapy for headache. *N Engl J Med* 1966;274:359–368.
5. Oken DE: Chronic renal diseases and pregnancy. A review. *Am J Obstet Gynecol* 1966;94:1023–1043.
6. Dalgaard OZ: Bilateral polycystic disease of the kidneys: A follow-up of 284 patients and their families. *Acta Med Scand* 1957;158:1–255.
7. Blantz RC: Effect of mannitol on glomerular ultrafiltration in the hydropenic rat. *J Clin Invest* 1974;54:1135–1143.
8. Navar LG, Bell PD, White RW, et al: Evaluation of the single nephron glomerular filtration coefficient in the dog. *Kidney Int* 1977;12:137–149.
9. Vintrup B: On the number, shape, structure, and surface area of the glomeruli in the kidneys of man and mammals. *Am J Anat* 1928;41:123–151.
10. Wesson LG: *The Physiology of the Human Kidney.* New York, Grune & Stratton, 1969, p 90.
11. Munck O: *Renal Circulation in Acute Renal Failure.* Oxford, Blackwell Scientific Publications, 1958.
12. Oken DE, Thomas SR, Mikulecky DC: A network thermodynamic model of glomerular dynamics: Application in the rat. *Kidney Int* 1981;19:359–373.
13. Oken DE: An analysis of glomerular dynamics in rat, dog, and man. *Kidney Int* 1982;22:136–145.
14. Oken DE: Theoretical analysis of pathogenetic mechanisms in experimental acute renal failure. *Kidney Int* 1983;24:16–26.
15. Brun C, Crone C, Davidsen HG, et al:

Renal interstitial pressure in normal and in anuric man: based on wedged renal vein pressure. *Proc Soc Exp Biol Med* 1956; 91:199–202.
16. Willassen Y, Ofstad J: Postglomerular vascular hydrostatic and oncotic pressures during acute saline volume expansion in normotensive man. *Scand J Clin Lab Invest* 1979;39:707–715.
17. Brenner BM, Troy JL, Daugharty TM, et al: Dynamics of glomerular ultrafiltration in the rat: II. Plasma flow dependence of GFR. *Am J Physiol* 1972;223:1184–1190.
18. Baylis C, Rennke HR, Brenner BM: Mechanisms of the defect in glomerular ultrafiltration associated with gentamicin administration. *Kidney Int* 1977;12:344–353.
19. Arendshorst WJ, Gottschalk CW: Glomerular ultrafiltration dynamics: Euvolemic and plasma volume-expanded rats. *Am J Physiol* 1980;239:F131–F186.
20. Källskog O, Lindbon LO, Ulfendahl HR, et al: Kinetics of glomerular ultrafiltration in the rat kidney. An experimental study. *Acta Physiol Scand* 1975;95: 293–300.
21. DiBona GF, Rios LL: Mechanism of exaggerated diuresis in spontaneously hypertensive rats. *Am J Physiol* 1978;235: F409–F416.
22. Wardle EN: Intravascular coagulation in experimental acute renal failure. Assessment by radio-fibrinogen technique. *Thromb Haemost* 1973;29:579–591.
23. Flores J, DiBona DR, Beck CH, et al: The role of cell swelling in ischemic tissue damage and the protective effect of hypertonic solute. *J Clin Invest* 1972;51:118–126.
24. McLachlan MSF, Davies RL, Leach KG: Diatrizoate levels in the kidney and lymph nodes in acute renal failure in the rat. *Nephron* 1974;13:443–454.
25. Solez K, Morel-Maroger L, Sraer JD: The morphology of "acute tubular necrosis" in man: Analysis of 57 renal biopsies and a comparison with the glycerol model. *Medicine* 1979;58:362–376.
26. Finckh ES, Jeremy D, Whyte HM: Structural renal damage and its relation to clinical features in acute oliguric renal failure. *Q J Med* 1962;31:429–446.
27. Sevitt S: Pathogenesis of traumatic uremia: A revised concept. *Lancet* 1959;2: 135–140.
28. Dalgaard OZ, Pedersen KJ: Renal tubular degeneration: Electron microscopy in ischaemic anuria. *Lancet* 1959;2:484–488.
29. Olsen TS: Ultrastructure of the renal tubules in acute renal insufficiency. *Acta Pathol Microbiol Scand [A]* 1967;71: 203–218.
30. Bohle A: Pathologische Anatomie des akuten Nierenversagens. *Verh Dtsch Ges Pathol* 1965;49:54–66.
31. Solez K, Morel-Maroger L, Sraer JD: The morphology of "acute tubular necrosis" in man: Analysis of 57 renal biopsies and comparison with the glycerol model. *Medicine* 1979;58:362–376.
32. Oken DE: Modern concepts of the role of nephrotoxic agents in the pathogenesis of acute renal failure. *Prog Biochem Pharmacol* 1972;7:219–247.
33. Olsen TS, Skjoldborg H: The fine structure of the renal glomerulus in acute anuria. *Acta Pathol Microbiol Scand* 1967;70: 205–214.
34. Levin ML, Simon NM, Herdson PB, et al: Acute renal failure followed by protracted, slowly resolving chronic uremia. *J Chronic Dis* 1972;25:645–651.
35. Oken DE: Pathogenetic mechanisms in acute renal failure, in Hook JB (ed): *Toxicology of the Kidney.* New York, Raven Press, 1981, pp 117–134.
36. Flamenbaum W: Pathophysiology of acute renal failure. *Arch Intern Med* 1973;131: 911–928.
37. Stein JH, Lifschitz MD, Barnes LD: Current concepts on the pathophysiology of acute renal failure. *Am J Physiol* 1978; 234:F171–F181.
38. Hollenberg NK, Adams DF, Oken DE, et al: Acute renal failure due to nephrotoxins: Renal hemodynamic and angiographic studies in man. *N Engl J Med* 1970;282: 1329–1334.
39. Reubi FC: The pathogenesis of anuria following shock. *Kidney Int* 1974;5:106–110.
40. Shaldon S, Rae AI, Rosen SM, et al: Renal circulation in acute renal failure, in Shaldon S, Cook C (eds): *Acute Renal Failure.* Oxford, Blackwell, 1964.
41. Hollenberg WK, Epstein M, Rosen SM, et al: Acute oliguric renal failure in man: Evidence for preferential renal cortical

ischemia. *Medicine* 1968;47:455–470.

42. Bricker NS: On the meaning of the intact nephron hypothesis. *Am J Med* 1969;46: 1–4.
43. Jensen JT: Renal angiography in acute anuria. *Scand J Urol Nephrol* 1981;S57: 19–26.
44. Hollenberg NK, Sandor T, Conroy M, et al: The transit of radioxenon through the oliguric human kidney: analysis by the method of maximum likelihood. *Kidney Int* 1973;3:177–185.
45. Ladefoged J, Winkler K: Hemodynamics in acute renal failure. The effect of hypotension induced by dihydralazine on renal blood flow, mean circulation time for plasma, and renal vascular volume in patients with acute oliguric renal failure. *Scand J Clin Lab Invest* 1970;26:83–87.
46. Edwards RM: Segmental effects of norepinephrine and angiotensin II on isolated renal microvessels. *Am J Physiol* 1983; 244:F526–F534.
47. Myers BD, Chui F, Hilberman M, et al: Transtubular leakage of glomerular filtrate in human acute renal failure. *Am J Physiol* 1979;6:F319–F325.
48. Anderson RJ, Linas SL, Berns AS, et al: Nonoliguric acute renal failure. *N Engl J Med* 1977;296:1134–1138.
49. Bhat JG, Gluck MC, Lowenstein J, et al: Renal failure after open heart surgery. *Ann Int Med* 1976;84:677–682.
50. Hilberman M, Myers BD, Carrie BJ, et al: Acute renal failure following cardiac surgery. *J Thorac Cardiovasc Surg* 1979;77: 881–888.
51. Powers S, Boba A, Stein A: The mechanism and prevention of distal tubular necrosis following aneurysmectomy. *Surgery* 1957;42:156–162.
52. Kountz SL, Tuttle KL, Cohn LH, et al: Factors responsible for acute tubular necrosis following lower aortic surgery. *JAMA* 1963;183:447–451.
53. Plaut ME, Schentag JJ, Jusko WJ: Aminoglycoside nephrotoxicity. Comparative assessment in critically ill patients. *Medicine* 1979;10:257–266.
54. Brater DC: Pharmacodynamic considerations in the use of diuretics. *Annu Rev Pharmacol Toxicol* 1983;23:45–62.
55. Chennavasin P, Seiwell R, Brater DC, et al: Pharmacodynamic analysis of the furosemide-probenecid interaction in man. *Kidney Int* 1979;16:187–195.
56. Hamilton RW, Gardner LB, Penn AS, et al: Acute tubular necrosis by exercise-induced myoglobinuria. *Ann Intern Med* 1972;77: 77–82.
57. Fuss M, Bagon J, Dupont E, et al: Parathyroid hormone and calcium blood levels in acute renal failure: With special reference to one patient developing transient hypercalcemia. *Nephron* 1978;20: 196–202.
58. Montgomerie JZ, Kalmanson GM, Guze LB: Renal failure and infection. *Medicine* 1968;47:1–32.
59. Dobbelstein H: Immune system in uremia. *Nephron* 1976;17:409–414.
60. Maher JF, Schreiner GE: Cause of death in acute renal failure. *Arch Intern Med* 1962;110:493–504.
61. Smits H, Freedman LR: Prolonged venous catheterization as a cause of sepsis. *N Engl J Med* 1967;276:1229–1233.
62. Wacker W, Merrill JP: Uremic pericarditis in acute and chronic renal failure. *JAMA* 1954;145:764–765.
63. Tyler HR: Neurological complications of acute and chronic renal failure, in Merrill JP (ed): *The Treatment of Renal Failure.* New York, Grune & Stratton, 1965, pp 315–337.
64. Eliahou HE, Modan B, Leslau V, et al: Acute renal failure in the community; an epidemiological study, in Friedman EA, Eliahou HE (eds): *Proc Conf on Acute Renal Failure,* US Dept of Health, Education, and Welfare publication no. (NIH) 74-608, 1973, pp 143–158.
65. Balch HH: The effect of severe battle injury and of post-traumatic renal failure on resistance to infection. *Ann Surg* 1955; 142:145–163.
66. Abbott WM, Abel RM, Beck CH, et al: Renal failure after ruptured aneurysm. *Arch Surg* 1975;110:1110–1112.
67. Baird RJ, Gurry JF, Kellam JF, et al: Abdominal aortic aneurysms: recent experience with 210 patients. *Can Med Assoc J* 1978;118:1229–1235.
68. Oken DE: Nosologic considerations in the nomenclature of acute renal failure. *Nephron* 1971;8:505–510.
69. Fine LG, Eliahou HE: Acute oliguric intrinsic renal failure: Diagnostic criteria and clinical features in 61 patients. *Isr J*

Med Sci 1969;5:1024–1031.
70. Brun CE, Knudsen OE, Raa Schou F: Influence of posture of kidney function; glomerular dynamics in passive erect position. *Acta Med Scand* 1945;122:332–341.
71. Miller PD, Krebs RA, Neal BJ, et al: Hypodipsia in geriatric patients. *Am J Med* 1982;73:354–356.
72. DeRubertis F, Michelis M, Beck N, et al: Essential hypernatremia due to ineffective osmotic and intact volume regulation of vasopressin secretion. *J Clin Invest* 1976; 50:97–111.
73. Baek S, Makabali GG, Bryan-Brown CW, et al: Plasma expansion in surgical patients with high central venous pressure (CVP); the relationship of blood volume to hematocrit, CVP, pulmonary wedge pressure, and cardiorespiratory changes. *Surgery* 1975;78:304–315.
74. Oken DE: Diagnosis and treatment of acute renal failure. *Mod Treat* 1969;6: 927–951.
75. Kerr DNS: Acute renal failure, in Black DAK (ed): *Renal Disease.* Oxford, Blackwell, 1972, p 452.
76. Loening S, Carson CC, Faxon DP, et al: Ureteral obstruction from Hodgkin's disease. *J Urology* 1974;111:345–349.
77. Geller SA, Lin C-S: Ureteral obstruction from metastatic breast carcinoma. *Arch Pathol* 1975;99:476–478.
78. Perrin J, Mousselon J, Bonnet P: Tumeurs secondaires de l'uretère. *J Urol Nephrol* 1964;70:381–385.
79. Lundberg WB, Cadman ED, Finch SC, et al: Renal failure secondary to leukemic infiltration of the kidneys. *Am J Med* 1977;62:636–642.
80. Reem GH, Vanamee P: Electrolyte disturbances associated with cancer. *J Chronic Dis* 1963;16:737–755.
81. Madias NE, Harrington JT: Platinum nephrotoxicity. *Am J Med* 1978;65:307–314.
82. Hall-Craggs M, Brenner DE, Vigorito RD, et al: Acute renal failure and renal tubular squamous metaplasia following treatment with streptozotocin. *Hum Pathol* 1982;13: 597–601.
83. Von Hoff DD, Penta JS, Helman LJ, et al: Incidence of drug-related deaths secondary to high-dose methotrexate and citrovorum factor administration. *Cancer Treat Rep* 1977;61:745–748.
84. Ultmann JE: Hyperuricemia in disseminated neoplastic disease other than lymphomas and leukemias. *Cancer* 1962;15: 122–129.
85. Pascal RR: Renal manifestations of extrarenal neoplasms. *Hum Pathol* 1980;11:7–17.
86. Kanwar YS, Manaligod JR: Leukemic urate nephropathy. *Arch Pathol* 1975;9: 467–472.
87. Kjellstrand CM, Campbell DC, Hartitizsch B, et al: Hyperuricemic acute renal failure. *Arch Intern Med* 1974;133:349–359.
88. DeFronzo FA, Humphrey RL, Wright JR, et al: Acute renal failure in multiple myeloma. *Medicine* 1975;54:209–223.
89. Koss MN, Pirani CL, Osserman EL: Experimental Bence Jones cast nephropathy. *Lab Invest* 1976;34:579–591.
90. Booth LJ, Smith EKM: Acute renal failure in multiple myeloma. *Can Med Assoc J* 1974;111:334–335.
91. Border WA, Cohen AH: Renal biopsy diagnosis of clinically silent multiple myeloma. *Ann Intern Med* 1980;93:43–46.
92. Myers GH, Whitten DM: Acute renal failure after excretory urography in multiple myeloma. *Am J Roentgenol Radiat Ther Nucl Med* 1971;113:583–588.
93. Appel GB, Neu HC: The nephrotoxicity of antimicrobial agents. *N Engl J Med* 1977; 296:663–670 and 722–728 and 784–787.
94. Girard J-P: Allergic reactions to antibiotics. *Helv Med Acta* 1972;36:3–22.
95. Grattan WA: Hematuria and azotemia associated with administration of methicillin. *J Pediatr* 1964;64:285–287.
96. Linton AL, Clark WF, Drieger AA, et al: Acute interstitial nephritis due to drugs. *Ann Intern Med* 1980;93:735–741.
97. Nessi R, Bonoldi GL, Redaelli B, et al: Acute renal failure after rifampicin: a case report and survey of the literature. *Nephron* 1976;16:148–159.
98. Gary NE, Dodelson R, Eisinger RP: Indomethacin-associated acute renal failure. *Am J Med* 1980;69:135–136.
99. Regester RF: The nephrotic syndrome and renal failure associated with use of nonsteroidal antiinflammatory drugs. *J Tenn Med Assoc* 1980;63:709–711.
100. Chatterjee GP: Nephrotic syndrome induced by tolmetin. *JAMA* 1981;246:1589.
101. Rudnick MR, Bastl CP, Elfenbein IB, et al: Cimetidine-induced acute renal failure.

Ann Intern Med 1982;96:180–182.
102. Agarwal BN, Cabebe FG, Hoffman BI: Diphenylhydantoin-induced acute renal failure. *Nephron* 1977;18:249–251.
103. Gelbart DR, Weinstein AB, Fajardo LF: Allopurinol-induced interstitial nephritis. *Ann Intern Med* 1977;86:196–198.
104. Bennett WM: Hazards of the appetite suppressant phenylpropanolamine. *Lancet* 1979;2:42–43.
105. Mullick FG, McAllister HA Jr, Wagner BM, et al: Drug-related vasculitis: clinicopathologic correlations in 30 patients. *Hum Pathol* 1979;10:313–318.
106. Cronin RE: Aminoglycoside nephrotoxicity: Pathogenesis and prevention. *Clin Nephrol* 1979;11:251–256.
107. Kampmann JP, Hansen M: Glomerular filtration rate and creatinine clearance. *Br J Clin Pharmacol* 1981;12:7–14.
108. Crockroft DW, Gault MH: Prediction of creatinine clearance from serum creatinine. *Nephron* 1976;16:31–41.
109. Burton JR, Lichtenstein NS, Colvin RB, et al: Acute renal failure during cephalothin therapy. *JAMA* 1974;229:679–682.
110. Olsen S, Asklund M: Interstitial nephritis with acute renal failure following cardiac surgery and treatment with methicillin. *Acta Med Scand* 1976;199:305–310.
111. Kleinknecht D, Kanfer A, Morel-Maroger L, et al: Immunologically mediated drug-induced acute renal failure. *Contrib Nephrol* 1978;10:42–52.
112. Brezin JH, Katz SM, Schwartz AB, et al: Reversible renal failure and nephrotic syndrome associated with non-steroidal anti-inflammatory drugs. *N Engl J Med* 1979; 301:1271–1273.
113. Textor SC, Gephardt GN, Bravo EL, et al: Membranous glomerulopathy associated with captopril therapy. *Am J Med* 1983; 74:705–712.
114. Chrysant SG, Dunn M, Marples D, et al: Severe reversible azotemia from captopril therapy: Report of three cases and review of the literature. *Arch Intern Med* 1983; 143:437–441.
115. Hricik DE, Browning PJ, Kopelman R, et al: Captopril-induced functional renal insufficiency in patients with bilateral renal-artery stenoses or renal-artery stenosis in a solitary kidney. *N Engl J Med* 1983; 308:373–376.
116. Curtis JJ, Luke RG, Whelchel JD, et al: Inhibition of angiotensin-coverting enzyme in renal-transplant recipients with hypertension. *N Engl J Med* 1983;308:377–381.
117. Osius TG, Hinman F: Dynamics of acute urinary retention: a manometric, radiographic and clinical study. *J Urol* 1963; 90:702–712.
118. Lepor H, Walsh PC: Idiopathic retroperitoneal fibrosis. *J Urol* 1979;122:1–6.
119. Charnock DA, Riddell HI, Lombardo LJ: Retroperitoneal fibrosis producing ureteral obstruction. *J Urol* 1961;85:251–257.
120. Sanders RC: Renal ultrasound. *Radiol Clin North Am* 1975;13:417–434.
121. Bosniak MA, Schweizer RD: Urographic findings in patients with renal failure. *Radiol Clin North Am* 1972;10:433–445.
122. Lessman RK, Johnson SF, Coburn JW, et al: Renal artery embolism: Clinical features and long-term follow-up of 17 cases. *Ann Intern Med* 1978;477–482.
123. Hoxie JH, Coggin CB: Renal infarction: Statistical study of two hundred and five cases and detailed report of an unusual case. *Arch Intern Med* 1940;65:587–594.
124. Regan FC, Crabtree EG: Renal infarction: a clinical and possible surgical entity. *J Urol* 1948;59:981–1018.
125. Goldsmith EI, Fuller FW, Lambrew CT, et al: Embolectomy of the renal artery. *J Urol* 1968;99:366–370.
126. Peterson NE, McDonald DF: Renal embolization. *J Urol* 1968;100:140–145.
127. Kassirer JP: Atheroembolic renal disease, in Strauss MB and Welt LG (eds): *Diseases of the Kidney.* Boston, Little, Brown & Co, 1971, pp 1039–1048.
128. Thurlbeck WM, Castleman B: Atheromatous emboli to the kidneys after aortic surgery. *N Engl J Med* 1957;257:442–447.
129. Ramirez G, O'Neill WM, Lambert R, et al: Cholesterol embolization, a complication of angiography. *Arch Intern Med* 1978; 138:1430–1432.
130. Smith MC, Ghose MK, Henry AR: The clinical spectrum of renal cholesterol embolization. *Am J Med* 1981;71:174–180.
131. Ho SW-C, Thatcher GN, Matz LR: Reversible renal failure due to renal cholesterol embolism. *Aust N Z J Med* 1982;12:531–533.
132. Richards AM, Eliot RS, Kanjuh VI, et al: Cholesterol embolism, a multiple system

disease masquerading as polyarteritis nodosa. *Am J Cardiol* 1972;15:696–707.

133. Birch DF, Fairley KF: Haematuria: glomerular or non-glomerular? *Lancet* 1979; 2:845–846.
134. Eliahou HE, Bata A: The diagnosis of acute renal failure. *Nephron* 1965;2: 287–295.
135. Oken DE: On the differential diagnosis of acute renal failure. *Am J Med* 1981;71: 916–920.
136. Handa SP, Morrin PAF: Diagnostic indices in acute renal failure. *Can Med Assoc J* 1967;96:78–82.
137. Miller TR, Anderson RJ, Linas SL, et al: Urinary diagnostic indices in acute renal failure. A prospective study. *Ann Intern Med* 1978;89:47–50.
138. Espinel CH, Gregory AW: Differential diagnosis of acute renal failure. *Clin Nephrol* 1980;13:73–77.

CHAPTER 7 Chronic Renal Failure in the Elderly: Diabetic Renal Disease in the Elderly

Jesse E. Hano

CHRONIC RENAL FAILURE

The functional and anatomical changes that occur in the aging kidney are in a sense a model of slowly progressive renal insufficiency; however, the loss of renal function is not clinically apparent and residual renal function is usually adequate. That there is a decrease in "renal reserve" in the elderly has been generally recognized, but the clinical characteristics and epidemiology of those individuals who develop chronic renal failure have not been delineated adequately. Few longitudinal studies characterizing the development of renal failure in a community are available. One such study in the United States examined 8641 people over an 8-year period, during which time 14 (0.2%) developed renal failure.[1] Of the 471 people 65 years of age or older, eight (1.7%) developed renal failure, whereas only six (0.8%) of the remaining 8170 under age 65 did so. This relationship of increasing renal failure with age is further amplified by the fact that 86.6% of those developing renal failure were over age 45. Similarly, the majority of patients with renal failure were over the age of 50 in reports from Scotland, Northern Ireland, Wales, and Finland.[2–5] Although some studies excluded candidates over 50 years of age, virtually all noted an increased mortality from renal failure with advancing age.[6–8]

Population studies have not determined whether the gradual loss of renal function with age is related to an increase in renal disease in the elderly or simply "senescent kidneys" affected by other adverse factors. In the 14 cases cited previously the initial examination 1 to 8 years prior to the diagnosis of renal failure did not yield a history of acute or chronic renal disease, although approximately 21% had proteinuria detected upon entrance into the study.[1] Other associations included congestive heart failure, coronary artery disease, hyperglycemia, hyperuricemia, and hypacusis. It seems unlikely that the latter finding is related to hereditary nephritis in this age group, and most likely represents otosclerosis from vascular disease and/or the effects of aminoglycoside antibiotics and loop diuretic usage. An increased frequency of urinary tract infection was noted in the group who developed renal failure,[1] and others have noted this to be an increasing association with death in the elderly.[7,9] However, it must be stated that most patients with a past history of urinary tract infection do not develop chronic renal failure. Interpretation of the above studies is hampered by the lack of a precise histologic diagnosis of the renal disease.

More recently renal biopsy data has been obtained from patients who presented with renal disease after 60 and up to 84 years of age.[10] In this study known systemic diseases such as diabetes mellitus and amyloidosis were excluded, and an adequate renal biopsy was required for inclusion in the protocol. Therefore, while the accuracy of the diagnosis of the renal disease was markedly improved, the patients studied may not be representative of the incidence of specific renal diseases in the elderly. Table 7-1 indicates the renal biopsy diagnosis and compares the incidence of acute and chronic renal failure in 115 patients.[10] Only 14 patients (12%) had chronic renal failure at initial presentation, and six of these, or 48% of the chronic renal failure group, had glomerulosclerosis. Further analysis of data presented in the text[10] indicated that an additional 19 patients from the acute renal failure category developed progressive renal insufficiency (Table 7-1). Thus, approximately 30% of all these patients sustained chronic renal failure over the 8 years of the study. Idiopathic crescentic glomerulonephritis accounted for the majority of progressive loss of renal function, and its overall incidence of 16.5% was about four times that seen in patients less than 60 years of age.[10] This unusually high incidence of rapidly progressive glomerulonephritis as well as the large numbers of elderly in other series[11–14] suggests that the aged may be prone to develop this entity. While it was not possible to track all of the patients from this report, it is clear that the most frequent causes of chronic renal failure included glomerulonephritis, glomerulosclerosis, and vasculitis (Table 7-1).

In contrast to the above results are the findings of a prospective survey to ascertain the number of patients with chronic renal failure who might benefit from renal replacement therapy.[3] The causes of renal failure in the over-60 age group are listed in Table 7-2. Renal failure was equally distributed between the sexes, but the causes were of somewhat different frequencies. Pyelonephritis was the most frequent diagnosis and occurred more commonly in females, whereas obstruction predominated in males and was the third most frequent cause of chronic renal failure. Nephrosclerosis and glomerulonephritis together with the two previous diagnoses accounted for more than 60% of the causes of renal failure in the elderly in this survey. Although the previously cited clinicopathologic study[10] and this survey are not comparable they do provide insight into the most common causes of chronic renal insufficiency in the elderly.

Obstructive uropathy, an exceedingly common disorder in the elderly, may present with varying degrees of renal insufficiency and may be of either acute or chronic onset. The incidence of benign prostatic

Table 7-1
Comparative Incidence of Acute and Chronic Renal Failure in Elderly Patients

Renal Biopsy Diagnosis	Total Patients	Acute Renal Failure (<2 months)	Chronic Renal Failure (>2 months)	Progressive Renal Failure
Idiopathic crescentic glomerulonephritis	19	17	2	11
Membranous glomerulopathy	15	–	–	2 died after renal failure; others had variable renal function
Minimal change nephrotic syndrome	9	–	–	–
Focal proliferative glomerulonephritis	7	1	–	–
Diffuse proliferative glomerulonephritis	5	4	1	–
Chronic glomerulonephritis	5	1	1	–
Membranoproliferative glomerulonephritis	2	–	–	2
Glomerulosclerosis	1	6	–	–
Vasculitis	6	3	–	1
Amyloidosis	5	2	–	–
Wegener's granulomatosis	4	4	–	3 variable
Interstitial nephritis	4	2	2	–

Data derived from Moorthy and Zimmerman.[10]

Table 7-2
Causes of Chronic Renal Failure in Patients over 60 Years of Age

Diagnosis	Incidence (%)	No. of Patients *Males*	*Females*	*Total*
Pyelonephritis	19.7	7	17	24
Nephrosclerosis	16.4	9	11	20
Postrenal causes	14.7	16	2	18
Glomerulonephritis	10.6	8	5	13
Urolithiasis	5.7	2	5	7
Polycystic disease	2.5	3	0	3
Diabetes mellitus	2.5	0	3	3
Collagen disease	0.8	0	1	1
Miscellaneous	0.8	1	0	1
Unknown	26.2	16	16	32
Totals		62	60	122

Data derived from McGeown.[3]

hypertrophy accounts for obstructive renal disease so commonplace in older men, and is attended by impaired renal function in 15% at the time of hospital admission.[15] Other studies of prostatism with chronic urinary obstruction have shown the glomerular filtration rate and renal plasma flow to be reduced to about two-thirds of the expected values for normal 60-year-old men.[16] Renal function was diminished further by the presence of infection. In a small proportion of patients presenting with uremia associated with prostatic obstruction, progressive renal insufficiency ensues despite relief of the obstruction.[15] This was observed in approximately 10% of such patients in another series.[17] Other causes of obstruction in the elderly included neurogenic bladder, carcinoma of the bladder, ureters, or other pelvic structures, calculi, blood clots, uterine prolapse, and retroperitoneal fibrosis.[18–21] While obstructive uropathy in the elderly may present in the classic manner with periods of anuria alternating with polyuria or with the polyuria of partial obstruction, progressive renal damage due to obstruction may not be associated with any of the usual symptoms.[22]

Multiple myeloma, a disease of the older population, has been associated with renal failure in about 55% of the patients[23]; chronic renal failure occurs commonly and generally carries a grave prognosis.[24] In a recent series of 24 patients presenting with severe renal failure with multiple myeloma, two thirds were over the age of 60, and only one had normal kidney function at the time of diagnosis only to develop renal failure later.[25] The diagnosis of renal insufficiency often precedes the diagnosis of multiple myeloma, and occasionally the diagnosis of myeloma may be established first by kidney biopsy.[26] In addition several patients received hemodialysis before myeloma was diagnosed. Patients may also present as acute renal failure in the absence of any precipitating or preexisting conditions (eg, known renal disease, nephrotoxic antibiotics, contrast media), and under these circumstances renal function is seldom regained.[27] Renal biopsy usually shows "myeloma kidney" characterized by tubular atrophy and precipitation of Bence Jones protein casts in the tubular lumen. Amyloid deposition is noted in about 25% of the biopsy and autopsy material.[25] Plasma cell infiltration may also be seen. Other factors such as nephrocalcinosis and hyperuricosuria may contribute to the renal damage, but renal failure in myeloma correlates with light chain disease and the presence of Bence Jones proteinuria.[28] Light chain toxicity to the tubules[29] and their intratubular precipitation[30] probably are the major causes of renal failure in myeloma.

Patients with light chain disease fail to regain renal function,[25] and renal failure remains the single most ominous prognostic factor in this disease. Despite this, if one prevents death from uremia in the myeloma patient by providing dialysis, the prognosis for the dialyzed group is similar to the myeloma patient without renal insufficiency. Survival at 1 year for myeloma patients on dialysis was 53% as compared to 66% in those not requiring chronic dialysis.[25] Therefore, chronic dialysis if indicated should not be withheld from the myeloma patient with renal failure. Furthermore, an occasional patient may be able to discontinue dialysis.[25,31]

Amyloidosis commonly presents as the nephrotic syndrome and is usually a complication of a systemic illness such as myeloma. Chronic renal failure represents a minority initial presentation of this disease. Primary amyloidosis of the kidney occurs predominantly in people over 60 years of age, and although its usual presentation is nephrotic syndrome, a small number are initially uremic. The diagnosis is usually established by renal biopsy, since there are few clues to the diagnosis other than heavy proteinuria. Some investigators report that 20% of their nephrotic patients over age 50 have primary renal amyloidosis.[32] Chronic renal failure usually appears late in the illness in the majority of patients and treatment appears to be of little value. Mortality ranges from 50% to 70% at 1 year with few long-time survivors on dialysis.[32,33]

Atheromatous renovascular disease occurs most often in the elderly and may present as atheromatous emboli or renal artery occlusion associated with renal insufficiency. A diagnosis of bilateral renal artery occlusion should be considered in the elderly presenting with drug-resistant hypertension and progressively declining renal function. A recent study revealed that nine of 30 patients with renal artery occlusion were 60 or more years old while the remaining 21 were over 50 years of age, and nearly one half had a serum creatinine above 1.5 mg/dL.[34]

All lesions in this age group were arteriosclerotic. Almost half of the patients undergoing surgical treatment obtained improved renal function, and about 90% had better control of their hypertension. In the ten patients considered high risk and not receiving operative therapy, there was a tendency toward progression of renal insufficiency and intractable hypertension.[34]

Atheroembolic disease may present as chronic renal failure, and most often is seen in the elderly male with extensive abdominal aortic atherosclerosis.[35] The primary renal lesion consists of cholesterol-rich emboli occluding the arcuate and interlobular arteries. These appear as biconvex, needle-like clefts in standard tissue preparations of skin, lymph nodes, bone marrow, muscle, and kidney.[35,36] Atheromatous embolization presents a characteristic picture that includes progressive renal function loss associated with one or more of the following: livedo reticularis, digital necrosis, retinal emboli, and episodic or persistent hypertension.[36] Most commonly this disease follows surgical manipulation of a severely diseased aorta or angiography. However, in some cases progressive renal failure may be the only manifestation of spontaneous development of atheromatous embolic disease[37] requiring renal biopsy to establish the diagnosis. This syndrome is usually associated with a relentless decline in renal function; however, the degree of renal failure may also be mild to moderate, and in some instances will improve with time or after dialysis treatment.[36] No specific therapy is available, and prevention in the elderly with severe atherosclerosis must be accomplished by careful operative technics on the aorta and its major branches and the avoidance of angiography whenever possible.

The development of renal failure associated with bacteriuria has been alluded to previously, but the mechanism responsible has not been defined. It is thought that bacteriuria in the elderly accelerates preexisting nephrosclerosis,[38] and in the absence of structural defects of the genitourinary tract does not appear to be associated with the appearance of renal failure.[39]

Several other diseases may cause chronic renal failure in the elderly. Polycystic renal disease is the sole hereditary disorder that may be encountered with significant frequency, but uremia with renal salt wasting due to medullary cystic disease has been reported.[40] Although hyperuricemia has been one of the correlates of renal insufficiency in the older patient, it alone does not impair renal function. Renal insufficiency occurring in the gouty patient appears to be more related to hypertensive vascular disease and other intrinsic renal disease.[41] Renal failure in the elderly may be the presenting feature of renal papillary necrosis syndromes, and is particularly associated with diabetes mellitus, infection, and urinary obstruction.[42]

DIABETIC RENAL DISEASE

Diabetic nephropathy resulting in end-stage renal disease accounts for approximately 25% of patients entering dialysis in the United States.[43] Most interest and research have centered on type 1 (insulin-dependent, juvenile onset) diabetes mellitus since death due to renal failure in the past has occurred in approximately one half of those patients having had the disease prior to age twenty.[44] It is commonly appreciated that the incidence of renal failure as a cause of death decreases as diabetes mellitus is acquired later in life and it accounts for less than 1% of the deaths in diabetics over age 60. Death in the older group is more commonly related to the macrovasculopathy of cardiovascular disease. Although emphasis has been placed on the renal complications of juvenile diabetes mellitus, type 2 (noninsulin-dependent, maturity onset) diabetes mellitus is the most prevalent form of the disease, occurring principally in the individual over middle age without a propensity for ketoacidosis and frequently obese. The nephropathy of type 1 and type 2 appears to be similar, and is histologically characterized predominantly by glomerulosclerosis with mesangial thickening and nodule formation, hyalinosis of afferent and efferent arterioles, and occasionally pyelonephritis.[45] Glomerulosclerosis is more common in the younger patient and is associated with proteinuria and nephrotic syndrome. The appearance of sustained proteinuria in type 1 diabetes mellitus is associated with advanced renal failure in half of the patients within 5 years of its onset. In older patients similar histologic findings at autopsy have not necessarily been associated with nephrotic syndrome, and on occasion there has been no clinical evidence of proteinuria.[44]

Recently the clinical characteristics of renal disease in maturity onset diabetes mellitus have been analyzed in a population in which the majority of the study subjects were over age 60.[46] Abnormal urinary protein excretion (>150 mg/24 h) occurred in half the patients often early after diagnosis. In the remainder protein excretion was generally greater than age-matched nondiabetic controls. Unlike type 1 patients albumin excretion was elevated early in the course of the type 2 disease (24%) even with normal total protein excretion. Excessive urinary excretion of albumin and high molecular weight proteins (>100,000) were the first manifestations of type 2 diabetic nephropathy.[46] Proteinuria in the older patient remained moderate and was in the nephrotic range in less than 4% of the patients. Proteinuria tended to be greater the longer the duration of diabetes mellitus, but half of the patients maintained normal protein excretion regardless of the duration of disease. Proteinuria persisted in most patients despite satisfactory control of blood sugar.

The glomerular filtration rate (GFR) was well maintained and was considered normal for age in 83% of patients with urinary protein excretion <150 mg/24 h and in 65% of the patients who exceeded that value. Only 9% had a GFR below 60 mL/min, and only one patient required dialysis out of the 510 who were followed from 1 to 8 years in this study.[46] Hypertension (present in 46% of the patients) correlated with increased urinary protein and reduced GFR. Almost 25% of the patients died from other causes during the period of observation. There were 90 patients with diabetes mellitus for 16 or more years out of which 38 had normal protein excretion, and 29 of these had a GFR above 80 mL/min, 16 of whom were diabetic for over 20 years. Renal biopsies in this study confirmed the similar histologic appearance of renal disease in both types of diabetes mellitus.[46]

Thus, the prognosis of diabetic nephropathy in the elderly appears relatively good as compared to that seen in type 1 disease. The progression of diabetic nephropathy may be slowed by better glucose control, adequate hypertension treatment, and prompt treatment of urinary tract infections.[46,47] However, longevity is determined more by the cardiovascular system in the elderly diabetic than by diabetic nephropathy. The role that newer oral agents might play in reducing diabetic nephropathy in the elderly awaits study.[48]

EVALUATION OF CHRONIC RENAL FAILURE

Clinical Since renal failure in the elderly is so commonly prerenal,[49] adverse reversible factors affecting the senescent kidney must be diligently searched for in the history and physical examination, eg, congestive heart failure, volume depletion, drug toxicity. While the elderly patient may present with one or more of the classic features of uremia, their presenting symptoms may be that of the underlying disorder that places the kidney at risk or they may be nonspecific such as nausea, vomiting, and weakness.[50] Weight loss and anorexia are sometimes the only complaints of uremia. Description of symptoms by the elderly varies remarkably, especially regarding dysuria, nocturia, incontinence, and prostatic symptoms, particularly in the institutionalized geriatric.[51] When present, the above symptoms, as well as polyuria and hematuria, may reflect conditions associated with chronic renal insufficiency. Accelerated hypertension or unexplained edema should prompt evaluation for chronic renal disease.

Laboratory The presence of proteinuria with excretion rates greater than 150 mg/24 h should not be ascribed to senile kidneys and values above 500 mg should be carefully evaluated. While red blood cell casts have been described infrequently in the elderly,[49] their presence indicates renal parenchymal disease. The serum creatinine underestimates the severity of renal impairment in the elderly, and some have recommended the blood urea nitrogen as a better screening indicator.[49] Anemia and bilaterally small kidneys on a plain film of the abdomen remain a reliable sign of chronic renal failure, although kidney size decreases with age.[50] Sonography has largely replaced excretory urography for excluding urinary tract obstruction and determining kidney size. Intravenous pyelography should be avoided in the elderly patient because of the adverse effects of contrast agents on renal function and their tendency to aggravate chronic renal failure. Isotopic renal blood flow studies are useful to screen for bilateral renal artery stenosis or renal artery embolization in the appropriate clinical setting. Arteriography should be reserved for those patients having a high probability of correctable vascular disease of the renal arteries. Finally, renal biopsy should be considered in the elderly patient with chronic renal failure of undetermined etiology.[10]

REFERENCES

1. Perlman LV, Kennedy BW, Hayner NS: Primary and secondary renal failure in a total community (Tecumseh, Michigan): preponderance in the elderly and possible antecedent factors. *J Am Geriatr Soc* 1974; 22:25–29.
2. Pendreigh DM, Howitt LF, MacDougall AI, et al: Survey of chronic renal failure in Scotland. *Lancet* 1972;1:304.

3. McGeown MG: Chronic renal failure in Northern Ireland, 1968–70 (A prospective survey). *Lancet* 1972;1:307–310.
4. Branch RA, Clark CW, Cochrane AL, et al: Incidence of uremia and requirements for maintenance hemodialysis. *Br Med J* 1971; 1:249–254.
5. Sourander L, Kasanen A, Pasternack A, Kaarsalo E: Uremia in the aged in South-Western Finland. *Scand J Soc Med* (Suppl) 1977;14:221–224.
6. Hood B, Falkheden T, Carlsson M: Trends and present pattern of mortality in chronic uremia. *Acta Med Scand* 1967;181:561–569.
7. Waters WE, Lond MB: Trends in mortality from nephritis and infections of the kidney in England and Wales. *Lancet* 1968;1:241–243.
8. Baruch Modan PH, Moore BP, Paz B: Mortality from renal disease in Israel. *J Chronic Dis* 1970;22:727–732.
9. Dontas AS, Kasviki-Charvati P, Papanayiotou PC, et al: Bacteriuria and survival in old age. *N Engl J Med* 1981;304: 939–942.
10. Moorthy AV, Zimmerman SW: Renal disease in the elderly: clinicopathologic analysis of renal disease in 115 elderly patients. *Clin Nephrol* 1980;14:223–229.
11. Montolin J, Darnell A, Torras A, et al: Acute and rapidly progressive forms of glomerulonephritis in the elderly. *J Am Geriatr Soc* 1981;29:108–116.
12. Beirne GJ, Wagnild JP, Zimmerman SW, et al: Idiopathic crescentic glomerulonephritis. *Medicine* 1977;56:349–381.
13. O'Neill WM Jr, Etheridge WB, Bloomer A: High dose corticosteroids. Their use in treating idiopathic rapidly progressive glomerulonephritis. *Arch Intern Med* 1979;139:514–518.
14. Bolton WK, Couser WG: Intravenous pulse methylprednisolone therapy of acute crescentic rapidly progressive glomerulonephritis. *Am J Med* 1979;66:495–502.
15. Beck AD: Benign prostatic hypertrophy and uremia: review of 315 cases. *Br J Surg* 1970;57:561–565.
16. Olbrich O, Woodford-Williams E, Irvine RE, et al: Renal function in prostatism. *Lancet* 1957;1:1322–1324.
17. Parsons FM: Chemical imbalance occurring in chronic prostatic obstruction: A preliminary survey. *Br J Urol* 1954;26:7–21.
18. Delano BG: Renal disease in the elderly. *Med Instrum* 1982;16:91–92.
19. Parsons V: What decreasing renal function means to aging patients. *Geriatrics* 1977; 32:93–99.
20. Mueller-Heubach E: Prolapsus uteri causing hydronephrosis. *J Am Geriatr Soc* 1969; 17:1055–1063.
21. Carter CB, Olicheny MJ, Westervelt FB Jr: Renal failure in the elderly. *South Med J* 1970;63:805–808.
22. Makamel E, Nissenkorn I, Boner G, et al: Occult progressive renal damage in the elderly male due to benign prostatic hypertrophy. *J Am Geriatr Soc* 1979;27:403–406.
23. Kyle RA: Multiple myeloma: review of 869 cases. *Mayo Clin Proc* 1975;50:29–40.
24. Cohen HJ, Rundles RW: Managing the complications of plasma cell myeloma. *Arch Intern Med* 1975;135:177–184.
25. Cosio FG, Pence TV, Shapiro FL, et al: Severe renal failure in multiple myeloma. *Clin Nephrol* 1981;15:206–210.
26. Border WA, Cohen AH: Renal biopsy diagnosis of clinically silent multiple myeloma. *Ann Intern Med* 1980;93:43–46.
27. Lazarus HM, Adelstein DJ, Herzig RH, et al: Long-term survival of patients with multiple myeloma and acute renal failure at presentation. *Am J Kidney Dis* 1983; 2:521–525.
28. DeFronzo RA, Cooke CR, Wright JR, et al: Renal function in patients with multiple myeloma. *Medicine* 1978;57:151–166.
29. Preuss HG: Effects on rat kidney slice function in vitro of proteins from the urines of patients with myelomatosis and nephrosis. *Clin Sci Molec Med* 1974;46:283–294.
30. Koss MN, Pirani CL, Osserman EF: Experimental Bence Jones cast nephropathy. *Lab Invest* 1976;34:579–591.
31. Brown WW, Hebert LA, Piering WE, et al: Reversal of chronic endstage renal failure due to myeloma kidney. *Ann Intern Med* 1979;90:793–794.
32. Ogg CS, Cameron JS, Williams DG, et al: Presentation and course of primary amyloidosis of the kidney. *Clin Nephrol* 1981; 15:9–13.
33. Kyle RA, Bayrd ED: Amyloidosis: Review of 236 cases. *Medicine* 1975;54:271–299.
34. Whitehouse WM Jr, Kazmers A, Zelenock GB, et al: Chronic total renal artery occlusion: Effects of treatment on secondary hy-

pertension and renal function. *Surgery* 1981;6:753–763.
35. Kassirer JP: Atheroembolic renal disease. *N Engl J Med* 1969;281:812–817.
36. Smith MC, Ghose MK, Henry AR: The clinical spectrum of renal cholesterol embolization. *Am J Med* 1981;71:174–180.
37. Varanasi UR, Moorthy AV, Beirne GJ: "Spontaneous" atheroembolic disease as a cause of renal failure in the elderly. *J Am Geriatr Soc* 1979;27:407–409.
38. Dontas AS, Papanayiotou P, Marketos SG, et al: The effect of bacteriuria on renal functional patterns in old age. *Clin Sci* 1968; 34:73–81.
39. Nicolle LE, Bjornson J, Hardeny GKM, et al: Bacteriuria in elderly institutionalized men. *N Engl J Med* 1983;309:1420–1425.
40. Swenson RS, Kempson RL, Friedland GW: Cystic disease of the renal medulla in the elderly. *JAMA* 1974;228:1401–1404.
41. Yu TF, Berger L: Impaired renal function in gout – its association with hypertensive vascular disease and intrinsic renal disease. *Am J Med* 1982;72:95–100.
42. Eknoyan G, Qunibi WY, Grissom RT, et al: Renal papillary necrosis: an update. *Medicine* 1982;61:55–73.
43. Friedman EA: Diabetic nephropathy: strategies in prevention and management. *Kidney Int* 1982;21:780–791.
44. Knowles HC Jr: Magnitude of the renal failure problem in diabetic patients. *Kidney Int* 1974;6(suppl):52–57.
45. Mauer SM, Steffes MW, Brown DM: The kidney in diabetes. *Am J Med* 1981;70: 603–612.
46. Fabre J, Balant LP, Dayer PG, et al: The kidney in maturity onset diabetes mellitus: a clinical study of 510 patients. *Kidney Int* 1982;21:730–738.
47. Mogenson CE: Progression of nephropathy in long-term diabetics with proteinuria and effect of intitial hypertensive treatment. *Scand J Clin Lab Invest* 1976;36:383–388.
48. Camerini-Davalos RA, Velasco C, Glasser M, et al: Drug-induced reversal of early diabetic microangiopathy. *N Engl J Med* 1983;309:1551–1556.
49. Kafetz K: Renal impairment in the elderly: a review. *J R Soc Med* 1983;76:398–401.
50. Rosen H: Renal disease in the elderly. *Med Clin North Am* 1976;60:1105–1119.
51. Jewett MAS, Fernie GR, Holliday PJ, et al: Urinary dysfunction in a geriatric long-term care population: prevalence and patterns. *J Am Geriatr Soc* 1981;29:211–214.

CHAPTER 8 Sodium and Water Disorders in the Elderly

Domenic A. Sica
Antonia Harford

Disorders of sodium metabolism are common occurrences in the hospitalized elderly patient. Fortunately, the disorders of hyponatremia (< 135 mEq/L) and hypernatremia (>145 mEq/L) are ones whose diagnosis and treatment are firmly grounded on established physiologic principles. This chapter will serve to describe the clinical settings, diagnosis, signs and symptoms, and the therapy of these disorders of tonicity as they apply to the elderly population. In this regard, a number of features exist which distinguish the occurrence of either hyponatremia or hypernatremia in the elderly patient from its presentation in a younger patient population.

INCIDENCE

Under basal conditions serum sodium values remain normal with advancing age if the elderly subjects are healthy.[1,2] Leask et al sampled randomly from a population of patients over the age of 65 who were residing at home. They observed neither an age nor a sex difference in the concentration of serum sodium (Table 8-1). These results were confirmatory of earlier studies by Wootton and King[4] and Roberts[5] which had also demonstrated normal serum sodium values in the elderly.

The normal sodium values found in healthy elderly subjects are in contradistinction to those found in institutionalized elderly subjects. In a series of 619 patients, newly hospitalized on a geriatric unit, serum sodium values were set at a lower level (135 to 138 mEq/L) and displayed a wider range.[2] Additional studies by

Table 8-1
Serum Sodium Values in Home-Dwelling Elderly

Age (yr)	No. (sex)	Sodium
65–74	95 (M)	140.5±3.1
>75	68 (M)	140.8±2.5
65–74	149 (F)	141.0±2.6
>75	133 (F)	140.9±3.0

Adapted from Leask et al.[3]

Sunderam and Manikar on patients in a geriatric department, performed over a 10-month period, showed that 77 patients (11.3%) had serum sodium values less than 130 mEq/L, and 31 patients (4.5%) had serum sodium values below 125 mEq/L.[6] In another series by Kleinfeld et al,[7] 160 patients in a chronic disease facility were randomly sampled for serum sodium values; their mean age was 72 years with 75% of the population exceeding 65 years of age. They defined hyponatremia as a value less than 135 mEq/L and found that 36 patients (22.5%) were below this value and that the mean determination in these 36 patients was 120 mEq/L (range 109 to 135 mEq/L).[7]

On initial appraisal, it would seem that the incidence of hyponatremia is particularly high in a hospitalized elderly population. In reality, the occurrence of hyponatremia among hospitalized patients is often merely an epiphenomenon of a wide variety of disease states, and its incidence is high regardless of the age of those under study. When defined as a value below the two standard deviation reference range, hyponatremia occurred in 15% of the patients in a large series reported by Flear and Gill[8] (Table 8-2). Other series have reported even higher incidence figures with Owen and Campbell[9] finding hyponatremia in 50% of 5000 patients and Bradham and Gadsden[10] in 36% of 1000 patients. These findings would then suggest that hyponatremia occurs in the elderly but it still remains to be determined whether this represents a predilection towards this electrolyte disturbance that is unique to the elderly or whether we are seeing its occurrence as the result of a higher incidence of disease, drug therapy, and hospitalization in the elderly.

There are no available studies that have examined the incidence of hypernatremia in the elderly. Despite this, it has been observed that hypernatremic dehydration often occurs in institutionalized elderly individuals reflecting their tendency to suffer free water losses yet be unable to successfully accomplish replacement.[11,12] In comparison to the incidence of hyponatremia (15% to 50%) in hospitalized patients,[8,9] hypernatremia is much less common, occurring in only 1% of a population (619 patients) studied by Hodkinson.[2]

PHYSIOLOGY

In man, there exists a physiologic system which maintains plasma osmolality and its principal determinant, plasma sodium, within a relatively narrow range. This system is quite efficient in maintaining plasma sodium between 135 and 145 mEq/L and plasma osmolality in a range of from about 275 to 295 mosm/kg. This flexibility is accomplished by a thirst-neurohypophyseal-renal feedback system which relies upon increases or decreases in total body water to counteract alterations in the plasma concentration of sodium or other solutes. This system is quite sensitive (1% to 2% threshold) and is characterized by a tight linkage between the plasma osmolality and the control of thirst and vasopressin secretion.[13] A

Table 8-2
Occurrence of Hyponatremia in 2852 Hospital Patients

Serum Sodium (mEq/L)	No. of Patients	% of Population
131–134	294	10.3
126–130	106	3.7
121–125	28	1.0
<120	7	0.2
Total	435	15.2

Study population was composed of all patients in whom plasma urea and electrolyte concentrations were requested over a 2-year period. Adapted from Flear and Gill.[8]

fall in plasma sodium to values below normal, termed *hyponatremia*, reflects either a relative or absolute excess of total body water. The converse disorder, termed *hypernatremia*, generally connotes a relative or absolute decrease in total body water. Of these two disorders hyponatremia is by far the more prevalent among the elderly though a number of physiologic aberrations exist which sensitize the elderly to the development of hypernatremia.

Thirst

The process of drinking occurs as part of a powerful behavioral drive which is largely *anticipatory* in nature. Under normal circumstances water intake exceeds its needs thereby suppressing any stimulus for thirst. If for some reason water is withheld, hypertonicity will develop in both the intra- and extracellular fluid compartments. This stimulates thirst and the ingestion of fluid rapidly returns body water to normal tonicity. Of the alterations that occur, the decrease in cell volume that accompanies hypertonicity is the most important stimulus to thirst. Gilman[14] demonstrated that following the administration of either hypertonic saline or urea to dogs, that the dogs drank nearly twice as much when given hypertonic saline. Though the rise in osmolality in the extracellular fluid compartment was similar in both instances, the extent of intracellular dehydration was likely to have been considerably greater with hypertonic saline which unlike urea is localized primarily to the extracellular space.[14]

An additional stimulus regulating thirst is that of extracellular volume depletion as might be seen with sodium depletion[15] or blood loss.[16] In this instance, arterial baroreceptors or receptors in the left atrium are stimulated which then transmit signals to CNS loci which then precipitate drinking. This mechanism operates only under conditions of severe volume loss and thirst would suggest that angiotensin II is not an effective dipsogen under most conditions where physiologic degrees of volume depletion are present. Previous experimental work that had demonstrated a role for angiotensin II as a dipsogen in rats[17] probably requires reinterpretation in humans since this animal species differs substantially from man as regards thirst stimulation when angiotensin II is increased.

The primary thirst disturbance in the elderly is *hypodipsia*. This most commonly results from an inability to express the sensation of thirst which is further compounded by the elderly being in situations where access to water is limited. The elderly develop a number of illnesses which limit their expression of a need for water; such is the case with cerebrovascular accidents, which depress the level of consciousness and immobilize the patient to an extent that severely limits their *personal* replacement of fluid losses. The occurrence of hypodipsia leading to hypernatremia is a known event in the incapacitated elderly patient but is not often considered in alert, elderly subjects who may have merely suffered a nonaphasia-producing cerebrovascular event. In fact, Miller et al have described six patients (aged 68 to 91 years) with prior nonaphasic cerebrovascular events who, despite full ability to communicate needs and the physical ability to obtain water, were still without thirst at a time when severe hyperosmolality was present (mean plasma osmolality 363 mosm/L).[18] Similar findings were observed by Mukherjee et al in the course of a 54-hour fluid deprivation study in six elderly patients (aged 65 to 91 years). Of these six patients only one experienced thirst despite a significant body weight loss during the study (range 2% to 4%). The sole patient who demonstrated a normal thirst response was also the only one with a normal osmoreceptor response to dehydration as well (Figure 8-1).[19] Both of these observations[18,19] suggest that hypodipsia is more common in the elderly population than might be expected.

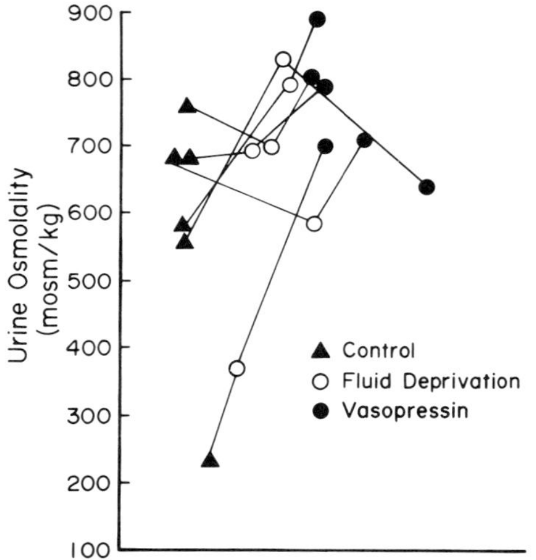

Figure 8-1 Changes in urine osmolality from control specimen (▲) to that after a minimum fluid deprivation period of 54 hours (○) and after the subsequent administration of 5 IU vasopressin in oil intramuscularly (●). (Reproduced with permission from Mukherjee et al.[19])

Control of Antidiuretic Hormone Release

The major stimulus for the secretion of antidiuretic hormone (ADH) is an increase in plasma osmolality with a rise of 1% in plasma osmolality being sufficient to stimulate secretion of ADH. Alterations in volume can override as well as modulate the control exerted by tonicity but seldom do so unless the volume loss exceeds 10%. A final control system based on nonosmotic stimuli to ADH secretion includes pain, emotion, stress, and cholinergic activity. A number of pharmacologic agents such as meperidine, morphine, or bariturates are utilized in clinical situations where nonosmotic stimuli are prevalent and may in and of themselves contribute to the release of ADH.

The ADH that enters the blood stream does so following its release from the posterior pituitary with its formation having occurred within the supraoptic and paraventricular nuclei of the hypothalamus. Once released, ADH circulates within the vascular space with a half-life of five to ten minutes. Its primary locus of action appears to be the basolateral surface of the collecting duct where, once it has been bound to receptors, there is initiated a sequence of steps which ultimately leads to increased permeability to water on the luminal surface of the collecting duct.

A number of anatomic and physiologic abnormalities exist in the control of ADH in the elderly. On initial appraisal, since there is a defect in urinary concentrating ability in the elderly,[20] it would seem that this could be explained by a defective release of ADH since there are data supporting the existence of such a defect. Rowe evaluated ADH release in six elderly subjects (aged 68 to 81 years) in response to the nonosmotic stimulus of assuming an upright posture from a previously supine position, and observed a relative insensitivity of ADH release in response to this baroreceptor stimulus.[21] Despite this observation, most remaining studies would suggest defective regulation by events which ordinarily either inhibit or stimulate ADH release. Miller,[22] utilizing an *in vitro* system of isolated hypothalamic-neurohypophyseal units, demonstrated that ADH release was greater under both basal and stimulated conditions in units obtained from aged rats. The amount of ADH in the posterior pituitary was consistently greater in the aged animals and at any level of osmotic stimulation the percentage of ADH released was also uniformly greater. These findings were expressed in the intact animals studied as an increase in basal levels of ADH. Analogous results have been obtained in studies performed by Helderman et al[23] in which elderly subjects (aged 52 to 66 years) and younger subjects (aged 22 to 48 years) were studied with stimuli known to increase (3% NaCl) and decrease (ethanol) ADH release. Despite a similar rise in serum osmolality following 3% NaCl, the older subjects increased plasma ADH by 450% whereas the younger subjects only increased ADH values by 250% (Figure 8-2). Osmoreceptor sensitivity (slope of plasma ADH *v* serum osmolality) was appreciably greater in the elderly. In this same study, when intravenous (IV) ethanol was administered, ADH was clearly inhibited to a lesser degree in the elderly patients. It is possible that the results of these studies[23] can be explained by alterations in the metabolic clearance of ADH, though studies performed by Engel et al[24] have shown that there is very little difference in the kinetic parameters defining ADH disappearance regardless of the age of the study subjects (11 subjects: age range 19 to 31 years; 4 subjects: age range 62 to 80 years). These observations suggest that ADH is present in the elderly and that provocative stimuli both accentuate its release and limit its suppressibility though the reasons for these observations are still unknown.

Renal Regulation of Water Excretion

Once the glomerular ultrafiltrate enters the proximal tubule (180 L filtrate/day) the process of fluid reabsorption begins. In the proximal tubule fluid reabsorption is *isosmotic;* demonstrating an intimate relationship to the tubular reabsorption of sodium. Some 60% of the solute and water entering the proximal tubule are ultimately absorbed within this nephron segment. Beyond the proximal tubule the intimate relationship between solute and water reabsorption is lost, with water absorption occurring largely independent of any solute resorbed.

Water resorption is linked to several factors the most important of which are the renal interstitial solute content, tubular fluid solute content, as well as tubular permeability to both water and solute with water permeability most closely correlating with the circulating level of ADH (Figure 8-3). The application of *countercurrent multiplication* principles allows for the progressive rise in interstitial osmolality to values of 1200 mosm/kg; this results primarily from the accumulation of NaCl and urea in this interstitial compartment. The mechanism of countercurrent multiplication requires solute impermeability–water permeability in one limb of the loop of Henle and the converse in the connecting limb. In man, the descending limb is highly water permeable–solute-impermeable and tubular fluid having entered this segment reaches an osmolality of 1200 mosm/kg by the bend of Henle's loop. As tubular fluid enters the ascending limb, solute is extracted in excess of water and tubular fluid osmolality declines substantially approaching values of 100 mosm/kg in the distal tubule. The subsequent reabsorption of water or its packaging as the final urine is largely determined by the prevailing levels of ADH. The capacity of ADH to facilitate the final reabsorption of water then largely dictates that ambient levels of ADH determine whether the final urine osmolality is either dilute or concentrated.

It has been observed since the studies of Lewis and Alving that the aged kidney has

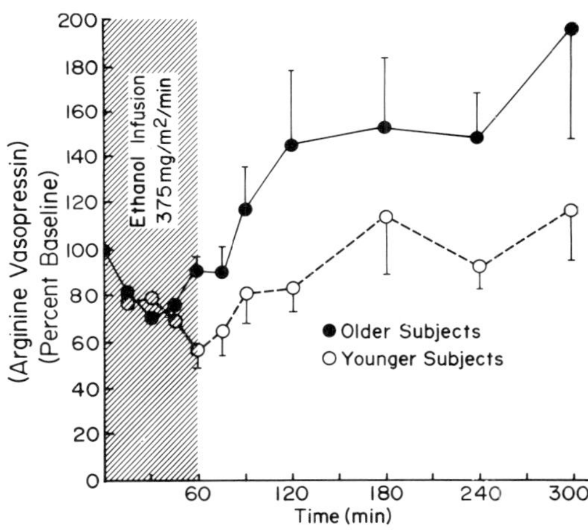

Figure 8-2 The response of plasma arginine vasopressin (AVP) to a 1-hour ethanol infusion (375 mg/m^2/min) in young (aged 22 to 48 years) and older (aged 52 to 66 years) subjects. The base-line value for both groups is that value obtained after overnight dehydration and is designated 100%. The maximal decline in AVP reached a nadir of 58 ± 7% of base-line at 60 minutes in the younger subjects. In the older subjects the nadir reached was only 71 ± 12% of the base-line at 30 minutes and a paradoxical rise in values was seen despite the continuing presence of ethanol. (Adapted with permission from Helderman et al.[23])

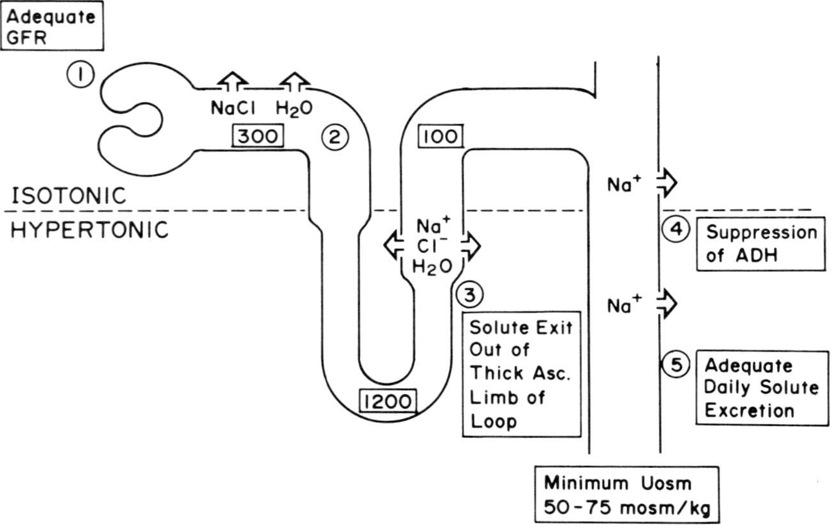

Figure 8-3 Representation of the sites (1–5) in the nephron critical to the development of an appropriately dilute urine.

distinct limitations in its ability to concentrate urine.[25] This finding has been confirmed on numerous other occasions both in man[26–28] and in the rat.[29] Most of these studies are open to some criticism since their conclusions were reached from cross-sectional studies which examined small numbers of patients often representing a chronically debilitated population.[25–28] Not until the carefully performed studies of Rowe et al[20] was there a patient sampling truly adequate for the assessment of urinary concentrating ability. Employing a longitudinal study design in a carefully screened cohort of male volunteers who were without concurrent medical illnesses, it was convincingly demonstrated following 12 hours of dehydration that elderly subjects were less able than young or middle-aged subjects to alter urinary volume or osmolality.

The actual cause of the concentrating defect in the kidney is unknown, though a number of possibilities exist (Table 8-3). These possibilities can be categorized as glomerular alterations, alterations in tubular responsivity to ADH, or as intrarenal factors.

Certain authors have attributed the decline in concentrating ability with age to the concurrent drop in GFR seen in the elderly.[26,28] Contrary to this, Row et al observed no correlation between the level of creatinine clearance and the maximum urinary osmolality possible following 12 hours of fluid deprivation[20] suggesting that although the decline in GFR undoubtedly contributes to the concentrating effect, it certainly is not the sole determinant.

Antidiuretic hormone levels are not decreased in the elderly.[21,23,30] Therefore, since adequate circulating levels of ADH exist, limited urinary concentrating ability should then reflect a defect intrinsic to the kidney. Lindeman et al administered submaximal doses of vasopressin (8 mU/h during water diuresis) to elderly subjects and found no age-related decline in the maximal urinary osmolality reached.[31] However, the maximum urinary osmolality attained with high-dose vasopressin is diminished in elderly subjects undergoing a water diuresis. Miller and Shock[27] administered IV vasopressin (0.5 mU/kg/body weight) to elderly subjects and younger subjects undergoing water diuresis. A clear negative correlation existed between the maximum urine/plasma (U/P) inulin ration obtained and age (younger group, mean age 34.6 years: U/P inulin 117; older group, mean age 73.3 years: U/P inulin 45).[27] This finding, whether due to a defect in medullary tonicity or to receptor alterations, suggests that the distal nephron's ability to perform maximal osmotic work is impaired despite an adequate supply of ADH.

It is very likely that an intrarenal mechanism serves as a major contributor to the observed concentrating defect. Nephron dropout occurs with aging, a phenomenon which causes an increase in the solute load to remaining nephrons leading to an osmotic diuresis. The solute and water loss which ensues from this osmotic diuresis then limits the absorption of NaCl and urea which are integral in the maintenance of medullary interstitial tonicity.[32] In addition, in studies performed by Nunez et al,[33] solute free water generation was deficient in elderly patients, possibly contributing to the inability to reach the medullary tonicity necessary for optimal urinary concentration. A final consideration in respect to optimization of medullary tonicity is that of the role of medullary blood flow. Anatomic studies in the aging kidney suggest a relative sparing of medullary vasculature from degenerative changes as compared to the cortical vessels.[34] Additionally, Hollenberg et al, utilizing xenon washout studies in prospective kidney donors (aged 17 to 76 years) to assess renal hemodynamics, found that there existed a *relative* increase in medullary blood flow.[35] Each of these latter observations would limit solute accumulation within the medullary interstitium and thereby limit the extent to which urine is concentrated.

A synthesis of the information on defective urinary concentrating ability is difficult. Whatever its etiology, it is likely to be multi-factorial with components based on diminished GFR and defects in the ability to develop an appropriate medullary interstitial gradient. Though the concentrating defect in the elderly is consistently observed it seldom is of sufficient magnitude to precipitate hypertonic volume depletion unless both a thirst defect and extrarenal fluid losses are superimposed on it.

The ability to generate free water (C_{H_2O}) and thereby dilute urine is critical in the avoidance of dilutional hyponatremia. A number of steps are important in order that solute-free water might be generated. An initial requirement is the adequate delivery of solute to the diluting regimen. This in turn necessitates sufficient renal perfusion and glomerular filtration to ensure adequate departure of solute from the proximal tubule [Figure 8-3: (1) and (2)]. Once filtrate has exited the proximal tubule it is necessary that it reach distal diluting sites whose functional intactness allows sodium removal and hence the generation of C_{H_2O} [Figure 8-3: (3)]. Finally, any solute-free water having been so generated must still escape reabsorption in the collecting duct in order to enter the final urine, which further necessitates the suppression of ADH or ADH-like substances [Figure 8-3: (4)].

Table 8-3
Physiologic Considerations in Disorders of Sodium Metabolism in the Elderly

Thirst
Hypodipsia[18,19]

Control of ADH Release
Increased levels in response to a hyperosmolar stimulus[23]
Decreased suppressibility with ethanol[23]
Baroreceptor insensitivity to positional change[21]
Increased capacity for release of ADH in isolated neurohypophyseal systems[22]
Normal disappearance kinetics of antidiuretic hormone[24]

Renal Regulation of Water Excretion
Decrease in glomerular filtration rate
Defect in free water clearance
Increased solute load/remaining nephron
Normal response to submaximal ADH infusion
Decreased maximal urinary osmolality to high-dose vasopressin
Relative increase in medullary blood flow
Defect in the generation of the medullary interstitial gradient

Even though a number of physiologic processes are necessary for optimal C_{H_2O}, the ability to excrete C_{H_2O} is ultimately limited by the amount of solute requiring urinary excretion. Urinary solute excretion is primarily a function of dietary sodium and protein intake with a representative solute load being 800 mosm/d [Figure 8-3: (5)]. With a minimum osmolality of 50 mosm/kg maximum daily urine output would be: (800 mosm/d)/50 mosm/L) = 16 L/d.

There have been few studies whose goal has been to assess C_{H_2O} in the senescent kidney. Studies performed to date suggest that a defect in C_{H_2O} exists in the elderly.[26,31] Lindeman et al water-loaded (20 mL/kg) young (mean age 31 years) and elderly subjects (mean age 84 years) and also found that young subjects reached urinary osmolalities of 52 ± 3 mosm/kg whereas the elderly subjects only attained osmolality values of 74 ± 6 mosm/kg.[31] An explanation for both the decreased C_{H_2O}[26,31] and the defect in minimum urinary osmolality[31] comes from events associated with the age-related drop in GFR. If C_{H_2O} is to be a useful clinical concept, it is important to realize that a decline in GFR will limit its absolute value regardless of a normal process of dilution beyond the glomerulus. Therefore, an accurate assessment of C_{H_2O} is only gained by factoring it by measured GFR (C_{H_2O}/100 mL GFR) which in the elderly should then provide the appropriate correction factor for the known decline in GFR seen with aging. A recalculation of data obtained by Lindeman, factoring for the diminished GFR in the elderly population, would then suggest that maximal C_{H_2O} is similar in both a young and an elderly population. Additional studies by Dontas et al[26] and Nunez et al[33] would suggest though, that the C_{H_2O} defect persists following correction for a lowered GFR but only in *elderly females.*

A cautionary note should be raised as regards the minimum urinary osmolality reached following water loading in the elderly. Prior work[31] would suggest a minimal (52 ± 3 mosm/kg *v* 74 ± 6 mosm/kg) yet significant defect, an explanation for which might then be rendered by phenomena associated with the age-related decline in total nephron mass. As nephron mass declines an increasing share of the workload is assumed by the remaining nephrons but only at the expense of the initiation of an osmotic diuresis in these same nephrons. This limits the minimum urinary osmolality that is attainable in any situation based on an almost obligatory solute excretion. With solute restriction (limited salt intake) in individuals with variable levels of azotemia, an improvement, in fact, occurs in the lowest level of urinary osmolality[36,37] reached, further supporting the belief that any defect affecting C_{H_2O} in the elderly is based on GFR changes alone.

SIGNS AND SYMPTOMS

The signs and symptoms of hyponatremia and hypernatremia are correlated both with the rate of change in the serum sodium value and with the absolute value obtained. In general, symptoms seldom develop unless the serum sodium value falls outside of the range of 130 to 145 mEq/L. Once outside this range, the predominant symptom complex observed is neurologic, relating to the inability of brain cells to accommodate quickly enough to stresses which rapidly change their cell volume. In the instance of hyponatremia, brain cell volume expands, leading to a picture of cerebral edema; whereas with hypernatremia brain cell volume initially diminishes, leading to a rapid shrinkage in CNS water content.

It cannot be overly stressed that the acuteness of the osmolality disturbance dictates the severity of its symptom complex. At its extreme, *symptoms* of disorientation or psychosis are present, while prominent neurologic events such as Cheyne-Stokes respiration or seizures may be *signs* of the severity of the change in osmolality. Some symptoms (Table 8-4) are quite easily attributed to hyponatremia, while others such as nausea, anorexia, or agitation are very difficult to separate from the natural progression of cerebrovascular and other degenerative illnesses in the elderly.

Arieff et al reviewed their experience with 66 patients on a renal consultation service, and observed a considerable difference in symptomatology and mortality between those patients with the acute onset of a serum sodium less than 128 mEq/L and those with a more gradual development of a similar serum sodium value (Table 8-5).[38] No such series of patients exists wherein the symptomatology and mortality of hyponatremia have been specifically addressed in an elderly population. It can be stated, though, that hyponatremia of a magnitude sufficient (<130 mEq/L) to suggest concern as to its etiology, is often entirely asymptomatic in the elderly. In the series of Kleinfeld et al,[7] 160 patients in a chronic disease facility were randomly sampled, and of the 36 observed with serum sodium values less than 135 mEq/L, nine were entirely asymptomatic and the symptoms observed in the remainder were often merely an accentuation of those symptoms otherwise attributable to an underlying disease state. Also, in a series of 77 newly hospitalized patients reported by Sunderam and Mankikar,[6] 39% of those observed to have serum sodium values less than 130 mEq/L had no symptoms attributable to hyponatremia. It would seem then, that it is necessary to maintain a high index of suspicion for hyponatremia in the elderly when addressing the etiology of otherwise innocuous systemic and CNS complaints such as anorexia, nausea, lethargy, or disorientation.

Table 8-4
Symptoms and Signs Associated with Hyponatremia

Symptoms	Signs
Nausea	Pathologic reflexes
Headache	Seizures
Muscle cramps	Coma
Anorexia	Pseudobulbar palsy
Agitation	Cheyne-Stokes respiration
Disorientation	
Psychosis	Hemiparesis

HYPONATREMIA

A low plasma sodium concentration can be ascribed to a number of causes with the majority of these being clearly separable by measurement of *serum osmolality*. This use of the serum osmolality as a diagnostic discriminator facilitates the partitioning of hyponatremia into hypertonic, isotonic, and hypotonic forms of the disorder. The hypotonic forms of hyponatremia are then

Table 8-5
Etiology and Mortality in 66 Patients with Serum Sodium of 128 mEq/L or Less

	Acute Hyponatremia	Chronic Hyponatremia	
		Symptomatic	*Asymptomatic*
No. of patients	14	25	27
Mortality	50%	12%	0
Volume overload	71%	4%	0
Chronic renal failure	0	12%	19%
Acute renal failure	23%	0	19%
Heart failure*	31%	28%	30%
SIADH	29%	36%	15%
Postoperative†	43%	8%	15%
Hypertension*	0	20%	19%

*Commonly associated with diuretic usage.
†Associated with use of 5% dextrose in water.
Adapted from Arieff et al.[38]

further divisible by employing an accurate clinical assessment of the patient's *extracellular fluid volume* (ECF). This categorization of hyponatremia can be successfully employed since the serum sodium value is merely a reflection of the concentration of sodium in water. Processes controlling sodium and water retention may operate independently; thus, hyponatremia as a hypotonic syndrome may occur with a body sodium content that is either increased, decreased, or seen as being clinically normal (Figure 8-4).

ISOTONIC HYPONATREMIAS

Pseudohyponatremia is one of the more common causes of isotonic hyponatremia. It occurs when the normal plasma water/plasma solids ratio (93/7) changes in favor of the accumulation of plasma solids. Lipids and proteins are the primary components of plasma solids with electrolytes being virtually excluded from this compartment; thus electrolytes are primarily localized to the aqueous phase of plasma. When lipids or proteins increase there occurs an expansion in circulating volume and a displacement of water that is manifest as an increase in solids/unit volume of plasma (Figure 8-5). Thus, the content of sodium (aqueous phase) diminishes in any such newly formed liter of plasma though there is no alteration in the concentration of this cation within the newly shrunken aqueous phase. Though routine automated chemistries would demonstrate a fall in serum sodium, serum osmolality would be normal since it is a colligative determination based on the actual concentration of solute (sodium) within its solvent (plasma water).

Multiple myeloma accounts for about 10% of hematologic malignancies. It is a disease absent from young patients with only 2% of the subjects in a series of 369 patients reported by Kyle being less than 40 years of age with a mean age in this series of 62 years.[39] Protein accumulation in myeloma causes a displacement of water sufficient to affect serum sodium only when values exceed 12 to 15 g%.[40] For this reason, on occasion when protein values are only moderately raised, an additional explanation has been necessary for the hyponatremia seen with myeloma.[41] In these cases, serum sodium values have been low but the chloride concentration has remained disproportionately high reflecting displacement of sodium intracellularly by the cationic myeloma proteins and the compensatory retention of chloride in the intravascular space. Another form of protein excess, benign monoclonal gammopathy, occurs in as many as 3% to 5% of individuals over the age of 70. Though its effects on sodium values await further characterization it is unlikely that gammopathies significantly affect serum sodium values since the rise in total protein seen with them is usually less than 1 g%.[42]

It is important to note that the methodology utilized in the measurement of serum sodium is not uniform since it is only when serum sodium is measured by flame photometry or indirect potentiometry that "pseudohyponatremia" occurs. Direct potentiometry, which measures the activity of sodium in the aqueous phase, gives serum sodium values consistent with those predicted by osmolality measurements.[43,44]

Lipid disturbances are also capable of leading to interpretative errors in serum sodium values when standard methodology is employed.[43,45] The pseudohyponatremia observed with hyperlipidemia correlates much better with the level of triglyceride elevation rather than that of cholesterol. In absolute terms, triglyceride values must exceed 1500 mg/dL prior to their affecting serum sodium measurement to an extent which exceeds that of the random error in measurement. Triglyceride elevations to this degree are distinctly uncommon in the elderly and when present frequently reflect a secondary metabolic disturbance. There are many such secondary disturbances including poorly controlled diabetes mellitus,[46] hypothyroidism,[47] uremia,[48]

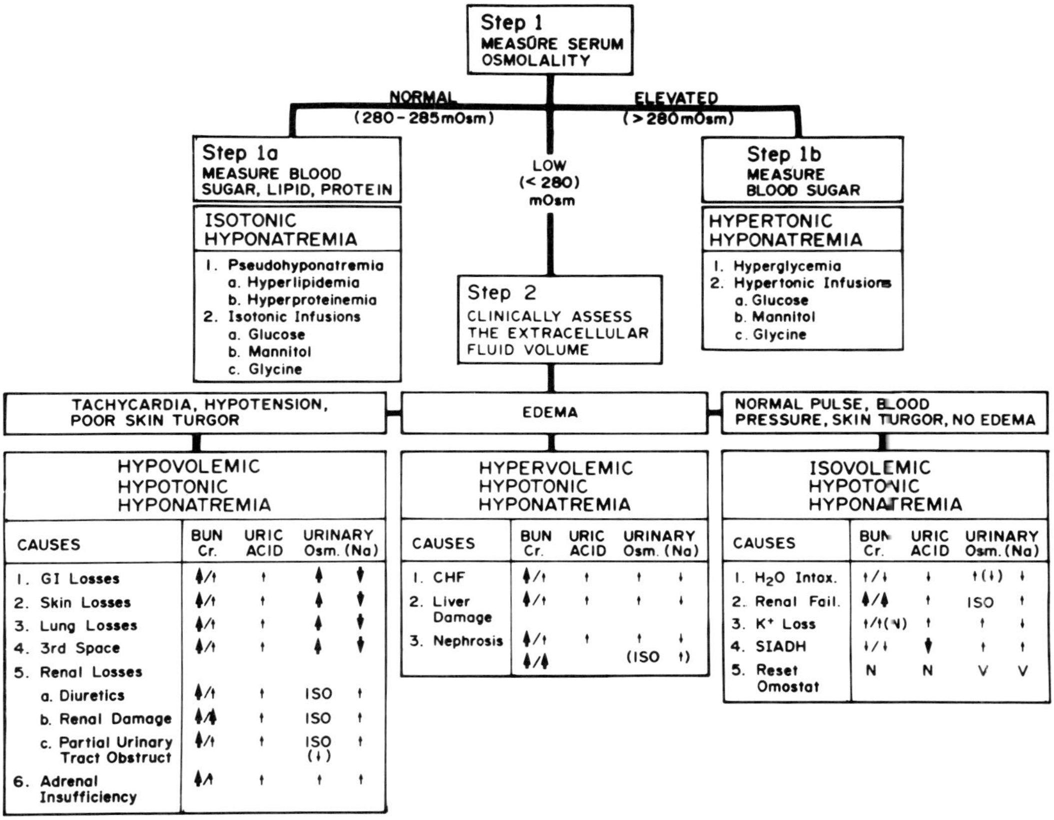

Step 1
MEASURE SERUM OSMOLALITY

NORMAL (280–285mOsm) | LOW (< 280) mOsm | ELEVATED (> 280mOsm)

Step 1a
MEASURE BLOOD SUGAR, LIPID, PROTEIN

ISOTONIC HYPONATREMIA

1. Pseudohyponatremia
   a. Hyperlipidemia
   b. Hyperproteinemia
2. Isotonic Infusions
   a. Glucose
   b. Mannitol
   c. Glycine

Step 1b
MEASURE BLOOD SUGAR

HYPERTONIC HYPONATREMIA

1. Hyperglycemia
2. Hypertonic Infusions
   a. Glucose
   b. Mannitol
   c. Glycine

Step 2
CLINICALLY ASSESS THE EXTRACELLULAR FLUID VOLUME

TACHYCARDIA, HYPOTENSION, POOR SKIN TURGOR

HYPOVOLEMIC HYPOTONIC HYPONATREMIA

CAUSES	BUN Cr.	URIC ACID	URINARY Osm.	(Na)
1. GI Losses	⇑/↑	↑	⇑	⇓
2. Skin Losses	⇑/↑	↑	⇑	⇓
3. Lung Losses	⇑/↑	↑	⇑	⇓
4. 3rd Space	⇑/↑	↑	⇑	⇓
5. Renal Losses				
a. Diuretics	⇑/↑	↑	ISO	↑
b. Renal Damage	⇑/⇑	↑	ISO	↑
c. Partial Urinary Tract Obstruct	⇑/↑	↑	ISO (↓)	↑
6. Adrenal Insufficiency	⇑/↑	↑	↑	↑

EDEMA

HYPERVOLEMIC HYPOTONIC HYPONATREMIA

CAUSES	BUN Cr.	URIC ACID	URINARY Osm.	(Na)
1. CHF	⇑/↑	↑	↑	↓
2. Liver Damage	⇑/↑	↑	↑	↓
3. Nephrosis	⇑/↑	↑	↑	↓
	⇑/⇑		(ISO	↑)

NORMAL PULSE, BLOOD PRESSURE, SKIN TURGOR, NO EDEMA

ISOVOLEMIC HYPOTONIC HYPONATREMIA

CAUSES	BUN Cr.	URIC ACID	URINARY Osm.	(Na)
1. H_2O Intox.	↑/↓	↓	↑(↓)	↓
2. Renal Fail.	⇑/⇑	↑	ISO	↑
3. K^+ Loss	↑/↑(N)	↑	↑	↓
4. SIADH	↓/↓	⇓	↑	↑
5. Reset Omostat	N	N	V	V

Figure 8-4 An approach to the diagnosis of hyponatremia. N = normal, ISO = isotonic, V = variable. Further details are in the text. (Adapted with permission from Narins RG, Jones ER, Stom EC, et al: Fluid-electrolyte diagnostic strategies. *Am J Med* 1982;72:496–520.

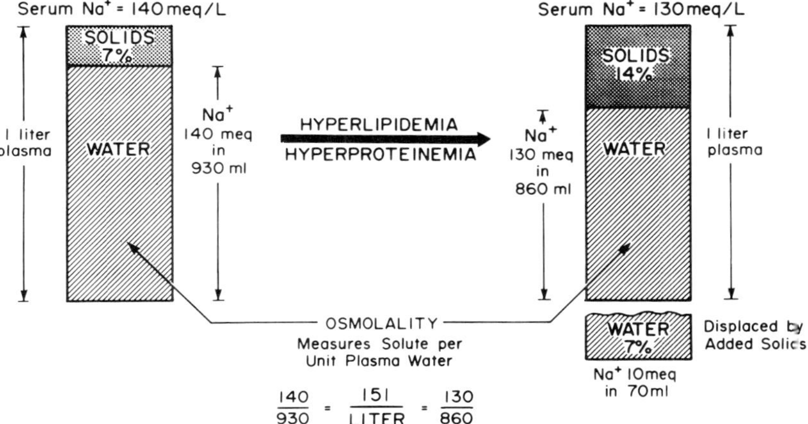

Figure 8-5 An approach to isotonic hyponatremia. An accumulation of solids displaces sodium-rich serum water. In this instance, the concentration of sodium is unchanged in the remaining serum water; but each liter of serum present contains less water and sodium. (Adapted with permission from Narins RG, Lazarus JM: The renal system, in Vandam LD, (ed): *To Make the Patient Ready for Anesthesia.* Menlo Park, Calif, Addison-Wesley Publishing Co, 1980.)

and/or alcohol.[49,50] Though the elderly patient can develop any of these disturbances he is particularly susceptible to the development of diabetes mellitus.

Isotonic solutions of mannitol or glucose initially remain extracellular when infused, where they result in a dilution of sodium. Their use is readily apparent, which facilitates etiologic determination of the hyponatremia.

HYPERTONIC HYPONATREMIAS

There are a number of substances which when present in excess are capable of acting as *effective osmoles*. That is, by the nature of their primarily extracellular location they develop an osmotic pressure gradient that requires movement of sodium free water from the intracellular compartment (isotonic) to the extracellular compartment (hypertonic by virtue of osmoles added). This flux of sodium free water normalizes ECF tonicity but only at the expense of diluting all electrolytes in the ECF space. Other substances such as methanol, ethanol, and urea are *ineffective osmoles* since when present in excess, they are found in total body water, and affect neither water distribution nor serum sodium concentration.[51]

The development of hypertonic hyponatremia is not limited to a particular age group. Despite this, certain facets of its inception are germane to the elderly. Of all the substances causing this entity, mannitol,[52] glucose,[53,54] glycine,[55-57] and glycerol[58] all are small molecular weight substances and therefore require only nominal elevations in their ECF concentration before leading to the development of a significant osmotic pressure gradient. The ultimate ECF concentration of any of these substances is dictated by their rate of administration or generation (glucose) and the capacity for their excretion by the kidney. Therefore, the most dramatic elevations in the levels of any of these substances occur when their use is superimposed on a background of renal failure. Such is the case for mannitol, which may be used in an attempt to promote a diuresis in oliguric conditions such as heart failure or acute renal failure.[52,59] This is also the case with glycine, a substance commonly used as an irrigation solution during transurethral resection of either the bladder or the prostate. As much as 20 L of isotonic glycine may be utilized during these procedures; though absorption may be variable it can be sufficient to lower serum sodium values to below 100 mEq/L.[56] Symptoms at this level of hyponatremia can include disorientation, confusion, and EKG abnormalities. The etiology of these symptoms is not entirely clear but may reflect the sudden intravascular volume expansion[55] or direct glycine toxicity[57] since plasma osmolalities are not dramatically increased. Glycerol is an agent primarily utilized to decrease intracerebral pressure elevations. At low dosages, liver metabolism controls its elimination (up to serum values of 0.15 mg/mL). When these serum values are exceeded, urinary elimination plays an increasingly prominent role. Glycerol accumulation can commonly lead to hyperosmolality which in at least some instances reflects the gluconeogenic properties of glycerol and the development of a nonketotic hyperglycemic state.[60] The most common cause of hyponatremia, as the result of localization of a hypertonic substance to the ECF space, is hyperglycemia. In general, for every increment of 62 mg/dL in the blood sugar, sufficient water is drawn into the intravascular compartment to lower serum sodium concentration by 1 mEq/L.[53] The occurrence of nonketotic hyperosmolar coma secondary to hyperglycemia is often cited as an example where the magnitude of the attendant blood sugar elevation is sufficient to significantly lower the plasma sodium concentration. In fact, patients presenting with such a nonketotic condition are often hypernatremic despite convincing elevations in blood sugar, reflecting the protracted osmotic diuresis that these patients suffer prior to hospitalization.[54] It is only when the rise in glucose concentration is rapid (hours to days) that significant decreases in serum sodium values occur.

HYPOTONIC HYPONATREMIA

The hypotonic forms of hyponatremia are most easily separated by a clinical assessment of the volume status of the patient. This form of hyponatremia does not occur unless there has been prior ingestion of water or the administration of hypotonic fluids since the body is incapable of losing sodium-containing fluids whose sodium content exceeds that found in blood.

Hypovolemic Hyponatremia

Volume depletion, in the presence of an unremitting water intake, is a common cause of hyponatremia. This decrease in total body salt and water content occurs in association with either nonrenal or renal losses of sodium. Nonrenal causes of sodium loss include the gastrointestinal (GI) tract (vomiting, diarrhea, biliary drainage), skin (burns, sweating), lungs (bronchorrhea), or via sequestration of plasma volume (ie, "third spacing") (pancreatitis, traumatized muscle, peritonitis).

In all of these situations a number of hormonal and hemodynamic forces come into play which, in turn, limit the ability to excrete ingested water. These effects of volume depletion on the evolution of hyponatremia are accomplished by altering renal water excretion, thirst, and possibly from fluctuations in potassium balance. First, the decrease in ECF volume leads to renal hypoperfusion, a decrease in GFR, an increase in proximal tubular salt and water absorption, and finally to a reduced delivery of water to the diluting segments, thereby limiting the quantity of free water that can be generated.[61] This decreased delivery of water to the diluting segment results in diminished urine volume and if sufficiently slowed can lead to an isotonic to slightly hypertonic urine even in the absence of ADH. This phenomenon has been demonstrated in diabetes insipidus patients administered hexamethonium to induce hypotension[62] and probably is the result of the fact that the collecting duct is not entirely impermeable to water in the absence of vasopressin if the passage of urine is sufficiently slowed.[63] Second, hypovolemia stimulates carotid sinus baroreceptors resulting in the release of ADH which further impairs the generation of free water. Of additional importance is the production of angiotensin II, as the result of volume contraction, which may then in addition stimulate thirst centers in the brain.

It should be noted in the hypovolemic patient that in addition to the telltale physical findings of decreased ECF volume (Table 8-6), that patients with extrarenal losses of sodium avidly conserve sodium in an attempt to reexpand ECF volume. Urine sodium concentration is typically low, less than 10 mEq/L, and urine osmolality high, greater than 400 mosm/kg. If the volume contraction is particularly severe the BUN/creatinine ratio will exceed 10/1 due to increased passive backdiffusion of urea in a low urine flow state.

Hyponatremia, due to volume depletion, may also result from inordinate renal sodium losses. This occurs primarily in three clinical situations, most commonly with diuretic use but also in mineralocorticoid deficiency as well as chronic renal

Table 8-6
Clinical Findings Useful in the Assessment of Extracellular Fluid Volume Status

Volume Contraction	Volume Expansion
Neck vein distension	Neck vein distension
Resting tachycardia or hypotension	Edema
Orthostatic tachycardia or hypotension	Ascites/pleural effusions
Diminished skin turgor	Cardiac summation gallop

disease, particularly when it involves the interstitium. Disruption of the renal architecture, as occurs with interstitial disease, will lead to impaired sodium reabsorption; this then results in decreased free water clearance by virtue of decreasing the GFR, increasing proximal tubular reabsorption, and by a volume contraction stimulus to ADH release. Patients with mineralocorticoid deficiency, due to Addison's disease, conserve sodium inefficiently owing to low aldosterone levels. The diluting defect in this disease is related to both the negative salt balance that occurs,[64] leading to a decrease in renal blood flow and GFR, and to the release of ADH[65] based on the nonosmotic stimulus of volume contraction.

Hyponatremia, associated with volume depletion due to diuretic usage, represents an important cause of hyponatremia in the elderly (Figure 8-6). In the series on hyponatremia in the elderly by Sunderam and Mankikar, of 77 patients with a serum sodium concentration below 130 mmol/L, approximately 65% had diuretics implicated.[6] Of additional concern is the fact that advanced age is an important risk factor in the development of diuretic-induced hyponatremia. In several series[66–69] the mean age of the involved patient was over 75 years, and this age-related bias appeared unrelated to the magnitude of consumption of such drugs in any particular age group. Why the elderly are particularly prone to this disturbance is unclear. Pressure-volume alterations provoking ADH release seem an unlikely explanation since ADH release is weakly stimulated by baroreceptor stimuli in the elderly,[21] and an age-related decrease in diluting ability is unlikely to be of sufficient magnitude to be considered causal.[70] Three mechanisms can be implicated as causes for severe hyponatremia due to diuretics: volume depletion, potassium depletion, and an inhibition of urinary dilution, the latter due to impaired sodium chloride reabsorption in the diluting segment.[70,71] Diuretic-induced hyponatremia occurs within the first several days of the initiation of therapy[72] at a time when fluid losses are the greatest. At this point a new level of sodium balance occurs which only worsens in the instance of a superimposed problem such as increased water intake, vomiting, or diarrhea (Figure 8-6). Although loop diuretics are known to cause hyponatremia, it is far more common with thiazide diuretics since they demonstrate little effect on urinary concentrating ability.[66,70,71] This occurs because loop diuretics are active at the thick ascending limb of the loop of Henle, and by restricting sodium reabsorption in this segment they limit the amount of solute available for maintenance of medullary tonicity. Thus, if ADH contributes to the development of diuretic-induced hyponatremia, in the case of loop diuretics, it does so by causing equilibration of urine against a medullary interstitial tonicity that is *less* than normal. Alternatively, thiazide diuretics act within the cortical segment of the distal tubule and have no effect within the medulla. Therefore, urinary concentrating ability is unaffected by their use, and if reason exists for the presence of ADH, greater defects in free water excretion can occur.[73]

Hypervolemic Hypotonic Hyponatremia (Figure 8-4)

Hyponatremia, in association with an increase in total body sodium content, occurs

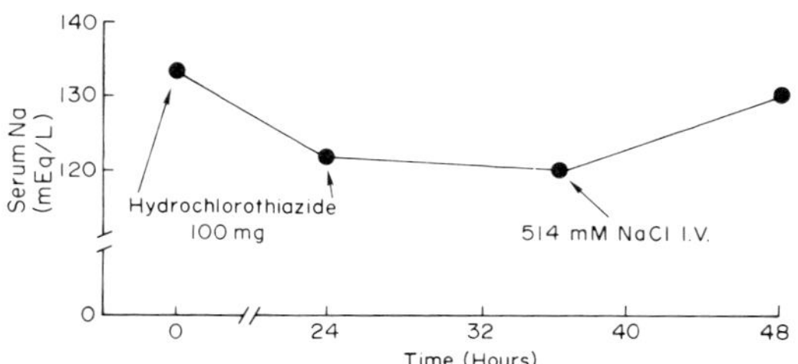

Figure 8-6 The effect of hydrochlorothiazide 100 mg/d for two days on serum sodium. Access to water was not limited. Urinary solute loss and retention of water accounted completely for the fall in serum sodium. Neurologic symptoms at 37 hours necessitated treatment with hypertonic saline. (Adapted with permission from Ashraf et al.[66])

in a limited number of clinical situations. These include hepatic cirrhosis, nephrotic syndrome, and advanced congestive heart failure. Although, in the instance of each of these disorders, total body water and sodium is in excess, the body behaves as if a decreased "effective" circulating plasma volume is present, with the kidney reacting as if it were hypoperfused. The kidneys then attempt to retain salt and water to increase their perfusion by increasing proximal reabsorption. Unfortunately this endeavor decreases distal delivery and limits free water excretion. This concept is supported by the observation that following the administration of mannitol (decreases proximal reabsorption) to congestive heart failure patients[74] or cirrhotics,[75] free water excretion increases.

An additional factor in these conditions that enters into the limitation in diluting ability is an excessive secretion and/or altered metabolic clearance of ADH. In cirrhosis, studies have shown that ADH levels are elevated[76,77] and that its metabolic clearance rate is diminished.[77] This multifactorial etiology for hyponatremia is not present in all cirrhotics, since it is only those cirrhotics with demonstrable edema and/or ascites who respond in an abnormal manner to the administration of free water.[78,79]

An excess of ECF volume frequently characterizes the nephrotic syndrome. This disease may also involve a defect in the kidney's perception of "effective circulating volume." It would seem that alterations in proximal tubular reabsorption are not as prominent in nephrotic syndrome since studies both in rats[80] and humans[81,82] suggest a more prominent role for more distal nephron structures or deep nephrons in sodium reabsorption in this setting. The extent of ADH involvement in the impaired renal diluting capacity of the nephrotic syndrome awaits further characterization.

Of the three disturbances leading to hypervolemic hyponatremia, advanced congestive heart failure is the one most common to the elderly. Though cardiac function normally declines with age, heart failure is not an expected manifestation of age alone. Rather, combinations of coronary artery disease, hypertensive heart disease, and/or valvular heart disease will facilitate the development of heart failure in the aged. Once present, heart failure leads to the activation of a number of compensatory humoral and hormonal responses with resulting diminution in renal blood flow (RBF) and preferential efferent arteriolar vasoconstriction. The net effect of these vascular alterations is a greater fall in RBF than GFR and an increase in the filtration fraction. Further hemodynamic translation of these events requires that the increased filtration fraction lead to increased peritubular protein concentration and the raised oncotic pressure in peritubular vessels then facilitates a heightened reabsorption of sodium and water along the length of the proximal tubule. A reduced availability of sodium and water for delivery to the diluting segment consequently limits the generation of free water. Substantiation of this postulate is available from studies in hyponatremic cardiac failure patients, a group of patients in whom the administration of either mannitol[74] or furosemide[83] results in conversion from a hypertonic to a dilute urine.

Early clinical observations based on improvement in water excretion in heart failure patients following the administration of ethyl alcohol[84,85] suggested a role for ADH in the genesis of diluting abnormalities. In many heart failure patients ADH levels are elevated,[86–88] at least in part as the result of high-pressure baroreceptors sensing a decrease in effective circulating blood volume thereby causing a nonosmotic release of ADH. In the assessment of ADH levels in heart failure patients the age of the patient is an important determinant of the plasma ADH concentration. In the study of Rondeau et al[88] it was shown that plasma ADH levels, both in normals and heart failure patients, rose steadily with increasing age though the patients with cardiac insufficiency as a group always had higher values. This observation, though of interest, appears unrelated to any facet of the cardiac disease, and remains unexplained.

In all of these conditions urine sodium values seldom exceed 20 mEq/L and urine osmolality is usually greater than 400 mosm/kg. As these diseases progress in severity two biochemical events mark their level of severity. First, there is a disproportionate rise of the BUN in relation to the serum creatinine. Second, with increasingly avid proximal tubular sodium reabsorption little sodium reaches the loop of Henle and there is a dissipation of the medullary interstitial gradient with the excretion of an isotonic urine. The combination of a low urine sodium with isotonic urine in these conditions suggests far advanced disease.

Isovolemic Hyponatremia (Figure 8-4)

Hyponatremia, in association with an apparently normal ECF volume on clinical examination, is almost always the result of excess circulating ADH. This form of hyponatremia has by convention come under the rubric of "syndrome of inappropriate secretion of antidiuretic hormone" (SIADH), though a number of additional etiologies exist which manifest similar pathophysiologic findings.

The primary pathophysiologic event which underlies this disorder is enhanced water reabsorption from the collecting duct attributable to the hormonal effects of *inappropriate* quantities of ADH. It should be emphasized that despite the presence of excess circulating ADH that hyponatremia does not occur unless in conjuction with the hormonal excess there occurs the ingestion of water.[89,90] Certain diagnostic clues based on the excess of ADH are both useful hints and a prerequisite to the diagnosis of SIADH (Table 8-7). The net result of this excess activity of ADH is an expansion of the ECF volume. Since only one third of that water retained is within the ECF space (two thirds is intracellular), overt signs of volume excess are typically absent. Instead, what is observed are the biochemical changes which follow the ECF volume expansion and concomitant rise in GFR. These include low values for BUN, creatinine and uric acid.[91]

The causes of SIADH are numerous and are listed in Table 8-8. The etiologic distinctions for SIADH are based primarily on whether there is an ectopic production of

Table 8-7
Criteria for the Diagnosis of SIADH*

1. Serum hypo-osmolality and hyponatremia
2. Urine osmolality less than maximally dilute
3. Matching of urine sodium intake with output
4. Absence of other causes of decreased diluting ability (endocrine dysfunction)
5. Improvement with water restriction

*SIADH = syndome of inappropriate secretion of antidiuretic hormone.

Table 8-8
Disorders Associated with SIADH

1. Tumors producing ADH
   a. Lung
      Oat-cell carcinoma
      Large-cell carcinoma
   b. Carcinoma of the duodenum, thymus, pancreas
   c. Carcinoma of the ureter
   d. Hodgkin's disease
   e. Myeloid leukemia
   f. Tuberculosis
2. Increased hypothalamic production of ADH
   a. Pulmonary
      Infection (viral, fungal, or bacterial)
      Positive pressure ventilation
      Acute respiratory failure
      Asthma
   b. Central nervous system
      Infection (meningitis of any etiology)
      Encephalitis
      Tumor (primary or metastatic)
      Traumatic (subdural hematoma or hemorrhage)
      Vascular (cerebral thrombosis or hemorrhage)
      Guillain-Barré syndrome, acute psychosis, stress
   c. Drugs
   d. Postoperative
   e. Idiopathic

the hormone, as seen with tumors, or whether it occurs as the result of an increase in the endogenous production of ADH. In the instance of increased endogenous production of ADH the provoking stimulus may arise from the pulmonary system, the CNS, or occur as a function of medication ingestion.

A number of tumors have been shown to be capable of the nonhypophyseal production of ADH. By far, the most common and best investigated is bronchogenic carcinoma, particularly of the oat cell variant, with ADH demonstrable both by bioassay and radioimmunoassay.[92,93] These assays have demonstrated the presence of the hormone both in tumor extracts[94] and more importantly, in tumor slices incubated with the appropriate amino acids,[95] therefore negating the possibility that ADH had nonspecifically adsorbed to the tumor. Vorherr et al have observed that bronchogenic carcinomas, among other tumors, are capable of production and secretion of ADH despite the absence of clinically detectable hyponatremia.[96] This indicates that clinically detectable SIADH is probably much less common than actual tumor-associated ADH production. Why tumors produce ADH is uncertain, though it is felt by some to represent a derepression of synthesis accompanying the malignant transformation. Though not a malignant condition, tuberculosis pulmonary tissue has been shown to be capable of the production of bioassayable ADH.[97] In this instance, nonspecific adsorption of circulating ADH to the involved tissue was not excluded, thereby raising a question as to the significance of these findings.

A number of other pulmonary diseases including pneumonia (Table 8-8),[98,99] acute respiratory failure,[100] asthma,[101] and positive pressure ventilation[102] may also be associated with SIADH. The mechanism of ADH release is uncertain but may involve varying degrees of stimulation of right atrial and ventricular stretch receptors, the result of anatomical-vascular distortions as they might occur with any of these pulmonary diseases. An extension of this postulate involves the hyponatremia seen with positive pressure ventilation[102,103] which may be attributed to a decrease in left atrial stretch. The change in distension then decreases afferent tone in the vagus with ADH consequently being released.[104]

A number of neuropsychiatric disturbances can promote the excessive release of ADH from the neurohypophysis. Of these, several are common to an elderly population including subdural hematomas[105] or hemorrhage[106] as well as cerebrovascular accidents which may result from either thrombotic or hemorrhagic phenomena (Table 8-8).[107] The exact means by which these events transmit a noxious stimulus for the release of ADH is unclear. Despite this, the clinical significance of these entities as causes of hyponatremia cannot be underestimated since their presence may contribute to further functional deterioration, of a reversible nature, in patients so afflicted.[108]

In clinical practice it is readily apparent that a large number of drugs manifest an ability to cause impaired excretion of water, a finding usually totally unrelated to the primary pharmacologic action of the drug. Drugs are capable of affecting water excretion by a number of mechanisms, all of which involve a disruption of the normal integrity of the thirst–ADH release–ADH action axis (Table 8-9). The fact that most geriatric populations are administered a wide range of pharmacologic agents puts them at particular risk for the development of medication-related side effects which in the case of certain of these drugs (Table 8-9) may result in severe degrees of hyponatremia. This is particularly so since certain of these medications have a particular usage profile that calls for their frequent use among the elderly.

Antidiuretic hormone or its analogues are utilized primarily in the therapy of diabetes insipidus, though the occasional use of vasopressin in the control of GI bleeding can lead to hyponatremia if concurrent free water administration is not

Table 8-9
Drugs Which Impair Free-Water Excretion

Antidiuretic Hormones (ADH)
Vasopressin
Oxytocin
Increased Release of ADH
Nicotine
Cyclophosphamide
Clofibrate
Barbiturates
Morphine
Chlorpropamide
Vincristine
Psychotropic drugs
Carbamazepine
Potentiation of Action of ADH
Chlorpropamide
Nonsteroidal anti-inflammatory drugs

carefully controlled.[109] Intravenous use of the antitumor alkylating agent, cyclophosphamide, must be undertaken with caution. Cyclophosphamide produces an ADH-like antidiuresis[110,111] that is particularly problematic, since this drug often requires the administration of large volumes of fluid to avert the development of cystitis. This complication can be minimized if the administered fluid is isosmotic saline rather than solutions primarily comprised of free water.

Chlorpropamide, a commonly employed oral hypoglycemic agent, is probably the most common cause of drug-induced SIADH. In some series its occurrence has been observed in up to 4% of the population under study.[112] Chlorpropamide is unique in that it is felt to act by potentiating the effect of existing ADH[113,114] and to possibly increase the release of ADH as well.[115] Its ADH-potentiating effect relates to an increase of the normal ADH-induced adenyl cyclase activity and resultant cAMP generation.[115] Regardless of the mechanism by which chlorpropamide induces hyponatremia, when it does occur it is most commonly observed in elderly patients.[112,116,117] In the series of five patients described by Weissman[112] to have had symptomatic hyponatremia caused by chlorpropamide, the age range was from 59 to 81 years. In a separate study Tanay et al[116] observed the occurrence of hyponatremia from chlorpropamide in two patients who were 74 and 62 years of age, respectively. The use of this agent in elderly patients may be particularly hazardous when additional reasons for defects in diluting ability exist (diuretic use or congestive heart failure) and may make for a situation wherein a significant risk of symptomatic hyponatremia exists.[112]

It has been known for some time that narcotics lead to an antidiuresis following their acute administration. In a number of animal species[118] as well as in man[119] morphine has been shown to directly stimulate the release of ADH. These findings are important since opiate use and toxicity is not uncommon in the elderly[120] being most commonly observed in situations requiring intensive pain management such as terminal malignancies, myocardial infarctions, or as a consequence of surgical procedures.[121] The ability of narcotics to stimulate ADH release is unquestioned; what requires further clarification is the extent of this release in an elderly population. Despite this the chronic use of morphine, with sizable quantities of free water, should be seen as a situation likely to lead to hyponatremia and contribute to increased patient morbidity in the elderly.

Psychotropic drugs are an additional cause of drug-induced hyponatremia in the elderly. In the institutionalized elderly patient, it has been estimated that almost 50% of these patients are chronically ingesting tranquilizers,[122] which then places them at considerable risk for any untoward effects associated with these agents. Hyponatremia has been reported with the drugs thiothixene,[123] fluphenazine hydrochloride,[124] amitriptyline hydrochloride,[125] phenothiazines,[126] and monoamine oxidase inhibitors.[127] There is little available information on how these agents cause hyponatremia, but two caveats need be raised as regards its occurrence. First, ADH excess has been reported in conditions of exacerbated psychosis, raising for consideration the role of any underlying psychosis in promoting ADH release.[128] Second, psychotropic drugs commonly manifest anticholinergic properties which can lead to dryness of the mouth[129] and thus aggravate preexisting tendencies towards compulsive water drinking. Such a possibility has been observed with the drug thioridazine. In this case, the kidney retained a normal ability to dilute, but hyponatremia occurred when the kidneys' diluting mechanism was overwhelmed by the excessive fluid load ingested.[130]

A final group of drugs suggested as possible factors in the development of hyponatremia are the nonsteroidal antiinflammatory drugs. These drugs, by virtue of their prostaglandin-inhibitory properties, can unmask the activity of ADH, by reducing what is a normal antagonism of cellular AHD effect exerted by prostaglandins.[131] Despite this, hyponatremia has been a rare occurrence following their use.[132] This may reflect the fact that these agents can directly inhibit ADH release[133] or that they maintain no place in water metabolism, since once ADH release[133] stops or levels are low, as occurs with any initial drop in plasma osmolality, tissue antagonism of ADH becomes meaningless.

The elderly patient is one in whom the potential for gradual organ failure often leads to a need for operative intervention. The occurrence of hyponatremia in the postoperative period is a very common phenomenon. Its occurrence is the result of increased release of ADH, a function of nonosmotic stimuli eliciting a release of ADH. A number of events, common to the operative procedure, serve as nonosmotic stimuli to ADH release including anxiety, surgery,[134,135] anesthesia,[135,136] and pain.

This release of ADH is probably accomplished by these stimuli decreasing parasympathetic tone in ascending afferents which in turn increases the release of vasopressin.[137] Because of this high nonsuppressible level of ADH, any fluid prescription utilized should be mindful of the likelihood of its retention; in view of this the excessive and prolonged postoperative administration of free water must be cautiously monitored.[121]

In rare instances, SIADH has no cause identified and is termed idiopathic. A number of these cases have occurred in elderly patients[138–140] suggesting that this entity may be more prevalent in this age group. As previously discussed, this could merely represent an extension of what are pre-existent age-related abnormalities in the regulation of ADH. Several studies have suggested increased plasma ADH activity in elderly patients when measured by bioassay[141,142] or radioimmunoassay[88] and others have demonstrated excessive responses to stimuli ordinarily designed to either inhibit or stimulate the release of ADH.[23] Despite these observations, the occurrence of idiopathic SIADH is very rare and becomes rarer still when one appreciates the fact that prolonged follow-up (>6 months) will sometimes reveal the presence of an occult tumor (frequently pulmonary) as the inciting factor.[143]

There are three additional disturbances which fall into the category of isovolemic hyponatremia but actually represent variants of it. These are hypothyroidism, reset osmostat, and primary polydipsia.

The reasons why hyponatremia occurs in myxedematous conditions are not entirely explained. Patients with hypothyroidism, whose volume status is normal, generally have minimal disturbances in maximal urinary diluting ability.[144,145] In advanced myxedema, urinary diluting ability is impaired for a number of reasons. Cardiac output is frequently diminished[146] activating baroreceptors which may stimulate the release of ADH. This decline in cardiac function may further contribute to decreased free water excretion by lowering the GFR. Renal hemodynamic and metabolic alterations can lead to a lowered GFR, increased proximal tubular reabsorption,[147] and ascending limb dysfunction,[148] all of which may further contribute to altered handling of water by the kidney. The interpretation of ADH values, obtained in myxedematous patients, is complicated since values are heterogeneous, being either elevated[149] or suppressed[150] despite cardiac function appearing as normal. This entity, hypothyroidism, is an important and necessary consideration as a contributing factor to otherwise unexplained hyponatremia in the elderly. The incidence of primary hypothyroidism increases with age[151] and its symptoms such as dry skin, constipation, lethargy, loss of mental activity, and arthralgias may be incorrectly attributed to the normal aging process. From a clinical perspective mild hypothyroidism seldom leads to hyponatremia; it is only when other factors are superimposed (pneumonia, pharmacologic agents) that the magnitude of the alteration in urinary diluting ability is sufficiently amplified to result in life-threatening hyponatremia.

In recent years, considerable attention has been directed toward an entity dubbed "reset osmostat." This finding is observed in patients with chronic debilitating illnesses such as tuberculosis, cancer, and malnutrition and is characterized by mild hyponatremia and hypo-osmolality with: (*a*) normal excretion of a water load, (*b*) hypertonic urine formation in response to hypertonic saline or dehydration, (*c*) no change in serum sodium following isotonic saline.[152,153] All of these events transpire around a plasma osmolality that is clearly hypotonic. This variant of hyponatremia is not progressive and is corrected following institution of therapy and resolution of the underlying illness. This resetting of the threshold for ADH release may simply be a variant of SIADH, reflecting the ability of nonosmotic stimuli to alter the osmotic threshold for release of ADH. Such nonosmotic stimuli are to be expected in the illnesses associated with the reset osmostat. An additional consideration as relates to the reset osmostat comes from the work of Flear and Singh.[154] They suggest that "sick cells" develop with these debilitating illnesses, and that the alterations in cell membrane permeability that ensue facilitate the loss of organic intracellular osmoles such as proteins, amino acids, creatinine phosphate, and metabolic intermediates.[154] Since osmolality must be equal between the cell exterior and the cell interior, plasma osmolality can be expected to fall by normal homeostatic mechanisms and result in hyponatremia.

Compulsive water drinking or psychogenic polydipsia is a behavioral disorder found most commonly in individuals suffering with psychiatric illnesses.[155,156] Typically, the kidney has the ability to eliminate vast quantities of solute-free water, so despite the polydipsia that these patients suffer from, it is a feat consuming much of one's energies to outdrink the normal excretory capacity of the kidney. For this reason these patients usually maintain a minimally depressed serum sodium and excrete copious quantities of dilute urine. It is only when an additional restraint is placed on water excretion, such as diuretic therapy[157] or cardiac disease, that the most severe degrees of hyponatremia, reaching life-threatening levels, will occur.

The elderly, not uncommonly, are placed in clinical situations where it is quite easy to overwhelm their water excretory capacity despite normal generation of solute-free water. First, their use of psychotropic drugs is high[122] and these agents can stimulate thirst by leading to a dry mouth.[130] Second, the ability to excrete solute-free water is limited by a poor dietary intake. Normal solute excretion is quite variable but may be about 800 mosm/d in a normal individual and is comprised primarily of KCl, NaCl, and urea. If the minimum urinary osmolality possible is 50 mosm/kg then the maximal daily urine volume is 16 L [(800 mosm/d)/(50 mosm/kg)=16 L/d]. If the daily solute load requiring excretion falls to 300 mosm, as may be the case in an elderly patient on a salt-restricted diet with limited protein intake, then the maximum urine volume is 6 L [(300 mosm/d)/(50 mosm/kg)]. It is optimistic to assume a minimum urinary osmolality of 50 mosm/kg for an elderly person. A more realistic value, in part due to the age-related decline in GFR, is probably 100 mosm/kg.[36,37] Recalculating [(300 mosm/kg)/(100 mosm/kg)], therefore, in this example, a maximum urinary output is 3 L/d as long as *no* ADH is present. Intake exceeding 3 L/d, in the case outlined, could lead to the rapid development of hyponatremia despite the only alteration being a change in dietary solute intake.

THERAPY

The therapy employed for hyponatremia is determined by several factors. These include the cause of hyponatremia, the level of hyponatremia, and the severity of the accompanying signs and symptoms. Once these determinants are established then the primary goal of increasing the serum sodium can be undertaken. In general, states of ECF volume and sodium excess necessitate the restriction of salt and water intake. Those individuals whose ECF volume is decreased require isotonic saline, with modification in the anion accompanying sodium being based on the acid-base status of the individual. In all hyponatremic patients, the level of concern for initiating therapy rises appreciably when neurologic symptoms are present or the plasma sodium is less than 110 to 115 mEq/L. In this instance, the most aggresive therapy available (hypertonic saline 3% or 5%) is called for, since it is in these settings that permanent neurologic damage or death may result.[38,66] The aim of using hypertonic saline is not to normalize the plasma sodium but rather to raise its concentration to >120 mEq/L, a level at which the patient should be relatively safe.

Specific Treatment of Causes of Hyponatremia

Before any treatment is instituted it must be established that isotonic hyponatremia, or so-called *pseudohyponatremia,* does not exist since specific therapy is not required for this disorder. In addition, in the case of hypertonic hyponatremia, most commonly seen with hyperglycemia, the implementation of water restriction or the infusion of hypertonic saline solutions will further increase an already elevated plasma osmolality with the potential for deleterious results. Correction of the hyperglycemia will eliminate the osmotic gradient established by the excess of intravascular glucose; thus solute-free fluid will re-enter the cellular compartment allowing serum sodium to once again normalize.

Hyponatremia which is attributed to hormonal deficiencies of glucocorticoids,[158,159] mineralocorticoids, or thyroid hormone[145,149] will be corrected with the replacement of the missing substance. When the reset osmostat is present, attempts at correcting the hyponatremia will prove fruitless unless the underlying debilitating illness is rectified.[153] In the instance of *primary polydipsia* it is necessary to restrict water intake until the plasma sodium has normalized. Once this has occurred the major problem is one of behavioral modification since it is an unlikely occurrence that simply altering a predisposing drug regimen, often comprised of psychotropic agents wtih anticholinergic properties, will eliminate the chance of future occurrence.

Hypovolemic Hyponatremia

Before the institution of any therapy for hyponatremia, the volume status of the patient needs to be assessed, so that a correct judgment might be rendered as to the necessity for either the administration of NaCl or for the restriction of the intake of water.

In the instance of hypovolemic hyponatremia the physical exam will suggest the presence of a total body water deficit (orthostasis, tachycardia, diminished skin turgor). The volume deficit can be replaced with isotonic saline or its equivalent until volume depletion is no longer evident. Of equal importance in the management of this condition is the determination of the route, renal or extrarenal, of sodium and water loss. Diagnostically, if the fractional excretion of sodium exceeds 1% in a setting of volume contraction, then there is presumptive evidence for a renal source of the volume deficit. Full correction of the sodium deficit should never be attempted in the early hours of therapy since too rapid a change back to normal may be harmful.[160-162] Instead, from one third to one half of the calculated deficit should be given over the initial six hours of therapy and the remainder given (orally or parenterally) over the following 24 to 48 hours.

Calculation of the sodium deficit can be obtained from the following formula:

$$Na^+ \text{ deficit} = P_{Na^+} \text{ deficit/L} \times \text{volume of distribution of } P_{Na^+} \quad (1)$$

Equation (1) is further clarified by realizing that despite the primarily extracellular location of sodium, the osmolality changes with hyponatremia occur throughout total body water (TBW) giving a volume of distribution for the deficit of 60% and 50% of lean body weight for men and women, respectively. Therefore:

$$Na^+ \text{ deficit} = (140 - \text{current } P_{Na^+} \times 0.6 \text{ lean body weight (kg)} \quad (2)$$

Applying equation (2) to a 80-kg man with a plasma sodium (P_{Na^+}) of 110 mEq/L (2° to vomiting and water ingestion) gives a sodium deficit of 1440 mEq.

$$Na^+ \text{ deficit} = (140 - 110) \times 0.6 \times 80 = 1440 \text{ mEq}$$

This can be corrected with either isotonic saline (155 mEq of Na^+/L) or 3% saline (513 mEq of Na^+/L), the latter being reserved for instances where neurologic symptoms are present. There is no established optimal rate of correction of plasma sodium though most authorities would suggest an hourly rate of rise of plasma sodium not to exceed 2 to 3 mEq/L and a goal of therapy not to correct the deficit completely but rather to bring the plasma sodium value into a range usually unassociated with symptoms:

$$Na^+ \text{ deficit} = (125 - 110) \times 0.6 \times 80 = 720 \text{ mEq} \quad (3)$$

Once the sodium value is at about 120 mEq/L further correction should be based on the results of serial serum measurements since these formulas do not take into account the presence of isosmotic fluid losses having preceded any therapy. The continuing appraisal of physical findings will also assist in determining the adequacy of the attempts at volume repletion.

Hypervolemic Hyponatremia

Hyponatremia found in association with edema represents an excess of both water and sodium with disproportionate retention of the former. Therefore, the administration of sodium in any form is generally contraindicated. Rather, therapy is directed toward increasing water and sodium excretion as well as limiting free-water ingestion. In addition, since these disorders (heart failure, cirrhosis, nephrosis) generally involve a decreased effective circulating plasma volume, a therapeutic strategy which corrects these disorders may improve renal perfusion and increase delivery of sodium and water to distal diluting sites. Thus, water and sodium excretion improve with the administration of digoxin and/or vasodilators to heart failure patients or when albumin is given to cirrhotics.

Diuretic therapy is frequently employed in the management of these disturbances, but the use of diuretics, particularly those acting at the loop, may also be of assistance in the correction of severe or symptomatic hyponatremia. This operates under the principle of the diuretic effecting a sodium and water loss by the kidney with only the sodium loss being replaced resulting in a predominantly negative water balance.[163] In this regard, since loop diuretics affect both urinary concentrating and diluting ability, by virtue of their action in the medulla, there will result an isosmotic urine without further lowering of plasma osmolality. Thiazides, on the contrary, act within the renal cortex and can directly lead to hyponatremia by causing a hypertonic urine.[66,73]

In some patients with severe congestive heart failure, cirrhosis, or renal failure who also have hyponatremia, neither water restriction nor loop diuretics are effective. In such patients either peritoneal or hemodialysis should be considered.[164] Recently, isolated ultrafiltration has also become available for the management of hyponatremia.[165] This process utilizes an extravascular filter and filtration pressures supplied by the patient's own blood flow. It avoids the deleterious hemodynamic consequences of hemodialysis and should gain wide applicability in the management of severe hyponatremia in the elderly.

Isovolemic Hyponatremia

In individuals with SIADH the cornerstone of therapy is *water restriction* and the removal of any easily defined inciting agents such as pain, stress, tumors, or administered pharmacologic agents. If the level of hyponatremia is not particularly severe (>125 mEq/L), then fluid restriction should suffice. This is accomplished by limiting fluid intake to 500 to 1000 mL/d and allowing the excess water to be eliminated by insensible losses.

Occasionally, the SIADH fails to resolve necessitating chronic water restriction. This frequently proves cumbersome and has led to attempts at therapy which rely on either an increase in solute excretion or an antagonism of the effects of ADH. An increase in solute excretion can generally be accomplished by supplying the patient with a high-salt, high-protein diet or by supplementing the diet with 30 to 60 g/d of urea.[166,167] The latter may cause GI side effects which may be the limiting factor in its use in the elderly. The success of this form of therapy relies on the fact that urine output is necessarily determined by the quantity of solute requiring excretion. If excess ADH is present such that an average urinary osmolality is 800 mosm/kg, and dietary intake presents the kidney with 800 mosm requiring excretion, then the obligatory urine output will be 1000 mL. Assuming no diminution in ADH activity, solute supplementation to the point of excreting 1600 mosm/d will require an output of 2000 mL of urine and thereby allow a liberalization of fluid intake.

In a similar manner as above, if means are available to lower ADH-induced urinary osmolality from 800 mosm/L to 400 mosm/L, then maintaining solute intake at 800 mosm/d would allow for urinary outputs of 2000 mL/d. This can be achieved by administering furosemide in dosages sufficient (40 to 80 mg/d) to retard NaCl abstraction from the thick ascending limb of Henle's loop and thereby lower the medullary tonicity against which ADH leads to osmotic equilibration.[168] An alternative is to employ agents such as demeclocycline[169] or lithium[170] to induce a state of partial nephrogenic diabetes insipidus by inhibiting the activity of ADH on the distal nephron. In general, demeclocyline (600 to 1200 mg/d) is the better agent, being more effective and better tolerated.[171]

When the suddenness of the hyponatremia precludes institution of conservative therapy by virtue of neurologic symptoms, rapid correction is required to avoid further neurologic dysfunction or death. This is usually achieved by administering fluids whose osmolality exceeds that present in the urine; the urine osmolality generally exceeds 300 mosm/kg in SIADH which then limits the usefulness of isotonic saline in raising plasma sodium values. Administering normal saline to the SIADH patient, who is already volume- expanded, transiently increases plasma sodium.[89] The saline load is promptly excreted, though, and not uncommonly in a smaller volume of urine than the fluid volume in which it was administered, sometimes actually further lowering the plasma sodium concentration.

The preferred sodium concentration for administration is usually hypertonic (3% or 5%). This is also excreted in the urine, but at an osmolality substantially lower than that of the infused solution, leading to greater free-water excretion than intake and an increment in plasma sodium. Though the amount of sodium administered is calculated to raise the serum sodium value to some arbitrary level [equation (3)] this disorder is actually one predominantly of water excess, which may be calculated as follows:

$$H_2O \text{ excess} = \%H_2O \times \text{total body weight} \times \left(1 - \frac{\text{measured } P_{Na^+}}{\text{normal } P_{Na^+}}\right) \quad (4)$$

Assuming a 70-kg man with SIADH whose plasma sodium value is 100 mEq/L:

$$H_2O \text{ excess} = 0.6 \times 70 \text{ kg} \times \left(1 - \frac{100}{140}\right)$$

$$42 \text{ kg} \times \frac{40}{140} = 12 \text{ L}$$

Total correction of the hyponatremia will eventually require the excretion of this quantity of excess body water. Administering hypertonic saline can rapidly elevate the plasma sodium concentration, but carries the risk of further volume expansion in a patient alreadly volume-expanded. This may be particularly dangerous in elderly patients, many of whom have marginal degrees of cardiac compensation. Arieff et al, employing the administration of hypertonic saline (3%) alone in the management of hyponatremia, found no such complications.[38] Despite this observation, the preferred regimen in the elderly should probably include furosemide as well as hypertonic saline.[38] This avoids the potential hazard of cardiac decompensation as well as improving upon the free-water clearance obtained with hypertonic saline alone.

REFERENCES

1. Shock NW: Physiological aspects of aging in man. *Annu Rev Physiol* 1961;23: 97–122.
2. Hodkinson HM: The electrolytes, urea and tests of renal function, in Hodkinson HM (ed): *Biochemical Diagnosis of the Elderly,* New York, John Wiley, 1977, pp 40–52.
3. Leask RG, Andrews GR, Caird FI: Normal values for sixteen blood constituents in the elderly. *Age Ageing* 1973;2:14–23.
4. Wootton ID, King EJ: Normal values for blood constituents: Inter-hospital differences. *Lancet* 1953;1:470–471.
5. Roberts LB: The normal ranges, with statistical analysis for seventeen blood constituents. *Clin Chim Acta* 1967;16: 69–78.
6. Sunderam SG, Mankikar GD: Hyponatremia in the elderly. *Age Ageing* 1983;12: 77–80.
7. Kleinfeld M, Casimir M, Borra S: Hyponatremia as observed in a chronic disease facility. *J Am Geriatr Soc* 1979;27:156–161.
8. Flear CT, Gill GV: Hyponatremia: mechanisms and management. *Lancet* 1981;2: 26–31.
9. Owen JA, Campbell DG: A comparison of plasma electrolyte and urea values in healthy persons and in hospital patients. *Clin Chim Acta* 1968;22:611–618.
10. Bradham GB, Gadsden RH: Electrolyte patterns for 1000 hospital patients. *Surg Gynecol Obstet* 1962;114:535–538.
11. Himmelstein DU, Jones AA, Woolhandler S: Hypernatremic dehydration in nursing home patients. *J Am Geriatr Soc* 1983;31: 466–471.
12. Mahowald JM, Himmelstein DU: Hypernatremia in the elderly: relation to infection and mortality. *J Am Geriatr Soc* 1981;29:177–180.
13. Robertson GL, Aycinena PR, Zerbe RL: Neurogenic disorders of osmoregulation. *Am J Med* 1982;72:339–358.
14. Gilman A: The relation between blood osmotic pressure, fluid distribution and voluntary water intake. *Am J Physiol* 1937;120:323–328.
15. McCance RA: Experimental sodium chloride deficiency in man. *Proc R Soc Lond* 1936;119:245–268.

16. Oatley K: Changes of blood volume and osmotic pressure in the production of thirst. *Nature* 1964;202:1341–1342.
17. Fitzsimons JT: Angiotensin, thirst, and sodium appetite: retrospect and prospect. *Fed Proc* 1978;37:2669–2675.
18. Miller PD, Krebs RA, Neal BJ, et al: Hypodipsia in geriatric patients. *Am J Med* 1982;73:354–357.
19. Mukherjee AP, Coni NK, Davison W: Osmoreceptor function among the elderly. *Gerontol Clin* 1973;15:227–233.
20. Rowe JW, Shock NW, DeFronzo RA: The influence of age on the renal response to water deprivation in man. *Nephron* 1976; 17:270–278.
21. Rowe JW, Minaker KL, Sparrow D, et al: Age-related failure of volume-pressure-mediated vasopressin release. *J Clin Endocrinol Metab* 1982;54:661–664.
22. Miller M: Vasopressin secretion in the aging rat, in *Abstracts of the Endocrine Society, 65th Annual Meeting,* San Antonio, Texas, June 8–10, 1983, p 253.
23. Helderman JH, Vestal RE, Rowe JL, et al: The response of arginine vasopressin to intravenous ethanol and hypertonic saline in man: the impact of aging. *J Gerontol* 1978;33:39–47.
24. Engel PA, Rowe JW, Minaker KL, et al: Effect of exogenous vasopressin on vaso pressin release. *Am J Physiol* 1984;246:E202–E207.
25. Lewis WH, Alving AS: Changes with age in the renal function of adult men. Clearance of urea, amount of urea nitrogen in blood, concentrating ability of kidneys. *Am J Physiol* 1938;123:505–515.
26. Dontas AS, Marketos G, Paparayiotou P: Mechanisms of renal tubular defects in old age. *Postgrad Med J* 1972;48:295–303.
27. Miller JH, Shock NW: Age differences in the renal tubular response to antidiuretic hormone. *J Gerontol* 1953;8:446–450.
28. Lindeman RD, Van Buren HC, Raisz L: Osmolar renal concentrating ability in healthy young men and hospitalized patients without renal disease. *N Engl J Med* 1960;262:1306–1309.
29. Bengele HH, Mathias RS, Perkins JH, et al: Urinary concentrating defect in the aged rat. *Am J Physiol* 1981;240:F147–F150.
30. Kirkland J, Lye M, Goddard C, et al: Plasma arginine vasopressin in dehydrated elderly patients. *Clin Endocrinol (Oxf)* 1984;20:451–456.
31. Lindeman RD, Lee TD, Yiengst HJ, et al: Influence of age, renal disease, hypertension, diuretics, and calcium on the antidiuretic responses to suboptimal infusions of vasopressin. *J Lab Clin Med* 1966;68:206–223.
32. Coburn JW, Gonick HC, Rubini ME, et al: Studies of experimental renal failure in dogs. I. Effect of 5/6 nephrectomy on concentrating and diluting capacity of residual nephrons. *J Clin Invest* 1965;44:603–614.
33. Nunez JFM, Iglesias CG, Roman AB, et al: Renal handling of sodium in old people: A functional study. *Age Ageing* 1978;7:178–181.
34. Takazakura E, Sawabu N, Handa A, et al: Intrarenal vascular changes with age and disease. *Kidney Int* 1972;2:224–230.
35. Hollenberg NK, Adams DF, Solomon HS, et al: Senescence and the renal vasculature in normal man. *Circ Res* 1974;34:309–316.
36. Kleeman CR, Adams DA, Maxwell MN: An evaluation of maximal water diuresis in chronic renal disease. I. Normal solute intake. *J Lab Clin Med* 1961;58:169–184.
37. Adams DA, Kleeman CR, Bernstein LH, et al: An evaluation of maximal water diuresis in chronic renal disease. II. Effect of variations in sodium intake and excretion. *J Lab Clin Med* 1961;58:185–196.
38. Arieff AI, Llach F, Massry SG: Neurological manifestations and morbidity of hyponatremia. *Medicine* 1976;55:121–129.
39. Kyle RA: Multiple myeloma–review of 869 cases. *Mayo Clin Proc* 1975;50:29–40.
40. Frick PG, Schmid JR, Kestler JH, et al: Hyponatremia associated with hyperproteinemia in multiple myeloma. *Helv Med Acta* 1966;33:317–329.
41. Murray T, Long W, Narins RG: Multiple myeloma and the anion gap. *N Engl J Med* 1975;292:574–575.
42. Axelsson U, Bachmann R, Hallen I: Frequency of pathological proteins (M-components) in 6,995 sera from an adult population. *Acta Med Scand* 1966;79:235–247.
43. Ladenson JH, Apple FS, Koch DD: Misleading hyponatremia due to hyperlipidemia: a method-dependent error. *Ann Intern Med* 1981;95:707–708.
44. Ladenson JH, Apple FS, Aguanno JJ, et al: Sodium measurements in multiple

myeloma: two techniques compared. *Clin Chem* 1982;28:2383–2386.

45. Steffes MW, Freier EF: A simple and pre cise method of determining true sodium, potassium, and chloride concentrations in hyperlipemia. *J Lab Clin Med* 1976;88: 683–688.
46. Bell JA, Hilton PJ, Walder G: Severe hyponatremia in hyperlipaemic diabetic ketosis. *Br Med J* 1972;4:709–710.
47. Nikkila EA, Kekki M: Plasma triglyceride metabolism in thyroid disease. *J Clin In vest* 1972;51:2103–2113.
48. Brunzell JD, Albers JJ, Haas LB, et al: Prevalence of lipid abnormalities in chronic hemodialysis. *Metabolism* 1977;26:903–910.
49. Ginsberg H, Olefsky J, Farquhar JW, et al: Moderate ethanol ingestion and plasma triglyceride levels: a study in normal and hypertriglyceridemic persons. *Ann Intern Med* 1974;80:143–149.
50. Baraona E, Lieber CS: Effects of ethanol on lipid metabolism. *J Lipid Res* 1979;20: 289–315.
51. Robinson AG, Loeb JN: Ethanol ingestion: commonest cause of elevated plasma osmolality? *N Engl J Med* 1971;284:1253–1255.
52. Borges HF, Hocks J, Kjellstrand CM: Mannitol intoxication in patients with renal failure. *Arch Intern Med* 1982;142:63–66.
53. Katz M: Hyperglycemia-induced hyponatremia: calculation of expected serum sodium depression. *N Engl J Med* 1973; 289:843–844.
54. Arieff AI, Carroll HJ: Nonketotic hyperosmolar coma with hyperglycemia: clinical features, pathophysiology, renal function, acid-base balance, plasma-cerebrospinal fluid equilibria and the effects of therapy in 37 cases. *Medicine* 1972;51: 73–94.
55. Norris HT, Aasheim GM, Sherrard DJ, et al: Symptomatology, pathophysiology and treatment of the transurethral resection of the prostate syndrome. *Br J Urol* 1973;45: 420–427.
56. Henderson DJ, Middleton RG: Coma from hyponatremia following transurethral resection of prostate. *Urology* 1980; 15:267–271.
57. Osborn DE, Rao PN, Greene MJ, et al: Fluid absorption during transurethral resection. *Br Med J* 1980;2:1549–1550.
58. Frank MS, Nahata MC, Hilty MD: Glycerol: A review of its pharmacology, pharmacokinetics, adverse reactions and clinical use. *Pharmacotherapy* 1981;1: 147–160.
59. Aviram A, Pfau A, Czaczkes W, et al: Hyperosmolality with hyponatremia caused by inappropriate administration of mannitol. *Am J Med* 1967;42:648–650.
60. Sears ES: Nonketotic hyperosmolar hyperglycemia during glycerol therapy for cerebral edema. *Neurology* 1976;26: 89–94.
61. Schrier RW, Bichet DG: Osmotic and nonosmotic control of vasopressin release and the pathogenesis of impaired water excretion in adrenal, thyroid, and edematous disorders. *J Lab Clin Med* 1981;98:1–15.
62. Kleeman CR, Maxwell MH, Rockney R: Production of hypotonic urine in humans in the probable absence of antidiuretic hormone (ADH). *Proc Soc Exp Biol Med* 1957;96:189–191.
63. Jamison RL, Buerkert J, Lacy FB: A micropuncture study of collecting tubule function in rats with hereditary diabetes insipidus. *J Clin Invest* 1971;50:2444- 2452.
64. Ufferman RC, Schrier RW: Importance of sodium intake and mineralocorticoid hormone in the impaired water excretion in adrenal insufficiency. *J Clin Invest* 1972; 51:1639–1646.
65. Boykin J, McCool A, Robertson G, et al: Mechanism of impaired water excretion in mineralocorticoid deficient dogs. *Clin Res* 1975;23:233A.
66. Ashraf N, Locksley R, Arieff A: Thiazide-induced hyponatremia associated with death or neurologic damage in outpatients. *Am J Med* 1981;70:1163–1168.
67. Houdent C, Gruber D, LeVasseur F, et al: Pathologie iatrogère due à l'association amiloride-hydrochlorthiazide. *Ann Med Interne (Paris)* 1976;127:628–631.
68. Roberts CJC, Mitchell JV, Donley AJ: Hyponatremia: Adverse effect of diuretic treatment. *Br Med J* 1977;1:210.
69. Abramow M, Cogan E: Clinical aspects and pathophysiology of diuretic-induced hyponatremia. *Adv Nephrol* 1984;13:1–28.
70. Fichman MP, Vorherr H, Kleeman CR, Telfer N: Diuretic-induced hyponatremia. *Ann Intern Med* 1971;75:853–863.
71. Kennedy RM, Earley L: Profound hyponatremia resulting from a thiazide-induced decrease in urinary diluting capacity in a

patient with primary polydipsia. *N Engl J Med* 1970;282: 1185–1186.

72. Booker JA: Severe symptomatic hyponatremia in elderly outpatients: the role of thiazide therapy and stress. *J Am Geriatr Soc* 1984;32:108–113.
73. Szatalowicz VL, Miller PD, Lacher JW, et al: Comparative effect of diuretics on renal water excretion in hyponatremic oedematous disorders. *Clin Sci* 1982;62:235–238.
74. Bell NH, Schedl HP, Bartter FC: An explanation for abnormal water retention and hypoosmolality in congestive heart failure. *Am J Med* 1964;36:351–360.
75. Schedl HP, Bartter FC: An explanation for and experimental correction of the abnormal water diuresis in cirrhosis. *J Clin Invest* 1960;39:248–261.
76. Bichet D, Szatalowicz V, Chaimovitz C, et al: Role of vasopressin in abnormal water excretion in cirrhotic patients. *Ann Intern Med* 1982;96:413–417.
77. Skowsky R, Riestra J, Martinez I, et al: Arginine vasopressin (AVP) kinetics in hepatic cirrhosis. *Clin Res* 1976;24:101A.
78. Klinger ER Jr, Vaamonde CA, Vaamonde LE, et al: Renal function changes in cirrhosis of the liver. *Arch Intern Med* 1970; 125:1010–1015.
79. Eisenmenger WJ, Blondheim SH, Bongiovanni AM, et al: Electrolyte studies on patients with cirrhosis of the liver. *J Clin Invest* 1950;291:1491–1499.
80. Bernard DB, Alexander EA, Couser WG, et al: Renal sodium retention during volume expansion in experimental nephrotic syndrome. *Kidney Int* 1978;14:478–485.
81. Gur A, Adefuin PY, Siegel NJ, et al: A study of the renal handling of water in lipoid nephrosis. *Pediatr Res* 1976;10: 197–201.
82. Grausz H, Lieberman R, Earley LE: Effect of plasma albumin on sodium reabsorption in patients with nephrotic syndrome. *Kidney Int* 1972;1:47–54.
83. Schrier RW, Lehman D, Zacherle B, et al: Effect of furosemide on free-water excretion in edematous patients with hyponatremia. *Kidney Int* 1973;3:30–34.
84. Lamdin E, Kleeman CR, Rubini M, et al: Studies on alcohol diuresis: II. The response to ethyl alcohol in certain disease states characterized by impaired water tolerance. *J Clin Invest* 1956;35:386–393.
85. Murdaugh HV: Production of diuresis in hyponatremia edematous states with alcohol. *J Clin Invest* 1956;35:726.
86. Riegger GAJ, Lieban G, Kochsick K: Antidiuretic hormone in congestive heart failure. *Am J Med* 1982;72:49–52.
87. Szatalowicz VL, Arnold PE, Chaimovitz C, et al: Radioimmunoassay of plasma arginine vasopressin in hyponatremic patients with congestive heart failure. *N Engl J Med* 1981;305:263–266.
88. Rondeau E, de Lima J, Caillens H, et al: High plasma antidiuretic hormone in patients with cardiac failure: influence of age. *Min Elec Metab* 1982;8:267–274.
89. Bartter FC, Schwartz WB: The syndrome of inappropriate secretion of antidiuretic hormone. *Am J Med* 1967;42:790–806.
90. Leaf A, Bartter FC, Santos RF, et al: Evidence in man that urinary electrolyte loss induced by Pitressin is a function of water retention. *J Clin Invest* 1953;32:868–878.
91. Beck LH: Hypouricemia in the syndrome of inappropriate secretion of antidiuretic hormone. *N Engl J Med* 1979;301:528–530.
92. Bower BF, Mason DM, Forsham PH: Bronchogenic carcinoma with inappropriate antidiuretic activity in plasma and tumor. *N Engl J Med* 1964;271:934–938.
93. Amatruda TT, Mulrow PJ, Gallagher JC, et al: Carcinoma of the lung with inappropriate antidiuresis. Demonstration of antidiuretic-hormone like activity in tumor tissue. *N Engl J Med* 1963;269:544–549.
94. Utiger RD: Inappropriate antidiuresis and carcinoma of the lung. Detection of arginine vasopressin in tumor extracts by immunoassay. *J Clin Endocrinol Metab* 1966; 26:970–974.
95. George JM, Capen CC, Phillips AS: Biosynthesis of vasopressin in vitro and ultrastructure of a bronchogenic carcinoma. *J Clin Invest* 1972;51:141–148.
96. Vorherr H, Massry SG, Utiger RD, et al: Antidiuretic principle in malignant tumor extracts from patients with inappropriate ADH syndrome. *J Clin Endocrinol Metab* 1968;28:162–168.
97. Vorherr H, Massry SG, Fallet R, et al: Antidiuretic principle in tuberculous lung tissue of a patient with pulmonary tuberculosis and hyponatremia. *Ann Intern Med* 1970;72:383–387.
98. Rosenow EC III, Segar WE, Zehr JE:

Inappropriate antidiuretic hormones secretion in pneumonia. *Mayo Clin Proc* 1972;47:169–174.

99. Thomas TH, Morgan DB, Swaminathan R, et al: Severe hyponatremia: a study of 17 patients. *Lancet* 1978;1:621–624.
100. Szatalowicz VL, Goldberg JP, Anderson RJ: Plasma antidiuretic hormone in acute respiratory failure. *Am J Med* 1982;72: 583–587.
101. Baker JW, Yerger S, Segar WE: Elevated plasma antidiuretic hormone levels in status asthmaticus. *Mayo Clin Proc* 1976; 51:31–34.
102. Sladen AM, Laver B, Pontoppidan H: Pulmonary complications and water retention in prolonged mechanical ventilation. *N Engl J Med* 1968;279:448–453.
103. Khambatta HJ, Baratz RA: IPPB, plasma ADH, and urine flow in conscious man. *J Appl Physiol* 1972;33:362–364.
104. Henry JP, Gauer OH, Reeves JL: Evidence of the atrial location of receptors influencing urine flow. *Circ Res* 1956;4:85– 90.
105. Maroon JC, Campbell RL: Subdural hematoma with inappropriate antidiuretic hormone secretion. *Arch Neurol* 1970;22:234–239.
106. Joynt RJ, Afifi A, Harbison J: Hyponatremia in subarachnoid hemorrhage. *Arch Neurol* 1965;13:633–638.
107. DeTroyer A, Demanet JC: Clinical, biological and pathogenic features of inappropriate secretion of antidiuretic hormone. *Q J Med* 1976;45:521–531.
108. Lester MC, Nelson PB: Neurological aspects of vasopressin release and the syndrome of inappropriate secretion of antidiuretic hormone. *Neurosurgery* 1981;8:735–740.
109. Sherman LM, Shenay SS, Cerra FB: Selective intra-arterial vasopressin: clinical efficacy and complications. *Ann Surg* 1979; 189:298–302.
110. Steele TH, Serpick AA, Block JB: Antidiuretic response to cyclophosphamide in man. *J Pharmacol Exp Therap* 1973;185: 245–253.
111. DeFronzo RA, Braine J, Colvin OM, Davis PJ: Water intoxication in man after cyclophosphamide therapy: time course and relation to drug activation. *Ann Intern Med* 1973;78:861–869.
112. Weissman P, Shenkman L, Gregerman RI: Chlorpropamide hyponatremia: drug-induced inappropriate antidiuretic- hormone activity. *N Engl J Med* 1972; 284:65–71.
113. Moses AM, Fenner R, Schroeder ET, Coulson R: Further studies on the mechanism by which chlorpropamide alters the action of vasopressin. *Endocrinology* 1982;111:2025–2030.
114. Murase T, Yoshida S: Mechanism of chlorpropamide action in patients with diabetes insipidus. *J Clin Endocrinol Metab* 1973; 36:174–177.
115. Moses AM, Numann P, Miller M: Mechanism of chlorpropamide-induced antidiuresis in man: Evidence for release of ADH and enhancement of peripheral action. *Metabolism* 1973;22:59–66.
116. Tanay A, Firemann Z, Yust I, et al: Chlorpropamide-induced syndrome of inappropriate antidiuretic hormone secretion. *J Am Geriatr Soc* 1981;29:334–336.
117. Fine D, Shedrovilsky H: Hyponatremia due to chlorpropamide: a syndrome resembling inappropriate secretion of antidiuretic hormone. *Ann Intern Med* 1970;72:83–87.
118. Haldar J: Release of antidiuretic hormone by morphine in rats: an *in vivo* and *in vitro* study. *Proc Soc Exp Biol Med* 1982;169: 113–120.
119. Schneiden H, Blackmore EK: The effect of nalorphine on the antidiuretic action of morphine in rats and men. *Br J Pharmacol* 1955;10:45–50.
120. Caradoc-Davies H: Opiate toxicity in elderly patients. *Br Med J* 1981;282:905–906.
121. Deutsch S, Goldberg M, Dripps RD: Postoperative hyponatremia with the inappropriate release of antidiuretic hormone. *Anesthesiology* 1966;27:250–256.
122. Stewart RB, May FE, Hale WE, et al: Psychotropic drug use in an ambulatory elderly population. *Gerontology* 1982;28: 328–335.
123. Ajlouni K, Kern MW, Tures JF, et al: Thiothixene-induced hyponatremia. *Arch Intern Med* 1974;134:1103–1105.
124. DeRivera JLG: Inappropriate secretion of antidiuretic hormone from fluphenazine therapy. *Ann Intern Med* 1975;82:811–812.
125. Luzecky MH, Burman KD, Schultz ER: The syndrome of inappropriate secretion of antidiuretic hormone associated with amitriptyline administration. *South Med J* 1974; 67:495–497.

126. Kimelman N, Albert SG: Phenothiazine-induced hyponatremia in the elderly. *Gerontology* 1984;30:132–136.
127. Peterson JC, Pollack RW, Mahoney JJ, et al: Inappropriate antidiuretic hormone: secondary to a monoamine oxidase inhibitor. *JAMA* 1978;239:1422–1424.
128. Dubovsky SL, Grabon S, Berl T, et al: Syndrome of inappropriate secretion of antidiuretic hormone with exacerbated psychosis. *Ann Intern Med* 1973;79:551–554.
129. Cohen IM: Complications of chlorpromazine therapy. *Am J Psychiatry* 1956;113: 115–121.
130. Rao KJ, Miller M, Moses A: Water intoxication and thioridazine (Mellaril[R]). *Ann Intern Med* 1975;82:61–63.
131. Gross PA, Schrier RW, Anderson RJ: Prostaglandins and water metabolism: a review with emphasis on in vivo studies. *Kidney Int* 1981;19:839–850.
132. Blum M, Aviram A: Ibuprofen induced hyponatremia. *Rheumatol Rehabil* 1980;19: 258–259.
133. Glasson P, Gaillard R, Riondel A, et al: Role of renal prostaglandins and relationship to renin, aldosterone, and antidiuretic hormone during salt depletion in man. *J Clin Endocrinol Metab* 1979;49:176–181.
134. Ukai M, Moran WJ, Zimmerman B: The role of visceral afferent pathways on vasopressin secretion and urinary excretion patterns during surgical stress. *Ann Surg* 1968;168:16–28.
135. Moran WH Jr, Miltenberger FW, Shuayb WA, et al: The relationship of antidiuretic hormone to surgical stress. *Surgery* 1964; 56:99–108.
136. Dudley HF, Boling EA, LeQuesne LP, et al: Studies on antidiuresis in surgery. Effects of anesthesia, surgery and posterior pituitary antidiuretic hormone on water metabolism in man. *Ann Surg* 1954;140:354–367.
137. Schrier RW, Berl T: Nonosmolar factors affecting renal water excretion. *N Engl J Med* 1975;292:81–88.
138. Crowe M: Hyponatremia due to syndrome of inappropriate antidiuretic hormone secretion in the elderly. *Ir Med J* 1980;73: 482–483.
139. Ditzel J: Hyponatremia in an elderly woman and inappropriate secretion of antidiuretic hormone. *Acta Med Scand* 1966; 179:407–416.
140. Goldstein CS, Braunstein, S, Goldfarb S: Idiopathic syndrome of inappropriate antidiuretic hormone secretion possibly related to advanced age. *Ann Intern Med* 1983;99: 185–188.
141. Golovchenko SF: Blood vasopressin concentration in patients of different age with hypertension. *Probl Endokrinol (Mosk)* 1979; 25:36–39.
142. Frolkis VV: Role of vasopressin in development of pathology of the cardiovascular system in old age. *Kardiologiia* 1976;16:103–110.
143. Martinez-Maldonado M: Inappropriate antidiuretic hormone secretion of unknown origin. *Kidney Int* 1980;17:554–567.
144. DiScala VA, Kinney MJ: Effects of myxedema on the renal diluting and concentrating mechanisms. *Am J Med* 1971;50: 325–335.
145. DeRubertis FR Jr, Michellis MF, Bloom ME, et al: Impaired water excretion in myxedema. *Am J Med* 1971;51:41–53.
146. Amidi M, Leon DF, DeGroot WJ, et al: Effect of the thyroid state on myocardial contractility and ventricular ejection rate in man. *Circulation* 1968;38:229–239.
147. Emmanouel DS, Lindheimer MD, Katz AI: Mechanism of impaired water excretion in the hypothyroid rat. *J Clin Invest* 1974;54: 926–934.
148. Michael UF, Kelley J, Alpert H, et al: Role of distal delivery of filtrate in impaired renal dilution of the hypothyroid rat. *Am J Physiol* 1976;230:699–705.
149. Skowsky WR, Kikuchi TA: The role of vasopressin in the impaired water excretion of myxedema. *Am J Med* 1978;64:613–621.
150. Macaron C, Famuyiwa O: Hyponatremia of hypothroidism: appropriate suppression of antidiuretic hormone. *Arch Intern Med* 1978;138:820–822.
151. Ingbar SH: The influence of aging on the human thyroid hormone economy. *Geriatr Endocrinol* 1978;5:13–21.
152. Miles AI, Needle MA: Fixed hyponatremia with normal responses to varying salt and water intake. *N Engl J Med* 1971;284: 26–28.
153. DeFronzo RA, Goldberg M, Agus ZA: Normal diluting capacity in hyponatremic patients: reset osmostat or a variant of the syndrome of inappropriate antidiuretic hormone secretion. *Ann Intern Med* 1976;84: 538–542.

154. Flear CTG, Singh CM: Hyponatremia and sick cells. *Br J Anaesth* 1973;45:976–994.
155. Barlow ED, DeWardener HE: Compulsive water drinking. *Q J Med* 1959;28:235–258.
156. Langgard H, Smith WO: Self-induced water intoxication without predisposing illness. *N Engl J Med* 1962;266:378–381.
157. Beresford HR: Polydipsia, hydrochlorthiazide and water intoxication. *JAMA* 1970; 214:879–883.
158. Bethune JE, Nelson DH: Hyponatremia in hypopituitarism. *N Engl J Med* 1965;272: 771–776.
159. Green HH, Harrington AR, Valtin H: On the role of antidiuretic hormone in the inhibition of acute water diuresis in adrenal insufficiency and the effects of gluco–and mineralocorticoids in reversing the inhibition. *J Clin Invest* 1970;49:1724–1736.
160. Norenberg MD, Leslie KO, Robertson AS: Association between rise in serum sodium and central pontine myelinolysis. *Ann Neurol* 1982;11:128–135.
161. Norenberg MD: A hypothesis of osmotic endothelial injury: a pathogenetic mechanism in central pontine myelinolysis. *Arch Neurol* 1983;40:66–69.
162. Laureno R: Central pontine myelinolysis following rapid correction of hyponatremia. *Ann Neurol* 1983;13:232–242.
163. Hantman D, Rossier B, Zahlman R, et al: Rapid correction of hyponatremia in the syndrome of inappropriate antidiuretic hormone secretion. *Ann Intern Med* 1973; 78:870–875.
164. Ayus JC, Olivero JJ, Frommer JP: Rapid correction of severe hyponatremia with intravenous hypertonic saline solution. *Am J Med* 1982;72:43–48.
165. Laver A, Saccagi A, Ronco C, et al: Continuous arteriovenous hemofiltration in the critically ill patient: clinical use and operational characteristics. *Ann Intern Med* 1983;99:455–460.
166. Decaux G, Unger J, Brimioulle S, et al: Hyponatremia in the syndrome of inappropriate secretion of antidiuretic hormone: rapid correction with urea, sodium chloride, and water restriction therapy. *JAMA* 1982; 247:471–474.
167. Decaux G, Brimioulle S, Genette F, et al: Treatment of the syndrome of inappropriate secretion of antidiuretic hormone by urea. *Am J Med* 1980;69:99–106.
168. Decaux G: Treatment of the syndrome of inappropriate secretion of antidiuretic hormone by long loop diuretics. *Nephron* 1983; 35:82–88.
169. DeTroyer A: Demeclocycline. Treatment for syndrome of inappropriate antidiuretic hormone secretion. *JAMA* 1977;237:2723–2726.
170. White MG, Fetner C: Treatment of the syndrome of inappropriate secretion of antidiuretic hormone with lithium carbonate. *N Engl J Med* 1975;292:390–392.
171. Forrest JN, Cox M, Hong C, et al: Superiority of demeclocycline over lithium in the treatment of chronic syndrome of inappropriate secretion of antidiuretic hormone. *N Engl J Med* 1978;298:173–177.

CHAPTER 9

Acid-Base Disorders in the Elderly

David A. Goodkin
Robert Waldman
Robert G. Narins

The functional reserve of normal kidneys and lungs is remarkably vast. Despite the inexorable toll which passing decades exact upon hundreds of thousands of nephrons and alveolar units, acid-base disturbances associated with aging are not the rule, but the exception. Healthy elderly individuals in fact maintain normal blood pH, P_{CO_2} and HCO_3^- levels under basal conditions. However, during the stress of an intercurrent illness or an atypical challenge upon systemic pH, the homeostatic balance routinely maintained by these senescent organs proves fragile. Before addressing in detail the limitations which the elderly face in responding to perturbations of acid-base metabolism, specific disturbances for which they are at particular risk, and the therapeutic interventions currently available, it is important to review the central tenets of normal acid-base physiology and a practical approach to the prompt recognition of simple and mixed disorders.

FUNDAMENTAL DEFINITIONS AND CONCEPTS

Normal blood hydrogen ion concentration is rigorously controlled between the narrow limits of 36 and 44 *nanoequivalents* (nEq) per liter, which corresponds to a pH range of 7.36 to 7.44. As shown by a rearrangement of the Henderson-Hasselbalch equation,[1] the prevailing ratio of P_{CO_2} to

HCO_3^- concentration determines the exact hydrogen ion concentration:

$$(H^+) = 24 \times (P_{CO_2}/HCO_3^-) \qquad (1)$$

Cellular metabolic and oxidative reactions produce ongoing daily loads of about 1 mEq fixed acid/kg body weight, and of approximately 20,000 mmol CO_2. Two essential functions of the kidneys are the resynthesis of bicarbonate, to offset that which is consumed by metabolic acid production, and the reabsorption of large quantities of bicarbonate filtered at the glomerulus, in order to preserve the serum concentration and body stores of this invaluable buffer. The lungs, of course, eliminate gaseous CO_2. Acid-base homeostasis thus entails constant elimination of protons and CO_2, at moderate rates, during periods of good health. During pathologic stresses, blood buffers immediately dampen adverse impacts upon pH, and the kidneys and lungs subsequently react with compensatory responses in HCO_3^- and P_{CO_2}, respectively.[2-4]

Metabolic acidosis defines a pathologic process wherein an excess of fixed acid accumulates and consumes bicarbonate. Referring to equation (1), it is clear that such a hypobicarbonatemic process will elicit an increase in blood hydrogen ion concentration. When this simple disorder causes pH to fall below normal, by definition an acidemic state exists. Alternatively, the hallmark of a primary metabolic alkalosis is a sustained increment in serum bicarbonate, which will mandate a decrease in the P_{CO_2}/HCO_3^- ratio and a decrease in blood H^+ concentration, and thus tend to beget an alkalemia (an abnormally high blood pH). These primary metabolic acid-base disorders will, as mentioned, stimulate compensatory responses. Brain-stem chemoreceptors are sensitive to changes in the pH of extracellular fluid; ventilation is adjusted to minimize acid-base derangements. Hence, respiration is increased in response to metabolic acidosis, and the secondary hypocapnia reduces the elevated P_{CO_2}/HCO_3^- ratio. This compensatory fall in P_{CO_2} returns blood acidity toward normal, but never fully eliminates the rise in hydrogen ion concentration induced by the primary hypobicarbonatemia. The alkalemia which develops during simple metabolic alkalosis prompts the CNS to inhibit respiration. A compensatory rise in P_{CO_2} then partially offsets the initial decrease in the P_{CO_2}/HCO_3^- ratio caused by hyperbicarbonatemia.

Simple metabolic acid-base disorders are readily detected once one grasps the significance of the directional change in serum bicarbonate and realizes that the compensatory change in P_{CO_2} should be of parallel direction. The degree of change in serum bicarbonate concentration induces a predictable magnitude of respiratory compensation. Table 9-1 summarizes the anticipated compensations for each of the simple acid-base disorders. In fact, failure to attain the expected change in P_{CO_2} indicates the presence of a concomitant primary respiratory disturbance, prompting the diagnosis of a complicated, or mixed, metabolic-respiratory disorder.

Respiratory acidosis and alkalosis result from primary hypercapnia or hypocapnia, respectively. Thus, it is a change in the numerator of the P_{CO_2}/HCO_3^- ratio which serves to alter blood H^+ concentration. The respiratory acid-base disorders evoke compensatory adjustments of serum bicarbonate concentration. Rapid, albeit relatively small changes in serum bicarbonate concentration are effected by release or adsorption of hydrogen ions by cellular and extracellular nonbicarbonate buffers. Release of protons stimulated by respiratory alkalosis reduces serum bicarbonate concentration, thereby ameliorating the alkalemia. Adsorption of protons provoked by respiratory acidosis generates new bicarbonate, thereby lessening the hypercapnia-induced acidemia. The degree of compensation is proportional to the change in P_{CO_2} and is highly predictable (Table 9-1). The renal response to primary respiratory disorders develops over 24 to 36 hours. The sustained hypo- or hypercapnia causes the kidney to further

Table 9-1
Expected Compensation for Simple Acid-Base Disorders

Disorder	Primary Defect	Compensatory Response	Magnitude of Expected Compensation
Metabolic			
Acidosis	$\downarrow\downarrow\downarrow HCO_3^-$	$\downarrow\downarrow P_{CO_2}$	$P_{CO_2} = 1.5(HCO_3^-)\ 8 \pm 2$
Alkalosis	$\uparrow\uparrow\uparrow HCO_3^-$	$\uparrow\uparrow P_{CO_2}$	P_{CO_2} increases 6 mmHg for each 10 mEq/L increase in HCO_3^-
Respiratory			
Acidosis			
Acute	$\uparrow\uparrow\uparrow P_{CO_2}$	$\uparrow HCO_3^-$	HCO_3^- increases 1 mEq/L for each 10 mmHg rise in P_{CO_2}
Chronic	$\uparrow\uparrow\uparrow P_{CO_2}$	$\uparrow\uparrow HCO_3^-$	HCO_3^- increases 3.5 mEq/L for each 10 mmHg rise in P_{CO_2}
Alkalosis			
Acute	$\downarrow\downarrow\downarrow P_{CO_2}$	$\downarrow HCO_3^-$	HCO_3^- decreases 2 mEq/L for each 10 mmHg fall in P_{CO_2}
Chronic	$\downarrow\downarrow\downarrow P_{CO_2}$	$\downarrow\downarrow HCO_3^-$	HCO_3^- decreases 5 mEq/L for each 10 mmHg fall in P_{CO_2}

shrink or expand bicarbonate stores and thereby augment the acutely induced changes in bicarbonatemia. Renal bicarbonate synthesis is stimulated by respiratory acidosis and bicarbonaturia and acid retention by respiratory alkalosis. Therefore, both the severity and the duration of a change in P_{CO_2} dictate the magnitude of the compensatory increment or decrement in serum HCO_3^-, as delineated in Table 9-1. If a patient with a respiratory acidosis generates more alkali than the increment predicted by the guidelines in Table 9-1, then a superimposed metabolic alkalosis must be present. A concomitant primary metabolic acidosis may be diagnosed should the serum bicarbonate prove lower than one would predict on the basis of the P_{CO_2}. An abnormal P_{CO_2} and an appropriate degree of metabolic response chemically define uncomplicated, primary respiratory acid-base disorders.

To this point, the criteria for diagnosis of the simple acid-base disorders, and of the mixed metabolic/respiratory disturbances, have been set forth. One broad category remains to be characterized: mixed metabolic disorders, where more than one factor influences the serum HCO_3^- concentration. Of course, there is no group of respiratory counterparts (ie, no "mixed respiratory disorders"), since a patient cannot simultaneously hypoventilate and hyperventilate. An understanding of the concept of the anion gap (AG) is indispensible to the recognition of mixed metabolic acid-base disorders.[5] Simply stated, the AG represents the difference between the serum sodium concentration and the sum of the serum chloride and bicarbonate concentrations:

$$AG = (Na^+) - (Cl^- + HCO_3^-) \qquad (2)$$

The AG in normal subjects equals 12 ± 2 mEq/L. It serves as an index of the total concentration of the extracellular fluid (ECF) anions which are not routinely measured by clinical laboratories. Albumin, phosphate, and sulfate normally account for most of these unmeasured anions. It is important to realize that the AG is a conceptual, diagnostic tool, but does not represent any actual "deficiency" of serum anions. The sum of all ECF cations always equals the sum of all ECF anions, as ECF electroneutrality is never lost. It is because clinical laboratories routinely measure almost all the positive charges by assaying sodium and potassium, but a lesser fraction of all the negative charges by analyzing for chloride and bicarbonate, that an apparent disparity in cations and anions is created.

Metabolic acidoses consume bicarbonate, and substitute more acidic anions. During a hyperchloremic acidosis, such as renal tubular acidosis or diarrhea, the lost alkali is replaced by an equal quantity of Cl^-. The AG is unchanged, because the sum of Cl^- and HCO_3^- is not altered. Accrual of strong acids other than HCl in the ECF will not affect the serum Cl^- level, while consuming HCO_3^-. An increased AG then reflects the drop in the sum of Cl^- plus HCO_3^-. Table 9-2 segregates the various etiologies of metabolic acidosis on the basis of their effects on the AG. When a high AG metabolic acidosis is the sole acid-base disorder present, a tight stoichiometry between the decrement in serum bicarbonate concentration (ΔHCO_3^-) and the increment in the AG (ΔAG) will exist.[5-7] For example, in typical lactic acidosis both the decrement in plasma HCO_3^- and the increment in AG will closely match the rise in blood lactate concentration. Loss of this stoichiometric equivalence between the ΔAG and the ΔHCO_3^- constitutes key evidence for the presence of a mixed metabolic acid-base disturbance.

Consider first the setting in which the ΔHCO_3^- exceeds the ΔAG. Some of the alkali consumed must have been replaced by Cl^-, since the increment in AG (reflective of the concentration of the non-HCl acid anion) is less than the ΔHCO_3^-. The diagnosis of a mixed high AG and hyperchloremic (normal AG) acidosis follows from the observation of this chemical profile. Any combination of the high AG/normal AG acidoses listed in Table 9-2 may prove contributory. The hyperchloremic acidosis component may result from compensation of yet another disorder, respiratory alkalosis. Table 9-3 outlines the com-

Table 9-2
Causes of Metabolic Acidosis

Elevated Anion Gap	Normal Anion Gap
Renal Failure	Hypokalemic Acidosis
	Renal tubular acidosis
Ketoacidosis	Proximal
Starvation	Distal
Diabetes mellitus	Buffer deficiency
Alcohol-associated	phosphate
Glycogenosis I	ammonia
Defects in gluconeogenesis	Diarrhea
	Posthypocapnic
Lactic Acidosis	Carbonic anhydrase inhibitors
	Acetazolamide
Toxins	Mafenide acetate
Methanol	Ureteral diversions
Ethylene glycol	Ureterosigmoidostomy
Salicylates	Ileal bladder
Paraldehyde	Ileal ureter
	Normal-Hyperkalemic Acidosis
	"Early" renal failure
	Hydronephrosis
	Addition of HCl, NH_4Cl, Arg•HCl,Lys•HCl
	Hypoaldosteronism

mon causes of mixed metabolic acidosis with $\Delta HCO_3^- > \Delta AG$. Also worth noting is the unusual set of circumstances wherein a pre-existing low AG prevents the apparent Δ AG from accurately portraying the accumulation of a pathologic acid anion. An example would be a patient with profound hypoalbuminemia who goes into shock and develops a lactic acidosis. If the low albumin concentration had covertly lowered this individual's "base-line" AG from 12 mEq/L to 5 mEq/L, then a subsequent lactate burden of 10 mEq/L would decrease the serum HCO_3^- from 24 mEq/L to 14 mEq/L, and increase the AG from 5 mEq/L to 15 mEq/L. When the physician compares the resultant chemical profile with reference normal values, the resultant ΔHCO_3^- of minus 10 mEq/L would exceed the apparent ΔAG of 3 mEq/L (15 mEq/L minus the presumed base-line AG of 12 mEq/L). Table 9-3 includes other causes of a low AG which might mask high AG

Table 9-3
Common Causes of High Anion Gap (AG) with Excessive Hypobicarbonatemia ($\Delta HCO_3 > \Delta AG$)

1. Mixed High AG and Normal AG Acidosis
   a. Renal-related causes
      Early chronic renal failure
      Uremic acidosis with proximal or distal renal tubular acidosis
   b. Diabetes mellitus
      Diarrhea and diabetic ketoacidosis (DKA)
      Hypoaldosteronism and DKA
      Repair of DKA
   c. Lactic acidosis complicating diarrhea or other causes of normal AG acidosis

2. High AG Acidosis Partially Masked by a Coexistent Cause of a Low AG
   a. Paraproteinemia/hypoalbuminemia
   b. Severe hyponatremia
   c. Bromide/iodide
   d. Hypermagnesemia

3. Combined High AG Metabolic Acidosis with Chronic Respiratory Alkalosis
   a. Cirrhosis of the liver
   b. Burns treated with mafenide
   c. Pulmonary-renal syndromes
   d. Salicylate toxicity

acidoses and cause an apparent $\Delta HCO_3^- > \Delta AG$. None of these entities are encountered often, but when present they can divert attention from the true magnitude of a dangerous organic acidosis.

A metabolic alkalosis complicating metabolic acidosis is the most common cause of a ΔHCO_3^- that is less than the ΔAG. Table 9-4 displays the causes of metabolic alkalosis and Table 9-5 sets forth the common causes of a ΔAG which exceeds the ΔHCO_3^-. Note that the confounding metabolic alkalosis may be a secondary response to a primary respiratory acidosis inducing compensatory hyperbicarbonatemia.

The second possible explanation for the finding of $\Delta HCO_3^- < \Delta AG$ is the occurrence of an elevation in AG which is not caused by a metabolic acidosis (see Table 9-5). There is no reason to expect any decrement in serum HCO_3^- when influences other than metabolic acidosis increase the AG. Such conditions arise during administration of high-dose antibiotics or sodium salts of organic acids (sodium lactate, citrate, or acetate)—unmeasured anion concentration and AG increase, without influence upon serum HCO_3^-. Hypomagnesemia, with the concomitant hypokalemia and hypocalcemia it often induces, leads to accompanying losses of chloride. The fall in serum Cl^-, without change in serum Na^+ or HCO_3^-, increases the calculated AG. Perhaps surprising is the fact that pure, simple metabolic alkalosis modestly increases the AG. Excess alkali buffers hydrogen ions away from plasma proteins, which in turn contribute to the circulating unmeasured anions. Nonacidotic high AG states are reviewed in greater detail elsewhere.[5,8,9]

In summary, mixed acid-base disorders may be diagnosed on the basis of chemical profiles which reveal inappropriate or absent compensatory reactions to primary disturbances, or loss of the equality between the increment in AG and decrement in serum HCO_3^- concentration which is known to exist during simple high AG metabolic acidosis.

Table 9-4
Causes of Metabolic Alkalosis

ECF Volume Contraction (Saline-responsive U_{Cl} < 10 mEq/d)	ECF Volume Normal-Expanded (Sale-unresponsive U_{Cl} > 10 mEq/d
GI Alkalosis Gastric losses (vomiting, nasogastric suction) Chloride diarrhea	Normotensive Alkaloses Bartter's syndrome Severe K^+ deficiency Hypercalcemia Refeeding edema
Renal Alkalosis Diuretic-induced Exposure to poorly reabsorbed anions (antibiotics, SO_4^{2-}, PO_4^{3-} Posthypercapnia	Hypertensive Alkaloses Primary aldosteronism Hyperreninemic syndromes 11- and 17-Hydroxylase deficiency Liddle's syndrome
Exogenous Alkali Baking soda ($NaHCO_3$) Antacids Na salts of organic acids (citrate, lactate, acetate) Contraction Alkalosis	Exposure to nonadrenal mineralocorticoid (carbenoxolone sodium, licorice, chewing tobacco)

Table 9-5
Common Causes of High Anion Gap (AG) with Blunted Hypobicarbonatemia ($\Delta HCO_3 < \Delta AG$)

1. Mixed High AG Metabolic Acidosis and Metabolic Alkalosis
   - *a.* Renal-related causes:
     - Uremic vomiting
     - Alkali therapy in uremia
     - Transfusion alkalosis in uremia
     - $Al(OH)_3$ plus sodium polystyrene sulfonate therapy in uremia
     - Diuretic administration in uremia
   - *b.* Diabetes mellitus:
     - DKA and vomiting
     - $NaHCO_3$ therapy of DKA
   - *c.* Lactic Acidosis
     - When complicated by various causes of metabolic alkalosis
2. Nonacidotic High AG plus Normo- or Hyperbicarbonatemia
   - *a.* Pure metabolic alkalosis
   - *b.* High-dose carbenicillin/penicillin
   - *c.* Dehydration
   - *d.* Administration of salts of organic acids: Na acetate, citrate, or lactate
   - *e.* Hypomagnesemia
3. Mixed High AG Metabolic Acidosis plus Respiratory Acidosis

ACID-BASE PHYSIOLOGY IN THE ELDERLY

The principles discussed to this point apply to the aged as well as to the young. Specifically, blood hydrogen ion concentration depends upon the P_{CO_2}/HCO_3^- ratio, with the kidneys striving to appropriately adjust the serum bicarbonate concentration while ventilatory responses regulate the P_{CO_2}. Advancing age progressively impairs the maximal level of function of both the pulmonary and renal systems. Airway compliance, expiratory muscle strength, and vital capacity all decrease with age, and arterial PO_2 falls more than 10% between the ages of 20 and 80.[10] Furthermore, lung elastic recoil is lost due to age-related changes in elastin, and forced expiratory volume in one second (FEV_1) is markedly reduced.[11] As detailed in other sections of this book, the kidneys are also profoundly influenced by advancing years. Briefly, there are substantial and progressive reductions in cortical mass, renal plasma flow per gram of remaining tissue, glomerular filtration rate (GFR), plasma renin (and, secondarily, aldosterone) levels, renal concentrating capacity, diluting capacity, and ability to conserve sodium.[12,13]

The fact that normalcy of acid-base status is maintained by the aged under resting conditions, despite the substantial extent of renal and pulmonary functional losses, is truly impressive. Shock and Yiengst studied the acid-base parameters of 152 ambulatory men ranging from 40 to 89 years of age.[14] They found that serum HCO_3^- and P_{CO_2} do not significantly change between these ages, and remain within normal limits. Serum pH is also maintained within the normal range, although there is a statistically valid correlation between advancing years and declining pH. The mean serum pH of 7.368 obtained from the 80- to 89-year-old men studied is significantly lower than the reference mean of 7.400 stated for 20- to 29-year-old men.

Although elderly persons therefore appear capable of eliminating their typical daily burdens of acid and CO_2, they cannot respond to nonphysiologic acid-base stresses with the speed or vigor of younger individuals. Two groups have investigated renal acidification in the elderly, following acute acid loading.[15,16] Both employed the standard oral ammonium chloride (NH_4Cl) test, wherein the subject ingests 0.1 g NH_4Cl (in capsular form) per kilogram of body weight, over 30 to 45 minutes. The normal kidney responds to the ensuing 2 to 5 mEq/L decrease in serum HCO_3^- by markedly increasing net acid excretion and lowering urinary pH to below 5.3, within 4 to 6 hours. In both of the studies cited, the elderly patients had normal base-line acid-base values, lowered urinary pH to <5.3 in response to acid loading, and increased their net urinary acid excretion rates. However, the cohorts over age 60 were able to excrete only *half* as much of the ingested acid as did the groups of subjects under age 35 in the 6 to 8 hours following the acid loading. When corrections for reduction in glomerular filtration rate (GFR) are introduced, the age-related differences in net acid excretion are abolished. To the extent that the GFR is an index of functional renal mass, then the impairment in renal acidification seen in the elderly is largely due to loss of nephrons. These studies also demonstrate age-related decreases in urinary ammonium excretion, despite normal serum levels of glutamine (the precursor for renal ammoniagenesis). Titratable acid excretion, on the other hand, is not diminished with aging. Agarwal and Cabebe find that younger subjects can lower their urinary pH to an appreciably greater degree than can the elderly,[16] suggesting a distal tubular pH-gradient defect in the older persons. Adler et al, however, found no significant difference in the minimum urinary pH achieved.[15]

It is interesting to note that both of these papers report lower total acid excretion by the older subjects than by the young during the control periods. Since their control blood hydrogen ion concentrations are stable and within normal limits, the elderly must produce less acid endogenously each day, or they are in a chronic state of positive hydrogen ion balance with ongoing consumption of intracellular buffers (eg, in bone). The latter explanation is less tenable, as it is not to be expected that fixed body buffers would undergo progressive titration in the face of normal serum HCO_3^- concentrations.

Another study examined the effect of prolonged, rather than acute, NH_4Cl-loading on geriatric acid-base status.[17] Six subjects under age 39 and six over age 64 received 0.08 g NH_4Cl/kg body weight (ie, 1.5 mEq H^+/kg) during each day of the study. All had base-line serum pH and HCO_3^- values that were normal. By 1 week of acid ingestion, all six young subjects had adapted to the ongoing load, and their pH and serum HCO_3^- values had returned to normal. The elderly subjects developed more severe decreases in blood pH and serum HCO_3^- concentration. Although the acid salt was administered to this group for 11 to 14 days, no subject over age 64 was able to raise his pH or HCO_3^- to his base-line level prior to discontinuation of the drug. Urinary chemistries were not determined. This evidence suggests that geriatric individuals are not only restricted in their ability to excrete single, acute acid loads, but that their capacity to adapt to an ongoing, less severe acid burden is deficient as well.

Rosen avers that elderly patients respond retardedly to alkali loads, in a manner which is similar to their reduced rate of response to acid loading.[18] Thus, it is likely that their sluggish bicarbonaturic response to either infusion or ingestion of alkali would predispose them to metabolic alkalosis.

Acute experimental challenges to the ventilatory responsiveness of geriatric subjects reveal, again, that the elderly do not react to acid-base insults as effectively as their juniors, notwithstanding their ability to maintain normal P_{CO_2} and pH values when unstressed. Kronenberg and Drage first reported that the ventilatory response to acute hypercapnia, induced by the use of a rebreathing bag, is significantly decreased in elderly men.[19] In 1981, Peterson et al examined this phenomenon in greater detail.[20] Healthy volunteers rebreathed a mixture of 6% CO_2 – 94% O_2. All subjects reached end-tidal P_{CO_2} values of 60mmHg, while P_{O_2} was maintained above normal to preclude hypoxic stimulation of ventilation. Ten subjects aged 65 to 79 attained a mean minute volume of only 34.6 L, which is significantly lower than the mean value of 48.7 L generated by nine 22- to 29-year-olds. Sophisticated study of compartmental ventilation (eg, rib cage displacements) by magnetometry, and of inspiratory muscular effort by measurement of airway occlusion pressures, revealed that neither diminished respiratory compliance nor muscular weakness accounts for the impaired ventilatory flow responses in the elderly. The authors conclude that the differences between the groups are caused by alteration of neural output to the respiratory muscles in the aged, rather than mechanical differences. It is unclear whether geriatric subjects have difficulty in chemoreception, in central processing of perceived stimuli to ventilation, or in the delivery of neuromuscular excitation. The response to artificially induced *hypo*capnia was not investigated.

In light of all the above experiments, it should be clear that elderly patients are vulnerable indeed to acid-base disorders. Regardless of the precise variety of acid-base perturbation, the geriatric patient can mount only limited responses by the kidneys and lungs to protect the blood pH. Thus, the physician must diagnose and treat such disturbances in this population most exigently. The principles of acid-base pathophysiology and diagnosis discussed earlier apply to all ages. Thus, meticulous attention must be paid to the pH, HCO_3^-, P_{CO_2}, and AG in order to assess the type and severity of disorder(s) present, regardless of the patient's age. However, certain diseases and other causes of acid-base disorders are particularly prevalent among the geriatric population; clinical approaches must be tailored accordingly. The following sections will explore acid-base issues specifically relevant to the elderly. The differential diagnoses set forth in Tables 9-2, 9-4, 9-7, and 9-8 include entities affecting the young, such as diabetic ketoacidosis, congenital disorders, and pregnancy, which are considered in general reviews[3-5] but will not be discussed in detail again at this time.

SPECIFIC ACID-BASE DISORDERS AFFLICTING THE AGED

Metabolic Acidosis (Table 9-2)

Hypokalemic, normal AG acidoses

Diarrhea Diarrhea is a common problem for the elderly, arising spontaneously or resulting from fecal impaction, chronic intestinal ischemia, laxative abuse, dietary changes, or malignancy.[21] Bicarbonate losses in the stool produce a normal AG acidification of the blood. Potassium lost in the stool often leads to hypokalemia which provides a diagnostic clue in cases where a diarrheal etiology is not readily apparent from the history and physical. Drugs which may produce diarrheal side effects are often prescribed for the elderly, including quinidine, ampillicin, erythromycin (its efficacy in treating legionnaire's disease has led to its renewed popularity as a geriatric antimicrobial) and the nonsteroidal anti-inflammatory (NSAI) agents. It bears emphasizing that NSAI agents now represent the most widely prescribed generic group of drugs,[22] and are taken by millions of aged arthritis sufferers. Studies have demonstrated the laxative-like effects of NSAI drugs, both in vitro[23] and in vivo.[24,25] The renal effects of these drugs also may contribute to metabolic acidosis, as will be discussed subsequently.

As is already evident from our consideration of diarrhea, numerous medicines can induce acid-base disturbances. Table 9-6 provides a list of potential offenders which are often taken by the aged.

Renal tubular acidosis Renal tubular acidosis (RTA) is characterized by a normal AG, and results from: (1) failure of the proximal tubule to reabsorb a sufficient proportion of the filtered HCO_3^- (proximal RTA), (2) inability of the distal tubule to generate and maintain a hydrogen ion gradient between tubular lumen and blood

Table 9-6
Medicines Which Predispose the Elderly to Acid-Base Disorders

Acid-Base Disorder	Effect
Metabolic acidosis	
Acetazolamide	Carbonic anhydrase inhibition
Amphotericin B	Renal tubular acidosis (RTA)
Antibiotics	Diarrhea
Aspirin	High AG
Laxatives	Diarrhea
NSAI*	Diarrhea; low renin/low aldosterone
Phenformin†	Lactic acidosis
Quinidine	Diarrhea
Streptozotocin	Lactic acidosis; RTA
Tetracycline (old)	RTA
Metabolic alkalosis	
Antacids	Exogenous alkali
Cancer chemotherapy	Vomiting
Carbenoxolone†	Stimulates distal H^+ secretion
Digoxin	Vomiting
Diuretics	Contraction; bicarbonate retention
Estrogens	Increase renin substrate/aldosterone
Theophylline	Vomiting
Respiratory acidosis	
Barbiturates	Respiratory center suppression
Benzodiazepenes	Respiratory center suppression
Ethclorvynol	Respiratory center suppression
Opiates	Respiratory center suppression
Respiratory alkalosis	
Aspirin	Respiratory center stimulation

*NSAI = nonsteroidal anti-inflammatory agents.
†Not prescribed in United States; used abroad.

(distal RTA), or, (3) deficiency of urinary buffer (ammonium or phosphate). Narins and Goldberg describe these pathophysiologic processes in much greater detail.[26] Several diseases which increase in incidence with advancing age may cause a proximal RTA: amyloidosis, lead nephropathy, multiple myeloma, and other hyperglobulinemic states. The use of ancient tetracycline may also cause proximal RTA. Amyloidosis, hyperparathyroidism, and hyperglobulinemic states may lead to distal RTA, as well as to proximal RTA. Systemic amyloidosis is simply and safely diagnosed by aspiration of subcutaneous abdominal fat for Congo red staining and examination.[27,28] This procedure is receiving increasing attention as the preferred alternative to gingival, rectal, or renal biopsy. Sjögren's syndrome is most prevalent in the elderly, and in many cases has been associated with distal RTA. Amphotericin B is a potent agent, used to treat systemic fungal infections in elderly immunocompromised patients. A secondary distal RTA very commonly complicates this therapy. Failure of ammoniagenesis with consequent normal AG metabolic acidosis is known to occur in the settings of gout and of progressive tubulo-interstitial nephropathies; the elderly are prone to develop both of these entities. Low renin states also contribute to tubular acidosis, but this variety is hyperkalemic, and hence will be discussed subsequently.

Carbonic anhydrase inhibition Glaucoma is present in 2% of all persons over the age of 40.[29] Acetazolamide beneficially lowers intraocular pressure, but by inhibiting renal carbonic anhydrase it also can effect a metabolic acidosis. Since acetazolamide is usually reserved for patients unresponsive to topical medication,[30] this side effect may preclude use of the drug, and thus make surgical intervention a necessity. Laser therapy of glaucoma is a new alternative which holds great promise.[31] Fortunately, it is unusual for serum HCO_3^- to fall below 18 mEq/L due to acetazolamide usage.[32]

Ureteral diversions Elderly patients may require ureteral transplantation because of neoplastic complications (pelvic exenteration, bladder resection, obstruction by tumor, postirradiation bladder pathology), tuberculous bladder contractures, complications of urinary reflux, or inflammatory disease of the lower urinary tract. Diversional procedures sometimes permit urine to come in contact with intestinal mucosa for extended periods. Bicarbonate is transported into the urine, in exchange for Cl^-, leading to metabolic acidosis. A reduction in serum HCO_3^- complicates 50% to 75% of ureterosigmoidostomies,[33] while ileal diversions are less apt to result in stasis. Creevy observes hyperchloremic acidosis in less than 20% of patients undergoing ureteroileal anastomosis.[34] When metabolic acidosis complicates a ureteral diversion, oral $NaHCO_3$ therapy is initiated first. Surgical revision often proves necessary, particularly if stasis begets infection in addition to acidosis.

Hyperkalemic, normal AG acidoses

Hydronephrosis Benign prostatic hypertrophy, bladder muscular weakness, and kidney stones frequently cause morbidity in the elderly,[18] and, together with the entities enumerated above as indications for ureteral diversion, predispose the aged to urinary tract obstruction. Some patients with obstructive uropathy develop a hyperkalemic distal RTA due to hyporeninemic aldosterone deficiency and/or defects in distal hydrogen and potassium secretion.[35] Treatment should be directed at the underlying cause.

Hypoaldosteronism and early renal failure Hypoaldosteronism may develop in the elderly due to primary adrenal insufficiency (eg, autoimmune disease) or secondary to defects in the renin-angiotensin axis. Histories of prolonged diabetes mellitus, hypertension, interstitial nephritis, and gout are all associated with hyporeninemic hypoaldosteronism.[36] In many cases the adrenals ultimately become unresponsive even to exogenous ACTH and angiotensin II infusion. Hyperkalemia and metabolic acidosis become manifest due to lack of aldosterone-stimulated distal tubular secretion of H^+ and K^+, in each of the hypoaldosteronemic conditions. Tubulo-interstitial diseases also damage the distal tubular secretory apparatus directly – ie, render the tubules unresponsive to mineralocorticoid stimulation. Furthermore, tubulo- interstitial pathology impairs ammoniagenesis, exacerbating the acidosis. Hyperkalemia also suppresses generation of ammonium buffer. Chronic analgesic and "moonshine" (illicit alcohol) abuse, in particular, are highly punishing to the medullary interstitium. As is the case in hypoaldosteronism, direct damage to the distal tubules results in elevation of serum potassium and decreases in serum HCO_3^- concentrations. Thus, a variety of causes of renal failure yield normal AG metabolic acidosis, early on.

As mentioned earlier, NSAI drugs are taken by many older patients. There are a growing number of case reports of NSAI-induced, normal AG acidosis.[37,38] Tubular dysfunction and hyporeninemia both appear to play significant roles. Patrono et al have demonstrated a stimulatory effect of prostacyclin on renin release in man, which is blocked by indomethacin.[39] This phenomenon may contribute to metabolic acidosis.

Patients suffering from inadequate distal tubular H^+ secretion deserve a trial of mineralocorticoid replacement (eg, 9α-fludrocortisone acetate 0.1–0.2 mg taken twice daily). NSAI agents should of course be discontinued. Bicarbonate or sodium polystyrene sulfonate (a potassium exchange resin) therapy may prove necessary.

Elevated AG acidoses

Advanced renal failure The high AG acidosis of uremia is well recognized, and results from the simultaneous occurrence of reduced glomerular filtration of phosphate, sulfate, and organic acids and failure of tubular acid secretion and bicarbonate generation. A multitude of chronic diseases (diabetes mellitus, hypertension, glomerulonephritides, etc) may ultimately cause the aging kidneys to fail. A prototypical mixed high AG and hyperchloremic metabolic acidosis ($\Delta HCO_3^- > \Delta AG$) is encountered during the transition from early tubulo-interstitial disease, which causes distal tubular dysfunction and a normal AG acidosis as discussed above, to full-blown renal failure wherein the accumulation of unmeasured anions is the predominate source of metabolic acidosis.

Lactic acidosis Cohen and Woods provide the definitive description of the biochemistry and classification of the lactic acidoses.[40] Two broad etiologic categories are drawn. Grossly impaired tissue oxygenation, due to clinically apparent hypoxia, hypoperfusion, or profound anemia, characterizes type A lactic acidosis. The type B label applies to all lactic acidosis conditions which lack this causative common denominator. Clearly, the elderly may fall prey to respiratory failure or cardiovascular collapse, with attendant type A lactic acidosis. An aged patient with a serious infection who suddenly develops lactic acidosis requires prompt intensification of therapy and observation, as frank shock is likely to follow. During the premonitory period of shock, tissue hypoperfusion yields lactate accumulation, while splanchnic and peripheral vasoconstriction temporarily support the normal blood pressure.

Type B lactic acidosis follows from a variety of diseases and intoxications which alter intracellular metabolism or lactate transport and uptake. Those specifically relevant to the elderly include diabetes mellitus, renal failure, hepatic failure, malignancies (lymphoma, leukemia, sarcoma), and ingestion of biguanide hypoglycemics, salicylates, or streptozotocin.

Lactic acidosis carries a most serious prognosis. Vigorous effort must be made to treat the underlying cause. If the arterial pH is below 7.20, we recommend sodium bicarbonate administration to avoid arrhythmias and cardiovascular collapse. Dichloroacetate (DCA) reduces lactate levels by stimulating the enzyme pyruvate dehydrogenase, which enhances consumption of the anion and bicarbonate generation. This may emerge as an important ancillary treatment. Seven patients with lactic acidosis showed significant acid-base and hemodynamic improvement following DCA administration in a recent study, but none survived their primary illness.[41] Reversal of underlying pathology must remain the paramount priority.

Ketoacidosis Prolonged starvation prompts fatty acid mobilization and conversion to acetoacetate and β-hydroxybutyrate. The brain can utilize these ketoacids as energy sources during states of glucose deficiency. Economic and physical disadvantages may tragically condemn the elderly to periods of starvation, which rarely will cause the serum HCO_3^- to fall below 17 mEq/L.[42] Although diabetic and alcohol-associated ketoacidoses are important disorders, they are not particularly prevalent among the geriatric set, and are reviewed elsewhere.[4,43,44]

Salicylates Salicylate intoxication poses a major threat to acid-base homeostasis in the elderly. Anderson et al emphasize that this malady remains undiagnosed for longer periods following hospital admission in older patients, resulting in a 30% major morbidity rate and a 25% mortality rate.[45] An elevated AG metabolic acidosis classically accompanies salicylate intoxication, due to accumulating serum salicylic acid, lactate, and ketones. A mixed metabolic acidosis/ respiratory alkalosis (P_{CO_2} lower than predicted in response to the metabolic acidosis alone) is commonly noted, due to aspirin-induced hyperventilation. However, Gabow et al observe that in patients who have ingested additional drugs, the respiratory status is highly variable.[46] Geriatric patients often become poisoned accidentally when taking aspirin for medical problems, while overt suicide attempts are frequently to blame in younger adults. The latter variety of salicylate intoxication is more readily diagnosed upon a patient's arrival at the hospital.[45]

Forced alkaline diuresis is the cornerstone of treatment. Care must be taken to avoid pulmonary edema or hypokalemia when treating elderly patients.[45] Dialysis proves effective in cases of massive overdose with profound acidemia.

Toxins Certain alcoholics are wont to ingest a range of toxic inebriants. Methanol, ethylene glycol, and paraldehyde are associated with high AG metabolic acidoses and CNS depression.[2,47,48] Elderly subjects are found only sporadically among the series describing these disorders.

Metabolic Alkalosis (Table 9-4)

Gastric alkalosis Prolonged vomiting or nasogastric suction are classic causes of metabolic alkalosis. Sodium bicarbonate is absorbed into the blood, concomitant with gastric secretion of HCl. Emesis or nasogastric suction causes loss of HCl from the gastric juice, removing the stimulus for pancreatic HCO_3^- secretion and resulting in a net gain in serum alkali. Volume and potassium losses contribute further to the generation and maintenance of the metabolic alkalosis. A number of factors pertain to the development of gastric alkalosis in the elderly. Medicinal side effects often include vomiting; many geriatric patients require theophylline, digoxin, or cancer chemotherapy, for example. Other notable causes of vomiting in the elderly include intestinal obstruction, inflamed viscus (appendicitis, cholecystitis), inner ear disorders (labyrinthitis, Meniere's disease), migraine headache, and conditions of increased intracranial pressure (cerebrovascular accident, tumor). Iatrogenic metabolic alkalosis ensues whenever nasogastric suction is prescribed without appropriate fluid management. Uremia often induces vomiting, and such patients may well manifest a mixed high AG metabolic acidosis and metabolic alkalosis ($\Delta HCO_3^- < \Delta AG$). Therapy for gastric alkalosis entails cautious volume repletion, potassium repletion, and treatment of the underlying cause. Marked alkalemia predisposes to arrhythmias, tetany, and cerebral vasoconstriction. Thus, intravenous administration of acid should be considered for a blood pH >7.55, especially in patients with associated acute or chronic renal failure.

Diuretics Congestive heart failure and hypertension very often prompt the prescription of diuretics for elderly patients. All diuretics except those sparing of potassium (amiloride, spironolactone, and triamterene) may cause hyperbicarbonatemia. Metabolic alkalosis is a common side effect, due to several mechanisms.[49,50] Hypovolemia stimulates aldosterone secretion, which augments renal H^+ excretion. Similarly, states of diminished effective arterial volume such as congestive heart failure or liver failure with ascites may cause hyperaldosteronemia and metabolic alkalosis. Volume contraction per se may increase the serum HCO_3^-. Diuretic-induced hypokalemia prompts intracellular H^+ movement (in exchange for K^+ extrusion into the ECF), which in turn stimulates renal tubular H^+ secretion. Furthermore, diuretics ensure a steady delivery to the distal tubule of Na^+, for exchange with H^+. It should be clear that elderly patients on diuretic therapy require close attention to volume, electrolyte, and acid-base status.

High-dose antibiotic therapy Massive doses of sodium penicillin or sodium carbenicillin have been reported to cause hypokalemic renal alkalosis during periods of avid sodium retention.[2,51] Antibiotic anions are poorly reabsorbed from the glomerular filtrate while the Na^+ filtered with the drug is actively reclaimed. A negative luminal charge tends to develop from this unbalanced reabsorption of positively charged particles. The electrochemical gradient now favors the secretion of H^+ and K^+. This hypokalemic alkalosis must be watched for in patients receiving digoxin, lest toxicity be rapidly precipitated.

Exogenous alkali Normally, the kidneys are able to excrete excess HCO_3^- and maintain acid-base homeostasis. Van Goidsenhoven et al reveal that prolonged administration of up to 20 mEq/kg/d of alkali evokes minimal change in serum HCO_3^- or blood pH in young, normal subjects, who mount an effective bicarbonate diuresis.[52] However, as discussed earlier, the elderly cannot respond to acid-base stresses as readily as the young. Settings which place an older patient at further risk of a metabolic alkalosis from exogenous base include volume depletion and renal insufficiency. Geriatric individuals may receive exogenous HCO_3^- in the form of antacids, baking soda, or $NaHCO_3$ given to treat metabolic acidosis. It should be remembered that each gram of baking soda contains 12 mEq of $NaHCO_3$. Thus, each teaspoon delivers 5 g or 60 mEq. Tums® contains $CaCO_3$, each tablet of which provides 10 mEq of alkali. Rolaids® is an admixture of $Al(OH)_3$ and $NaHCO_3$, which yields 4.6 mEq of alkali per tablet; Alka-Seltzer® combines sodium and potassium bicarbonate, providing 15 mEq of alkali per tablet. Thus, the dyspeptic octagenarian has ample opportunity to abuse bicarbonate given the wide availability of these over-the-counter preparations. Lactic acidosis and ketoacidosis cause accumulation of anions (lactate, acetoacetate, β-hydroxybutyrate) which are metabolized to HCO_3^- when the underlying abnormality is resolved. Overzealous $NaHCO_3$ therapy, combined with endogenous conversion of pathologic anions to HCO_3^-, may yield a dangerous "overshoot" alkalemia, and is to be avoided. Salts of organic acids also may evoke metabolic alkalosis. Lactate, acetate, gluconate, and citrate are given as calcium salts to treat osteopenia in the aged. Multiunit blood transfusion imposes a citrate load which can yield clinically significant metabolic alkalosis.[53]

Mineralocorticoid excess Mineralocorticoids stimulate distal tubular Na^+ reabsorption, and secretion of H^+ and K^+. The intracellular shift of H^+ induced by hypokalemia increases the already-elevated rate of tubular H^+ secretion, and hence the degree of alkalosis. High renin states lead to pathologic increases in the rate of adrenal aldosterone secretion.

Hyperreninemia in the elderly is often the result of atherosclerotic stenosis of the renal artery or malignant hypertension. Estrogen therapy (eg, for osteoporosis) increases renin substrate. Primary aldosteronism, due to an adrenal adenoma (Conn's syndrome) or bilateral cortical adrenal hyperplasia, usually appears between the ages of 30 and 50. Of less relevance to the elderly are the inherited aldosterone-related disorders which lead to metabolic alkalosis: Bartter's syndrome, Liddle's syndrome, and 11- and 17-hydroxylase deficiencies. Glycyrrhizinic acid stimulates tubular aldosterone receptors, and can thereby cause sodium retention and hypokalemic metabolic alkalosis. This syndrome occurs in rare instances, following ingestion of large quantities of licorice, which contains this steroid.[54] Carbenoxolone is a hydrolytic product of glycyrrhizinic acid, used abroad in the drug therapy of gastric ulcer. It, too, possesses aldosteronelike properties and may lead to metabolic alkalosis.

Several approaches prove beneficial in the treatment of metabolic alkalosis associated with mineralocorticoid excess. If possible, the inciting process should be eliminated (eg, discontinuation of licorice, repair of renal artery stenosis, adrenal resection). Spironolactone, an aldosterone antagonist, may be employed to medically ablate the excess mineralocorticoid effects. Correction of hypokalemia will elicit a return to the ECF of hydrogen ions which had shifted intracellularly, lowering blood pH and slowing further tubular H^+ secretion. Since states of primary hyperreninemia or primary aldosteronism generate mild volume expansion and, ultimately, normal to high Na^+ excretion in the urine, saline administration will prove ineffective in treating the associated metabolic alkalosis.

Miscellaneous Hypercalcemia, without hyperparathyroidism, has been associated with enhanced renal bicarbonate reabsorption and metabolic alkalosis, though not all investigators are in agreement on this matter.[55] Malignancy, immobilization, and thiazide ingestion all cause hypercalcemia in the elderly. Carbohydrate ingestion by a starving person induces a mild metabolic alkalosis[55] by mechanisms which are not well understood.

Respiratory Acidosis (Table 9-7)

The elderly are vulnerable to each and every cause of respiratory acidosis included in Table 9-7. Chronic obstructive pulmonary disease is particularly prevalent in the geriatric population. Further, these patients may prove exquisitely sensitive to the respiratory side effects of sedatives. While review of the diagnosis and therapy of the individual respiratory disturbances

Table 9-7
Causes of Respiratory Acidosis

CNS Depression	Impaired Motions of Ventilation
Sedatives	Neuropathy
Cerebrovascular accident	Myopathy
Trauma/surgery	Kyphoscoliosis
Tumor	Crush or flail chest
	Pleural effusion
Airway Pathology	Pneumothorax
Chronic obstructive disease	
	Miscellaneous
Acute spasm	Cardiopulmonary arrest
Severe pneumonia	Ventilator malfunction
Severe pulmonary edema	Sleep disorders
Foreign body	
Tumor	

is best relegated to the pulmonary textbooks, certain acid-base principles should bear directly on management decisions.

Progressive acidemia can prove fatal. Signs of worsening acidemia include vomiting, obtundation, coma, and impaired cardiac contractility. Compromise of cardiac output may precipitate lactic acidosis, worsening the blood pH, and further lowering the threshold for ventricular fibrillation. Observation of the clinical manifestations of severe acidemia militates for mechanical ventilation, as does fatigue, for a patient not improving with less invasive care. A simultaneous metabolic acidosis also weighs in favor of earlier intubation, to avoid a sudden, fatal fall in blood pH. If a mixed metabolic alkalosis/respiratory acidosis is present, the patient's potassium status must be addressed. As noted, substantial losses of potassium often accompany significant metabolic alkaloses; hypokalemic myopathy may underlie the observed respiratory compromise. Finally, the physician should keep in mind that elderly subjects lack the ventilatory response to hypercapnia shown by younger subjects, as discussed earlier. This leaves even less margin of safety for observation and conservative management.

Respiratory Alkalosis (Table 9-8)

Most of the diagnoses shown in Table 9-8 bear consideration when investigating the cause of respiratory alkalosis in an aged patient. Pregnancy, progesterone excess, and analeptic overdosage are obviously unlikely in this setting. Pulmonary embolism and salicylate intoxication must be aggressively ruled out, because both are common, potentially lethal, readily diagnosed, and mandate acute treatments which will often prove highly beneficial.

As is the case for the respiratory acidoses, the individual causes of respiratory alkalosis determine the specifics of treatment, but certain generalizations are valid. It is prudent to evaluate the serum potassium, calcium, magnesium, phosphate, and the medication history when faced with a case of respiratory alkalosis. Hypokalemia, hypomagnesemia, and cardiac glycosides all increase the chances that alkalemia will induce arrhythmias or tetany. Cardiac conduction abnormalities and digoxin toxicity also worsen in the presence of hypocalcemia. Each of these factors therefore increases the urgency to correct the alkalosis, and necessitates repletion of the deficient cation. Severe respiratory alkalosis increases intracellular pH, as well as extracellular pH, and thereby stimulates the enzyme phosphofructokinase. The rapid phosphorylations which ensue can cause marked intracellular shifts of phosphate, and life-threatening hypophosphatemia. Hence the need to assess the serum phosphate, and replete as necessary.

Table 9-8
Causes of Respiratory Alkalosis

CNS Etiologies	Hypoxemia
Anxiety	Hepatic Insufficiency
Cerebrovascular accident	Salicylate Intoxication
Tumor	Analeptic Intoxication
Encephalitis	Progesterone Excess
Encephalopathy	Catecholamine Excess
Lung Disorders	Endotoxemia
Pulmonary embolism	Pregnancy
Pneumonia	Hyperthyroidism
Mild pulmonary edema	Inappropriate Artificial Ventilation
Mild restrictive disease	
Mild airway constriction	

REFERENCES

1. Kassirer JP, Bleich HL: Rapid estimation of plasma carbon dioxide from pH and total carbon dioxide content. *N Engl J Med* 1965; 272:1067–1068.
2. Emmett M, Narins RG: Clinical use of the anion gap. *Medicine* 1977;56:38–54.
3. Narins RG, Emmett M: Simple and mixed acid-base disorders: a practical approach. *Medicine* 1980;59:161–187.
4. Narins RG, Jones ER, Goodkin DA, et al: Metabolic acid-base disorders, in Arieff AI, DeFronzo RA (eds): *Fluid, Electrolyte and Acid-Base Disorders.* New York, Churchill Livingstone, 1984.
5. Goodkin DA, Krishna GG, Narins RG: Role of the anion gap in detecting and managing mixed metabolic acid-base disorders. *Clin Endocrinol Metab* 1984; in press.
6. Osnes J, Hermansen L: Acid-base balance after maximal exercise of short duration. *J Appl Physiol* 1972;32:59–63.
7. Narins RG, Bastl CP, Rudnick MR, et al: Acid-base metabolism, in Gonick HC (ed): *Current Nephrology.* New York, John Wiley & Sons, 1982, pp 79–130.
8. Androgué HJ, Brensilver J, Madias NE: Changes in the plasma anion gap during chronic metabolic acid-base disturbances. *Am J Physiol* 1978;235:F291–F297.
9. Madias NE, Ayus JG, Androgué HS: In creased anion gap in metabolic alkalosis: the role of plasma-protein equivalency. *N Engl J Med* 1979;300:1421–1423.
10. Fleischer WR: Laboratory assessment of acid-base imbalance. *Geriatrics* 1974;29: 96–104.
11. Brandsteller RD, Kazemi H: Aging and the respiratory system. *Med Clin North Am* 1983;67:419–431.
12. Rowe JW: The influence of age on renal function. *Resident Staff Physician* 1978; 24:49–55.
13. Tinetti ME: Effects of stress on renal function in the elderly. *J Am Geriatr Soc* 1983;31:174–181.
14. Shock NW, Yiengst MJ: Age changes in the acid-base equilibrium of the blood of males. *J Gerontol* 1950;5:1–4.
15. Adler S, Lindeman RD, Yiengst MJ, et al: Effect of acute acid loading on urinary acid excretion by the aging human kidney. *J Lab Clin Med* 1968;72:278–289.
16. Agarwal BN, Cabebe FG: Renal acidification in elderly subjects. *Nephron* 1980;26: 291–295.
17. Hilton JG, Goodbody MF, Kruesi OR: The effect of prolonged administration of ammonium chloride on the blood acid-base equilibrium of geriatric subjects. *J Am Geriatr Soc* 1955;3:697–703.
18. Rosen H: Renal disease in the elderly. *Med Clin North Am* 1976;60:1105–1119.
19. Kronenberg RS, Drage CW: Attenuation of the ventilatory and heart rate responses to hypoxia and hypercapnia with aging in normal men. *J Clin Invest* 1973;52:1812–1819.
20. Peterson DD, Pack AI, Silage DA, et al: Effects of aging on ventilatory and occlusion pressure responses to hypoxia and hypercapnia. *Am Rev Respir Dis* 1981;124: 387–391.
21. Samiy AH: Clinical manifestations of disease in the elderly. *Med Clin North Am* 1983;67:333–344.
22. Clive DM, Stoff JS: Renal syndromes associated with nonsteroidal antiinflammatory drugs. *N Engl J Med* 1984;310:563–572.
23. Gullikson GW, Sender M, Bass P: Laxative-like effects of nonsteroidal anti-inflammatory drugs on intestinal fluid movement and membrane integrity. *J Pharmacol Exp Ther* 1982;220:236–242.
24. Ward JR, Bolzan JA, Brame CL, et al: Sodium meclofenamate (Meclomen®) dose determining studies. *Curr Ther Res* 1978;23:S60–S65.
25. Zuckner J, Baldassare A, Harris GS, et al: Sodium meclofenamate (vs placebo) in the treatment of rheumatoid arthritis. *Curr Ther Res* 1978;23:S66–S71.
26. Narins RG, Goldberg M: Renal tubular acidosis: pathophysiology, diagnosis and treatment. *DM* 1977;23:3–66.
27. Livbey CA, Skinner M, Cohen AS: Use of abdominal fat tissue aspirate in the diagnosis of systemic amyloidosis. *Arch Intern Med* 1983;143:1549–1552.
28. Westermark P: Diagnosis and characterization of systemic amyloidosis by biopsy of subcutaneous abdominal fat tissue. *Intern Med Specialist* 1984;5:154–160.
29. Victor M, Adams RD: Common disturbances of vision, ocular movement, and hearing, in Isselbacher KS, Adams RD, Braunwald E, et al (eds): *Principles of In-*

ternal Medicine. New York, McGraw-Hill, 1980, pp 101–110.
30. Bienfang DC: Ophthalmologic problems, in Branch WT, Jr (ed): *Office Practice of Medicine.* Philadelphia, WB Saunders, 1982, pp 1065–1085.
31. Jacobs IH, Cinotti AA: Laser therapy of glaucoma. *J Med Soc NJ* 1980;77:187–189.
32. Narins RG, Gardner LB: Simple acid-base disturbances. *Med Clin North Am* 1981; 65:321–346.
33. Schwartz WB, Kassirer JP: Effects of ureteral transplantation, in Strauss MB, Welt LG (eds): *Diseases of the Kidney.* Boston, Little Brown & Co, 1963, pp 759–768.
34. Creevy CD: Renal complications after ileal diversion of the urine in non-neoplastic disorders. *J Urol* 1960;83:394–397.
35. Battle DC, Arruda JAL, Kurtzman NA: Hyperkalemic distal renal tubular acidosis associated with obstructive uropathy. *N Engl J Med* 1981;304:373–380.
36. DeFronzo RA: Hyperkalemia and hyporeninemic hypoaldosteronism. *Kidney Int* 1980;17:118–134.
37. Tan SY, Shapiro R, Franco R, et al: Indomethacin-induced prostaglandin inhibition with hyperkalemia: a reversible cause of hyporeninemic hypoaldosteronism. *Ann Intern Med* 1979;90:783–785.
38. Warren SE, Mosley C: Renal failure and tubular dysfunction due to zomepirac therapy. *JAMA* 1983;249:396–397.
39. Patrono C, Pugliese F, Ciabattoni G, et al: Evidence for a direct stimulatory effect of prostacyclin on renin release in man. *J Clin Invest* 1982;69:231–239.
40. Cohen RD, Woods HF: *Clinical and Biochemical Aspects of Lactic Acidosis.* Oxford, Blackwell Scientific Publications, 1976.
41. Stacpoole PW, Harman EM, Curry SH, et al: Treatment of lactic acidosis with dichloroacetate. *N Engl J Med* 1983;309: 390–396.
42. Cahill GF: Ketosis. *Kidney Int* 1981;20: 416–425.
43. Levy LJ, Duga J, Girgis M, et al: Ketoacidosis associated with alcoholism in nondiabetic subjects. *Ann Intern Med* 1973; 78:213–219.
44. Cooperman MT, Davidoff F, Spark R, et al: Clinical studies of alcoholic ketoacidosis. *Diabetes* 1974;23:433–439.
45. Anderson RJ, Potts DE, Gabow PA, et al: Unrecognized adult salicylate intoxication. *Ann Intern Med* 1976;85:745–748.
46. Gabow PA, Anderson RS, Potts DE, et al: Acid-base disturbances in the salicylate-intoxicated adult. *Arch Intern Med* 1978; 138:1481–1484.
47. Parry MF, Wallach R: Ethylene glycol poisoning. *Am J Med* 1974;57:143–150.
48. Bennett IL Jr, Freeman HC, Mitchell GL Jr, et al: Acute methyl alcohol poisoning: a review based on experiences in an outbreak of 323 cases. *Medicine* 1953;32: 431–463.
49. Rose BD: *Clinical Physiology of Acid-Base and Electrolyte Disorders.* New York, McGraw-Hill, 1984.
50. Garella S, Chang BS, Kahn SI: Dilution acidosis and contraction alkalosis: review of a concept. *Kidney Int* 1975;8:279–283.
51. Brunner FP, Frick PG: Hypokalemia, metabolic alkalosis, and hypernatremia due to "massive" sodium penicillin therapy. *Br Med J* 1968;4:550–552.
52. VanGoidsenhoven GM-T, Gray OV, Price AV, et al: The effect of prolonged administration of large doses of sodium bicarbonate in man. *Clin Sci* 1954;13:383–401.
53. Litwin MS, Smith LL, Moore FD: Metabolic alkalosis following massive transfusion. *Surgey* 1959;45:805–813.
54. Conn JW, Rovner DR, Cohen EL: Licorice-induced pseudoaldosteronism. *JAMA* 1968;205:492–496.
55. Cogan MG, Rector FC Jr, Seldin DW: Acid-base disorders, in Brenner BM, Rector FC Jr (eds): *The Kidney.* Philadelphia, WB Saunders Co, 1981, pp 841–907.

CHAPTER 10

Calcium, Phosphorus, and Magnesium Disorders in the Elderly

Lakhi M. Sakhrani
Shaul G. Massry

Abnormalities in divalent ion homeostasis are encountered in elderly individuals, and defects at multiple levels of their regulation are evident. These disturbances are listed in Table 10-1. It should be emphasized that most of these changes are modest. The mechanisms underlying these derangements are not fully explored as of yet.

CHANGES IN CALCIUM HOMEOSTASIS

Serum Calcium

A number of studies have shown no difference in total serum calcium in elderly individuals compared to healthy young subjects.[1–3] On the other hand, large population studies by Keatings et al[4,5] demonstrated a steady decline in total plasma calcium concentration with aging in men but not in women. This fall in total serum calcium is relatively small so that by the age 80 years, the levels are lower by 0.3 mg/dL than the corresponding values in a 20-year-old person. Parallel with this, the authors noted a fall in serum albumin in both elderly males and females. Using calculations of corrected calcium based on the total serum calcium and albumin, they suggested that diffusible calcium may decrease with age in men but increase with

Table 10-1
Disorders of Ca, P, and Mg Homeostasis in the Elderly

1. Mild decrease in serum calcium levels
2. Elevated serum PTH levels
3. Reduced blood levels of 25-hydroxyvitamin D and 1,25-dihydroxyvitamin D
4. Impaired intestinal calcium absorption
5. Mild decrease in serum phosphate
6. Decreased maximal tubular reabsorption of phosphate

age in women. A similar decline in total serum calcium concentration with age in men has also been observed by others.[6] On the other hand, Roberts[7] has reported the opposite trend, namely, that total serum calcium concentration declines with age only in women and not in men.

The data on the effect of aging on the concentration of ionized calcium are limited. A mild decrease (10%) in the serum levels of ionized calcium after the age of 40 has been reported.[3,8]

Serum Parathyroid Hormone Levels

Aging is accompanied by an elevation in serum levels of serum parathyroid hormone (PTH) levels in most patients.[1,2,9] However, in one study of healthy elderly subjects living at home, the levels of the hormone were normal. Assays which detect the C-terminal fragment of PTH show an approximately twofold increase in circulating levels of PTH beginning after age 50.[1,3,6,9,10] Elderly women appear to have higher PTH levels than elderly men.[3] It should be noted that glomerular filtration rate (GFR) declines with age after the middle of the fourth decade. At that time a linear decrease of 8 mL/min/1.73m^2 per decade develops.[11] Since the kidney is an important organ for clearing the C-terminal fragment of PTH,[12,13] it would be expected that as renal function declines, the concentrations of the fragment in the blood increase. In addition, it has been shown that secondary hyperparathyroidism develops as renal insufficiency ensues[14] and it is plausible that hyperactivity of the parathyroid glands also contributes to the elevated blood levels of PTH in the elderly. Indeed, the elevated PTH levels associated with aging are not due entirely to diminished clearance of the C-terminal fragment of PTH since the N-terminal fragment of PTH is also elevated.[2,9] Furthermore, concomitant with the increase of serum PTH levels in the elderly, nephrogenous cAMP levels are also increased demonstrating the biological activity of the elevated levels of the hormone.[1]

Although it has been postulated that the elevated serum levels of PTH in the elderly are due to declining renal function,[15] other factors may also be operative. It has been suggested that phosphate retention may play a role in the secondary hyperparathyroidism of aging,[15] but the available data do not provide strong support for this hypothesis.[9] Indeed, serum levels of phosphate are unusually low.[3] Alterations in vitamin D metabolism discussed below may participate in the genesis of the secondary hyperparathyroidism of aging.

It is evident from this discussion that the interpretation of an elevated serum level of PTH should take into consideration the age of the patient. This is particularly important during an evaluation of primary hyperparathyroidism. The latter disease is frequent in elderly patients,[16] and the mere finding of an elevated serum PTH level does not necessarily indicate the presence of a parathyroid adenoma.

Vitamin D Metabolism

Numerous studies have been done to assess serum levels of 25-hydroxyvitamin D [25(OH)D] in the aging population. Elderly individuals living at home have been reported to have both normal[2,17] and low[18] plasma levels of 25(OH)D. However, geriatric patients either in institutions for the aged or geriatric wards consistently have low serum concentration of 25(OH)D. This is not due to diminished vitamin D–binding globulin, which is in fact increased in the elderly.[19] A number of explanations have been offered for the low serum levels of 25(OH)D in the aged. First, lack of exposure to sunlight appears to be an important factor.[20] Second, dietary deficiency of vitamin D is common in the elderly,[18,20,21] and this may be the predominant factor in some individuals.[21] Third, evidence has been presented that the conversion of vitamin D to 25(OH)D is modestly impaired in elderly patients.[22] This impairment is not the result of failure to absorb vitamin D but rather reflects a diminished 25-hydroxylase activity in the liver since the serum levels of 25(OH)D do not increase appropriately after the subcutaneous administration of vitamin D. Malabsorption of vitamin D may also be present and contribute to the deficiency of 25(OH)D.[23] However, such a defect, if present, should easily be overcome, since serum levels of 25(OH)D could be increased after treatment with large oral vitamin D supplements.[24,25] The latter approach is therefore a useful means of treating elderly individuals with 25(OH)D deficiency. Ultraviolet radiation with fluorescent tubes also increases serum levels of 25(OH)D in the elderly but may not be convenient or practical.[25,26] Little is presently known on the effect of aging on cholecalciferol synthesis by the skin.

The information on the effect of aging on circulating levels of 1,25-dihydroxyvitamin D [1,25$(OH)_2$D] is limited. The serum levels of this metabolite have been found to be low-normal[27] or frankly low[28,29] in elderly patients. The decrease in the plasma concentration of 1,25$(OH)_2$D may be due to either impaired conversion of 25(OH)D to 1,25$(OH)_2$D by the kidney or to enhanced catabolism of 1,25$(OH)_2$D. Experiments in rats show that renal 25 OHD-1-α-hydroxylase activity declines with aging,[30,31] and such a decline in the activity of the enzyme may be related to a diminished renal mass or to changes in factors that normally stimulate the activity of this enzyme. Administration of PTH to elderly osteopenic and nonosteopenic individuals has resulted in a rise in the serum levels of 1,25$(OH)_2$D from low basal values to normal levels,[29,32] suggesting that the low basal values might be due to changes in factors that normally stimulate renal 25(OH)D-1-α-hydroxylase activity. To reconcile these data with the observations that elderly subjects have elevated serum levels of PTH, one must assume that greater increments in serum PTH are required to normalize the serum levels of 1,25$(OH)_2$D.

Intestinal Calcium Absorption

Intestinal calcium absorption decreases with age and the decline becomes evident after the age of 60 years and continues into the tenth decade.[28,33–35] Although generalized defects in intestinal absorption for many compounds have been demonstrated in the elderly,[36] the defect in calcium absorption seen in the elderly is not due to this malabsorption syndrome.

Studies of calcium absorption utilizing oral calcium 47 (^{47}Ca) show a normal rise in plasma ^{47}Ca at 1 hour but a subsequent decline; this is contrary to the pattern seen in malabsorption in which a delay in the appearance of ^{47}Ca is seen after an oral dose with only a minimal subsequent decline.[34] Gallagher et al[28] also noted that the decreased intestinal absorption of calcium seen in the elderly is not due to a generalized absorptive defect. They noted a good correlation between serum 1,25$(OH)_2$D levels and calcium absorption; furthermore, calcium absorption increased with administration of this active metabolite of vitamin D. These observations suggest that reduced levels of 1,25$(OH)_2$D in the elderly are most likely responsible for any defect in intestinal calcium absorption. In postmenopausal women, estrogen lack may also contribute to the calcium malabsorption since administration of estrogen leads to an improvement in this defect.[37] This favorable response is thought to be secondary to increased serum levels of $1,25(OH)_2D$ seen after estrogen administration.[37]

In young individuals, the intestinal calcium absorption displays an adaptive increase when they are placed on a low calcium diet. In the elderly individual, however, not only is the basal calcium absorption by the gut impaired but the adaptive increase in calcium as the result of a low dietary calcium intake is also markedly blunted.[28,38]

Serum Calcitonin Levels

Calcitonin levels in the serum have been found to decrease with aging.[15,39,40] It has been suggested that a further decline in serum calcitonin levels occurs after the menopause because of the importance of estrogens in stimulating the secretion of calcitonin.[27] Indeed, the administration of estrogen has been shown to increase the serum levels of calcitonin in postmenopausal women.[27]

CHANGES IN PHOSPHATE HOMEOSTASIS

Limited information is available concerning phosphate homeostasis associated with aging. The concentrations of serum inorganic phosphorus are affected both by age and sex. In men, serum phosphorus levels decline with age with the levels being less by 0.5 mg/dL at the age of 80 when compared to 20- to 30-year-old subjects.[4,5] In healthy normal women, serum phosphorus falls between the ages of 30 and 40 years only to gradually increase by age 80; the resulting serum concentrations of phosphorus are then similar to those found in 20-year-old women.[4] In ambulatory female patients, however, no change in serum phosphorus with aging is seen.[5]

The renal tubular maximum phosphate reabsorption (Tm_P) is reduced in elderly individuals,[1,15,18] and this may explain the changes in serum phosphorus concentrations in old men. The decrease in Tm_P is most likely due to the increase in serum PTH levels. However, an intrinsic renal defect in phosphate reabsorption unrelated to serum PTH status is an additional possibility. Indeed, in old rats, tubular reabsorption of phosphate is lower than in young animals, and this difference is independent of PTH.[41] The renal response to a low phosphorus diet in the elderly is not well characterized. Studies in animals, however, indicate that the renal adaptation to dietary phosphorus restriction, manifested by enhanced renal tubular reabsorption of phosphorus, is intact in old animals.[42,43]

Intestinal absorption of phosphorus in elderly patients is not well delineated nor is the response to a low dietary phosphorus diet. However, animal studies show that the intestinal absorption of phosphorus is not augmented in old animals compared to young animals when phosphorus is restricted in the diet.[30] This is not surprising since the adaptive increase in gut absorption of phosphorus depends on serum $1,25(OH)_2D$ which is decreased with aging.

CHANGES IN MAGNESIUM HOMEOSTASIS

No significant change in serum magnesium is seen with aging either in men or women.[4] However, in women erythrocyte magnesium content increases after the menopause[44] and this phenomenon may be related to decreased estrogen levels. At present no information is available on the renal and intestinal handling of magnesium in the aged.

ACKNOWLEDGMENT

Ms Joann Little provided secretarial assistance in the preparation of this manuscript.

REFERENCES

1. Insognia KL, Lewis AM, Lipinski BA, et al: Effect of age on serum immunoreactive parathyroid hormone and its biological effects. *J Clin Endocrinol Metab* 1981;53: 1072–1075.
2. Petersen MM, Briggs RS, Ashby MA, et al: Parathyroid hormone and 25-hydroxyvitamin D concentrations in sick and normal elderly people. *Br Med J* 1983;287:521–523.
3. Wiske PS, Epstein S, Bell NH, et al: Increases in immunoreactive parathyroid hormone with age. *N Engl J Med* 1979; 300:1419–1421.
4. Keatings FR Jr, Jones JD, Elveback LR, et al: The relation of age and sex to distribution of values in healthy adults of serum calcium, inorganic phosphorus, magnesium, alkaline phosphatase, total proteins, albumin and blood urea. *J Lab Clin Med* 1969;73:825–834.
5. Keatings FR, Jones JD, Elveback LR: Distribution of serum calcium and phosphorus values in unselected ambulatory patients. *J Lab Clin Med* 1969;74:507–514.
6. Roof BS, Piel CR, Hausen J, et al: Serum parathyroid hormone levels and serum calcium levels from birth to senescence. *Mech Ageing Dev* 1976;5:289–304.
7. Roberts LB: The normal ranges with statistical analysis for seventeen blood constituents. *Clin Chim Acta* 1967;16:69–89.
8. Roof BS, Gordon GS: Hyperparathyroid disease in the aged, in Greenblatt RB (ed): *Geriatric Endocrinology and Aging.* New York, Raven Press, 1978, p 36.
9. Gallagher JC, Riggs LB, Jerpbak CM, et al: The effect of age on serum immunoreactive parathyroid hormone in normal and osteoporotic women. *J Lab Clin Med* 1980; 95:373–385.
10. Fijita T, Ohata M, Ota K, et al: Aging and parathyroid hormone secretion. *J Gerontol* 1976;31:523–529.
11. Rowe JW, Andres RA, Tobin FD, et al: The effect of age on creatinine clearance in man. A cross sectional and longitudinal study. *J Gerontol* 1976;31:155–163.
12. Freitag J, Martin KJ, Hruska KA, et al: Impaired parathyroid hormone metabolism in chronic renal failure. *N Engl J Med* 1978;298:29–32.
13. Arnaud CD: Hyperparathyroidism and renal failure. *Kidney Int* 1973;4:89–95.
14. Slatopolsky E, Gaglar S, Pennell JP, et al: On the pathogenesis of hyperparathyroidism in chronic experimental renal insufficiency in the dog. *J Clin Invest* 1971;50: 492–499.
15. Berlyne M, Ben-ari J, Kushelsisky A, et al: The etiology of senile osteoporosis: Secondary hyperparathyroidism due to renal failure. *Q J Med* 1975;44:505–521.
16. Mundy GR, Cove DH, Fisher R: Primary hyperparathyroidism: Changes in the pattern of clinical presentation. *Lancet* 1980; 1:1317–1320.
17. Toss G, Almquist S, Larsson L, et al: Vitamin D deficiency in welfare institutions for the aged. *Acta Med Scand* 1980;208:87–89.
18. Amdahl, JL, Garry PJ, Hunsaker LA, et al: Nutritional status in a healthy elderly population: Vitamin D. *Am J Clin Nutr* 1983;36:1125–1233.
19. Barragry JM, Corless D, Auton J, et al: Plasma vitamin D binding globulin in vitamin D deficiency, pregnancy and chronic liver disease. *Clin Chim Acta* 1978;87: 359–365.
20. Corless D, Gupta SP, Sattar DA, et al: Vitamin D status of residents of an old people's home and long stay patients. *Gerontology* 1978;25:350–355.
21. Nayal AS, MacLennan WJ, Hamilton JC, et al: 25-hydroxy-vitamin D, diet and sunlight exposure in patients admitted to a geriatric unit. *Gerontology* 1978;24: 117–122.
22. Rushton C: Vitamin D hydroxylation in youth and old age. *Age Ageing* 1978;7:91–95.
23. Corless D, Beer M, Boucher BJ, et al: Vitamin D status in long stay geriatric patients. *Lancet* 1975;1:1404–1466.
24. Somerville PJ, Lien JWK, Kaye M: The calcium and vitamin D status in an elderly female population and their response to administered supplemental vitamin D_3. *J Gerontol* 1977;32:659–663.
25. Toss G, Andersson B, Diffey L, et al: Oral vitamin D and ultraviolet radiation for the prevention of vitamin D deficiency in the elderly. *Acta Med Scand* 1982;212: 157–161.
26. Corless D, Gupta SP, Surtula S, et al: Response of plasma 25-hydroxyvitamin D to ultraviolet irradiation in long stay geriatric

patients. *Lancet* 1978;2:649–651.
27. Stevenson JC, Abeyasekera G, Hillyard CJ, et al: Calcitonin and the calcium regulating hormones in post-menopausal women: Effect of estrogens. *Lancet* 1981;1:693–695.
28. Gallagher JC, Riggs BL, Eisman J, et al: Intestinal calcium absorption and serum vitamin D metabolites in normal subjects and osteoporotic patients. Effect of age and dietary calcium. *J Clin Invest* 1979;64:729–736.
29. Sorenson OH, Lumholtz B, Lung B, et al: Acute effects of parathyroid hormone on vitamin D metabolism in patients with the bone loss of aging. *J Clin Endocrinol Metab* 1982;54:1258–1261.
30. Armbrecht HJ, Zenser TV, Davis BB: Effect of age on the conversion of 25-hydroxyvitamin D_3 to 1,25 dihydroxyvitamin D_3 by kidney of rat. *J Clin Invest* 1980;66:1118–1123.
31. Horst RL, DeLuca HF, Jorgensen NA: The effect of age on calcium absorption and accumulation of 1,25 dihydroxyvitamin D_3 in intestinal mucosa of rats. *Metab Bone Dis Relat Res* 1978;1:29–33.
32. Riggs BL, Hamstra A, DeLuca HF: Assessment of 25-hydroxyvitamin D-1-hydroxylase reserve in postmenopausal osteoporosis. *J Clin Endocrinol Metab* 1981;53:833–835.
33. Alvezaki CC, Ikkos DC, Singhelakis P: Progressive decrease of the intestinal calcium absorption with age in normal man. *J Nucl Med* 1973;14:760–762.
34. Avioli L, McDonald JE, Sook WL: The influence of age on the intestinal absorption of ^{47}Ca in women and its relation to ^{47}Ca absorption in postmenopausal osteoporosis. *J Clin Invest* 1965;44:1960–1967.
35. Bullamore JR, Gallagher JC, Wilkinson R, et al: Effect of age on calcium absorption. *Lancet* 1970;1:535–537.
36. Montgomery RD, Haeney MR, Ross IN, et al: The aging gut: A study of intestinal absorption in relation to nutrition in the elderly. *Q J Med* 1978;57:197–211.
37. Gallagher JC, Riggs BL, DeLuca HF: Effect of estrogen on calcium absorption and serum vitamin D metabolites in postmenopausal osteoporosis. *J Clin Endocrinol Metab* 1980;51:1359–1364.
38. Ireland P, Fordtran JS: Effect of dietary calcium and age on jejunal calcium absorption in humans studied by intestinal perfusion. *J Clin Invest* 1973;52:2672–2681.
39. Deftos LJ, Weisman MH, Williams GH, et al: Influence of age and sex on plasma calcitonin in human beings. *New Engl J Med* 1980;302:1351–1353.
40. Samaan NA, Anderson GD, Adam-Mayne ME: Immunoreactive calcitonin in the mother, neonate, child and adult. *Am J Obstet Gynecol* 1975;121:622–625.
41. Caverzasio J, Bonjour JP, Fleisch H: Tubular handling of Pi in young growing and adult rats. *Am J Physiol* 1982;11:F705–F710.
42. Armbrecht HJ, Zenser TV, Gross CJ, Davis BB: Adaptation to dietary calcium and phosphorous restriction changes with age in the rat. *Am J Physiol* 1980;239(Endocrinol Metab 2):E-322–327.
43. Steele TH, DeLuca HF: Influence of dietary phosphorous on renal phosphate reabsorption in the parathyroidectomized rat. *J Clin Invest* 1976;57:867–874.
44. Henrotte JG, Benech A, Pineau M: Relationship between blood magnesium content and age in a French population, in Cantin M, Seelig MS (eds): *Magnesium in Health and Disease.* New York, Spectrum Books, 1980, pp 930–934.

CHAPTER 11 Bone Disease and the Elderly

Helen E. Gruber
Nachman Brautbar

The increase in the number of elderly patients in our population calls for intensified research toward a better understanding of, and more effective therapy for, bone disease of the elderly. This chapter will focus upon three major bone disorders frequently seen in the elderly patient: osteoporosis, Paget's disease, and osteomalacia. Although patients may be elderly when they consult their physician for skeletal problems arising from osteoporosis or Paget's disease, we now know that these bone disorders began many years earlier.

The last few decades have marked definite progress in our understanding of metabolic bone disease and bone physiology. Due to space limitations, we cannot cite all the important literature relevant to bone aging and bone disease of the elderly. Rather, we have chosen to present a general background upon which to discuss the recent data and important clinical studies which advanced our current understanding of bone physiology and the etiology and treatment of bone diseases.

The recent development of bone biopsy technics as well as specific histologic and tissue culture methods have provided tools with which to examine cellular and dynamic aspects of bone formation and bone resorption. Bone mineral analysis and neutron activation analysis allow direct assessment of both localized bone mass and total skeletal calcium content. In addition, calcium absorption and the important bone-related hormones—parathyroid hormone (PTH), calcitonin, and the vitamin D metabolites—can now be readily measured. However, in spite of these sophisticated analytical technics, many important and fundamental questions about normal bone physiology and mineral metabolism remain unanswered. Among such questions are those which concern the bone changes of normal aging. Thus it is necessary that our discussion begin with a summary of the normal skeletal changes known to accompany aging.

AGE-RELATED CHANGES IN NORMAL BONE

In general, one of the classic characteristics of aging is a decrease in adaptive capabilities. The aging process is associated with many changes in hormone secretory rates, secretion and response patterns, changes in target tissue sensitivity to hormones, and changes in protein synthesis and enzymatic activities.[1,2] Given such broad changes, it is not surprising that age-related alterations in cellular, biochemical, and physiologic functions of bone can result in a varied spectrum of bone problems.

Age-Related Changes in Bone Mass

The most evident change in bone seen with increasing age is a decrease in skeletal mass. Termed *osteopenia* this physiologic loss of bone mass appears to have been a problem even in prehistoric man.[3-6] Bone loss with aging has been documented by a variety of technics which have evaluated bone mass at a number of different skeletal sampling sites. Cortical bone in both the radius and the metacarpals appears to have been the best studied in this respect. Nordin has presented data on cortical thickness and total diameter of the metacarpal which show that in females bone loss has begun by the middle of the fourth decade, whereas values in males do not show a significant loss until 70 years of age.[7] As recently reviewed by Mazess,[8] cortical loss in the radius in males and females was generally detected at 40 to 45 years of age; the cortical loss rate reported for normal males ranged from 3% to 5% per decade; in females, the loss rate ranged from 2% to 9% per decade.[9-13] Similar bone loss patterns have been reported using radiographic measurement technics.[14,15] As generally noted in the older literature, bone changes in the female become most evident at and following the menopause. Using photon absorptiometric measurement of the radius, Johnston et al have fitted an exponential loss curve to a few of their patients who were studied over a number of years.[16] If this model proves accurate, the amount of initial bone mass present in a patient (which may have a genetic determination),[17,18] the age at onset of bone loss, and the rate at which bone is lost are all important factors serving to determine the ultimate magnitude of bone loss.

Recently Riggs et al have presented data which document changes that occur in bone mineral density of the spine and proximal femur with aging.[19] For normal women, regression of bone mineral density and age was both negative and linear. The overall decrease in bone density during life was 58% in the femoral neck, 53% in the intertrochanteric area of the femur, and 42% in the lumbar spine. For normal men a negative and linear regression existed as well, but the rate of loss was only two thirds of that seen in women for the femoral neck and intertrochanteric femur, and only one fourth of that seen in women for the lumbar spine. Riggs et al have also presented data showing that in normal women vertebral bone loss begins in *young adulthood* and does not accelerate until the immediate postmenopausal period.[20] In contrast, appendicular bone loss did not occur until age 50, accelerated from ages 51 to 65, and then decelerated slightly after 65 years of age. Overall, in the patients studied, bone loss was 47% for vertebrae,

30% for the midradius, and 39% for the distal radius. Vertebral and appendicular bone loss was minimal or insignificant in normal men. By age 60, 50% of the normal women studied (and virtually all women by age 85) demonstrated vertebral bone mineral density values below the maximum values used to confirm clinically evident osteoporosis. These subjects might then be considered to have asymptomatic osteoporosis.

Another quantitative technic that has been increasingly used to assess skeletal mass is the measurement of total body calcium (TBCa) using neutron activation analysis. This method provides a direct measure of total skeletal mass since 98% to 99% of the body's calcium is stored in the skeleton.[21] A high correlation has been demonstrated between TBCa (measured by neutron activation analysis) and bone calcium mass (as measured with gamma photon absorptiometry) at a number of sites including the radius, ulna, and humerus.[22] Rates of change for bone calcium mass in the radius, ulna, and humerus have been reported to be similar but change rates at these sites proved to be relatively more rapid than simultaneously measured changes in TBCa.[22] Cohn et al have evaluated TBCa in 79 subjects ranging in age from 30 to 90 years.[23] The average TBCa loss rate in women was 0.37% per year before menopause (50 years), and 1.1% per year after menopause. In men, the average TBCa loss rate was 0.7% per year after the age of 50. These data indicate that the average female in the 30–to 54-year age range loses 3.8 g/Ca/yr, primarily as the result of skeletal calcium loss. After the age of 55, the average female loses 7.6 g/Ca/yr. The average loss for men during the period from 50 to 90 years is 7 g/Ca/yr. Between the ages of 30 to 80, on the average a woman will lose approximately 28% of the TBCa that may have been originally present in her skeleton at age 30, whereas a man will lose only 20% of the calcium originally present at age 30.

Age-Related Changes in Bone at the Histologic Level

Bone is constantly undergoing remodelling, or turnover, even in an adult. Bone resorption and bone formation normally occur simultaneously. New bone matrix is produced by *osteoblasts*, which are well-differentiated cells seen on the surface of *osteoid*, the organic matrix of bone prior to its mineralization. Osteoblasts become entrapped in the matrix that they produce and are then termed *osteocytes*. The osteocyte cell population is interconnected throughout the bone matrix by fine cellular processes. Following secretion of bone matrix by osteoblasts, it is necessary that this be converted to mature osteoid prior to the initiation of mineralization. This maturation of osteoid follows the loss of proteoglycan and the formation of intermolecular cross links. At this stage the mineralization process begins. Both mineralization and bone formation rates can be determined by the analysis of tetracycline-labeling studies. Most tetracycline antibiotics form stable tetracycline-calcium chelates which fluoresce intensely at wavelengths readily examined with a fluorescence microscope. These chelates only form at sites of new bone formation where the bone contains 20% or less of its maximum mineral content. These chelates remain in the bone until it is eventually resorbed. Administration of two doses of tetracycline separated by a known time interval allows for the determination of the bone apposition rate (the micra of new bone matrix formed per day). The rate of osteoid maturation (in percent per day) can then be calculated by dividing the apposition rate by the osteoid width. During normal bone remodelling, and more so during times of calcium stress, bone is resorbed by *osteoclastis*, large multinucleate mature cells, rich in lysosomes. These cells can be readily identified in histologic sections by either their acid phosphatase content or by the criterion of multiple nuclei, though the demonstration of acid phosphatase activity is a more sensitive indicator of the presence of osteoclasts. Sites of present or past osteoclast activity may be identified by a scalloped or crenated edge on the bone surface, the result of the resorptive properties peculiar to osteoclasts.

Histologic changes in bone with aging have been documented by a number of investigators.[24–30] Meunier et al[30] found that male subjects showed a linear decrease in trabecular bone volume with increasing age. At age 80 years, the average male had lost 27% of the trabecular bone volume he had at age 20. Female subjects showed a slow decrease until age 50 years, a more rapid decrease from age 50 to 69 years, and a slower decrease after age 69. At age 80, the average female had lost 41% of the trabecular bone she had at age 20. No correlation was found between osteoid volume and age.[25] Likewise, no significant changes with increasing age have been found for the fraction of the trabecular surface covered with osteoid[26] or resorbing surface.[25] Lips et al[28] have found a significant decrease with increasing age for the mean wall thickness of trabecular bone packets. These bone packets represent the quantity of bone formed at a bone-forming site. Lips et al propose that this decrease in wall thickness, which they believe corresponds to a decrease in bone formation with aging, may in part explain physiologic senile osteopenia.

Age-Related Chemical Changes in Bone

Few studies have looked for changes in the chemical composition of bone with increasing age.[14] Some groups have documented unchanged calcium and phosphorus content[31] while others have reported a significant increase in calcium content with increasing age.[32,33] Conflicting reports have described changes in bone collagen with age: with one group finding increased collagen with age in lumbar vertebrae.[34] Other studies have noted that collagen content in the femora[35,36] remains unchanged[14–37] or decreases significantly with age.[35,36]

AGE-RELATED CHANGES IN ENDOCRINOLOGY RELEVANT TO BONE PHYSIOLOGY

Interpretation of biochemical findings in the elderly can be difficult. Increased BUN, low plasma calcium and, in women, increased plasma phosphate have all been reported to occur with aging.[38] Age-related changes have been documented for two hormones that are very important in bone physiology, PTH, and calcitonin. In normal women aged 20 to 90 years serum immunoreactive PTH (iPTH) increases significantly with aging, although Gallagher et al[39] report much less of an increase than have Berlyne et al.[40] This increase may represent increased PTH secretion, increased carboxy-terminal fragment production, reduced PTH clearance from the circulation, or a combination of these factors.[39] Serum calcitonin levels decrease with increasing age[41,42] and levels are lower in women than in men.[43]

Little information is currently available describing age-related changes in the vitamin D metabolites. Some data suggest that a decline in 25-hydroxyvitamin D [25(OH)D] and 1,25-dihydroxyvitamin D [1,25$(OH)_2$D] synthesis occurs with age.[44] Gallagher et al[44] propose that in normal elderly subjects the level of the 1-α-hydroxylase enzyme in the renal cortex decreases. This could lead to low serum 1,25$(OH)_2$D levels, decreased intestinal calcium absorption, and the resulting hypocalcemia may subsequently stimulate secretion of PTH. A decrease in the conversion of 25(OH)D to 1,25$(OH)_2$D may also play a role. Recent data by Epstein et al state that although 1,25$(OH)_2$D declines with age in both men and women, no significant decrease occurs in 25(OH)D.[45] In their study population serum inorganic phosphate was found to decrease significantly only in males. Total serum calcium and alkaline phosphatase increased significantly in females. The authors concluded that the primary defect with aging was a decreased formation of 1,25$(OH)_2D$ which then leads to decreased calcium absorption and increased PTH.

The reduced 1,25$(OH)_2D$ levels seen with aging may contribute to the impaired calcium absorption seen in the elderly. Decreased calcium absorption and possibly a loss of adaptation with increasing age have been reported by a number of investigators.[46,47] Heaney et al have found that untreated postmenopausal women show mean remodelling rates (measured with calcium kinetic methods) of 0.387 g/Ca/d for accretion and 0.425 g/Ca/d for resorption.[48] Their computed skeletal balance was −0.038 g/Ca/d. Premenopausal women exhibited accretion rates of 0.337 g/Ca/d and resorption rates of 0.358 g/Ca/d.

These changes in the important bone-related hormones have even greater impact because they are all closely interrelated to the homeostatic mechanisms controlling calcium metabolism. In addition, in the female the advent of the menopause causes many changes not only because of the associated decrease in estrogen levels themselves, but also because of the effect decreased estrogen levels are believed to have on bone physiology and bone-related hormones. Estrogen deficiency has been hypothesized to cause increased calcium release from bone which in turn causes decreased PTH levels, decreased conversion of 25(OH)D to 1,25$(OH)_2D$, and decreased 1,25$(OH)_2D$ production with the latter resulting in decreases in intestinal calcium absorption.[49] There is also evidence that estrogen deficiency itself decreases 25(OH)D-1-α-hydroxylase activity.[50] The effects of aging on reproductive function in women have recently been reviewed by Judd and Korenman[51] and Judd.[52] Young and Nordin[53] identified increased plasma and urinary levels of calcium and phosphorus in postmenopausal women. Excellent general reviews of menopausal changes in calcium balance[54,55] and changes in bone remodelling following the menopause[48] have been presented by Heaney et al.

Plasma bone Gla protein has recently been reported to decline with age and to be significantly correlated with creatinine clearance.[56] However, no correlation was found between Gla and age or between Gla and age when corrections were made for creatinine clearance. Catherwood et al[56] concluded that aging per se does not cause changes in plasma bone Gla protein.

OSTEOPOROSIS

Diagnosis

Osteoporosis, the principal cause of fractures in the elderly, affects one out of every four postmenopausal women in North America. Osteoporosis is characterized by a decreased bone volume within a normal periosteal perimeter, and in patients presenting with a compression fracture of the spine can best be diagnosed be a sequence which answers the following questions[57]: (1) Was the fracture "atraumatic," ie, was the mechanical stress involved less than the amount expected to produce such a fracture? (2) Does the patient exhibit generalized osteopenia (indicated by photon absorptiometry, decreased TBCa, radiologic evidence of other atraumatic fractures, and a history of increased fracture susceptibility)? (3) If a bone biopsy is possible, can osteomalacia be excluded, or can serum chemistry values rule out osteomalacia? If the answer to each of these questions is "yes," then a diagnosis of generalized axial osteopenia is warranted. The next step is to exclude causes of osteopenia other than osteoporosis. Table 11-1 summarizes the classification of osteoporosis and lists tests and results commonly used for diagnosis. If no evidence of secondary osteoporosis can be found for the patient, then the diagnosis becomes primary osteoporosis. Among cases of osteoporosis recently reviewed, 80% proved to be primary, and 95% of

Table 11-1
Osteoporosis: Classification and Tests Frequently Used for Diagnosis*

	Test or Comment	Results†
A. Primary Osteoporosis		
1. Idiopathic:		
a. Juvenile	Isolated or one or sometimes more than one child within a family may be affected	–
b. Young adults	Urine hydroxyproline	↑
2. Postmenopausal	Exclude other causes of osteoporosis	–
3. Senile‡	Excluded other causes of osteoporosis in patients 65 years old or more	–
B. Secondary Osteoporosis (Secondary to heritable or acquired abnormalities)		
1. Marfan's syndrome	Arm and leg length	↑
2. Morquio's syndrome	Serum hexosamine	↑
3. Homocystinuria	Urine homocysteine	↑
4. Osteogenesis imperfecta tarda	Platelet factor 3 activity	↓
5. Hypophosphatasia, adult form	Urine phosphoethanolamine	↑
6. Werner's syndrome	Obvious clinical features	–
7. Lactase deficiency	History; milk intolerance	–
8. Male hypogonadism (eg, Klinefelter's syndrome)	Serum testosterone	↓
9. Gut malabsorption	Serum 25-(OH)D	↓
	Serum PTH	↑
	Serum alkaline phosphatase	↑
	Urine Ca	↓
	Serum Ca	↓
	Serum PO_4	↓
10. Renal Ca Leak (renal hypercalciuria)	Urine cAMP	↑
11. Renal tubular acidosis, type 2	Serum CO_2	↓
12. Cirrhosis: Laennec's or biliary	Liver function tests	↓
13. Immobilization	Urine hydroxyproline	↑
14. Multiple myeloma§	Serum myeloma protein	↑
15. Low serum PO_4	Serum P	
a. Renal PO_4 leak‖ associated with low PO_4, high serum 1,25 and hypercalciuria	Serum P	↓
	PTH	↓
	Urine Ca	↑
b. Renal PO_4 leak associated with low serum PO_4, low serum $1,25(OH)_2D$ without hypercalciuria	Serum P	↓
	Urine Ca	↓
c. Treatment with PO_4 binders (eg, aluminum carbonate)	Serum P	↓
	PTH	↓
	Urine Ca	↑
16. Selective deficiency of $1,25(OH)_2D$ (adult onset)	Serum Ca	↓
	Serum P	↓
	PTH	↑
	Response to $1,25(OH)_2D$ treatment	nl
17. Anticonvulsant drugs	History	–
18. Female hypogonadism (eg, oophorectomy or Turner's syndrome)	Urine estrogen	↓
19. Cushing's syndrome	Serum cortisol	↑
20. Thyrotoxicosis	T_3, T_4	↑
21. Chronic alcoholism	History	–
22. Diabetes¶	Fasting blood sugar	↑
23. Chronic heparin treatment	History	–
24. Systemic mastocytosis (urticaria pigmentosa)	Physical examination	–
25. Chronic obstructive pulmonary disease	Pulmonary function tests	↓
26. Mild vitamin D deficiency (eg, patients > 70 years of age)	Serum 25-OH-D	↓

*Use is dictated by two criteria: (1) if the test discloses a readily treatable disease even if not common, and (2) the test is most likely to disclose an abnormality largely because the corresponding disease is relatively common. From Gruber and Baylink.[57]

these were in a group comprised of postmenopausal and senile individuals.[57]

Radiologic Features

The radiologic features of osteoporosis can be a valuable diagnostic tool[58-60] (Figures 11-1 and 11-2). Diffuse radiolucency is a general feature of osteoporotic bone. This results from decreased vertebral bone mass which in turn is due to thinned cortices and loss of trabecular bone (Figure 11-1). Other characteristic features include: (1) accentuation of vertical trabeculae, largely because of disappearance of horizontal trabeculae; (2) thinning of the vertebral cortex, originally described as resembling a "pencil thin line" by Albright et al[61]; (3) wedging of vertebral bodies, especially thoracic vertebrae (Figures 11-1 and 11-2); (4) biconcavity or "codfishing" of vertebral bodies in the lumbar region (Figure 11-2). The bony involvement of multiple myeloma is usually manifested by distinct lytic lesions on x-ray film, but if diffuse involvement is present, myeloma can be mistaken for osteoporosis. Thus, it is important that evaluation of patients with osteopenia include serum protein electrophoresis as a *screening* measure since myeloma occurs with some degree of frequency in the elderly.

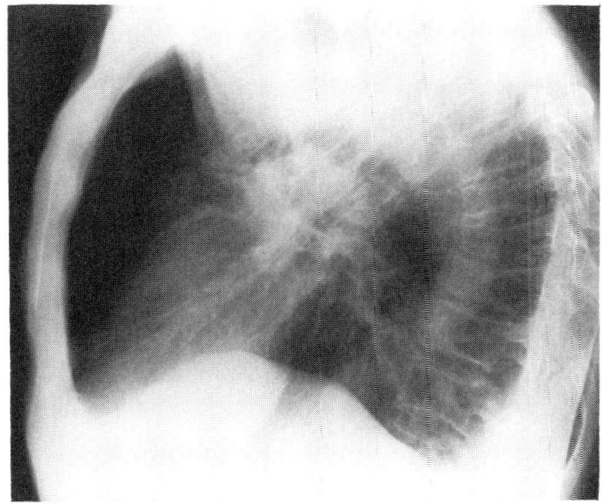

Figure 11-1 Lateral radiogram of the spine of an osteoporotic patient showing marked kyphosis, codfishing of lumbar vertebrae, anterior wedging of dorsal vertebrae, and prominent cortices. (Courtesy of Dr David J. Baylink.)

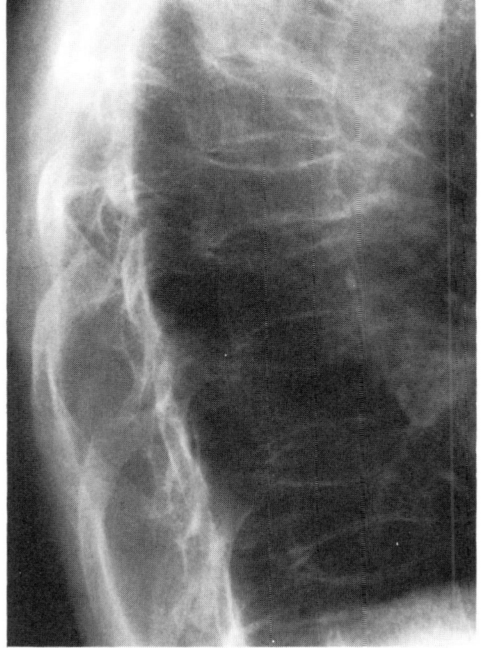

Figure 11-2 Lateral radiogram of the spine of an osteoporotic patient with prominent anterior wedging and codfishing. (Courtesy of Dr David J. Baylink.)

Clinical Tests and Bone Mineral Content

Laboratory findings on patients with primary nonheritable osteoporosis are in general normal. However, some tests for heritable primary osteoporosis may prove diagnostic. Certain laboratory findings with secondary osteoporoses may also be diagnostically useful (Table 11-1, section B).

†These changes indicate the changes that may occur, and do not preclude the possibility of no change. ↑ = increase, ↓ = decrease.
‡Encountered in patients over 65 years of age.
§May present or be associated with clinical osteoporosis.
‖In general, we find that when serum phosphorus is markedly decreased, the patient develops osteomalacia; when phosphorus is only modestly decreased, the patient develops osteoporosis.
¶Conflicting data on whether diabetes is associated with osteopenia.

Bone mineral content (BMC) of the radius as determined by photon absorptiometry can be useful in the identification of appendicular osteopenia.[16] A BMC measurement of the radius, corrected for bone width, which is two SD or more below the mean for normal age—and sex-matched subjects, *always* indicates appendicular osteopenia.[57] It is important to note that a normal BMC in the appendicular skeleton does not exclude osteopenia of the axial skeleton, and patients with seven or more vertebral fractures may demonstrate a normal BMC of the radius. However, the majority of patients with a low BMC also have axial osteoporosis. Therefore a low BMC of the appendicular skeleton usually indicates appendicular osteopenia and the likelihood of the same in the axial skeleton; a normal BMC in the appendicular skeleton *does not exclude* osteopenia in the axial skeleton.

Bone Histologic Findings

Osteoporotics display a great diversity with respect to cortical thickness and porosity, trabecular pattern and bone volume, and formation and resorption of bone.[27,62] A recent study by Whyte et al[63] confirmed this heterogeneity of bone features in a population of 25 postmenopausal subjects. Some patients showed normal or even elevated bone turnover while others showed low rates of bone formation. Similar results were found by Meunier et al in an earlier study.[27] In a corollary study quantitative bone biopsy results from patients with osteoporosis associated with pregnancy and lactation[64] were also found not to be significantly different from normal values, again pointing to the heterogeneous nature of this disorder. Despite this, mean wall thickness of trabecular bone packets in biopsies from postmenopausal osteoporotic patients is reduced compared to controls[65]; this provides further evidence that a decrease in bone formation may be a major factor contributing to bone loss in osteoporosis.

Only one study has addressed the extremely important task of determining osteoblast and osteoclast cell activities in postmenopausal osteoporotic subjects.[66] Although osteoclasts are not numerous in the iliac crest of postmenopausal osteoporotics, the individual osteoclast activity (calculated in terms of square millimeters of bone resorbed per osteoclast cell unit per day) is greater than the osteoblast activity (calculated in terms of square millimeters of matrix deposited per cell per day). Since the major determinants influencing bone formation and bone resorption are osteoblast number and osteoclast cell activity, respectively, the above finding is clearly weighted in favor of a state of increased resorption.

Endocrinology of Osteoporosis

This topic has recently been addressed in an excellent review by Johnston and Epstein.[67] Osteoporotic patients have been reported to have high, normal, or low PTH values,[39,40,62,68–71] although differences between the two commonly used radioimmunoassay systems (carboxy- and amino-terminal methods) must be taken into account in such comparisons. Patients with elevated PTH levels show significantly increased numbers of osteoclasts and forming surface in bone biopsy histology.[72] Among the classes of osteoporosis only a minority of postmenopausal osteoporotic females appear to have elevated PTH levels[39]; thus the exact role of PTH in the etiology of postmenopausal osteoporosis remains unclear.

The calcitonin response in postmenopausal osteoporosis to calcium stimulation was recently evaluated by Taggart et al.[73] Immunoreactive calcitonin levels increased significantly from base line in normal subjects ten and 20 minutes after a calcium infusion. However, calcitonin levels in osteoporotics did not change significantly at any time during a similar calcium infusion. These data are consistent with a decreased calcitonin response to calcium infusion in postmenopausal osteoporosis.[74] Such a calcitonin deficiency observed with increasing age may also be involved in the development of osteoporosis.[40,43,49,52]

Two studies report that serum 25(OH)D levels are not significantly different from normal in postmenopausal osteoporosis,[44,71] and one study reports that levels are significantly elevated compared to age-matched controls.[75] However, serum $1,25(OH)_2D$ levels were significantly lower in postmenopausal osteoporotics,[44,76,77] suggesting that there may exist an impaired conversion of 25(OH)D to $1,25(OH)_2D$. The mean decrease in $1,25(OH)_2D$ levels in postmenopausal osteoporosis was 25%, a level believed by some to account for the observed decrease in calcium absorption. This explanation appears particularly plausible since calcium absorption and $1,25(OH)_2D$ were significantly correlated within the normal range of values for $1,25(OH)_2D$ and because a dose of 0.4 μg/d of synthetic $1,25(OH)_2D$ was able to correct the impaired calcium absorption.[44,49] Despite this, in two additional studies there has been a failure to confirm the observation of lowered $1,25(OH)_2D$ levels in osteoporosis.[78,79] An additional observation by Slovik et al[79] notes that whereas normal subjects respond to a 24-hour infusion of human 1-34 PTH by nearly doubling their serum 1,25 levels, untreated osteoporotic patients showed no significant changes. This finding adds to the complexity inherent in the interpretation of $1,25(OH)_2D$ level in states of disordered mineral metabolism such as osteoporosis.

Calcium absorption is decreased in postmenopausal osteoporosis,[44] probably to the extent that it contributes significantly to the negative calcium balance seen in the elderly and postmenopausal osteoporotic patient.[49] Decreased calcium absorption is greatest in those patients whose diets are relatively low in calcium content.[50]

Bone Gla protein (the γ-carboxyglutamic acid-containing protein of bone) is receiving increased attention in bone research. Price et al[80] have found that plasma levels of this protein are significantly elevated above normal in osteoporotic patients. Urinary excretion of Gla is also elevated in osteoporosis.[81] Further studies are necessary to more completely define the meaning of plasma and urinary Gla levels in the development of osteoporosis.

It has recently been proposed that postmenopausal osteoporosis could involve an uncoupling effect of estrogen deficiency superimposed on the age-related decrease in the ability to effectively couple bone formation and bone resorption.[82] "Coupling" is a generalized counterregulatory phenomenon where an initial increase in bone resorption (such as is initiated by PTH) is followed by a secondary, nearly equal, increase in bone formation.[83,84] The net effect of this coupling is to reduce or minimize the bone loss that the resorptive agent or calcium stress would have produced if it had proceeded unchecked. Bone resorption and formation are thus interrelated processes, and since bone is constantly undergoing turnover, the balance between coupling and the endocrine mechanisms which are necessary to mobilize calcium is a finely tuned one. Thus, uncoupling could have serious consequences, especially when superimposed upon the age-related changes in bone and bone-regulating hormones which have been discussed previously.

Changes in the Chemical Composition of Bone in Postmenopausal Osteoporosis

Birkenhager-Frenkel has reported decreased collagen content[85] and decreased calcium/phosphorus[86] in bone from the iliac crest of osteoporotics. Additional studies have reported calcium to be decreased[87] or normal.[88] Matrix hydroxyproline has also been reported to be decreased.[89] An evaluation of bone matrix and mineral abnormalities by Burnell et al[90] has recently shown that osteoporotics display variable percentages of bone mineral and hydroxyproline in the bone matrix. Of those minerals examined, CO_3 and Ca/P were decreased while Na and Mg were increased. Four groups with different chemical composition of the iliac crest bone were identified: (1) a group with decreased matrix hydroxyproline and normal percentage of mineral, (2) a group with decreased matrix hydroxyproline and decreased percentage of mineral, (3) a group with normal matrix hydroxyproline and normal percentage mineral, and (4) a group with normal matrix hydroxyproline and decreased percentage of mineral. It is obvious that these studies dictate considerable latitude in the interpretation of matrix and mineral abnormalities in osteoporotics.

Therapy

The main goal in the treatment of osteoporosis is correction of low bone mass: This will prevent the complications of fracture, pain, and deformity.[91] Sometimes single agents can achieve this goal, but combination therapy may increase bone mass more readily. Baylink et al[91] stress the importance of suiting therapy to the severity of the osteoporosis: Prevention of further loss, and a modest increase in bone mass, if possible, may be well suited for patients with mild osteoporosis, whereas patients with moderate to severe bone loss require more than simply arresting bone loss. Patient evaluation during therapy is also important. Annual spinal x-ray films and bone photon absorptiometry measurements of the radius when available are recommended. Sodium fluoride therapy should be monitored by measurement of serum alkaline phosphatase; agents which decrease bone resorption should be followed with measurements of urinary hydroxyproline/milligram creatinine, a parameter which generally decreases in proportion to the decrease in bone resorption.

Estrogen therapy Conjugated estrogen is recommended at doses of 0.3 mg/d,[75] 0.625 mg/d,[92] or 1.25 mg/d,[91] (cyclically), or ethinyl estradiol (25 μg/d) or mestranol (25 μg/d) administered in 21-day cycles and withdrawn for ten days.[93] These can be used with oral calcium supplementation of 1000 mg/d. If clinical progression and additional fractures occur, the estrogen dose can be doubled from 0.625 mg/d, and a progestational agent, such as medroxyprogesterone acetate (10 mg/d) or norethindrone (5 mg/d) can be given for ten to 13 days of each month.[93] The potential for the development of endometrial carcinoma is a concern with estrogen therapy, although Gordon[94] believes that the doses of estrogen needed to correct postmenopausal bone loss are lower than those seen to be associated with cancer.

Although there is still uncertainty about its therapeutic usage,[95,96] estrogen appears to act by decreasing bone resorption (possibly by decreasing bone responsiveness to PTH) and thus slowing bone loss.[97] Several clinical studies have shown a slowing of bone loss in postmenopausal patients treated with estrogen.[16,97–100] Estrogen therapy has been shown to increase both serum $1,25(OH)_2D$ levels and calcium absorption.[101] Postmenopausal women treated with a mean estrogen dose of 0.0188 mg equivalents of ethinyl estradiol showed calcium accretion and resorption levels identical with premenopausal women.[48]

A synthetic steroid (tibolone) was reported to be effective in the prevention of bone loss in a British study by Lindsay et al.[102] High calcium intake supplemented by hormonal treatment has been reported to increase calcium retention in osteoporotic patients.[103] Combination therapy with estrogens and gestagen has been reported to produce an average 3% per year increase in mineral content.[104] Lindsay et al believe that the effects of estrogen may be long-lived, persisting for as long as 5 to 10 years.[105]

Marshall et al found that although estrogens decreased metacarpal bone loss,[106] they tended also to inhibit bone formation and did not entirely prevent vertebral compression fractures; this may be explained in part by reason of the estrogens not having corrected the negative calcium balance in patients with some degree of calcium malabsorption.[107] Nordin has cautioned that estrogen therapy is not without risk and should not be given to women over age 65 and in particular not to patients with ischemic heart disease or a prior history of thromboembolism.[108]

Calcitonin The ability of calcitonin to inhibit bone resorption makes this hormone an attractive candidate for a therapeutic role in the treatment of postmenopausal osteoporosis. Several short-term studies of calcitonin use and postmenopausal osteoporosis have been reported: Milhaud and Talbon[109] followed patients for more than 6 months; Rasmussen et al[110] evaluated nine patients on oral phosphate and calcitonin for 6 months, and Agrawal et al[111] studied nine patients on calcitonin, vitamin D_2, and calcium for 2 years. Recent results from a larger 2-year double-blind clinical study showed an initial positive effect (increased TBCa) when 100 Medical Research Council (MRC) units of salmon calcitonin per day were administered for 12 to 18 months; this was followed by a subsequent decline in response.[112] Iliac crest bone biopsies showed a significantly greater percent of total bone area in treated compared to control patients at 2 years and a significant decrease in percent resorbing surface in treated patients when evaluated by paired difference from base line. Calcitonin appeared relatively free from side effects; the main concern in its use is the necessity for parenteral administration.

Anabolic steroids Several short-term studies have suggested a potential therapeutic benefit for postmenopausal osteoporosis from the use of synthetic anabolic steroids.[113–115] Recent trials of methandrostenolone indicated a persistent increase of some 2% in TBCa over the 24 to 26 months of treatment.[116,117] Recent trials of the anabolic steroid stanozolol documented 4.4% increases from base line in TBCa in patients receiving 2 mg stanozolol three times a day for 3 of every 4 weeks.[118] Treated patients showed a decrease in urinary calcium, an increase in total urinary cAMP and a decrease in iPTH. Side effects included an increase in SGOT, increase in facial hair, ankle edema, hoarseness, and/or acne.

Sodium fluoride* The most prominent effect of fluoride on the skeleton is an increase in bone formation, uncoupling bone so that formation is favored over resorption.[119–121] Fluoride increases both the number and the activity of osteoblasts but in addition it impairs mineralization.[119,120] Axial bone mass is increased with fluoride therapy.[122,123] Total serum alkaline phosphatase and the nondialyzable fraction of urinary hydroxyproline increase significantly with fluoride treatment.[92,124] Combination treatment with sodium fluoride, vitamin D, and calcium has been shown to retard the development of vertebral compression fractures, especially after 2 years of such therapy.[121,125–127] Recent in vitro work has shown fluoride capable of increasing the proliferative rate of bone cells and in particular enhancing the effect of parathyroid extract to increase such bone cell proliferation.[128]

Although many investigators feel that the benefits of sodium fluoride use justify its inclusion in therapeutic regimens, serious issues attend its use: (1) 50% of treated patients exhibit significant side effects (synovitis, recurrent vomiting, anemia from gastrointestinal (GI) bleeding, painful plantar fasciitis); (2) development of osteomalacia is a serious concern; this may be lessened with concurrent vitamin D and calcium supplementation; (3) fluoridic bone possesses increased

*Not approved by the Food and Drug Administration. Research protocols commonly use 45 to 60 mg/d with calcium supplementation.[93]

crystallinity and a decreased elasticity; thus it may not have normal strength.[129]

Vitamin D metabolites Because 1,25-$(OH)_2D$ increases calcium absorption and because of the demonstrated low calcium absorption and 1,25$(OH)_2D$ levels in osteoporotics,[44,76,77] interest has recently been focused on use of this metabolite in the therapy of osteoporosis. Therapeutic results have not been uniformly successful with this agent. Christiansen et al[130] have found a 2% decrease in forearm cortical BMC in osteoporotic subjects treated with 1,25$(OH)_2D$ for 1 year (0.25 μg/d). More encouraging have been the results of Gallagher et al, who reported an increase in calcium absorption in 17/20 osteoporotic patients treated with 0.4 μg/d of 1,25$(OH)_2D$ for seven days.[131] However, with prolonged treatment the beneficial effect of this increased calcium absorption appears to decline.[132]

Vitamin D administration appears to have an adverse effect on the rate of development of spinal fractures.[133] Also, vitamin D alone or in combination with estrogens or sodium fluoride does not appear to impart additional therapeutic benefit to the osteoporotic.[134]

1-α-(OH)D therapy has been reported to either increase[135,136] or to have no effect[119] on BMC. Such a lack of an effect following 1-α-(OH)D treatment may also be seen based on evaluation of metacarpal bone loss and/or the deterioration demonstrated on spinal x-ray films.[137]

Other combined treatment studies Aloia et al have investigated in nine postmenopausal patients the value of a therapeutic regimen combining estrogen, fluoride, and calcium.[138] Significant positive slopes were found for TBCa and BMC with this combination therapy. Neutron activation analysis of the central third of the skeleton of osteoporotic patients who were receiving sodium fluoride and/or estrogen showed a mean increase in the calcium bone index of 5 ± 2% (SEM) compared to a negligible loss of 0.4 ± 1.9% for controls. The utilization of sodium fluoride therapy for 3 years has been associated with a significant increase in bone mineral, but in 6 patients studied who received bone biopsies there was concomitant histologic evidence of fluorosis.[139]

Other agents: Diphosphonates and PTH Diphosphonates are attractive agents for the treatment of osteoporosis since they have been shown to slow bone resorption. However, they also slow bone turnover[140] and inhibit hydroxyapatite crystal formation and dissolution. Ethane-1-hydroxy-1,1-diphosphonate (EHDP) treatment for 3 months resulted in secondary hyperparathyroidism and a hyperphosphatemia which contributed to a decreased serum ionized calcium. Bone biopsies also showed an increase in osteoid.[141] Another study documented a reduction in overall bone turnover, bone resorption, and mineralization.[142,143]

Since mild PTH exposure has been noted to have a net anabolic effect on the skeleton, PTH has also been evaluated in the therapy of osteoporosis. Treatment with the 1-34 synthetic fragment of human PTH increased the number of bone apposition sites in a small study.[144] Resorbing surface and the number of osteoclasts also increased, suggesting a future role for combining this therapy with agents which shorten osteoclast life span or activity. Parsons et al[145] showed an increase in trabecular bone volume in nine of ten patients treated with the 1-34 synthetic fragment of human PTH. This study also showed an increase in osteoid surface and an increase in intestinal calcium absorption whenever there was a demonstrated improvement in calcium balance.[145]

The importance of calcium in nutrition Along with appropriate exercise, calcium content of the diet is an issue which has perhaps received less attention than it deserves. In a recent editorial discussing the issue of calcium intake requirements and bone mass in the elderly,[146] Heaney stressed that recent evidence has shifted in favor of a more prominent role for calcium in the protection of bone mass and in the prevention of fractures. The currently recommended daily calcium allowance of 800 mg is probably too low, although what an optimum intake should be is still unknown. Marcus[147] has also recently commented on the interrelationship of endocrinology and nutrition in the maintenance of skeletal mass, and suggests a calcium intake for women of 1500 mg/d at the time of menopause. Although achieving a calcium intake of 1000 to 1500 mg/d may be difficult for some elderly patients, calcium intake can be supplmented in a tablet form.* It is generally believed that calcium supplementation has a beneficial effect on bone loss, but that this effect is less than that provided by other therapies.[93] The use of calcium as sole therapy in osteoporosis is relatively safe and best dictated in the individual patient by the severity of the disease process and fracture incidence. Other recent studies have dealt in greater detail with the issue of calcium[2,93] and phosphate[2] intake.

OSTEOMALACIA

Diagnosis

Certain physiologic processes in bone such as the mineralization rate and the rate of osteoid maturation serve as defense mechanisms in the scheme of calcium and phosphorus homeostasis. Osteomalacia is a disorder in which there is defective mineralization of newly laid down bone matrix. Assessment of a bone biopsy only by evaluation of structural osteoid features is frequently not sufficient to make a diagnosis of osteomalacia since many high turnover, or hyperosteoid states exist. These conditions demonstrate an increase in osteoid surface and area[57,148] but the lack of mineralization is really a reflection of a high rate of osteoid production exceeding the capacity for mineralization. The definitive characteristic of osteomalacia is an abnormal tetracycline incorporation such that the mineralization lag time (the time between the formation of osteoid and its mineralization) is clearly prolonged. When a bone biopsy from an osteomalacic patient is labeled with tetracycline (administration of two oral doses of tetracycline separated by a known time interval) and examined by fluorescence microscopy, widened, smudged single labels may be evident (Figures 11-3 and 11-4) or, if mineralization has ceased completely, no tetracycline label may be discernible. Common causes of adult-onset osteomalacia are listed in Table 11-2. This compilation is not all inclusive because new causes of osteomalacia are constantly discovered as our understanding of vitamin D and mineral metabolism expands. As can be seen from Table 11-2, osteomalacia can be present in a wide spectrum of clinical disorders. Recent evidence has shown that osteomalacia is not as common as previously believed in patients presenting with compression fractures of the spine; only about 5% of patients with axial osteopenia will have osteomalacia when a bone biopsy is performed.[57]

Radiologic Features

Radiologically, osteomalacia has either a normal appearance or osteopenia is evident.[149] The radiologic hallmark of severe osteomalacia is a localized area of linear rarefaction; such pseudofractures, termed Looser's zones or Milkman's fractures, represent areas where healing has been impaired by the bone mineralization defect. The radiologic appearance of these zones can be variable.[150] Looser's zones

---

*Seeman and Riggs[93] have provided the following useful information: A normal diet excluding dairy products contains 300 mg elemental calcium. 8 oz of milk provides 240 mg elemental calcium and five slices of American cheese contains 600 mg calcium. Medicinal tablet calcium content for commonly used products are: calcium carbonate, 650 mg = 250 mg elemental calcium; calcium gluconate, 650 mg = 58.5 mg elemental calcium; calcium lactate, 650 mg = 94.5 mg elemental calcium.

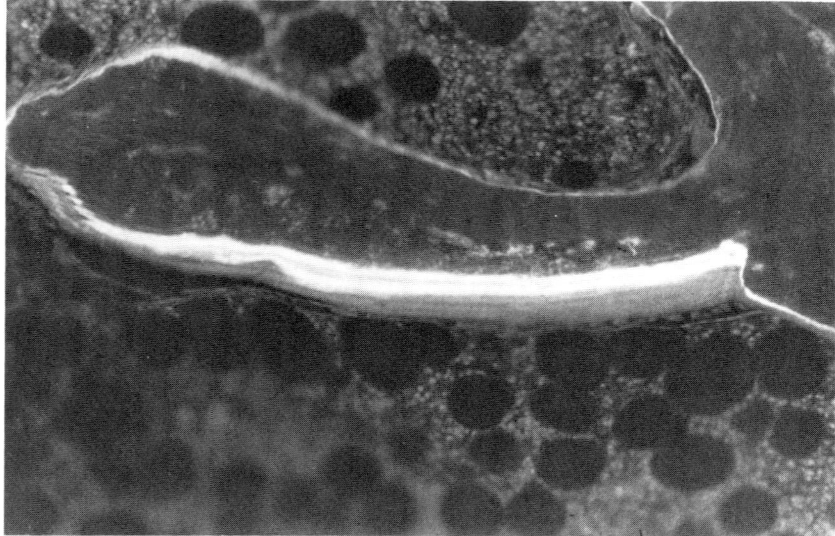

Figure 11-3 Anterior iliac crest biopsy from a patient who received two courses of tetracycline prior to biopsy. When examined unstained with fluorescence microscopy, double labels show that this site of bone formation was active when both the first and second courses of antibiotic were given (methacrylate embedment, 7 μ, $\times$ 185).

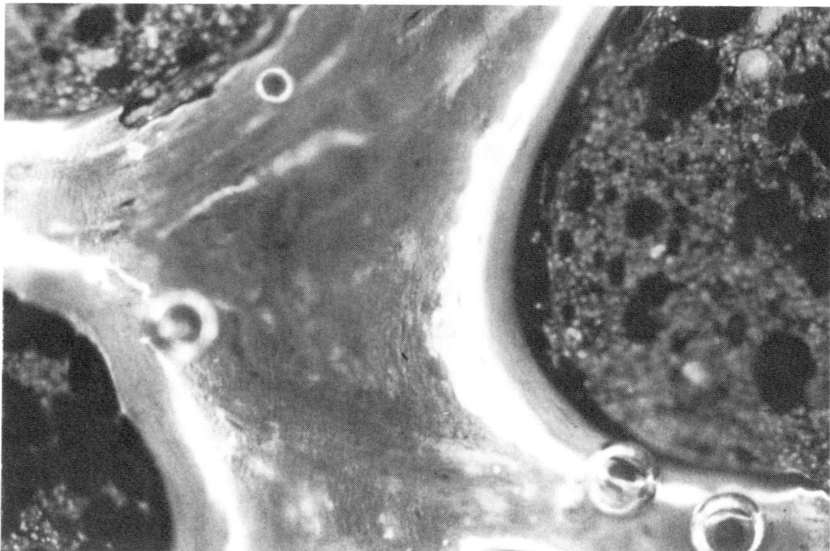

Figure 11-4 Anterior iliac crest biopsy from a patient with a mineralization defect. Although two courses of tetracycline were administered prior to biopsy, only one broad band of fluorescence is evident (methacrylate embedment, 7 μ, $\times$185).

Table 11-2
Causes of Osteomalacia in the Adult

1. Associated with vitamin D:
   a. Inadequate exposure to sunlight
   b. Inadequate absorption of D_2 from gut
   c. Hepatic disease impairing conversion of vitamin D_2 to $25(OH)D_2$ and/or vitamin D_3 to $25(OH)D_3$
   d. $1,25(OH)_2$ vitamin D deficiency (renal failure)
   e. Small intestinal diseases impairing absorption
   f. Anticonvulsant therapy ($25(OH)D_2$ deficiency)
2. Moderate to severe hypophosphatemia*
   a. Induced by phosphate binders
   b. Resulting from reduced renal phosphate reabsorptive capacities (hyperparathyroidism, primary and secondary renal tubular disorders)
   c. Soft tissue tumors
   d. Hemodialysis
   e. Alcoholism
   f. Other causes: acidosis, diabetic ketoacidosis, severe third-degree burns, gout
3. Other causes
   a. Fluoride therapy
   b. Treatment with some diphosphonates
   c. Decreased renal function and renal failure
   d. Total parenteral nutrition
   e. Antacids

*Corry and Lee[152] provide a complete discussion of clinical disorders associated with hypophosphatemia.

commonly occur in the scapula, pelvis, proximal long bones, and ribs.[38] Distinct in appearance from the microfractures that can occur in Paget's disease, Looser's zones commonly occur on the concavity of long bones.[38]

An additional feature of advanced osteomalacia is a blurred, fuzzy appearance of trabeculae in the vertebral bodies.[151] In addition, in patients past 70 years of age with both osteomalacia and osteoporosis, plastic deformities have been noted.[151]

Clinical Features and Bone Mineral Content

Bone pain and tenderness as well as lower extremity proximal muscle weakness are the predominant symptoms in osteomalacia; muscle weakness when present may vary in severity from the patient's complaint of difficulty in moving about to an obvious waddling gait.[38] Bone mineral content measurements are variable ranging from high to low values, but in most instances are usually normal,[151,152] and thus do not offer diagnostic distinction for osteomalacia.

Most elderly patients with osteomalacia will exhibit low serum calcium and/or low serum phosphate; alkaline phosphatase may be high or low. However, a few patients who do not show these biochemical changes will exhibit osteomalacia when a bone biopsy is examined with prior tetracycline labeling.[38,150] In cases of severe vitamin D deficiency, serum calcium, phosphate, and 25(OH)D values are low, leading to elevations in PTH and subsequent elevations in the bone isoenzyme of serum alkaline phosphatase. Urine calcium excretion will generally be depressed. Baylink[151] believes that there exist two syndromes of hypophosphatemia which may result in osteomalacia: (*a*) hypophosphatemia and high urine calcium (resulting from the increased $1,25(OH)_2D$ response to hypophosphatemia), and (*b*) hypophosphatemia without high urine calcium (such patients may have tubular resorptive abnormalities for phosphate and low 1-α-hydroxylase activity). Frame and Parfitt[150] also state that in osteomalacia urine calcium is usually low but that in certain instances hypercalciuria may be present such is the case with phosphate depletion or renal tubular acidosis.

Bone Histologic Findings

Advanced osteomalacia shows increased osteoid area, widened osteoid seams, and increased osteoid surface. The resorbing surface may be normal or increased, depending on the etiology. Marrow fibrosis may be present or absent.[153] As previously mentioned, histologic identification of osteomalacia depends on the detection of abnormal mineralization by tetracycline labeling (Figures 11-3 and 11-4). Advanced osteomalacia will show increased lag time for mineralization, an increase in the percentage of the mineralizing front labeled by tetracycline, or, in extreme cases actual absence of tetracycline incorporation due to cessation of mineralization. Hypocalcemia can serve as a stimulus for the development of secondary hyperparathyroidism. The additional effects of this increased PTH activity might then be seen on bone biopsy as an increase in osteoclast number and an increase in bone resorption.

Endocrinology of Osteomalacia

Osteomalacia in the geriatric patient often is multifactorial reflecting various combinations of abnormalities in the kidney, liver, or GI systems that occur with aging. The biochemical features accompanying osteomalacia can be complex. In the elderly patient, poor vitamin D intake, reduced exposure to sunlight, decreased renal function, and decreased calcium absorption may all be important factors in the development of osteomalacia. In addition, other conditions or complications can be implicated in osteomalacia; these include treatment with diphosphonates, fluoride, dialysis, and anticonvulsant therapy. Malabsorptive complications following intestinal resection or due to other intestinal problems (intestinal diverticula, Crohn's disease,[154] and hepatic or gallbladder problems leading to decreased bile salts may also culminate in an osteomalacic picture. Certain mesenchymal tumors lead to hypophosphatemia and thus osteomalacia. In most of these conditions, abnormalities in vitamin D metabolism and/or the action of vitamin D metabolites can be invoked; this mechanism is seen to play an increasingly important role as an improved understanding of the vitamin D system develops and more accurate assay technics become available with which to quantitate changes in vitamin D metabolites. Some of the mechanisms involved in many of the conditions mentioned above are complex and have recently been reviewed by Smith,[38] and Dent and Stamp.[154] Norman has recently reviewed vitamin D metabolism and its effects on calcium and phosphorus absorption.[155]

Therapy

Therapy for osteomalacia can be particularly rewarding and should be directed to the cause of the mineralization problem. Numerous therapeutic regimens are possible but any dose used should be tailored to the individual patient. Elderly patients with gluten-sensitive enteropathy respond well to gluten-free diets, 100,000 IU vitamin D_2/d,* and 2 g calcium/d.[151] Baylink[151] reports that patients so treated may show healing of pseudofractures, decrease in skeletal pain and fatigue, and weight gain. However, as mentioned below, long-term vitamin D therapy should be closely monitored by determining urinary calcium excretion (not to exceed 150 mg/d), with appropriate dose reductions or discontinuation when urinary calcium is either elevated or shows a continuous increase. Therapeutic trials of 50,000 IU vitamin D_2/d for 1 or 2 months will not, in most cases, produce vitamin D toxicity.[151]

Vitamin D-deficiency osteomalacia can exhibit a rapid improvement with vitamin D therapy. Muscle strength may increase in a few days; however, it has been reported that skeletal pain may worsen temporarily early in therapy.[38] Serum alkaline phosphatase and total urinary hydroxyproline may increase temporarily. There is a fall in PTH and an increase in serum phosphorus[156] and there may be an early decrease in both serum and urinary calcium. The latter may remain low until healing has progressed.[150]

*One milligram of vitamin D_2 is equivalent to 40,000 IU.[38]

Most authorities advise initiation of vitamin D therapy at doses below the expected maintenance dose. Barzel[157] suggests that 2 to 3 weeks of base-line therapy should occur before a tenfold dose increase is started. Frame and Parfitt[150] suggest that incremental doses should be no greater than one fourth the initial dose, or 0.25 mg, whichever is smaller. The interim period between dose increments should be long enough to allow detection of alkaline phosphatase and roentgenographic response.[150] As previously mentioned, pharmacologic doses require careful patient monitoring to avoid vitamin D intoxication; repeated weekly values for serum calcium, phosphorus, alkaline phosphatase, total protein, BUN, and creatinine and 24-hour urinary calcium, phosphate, and creatinine are recommended.[150]

Baylink[151] advises that when urinary calcium exceeds 200 mg/d, vitamin D therapy should be stopped because of the concern that renal stone formation (at urinary calcium levels greater than 250 mg/d in females and 300 mg/d in males) may be precipitated. In addition, hypercalciuria can precede the development of hypercalcemia. Any such rise in serum calcium is felt to be the most important complication that may result from vitamin D therapy.

Osteomalacia due to phosphate deficiency can ordinarily be treated with oral administration of 500 mg neutral phosphate four times a day (Neutrophos is a Na- and K-containing neutral phosphate salt; Neutrophos K contains no Na).[151] Higher doses may sometimes become necessary but are frequently accompanied by diarrhea when doses exceed 2 g/d. Patients with phosphate deficiency in combination with low serum $1,25(OH)_2D$ levels should also be treated with vitamin D to avoid any decrease in serum calcium. (It has been proposed that by increasing serum calcium to borderline high values that PTH will be depressed and the renal tubular maximum phosphate reabsorption [Tm_P] increased.[151])

The time necessary to reach maximum vitamin D effect varies with the preparation used: 4 to 10 weeks for vitamin D_2, 4 to 20 weeks for $25(OH)D_3$, and 0.5 to 1 week for $1,25(OH)_2D_3$.[150] The effects of vitamin D may also persist after cessation of therapy and are also variable: 6 to 18 weeks for vitamin D_2, 4 to 12 weeks for $25(OH)D_3$, and 0.5 to 1 week for $1,25(OH)_2D_3$. Likewise, the relative potency of the various preparations has been rated as follows: vitamin D_2, 1; $25(OH)D_3$, 2; $1,25(OH)_2D_3$, 20.[150] Brautbar et al state that the biological half-life of vitamin D following large doses is approximately 3 months.[158] These authors also stress that there is great individual variability in dosages tolerated before the appearance of toxicity.

In a recent review on the clinical management of osteomalacia, Avioli suggests a vitamin D dose of 400 IU/d for the management of osteomalacia resulting from dietary deficiency of vitamin D. In cases of vitamin D-resistant rickets, as much as 500,000 IU/d may be needed. Monthly monitoring of 25(OH)D is important in patients who are taking more than 25,000 to 50,000 IU/d.[159] In cases involving large doses of phosphate-binding antacids, Avioli recommends a change to a preparation such as calcium carbonate, which might then avoid the effects of any further alteration in phosphate homeostasis.

Baylink believes that vitamin D therapy will be adequate for any type of vitamin D deficiency osteomalacia,[151] and suggests the following therapeutic regimens: (1) nutritional deficiency: 1000 IU/d for 6 to 12 months, or 50,000 IU/d for 2 to 3 months; (2) in liver disease: 5000 to 10,000 IU/d; (3) in renal failure: 50,000 IU/d or more (or 50 μg/d 25(OH)D or 0.5 μg/d $1,25(OH)_2D$.

Calcium and Nutrition

It has been recommended that all patients with vitamin D deficiency osteomalacia maintain an adequate intake of calcium. This means inclusion of at least 800 mg/d calcium in their diet, and possibly even 1500 mg/d in order to promote healing of the osteomalacia.[151] In the geriatric population, this may be extremely important when one considers the possibility of poor diet. Other important factors in the elderly in respect to osteomalacia are the possibilities of low vitamin D intake and decreased exposure to sunlight.[2,157]

PAGET'S DISEASE

Paget's disease is the second most common disease of bone in the elderly and a disorder for which current findings provide new insight. Paget's disease is a localized bone disease which often results in marked skeletal deformities by the time the patient consults a physician. First described in 1876 by Sir James Paget under the name "osteitis deformans," this condition now bears his name and is usually diagnosed in patients older than 40 or 50 years of age. As in the case of osteoporosis, this again is a disease in which bone changes have been occurring for decades prior to patient presentation. The incidence of Paget's disease is estimated to be about 3% in persons over the age of 40; incidence increases with age and is estimated to be 5% to 11% for persons in their 90s.[160,161]

Paget's disease is common in Anglo-Saxon countries but rare in India, China, Japan, the Middle East, Africa, and Scandinavia. A hereditary component may exist in Paget's disease; some feel a simple mendelian autosomal dominant inheritance pattern is present, while others postulate a sex-linked recessive transmission.[162] Singer reports finding a family history of Paget's disease in 16% (9/55) of patients.[160] Evidence for a linkage between Paget's disease and the HLA system suggests the possibility of a predisposing factor located on chromosome 6.[162]

Diagnosis and Radiologic Features

Radiologic features are an important element in the differential diagnosis of Paget's disease although they may vary depending on the stage of the disease. Commonly involved sites are the spine, pelvis, and femoral head. The sacrum is involved in 56% of cases and the other portions of the spine in 50% of cases.[163] Walpin and Singer report that the lumbar vertebrae are affected more frequently than the thoracic or cervical vertebrae.[163] Extensive skeletal involvement is unusual. Symptomatic patients commonly complain of both pain and bony deformities. In patients with Paget's disease and degenerative arthritis, pain may be quite severe and arthritic complications may remain a significant problem even when Paget's disease has been adequately controlled.

A skeletal deformity is often apparent in the skull. One of the earliest (asymptomatic) skull features is a circumscribed radiolucent region which may persist for years (osteoporosis circumscripta). At a later stage, the skull becomes enlarged, usually more so in the occipital and frontal regions.[160] New bone is added to the outer table of the skull and the entire calvarium becomes coarsely thickened with a "cotton wool" appearance on x-ray film.[157,160] Basilar invagination can occur but usually does not produce neural compression. However, involvement of the temporal bone and ossicle can result in either hearing impairment or actual loss.[164] Maxillary and periodontal involvement can also occur leading to loss of the lamina dura and displacement of teeth.

The spine is a commonly involved site (Figure 11-5). Pain may be present; the early lesion sometimes resembles osteoporosis. Vertebrae show thickened margins and coarse central vertical striations. Compression fractures and compression of the spinal cord and nerve roots may also occur.

Cortical thickening and coarse trabecular patterns are present in the pelvis

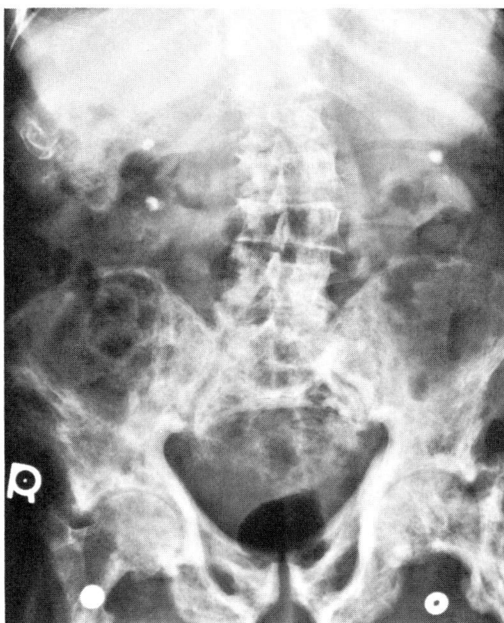

Figure 11-5 Roentgenogram of the pelvis and lumbar spine of a patient with Paget's disease. Vertebral margins and pelvic cortices are thickened. (Courtesy of Dr Frederick R. Singer.)

(Figure 11-5). Degenerative joint disease of the hip may develop after a long period. In long bones, the lytic wedge, the progressing front of bone resorption, resembles an arrowhead or the tip of a flame. This is often considered a classic presentation of Paget's disease.

Two biochemical measurements, serum alkaline phosphatase (which provides an index of osteoblast activity) and urinary hydroxyproline (which reflects bone resorption), are useful in the diagnosis of Paget's disease. Alkaline phosphatase is elevated and usually shows a good correlation with the radiologic extent of the disease.[165] Twenty-four-hour urinary hydroxyproline correlates well with serum alkaline phosphatase in Paget's disease.[166-168] Barzel[157] believes that the discovery of radiologic features typical for Paget's disease as well as increased alkaline phosphatase (in the absence of liver disease) are adequate to diagnose Paget's disease. Despite this any patient's history and data should still be carefully evaluated since neoplasia can sometimes present with similar features and may coexist with Paget's disease.[169] In addition, malignant changes in Paget's disease itself have been observed.[160]

Clinical Features and Endocrinology

Many patients are asymptomatic and Paget's disease may be detected during the course of radiologic evaluation for other reasons. Elderly patients with advanced disease may present with pain, deformity (midshaft bowing and thickening of the tibia, enlarged skull and clavicular involvement), nerve compression, or fractures. Cardiac output can be elevated.[166] Any increase in organ blood flow is proportional to the severity of the disease.[170] Henley et al[171] have found cardiovascular abnormalities in 32 out of 39 patients. Abnormalities included systemic hypertension, ischemic heart disease, cardiac enlargement, as well as valvular and/or arterial calcification.

Paget's disease is a localized disease and may affect many sites. Patients rarely develop a new lesion; rather, involvement at a site becomes more extensive. The enlarged bone seen in advanced cases is the end result of many years of disease activity; the earliest stages advance slowly and are characterized by bone loss. On occasion, lytic lesions may be observed on top of new bone formation.

When the resorptive phase of the disease dominates, there is a tendency for urinary calcium excretion to be elevated.[161] Similarly, acid phosphatase may be elevated in relation to increased bone resorption.[167]

Other biochemical changes in Paget's disease have recently been reviewed by Russell et al.[172] Urinary excretion of hydroxylysine and collagen-derived glycosides are increased. Both Gla[172,173] and proline iminopeptidase levels are elevated.[172]

The highest levels of PTH are found in patients with the most severe disease.[172] This increase may be due to secondary hyperparathyroidism resulting from an increased need for calcium by the involved skeletal sites.[174] Elevated PTH may contribute to increased bone turnover that may be seen in biopsies from noninvolved sites.

Changes in the Chemical Composition of Bone

Krane et al[175] found no significant difference in amino acid composition of bone in Paget's disease compared with normal bone. Likewise, the ratio of hydroxylysine to 4-hydroxyproline was not significantly different from normal. One report has documented a relative increase of a minor cross link, hydroxylysine or leucine, in bone from patients with Paget's disease.[176]

Histologic and Ultrastructural Features

Histologically, Paget's disease is characterized by three phases.[177] In the osteolytic phase, bone resorption is the prominent feature and is initially accompanied by marked hypervascularization. A period of very active bone formation and resorption follows. This is sometimes called the "mixed phase." When remodelling is extremely disordered, a characteristic mosaic of cement lines is present (Figure 11-6). Woven bone and fibrosis may also be present. The final sclerotic phase is characterized by decreased vascularity and fibrosis. Resorption may decrease and the bone may become denser and less vascular.

Although quantitative histology may be difficult to interpret in Paget's disease because of heterogeneity in involved sites, Meunier's studies[178] have documented increased bone area, resorbing and forming surfaces, and osteoid area. The rate of

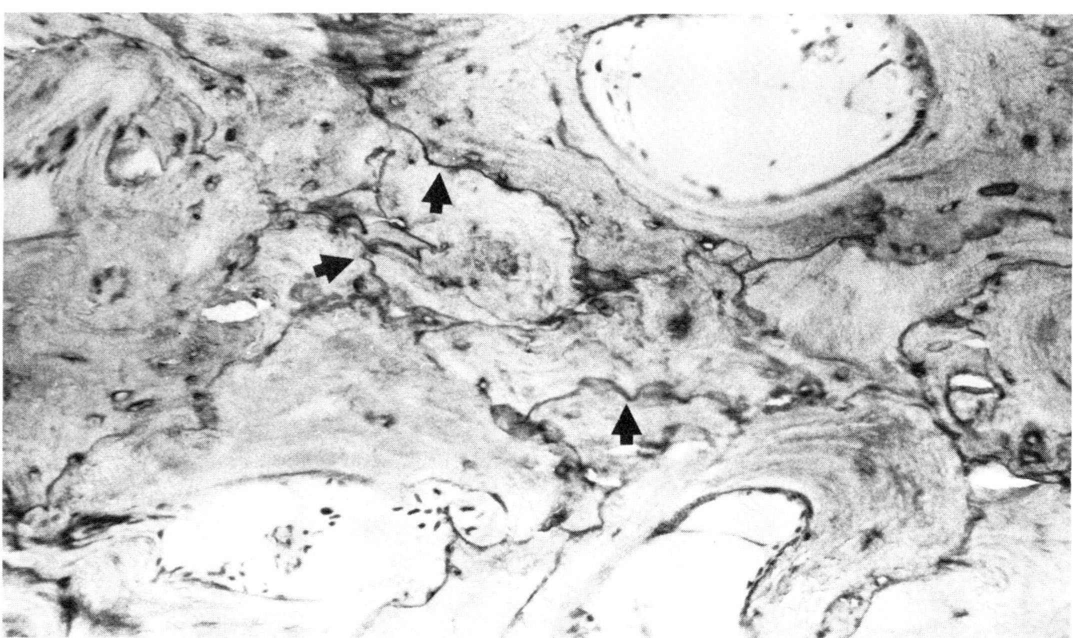

Figure 11-6 Anterior iliac crest bone biopsy from a patient with Paget's disease. The mosaic pattern of the cement lines (arrows) indicates the irregular bone remodeling in this disease (methacrylate embedment, toluidine blue stain, 5 μ, $\times$ 190).

matrix formation and the number of osteoclasts are elevated. Noninvolved bone can also show an abnormal increase in resorbing surface and a decrease in osteoid width, but the bone formation rate and bone area are normal.[178]

One of the most interesting cellular findings in Paget's disease is the recent discovery of nuclear inclusions in osteoclasts (Figure 11-7).[179-182] Most inclusions do not resemble intact viral bodies but rather appear like the viral nucleocapsid. This finding suggests that a virus may play a role in Paget's disease. These inclusions contain antigenic matter, or material capable of producing immunologic cross reactions to the measles group of viruses. Rebel et al have reported positive indirect immunofluorescence results for osteoclasts reacting with antimeasles antibodies.[183] Mills et al have documented a positive reaction of sera containing respiratory syncytial virus antibodies and osteoclasts cultured from patients with Paget's disease.[184]

These ultrastructural and immunocytologic data favor a viral etiology for Paget's disease. The appearance of symptoms long after any primary infection and the chronic development of the disease support the concept of a slow virus etiology. Mills has also recently shown that giant cell tumors contain nuclear inclusions morphologically identical with the 12- to 15-nm tubules characteristically seen in osteoclast nuclei in Paget's disease.[185]

Therapy

Asymptomatic patients usually require no treatment, but Singer recommends treatment for patients with severe bone pain in involved areas, cardiac failure related to high output, hypercalcemia (due to patient immobilization), and recurrent renal stones due to hypercalcemia.[160] Possible candidates for therapy due to advanced disease include patients with multiple fractures in affected sites with either nerve compression or onset in a site prone to a disabling deformity (in order to prevent complications in younger patients), or to aid patients preparing for orthopedic

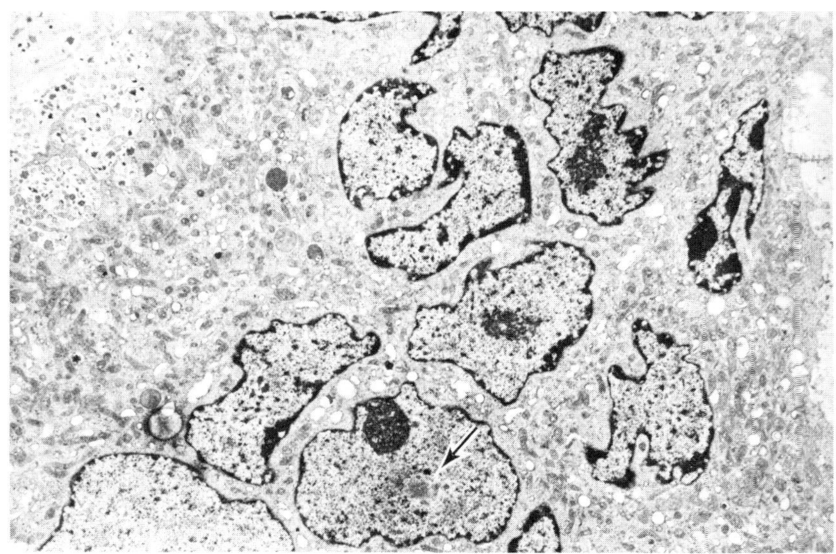

Figure 11-7A Electron micrograph of an osteoclast from a patient with Paget's disease. Ruffled border (upper left) and a large number of nuclei are apparent. A typical nuclear inclusion is present in the nucleus in the lower center (arrow) (× 5000; courtesy of Dr Barbara G. Mills).

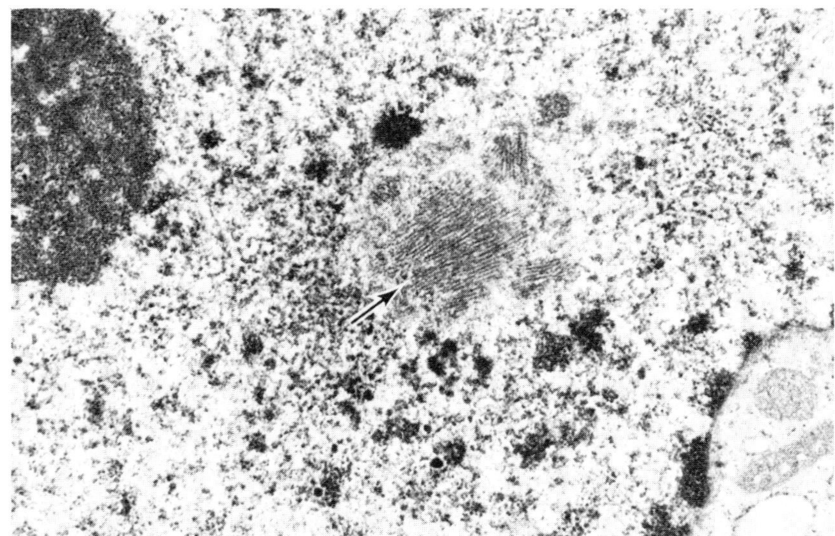

Figure 11-7B At higher resolution, the osteoclast nucleus shown in Figure 11-7A contains typical filaments of nuclear inclusions seen in Paget's disease. There is no attachment with the nucleolus and no membrane is associated with the inclusion (× 30,000; courtesy of Dr Barbara G. Mills).

surgery. This latter application may help to avoid complications due to severe bleeding which may occur due to the increased vascularity of Paget's disease.[160] The therapeutic principle involved in treatment of Paget's disease is achievement of an inhibition of osteoclast activity. In the strict sense, such therapy is probably only suppressive and does not truly cure the disorder.

Calcitonin Many clinicians believe that calcitonin affords the best therapy for Paget's disease. Recent work by Chambers[186] has documented the rapid, sensitive osteoclast response to calcitonin. When calcitonin is added to an in vitro preparation of osteoclasts, these cells show complete cessation of pseudopodial activity within minutes; such inhibition lasts as long as the cells remain viable.[186]

For Paget's disease calcitonin is usually given as 50 units salmon calcitonin daily, or three times a week, by subcutaneous injection. In severe cases involving advanced disability or neurologic impairment, a dose of 100 units daily, which is reduced to 50 units three times a week after appearance of response, is recommended by Avramides.[187] Patients generally experience a decrease in bone pain, sometimes as early as the first few weeks of therapy. Such relief is usually maximal by 3 to 6 months of therapy. Two thirds of patients may show relief of neurologic complications, though improvement is usually only partial. Walpen and Singer report reversal of severe paraparesis using calcitonin.[163] Some workers have documented radiologic improvement of a dose-related nature to long-term calcitonin therapy.[188] One study has documented increased TBCa prior to therapy and a decrease in TBCa during calcitonin therapy.[189] Treatment with calcitonin (and also with etidronate disodium, see below) produces a reduction in cardiac index in most patients.[171]

Singer et al have described three types of patient response to calcitonin therapy[160]: (1) complete biochemical and clinical remissions; (2) a larger group shows an early decrease in bone turnover but does not normalize as therapy continues; (3) an initial response but as therapy proceeds a return to pretreatment biochemical and clinical features.

The clinical effects of calcitonin therapy in Paget's disease include relief of bone pain, decrease of elevated skin temperature over affected sites, reduction of the elevated cardiac output, reversal of neurologic problems, stabilization of hearing loss, and improved mobility.[190] In addition, osteoclast number is reduced. On the average, there is a 50% decrease in serum alkaline phosphatase and urine hydroxyproline compared to pretreatment values. The advantages of calcitonin are that it is rarely toxic, has mild, infrequent side effects (nausea, facial flushing, polyuria, diarrhea, and rarely tetany), and results in radiologically demonstrable improvement. Calcitonin is generally recognized as the only therapy for Paget's disease that achieves the latter. Patients with high titers of antisalmon calcitonin antibodies usually show resistance to long-term therapy. The issue of the development of resistance to calcitonin was previously mentioned in relation to calcitonin's use in the treatment of osteoporosis. The loss of effectiveness of salmon calcitonin has received much recent interest[191] but is still difficult to interpret. Resistance has been seen in some patients who do not show calcitonin antibodies.[190] Patients who have developed resistance to salmon calcitonin have been reported to be effectively treated with human calcitonin (0.5 mg/d).[191–193]

Disadvantages of calcitonin therapy include the problem of the development of resistance, its subcutaneous route of administration, and its expense.

Etidronate disodium (EHDP) EHDP belongs to the class of compounds called diphosphonates, bone-seeking compounds with P-C-P bonds which have effects resembling pyrophosphate. Diphosphonates act to retard precipitation of calcium phosphate from solution and to slow the growth and dissolution of hydroxyapatite crystals. They also reduce bone resorption. The critical problem in EHDP therapy is to find a dose which will effectively suppress resorption without impairing mineralization and bone formation.[166]

EHDP has been in use for treatment of Paget's disease for a shorter time than has calcitonin. Wallach states that in the average patient with extensive skeletal disease, EHDP in a dose of 5 mg/kg/d produces effects similar to those attained with calcitonin.[194] In responsive patients, the clinical and biochemical response is usually complete within 6 months and some 25% to 50% of the patients may have a prolonged remission lasting months to years. Others will show a return to initial biochemical features within 1 year. Fromm et al report that doses of 10 to 20 mg/kg/d produced osteomalacic changes in bone with some patients experiencing unchanged or worsening bone pain.[195] EHDP can also increase the renal tubular maximum for phosphate and thus lead to hyperphosphatemia.[196]

EHDP has the advantage of oral administration and of being less expensive than calcitonin, but its main value is as a secondary form of therapy, particularly if there are obvious osteolytic lesions. However, in addition to some patients experiencing increased bone pain, high doses can result in fractures due to the induced mineralization defect. Adverse radiologic lesions have also been noted in some EHDP-treated patients. Wallach advises that one avoid EHDP therapy in patients with extensive bone resorption and in patients with few active foci who require treatment because of the location of the lesion.[194] A possibly beneficial therapy combining calcitonin and EHDP is under investigation.[197]

Other diphosphonates Dichloromethane diphosphonic acid (Cl_2MDP, clodronate disodium) has been used in a few recent trials. Two studies report that patients receiving 1600 mg/d for 6 months showed decreased urinary hydroxyproline, serum alkaline phosphatase, urinary calcium, and decreased numbers of osteoclasts.[198,199] Mineralization was not impaired.[199] A lower dose of 400 mg/d may also be useful.[199,200]

A second diphosphonate, APD (AHPDP) (3-amino-1-hydroxypropylidene)-1,1-bisphosphorate), has also been used in a few trials as therapy for Paget's disease. Frijlink et al found that a dose of 30 μmol/kg/d corrected biochemical values.[201] APD therapy has been noted to cause a rise in PTH and $1,25(OH)_2D_3$ coupled with an increase in net calcium absorption.[202] Two side effects of APD therapy are transient fever (noted in 40% of the patients) and transient decrease in peripheral lymphocyte count (50% below base-line values).

Other therapies Fluoride has been used in the past in the treatment of Paget's disease[203] but today is not considered to be a preferred therapeutic modality. Mithramycin has also been used[204] and acts via a toxic action on osteoclasts similar to its toxic action on neoplasms. However, severe GI, hepatic, and renal reactions are associated with this potentially lethal drug (including severe anorexia with or without vomiting, and increased levels of SGOT, BUN, and serum creatinine).[160,194]

SUMMARY AND DIRECTIONS FOR FUTURE RESEARCH

1. Many age-related changes occur in bone and in the endocrine systems interacting with bone to achieve calcium homeostasis.
2. Interpretation of biochemical and hormonal findings in the elderly patient can be difficult due to changes associated with aging and/or complications from coexisting conditions.
3. Interpretation of bone changes apparent on bone biopsy requires that one remember that the alterations seen are the result of processes taking many years, whereas clinical and biochemical findings represent measurements made at a single point in time.
4. Bone histology shows that postmenopausal osteoporosis is a very heterogeneous condition; it is unlikely that one therapeutic modality will effectively treat postmenopausal osteoporotics. The status of osteoblast and osteoclast cell number as well as cell activities should be considered when selecting therapy. It is hoped that future clinical investigations will lead to the development and implementation of reliable biochemical markers to provide information on bone formation and resorption without the need for invasive technics.

REFERENCES

1. Bartuska DG: Physiology of aging: Metabolic changes during the climacteric and menopausal periods. *Clin Obstet Gynecol* 1977;20:105–112.
2. Avioli LV: Aging, bone, and osteoporosis, in Korenman SG (ed): *Endocrine Aspects of Aging.* New York, Elsevier Biomedical, 1982, pp 199–230.
3. Dewey JR, Armelagos GJ, Bartley MH: Femoral cortical evolution in three Nubian archeological populations. *Hum Biol* 1969;41:13–28.
4. Perzigian AJ: The antiquity of age-associated bone demineralization in man. *J Am Geriatr Soc* 1973;21:100–105.
5. VanGerven DP, Armelagos GJ, Bartley HM: Roentgenographic and direct measurement of femoral cortical involution in a prehistoric Mississippian population. *Am J Phys Anthropol* 1969;31:23–38.
6. Posner AS, Thompson DD, Blumenthal NC, et al: Comparison of apatite in osteoporotic and non-osteoporotic human bone, abstracted in *Transactions of the 29th Annual Meeting of the Orthopaedic Research Society,* 1983, Anaheim, Calif, p 144.
7. Nordin BEC: Clinical significance and pathogenesis of osteoporosis. *Br Med J* 1971;1:571–576.
8. Mazess RB: On aging bone loss. *Clin Orthop* 1982;165:239–252.
9. Boyd RM, Cameron EC, McIntosch H, et al: Measurement of bone mineral content *in vivo* using photon absorptiometry. *Can Med Assoc J* 1974;111:1201–1205.
10. Goldsmith NF, Johnston JO, Picetti, et al: Bone mineral in the radius and vertebral osteoporosis in an insured population. *J Bone Joint Surg [Am]* 1973;55A:1276–1293.
11. Mazess RB, Cameron JR: Bone mineral content in normal US whites, in Mazess

RB (ed): *International Conference on Bone Mineral Measurement.* US Dept of Health, Education, and Welfare publication No. (NIH) 75-683, 1974.
12. Meema HE, Meema S: Compact bone mineral density of the normal human radius. *Acta Radiol Oncol Radiat Phys Biol* 1978;17:342–352.
13. Smith DM, Khairi M, Johnston CC Jr: The loss of bone mineral with aging and its relationship to risk of fracture. *J Clin Invest* 1975;56:311–318.
14. Dequeker J: Bone and ageing. *Ann Rheum Dis* 1975;34:100–115.
15. Garn SM, Rohmann GG, Wagner B, et al: Population similarities in the onset and rate of adult endosteal bone loss. *Clin Orthop* 1969;65:51–60.
16. Johnston CC Jr, Norton JA, Khairi RA, et al: Age-related bone loss, in Barzel U (ed): *Osteoporosis II.* New York, Grune & Stratton, 1979, pp 91–100.
17. Smith DM, Nance WE, Kang KW, et al: Genetic factors in determining bone mass. *J Clin Invest* 1973;52:2800–2808.
18. Johnston CC Jr, Hui S, Wiske P, et al: Bone mass at maturity and subsequent rate of loss as determinants of osteoporosis, in DeLuca HF, Frost H, Jee WS, et al (eds): *Osteoporosis: Recent Advances in Pathogenesis and Treatment.* Baltimore, University Park Press, 1981, pp 285–291.
19. Riggs BL, Wahner HW, Seeman E, et al: Changes in bone mineral density of the proximal femur and spine with aging. Differences between postmenopausal and senile osteoporosis syndromes. *J Clin Invest* 1982;70:716–723.
20. Riggs BL, Wahner HW, Dunn WL, et al: Differential changes in bone mineral density of the appendicular and axial skeleton with aging: Relationship to spinal osteoporosis. *J Clin Invest* 1981;67:328–355.
21. Chesnut CH III, Nelp WB, Baylink DJ, et al: Effect of methandrostenolone on postmenopausal bone wasting as assessed by changes in total bone mineral mass. *Metabolism* 1977;26:267–277.
22. Manzke E, Chesnut CH III, Wergedal JE, et al: Relationship between local and total bone mass in osteoporosis. *Metabolism* 1975;24:605–615.
23. Cohn SH, Vasewani A, Zanzi I, et al: Changes in body chemical composition with age measured by total-body nuetron activation. *Metabolism* 1976;25:85–95.
24. Malluche H, Meyer W, Sherman D, et al: Quantitative bone histology in 84 normal American subjects. Micromorphometric analysis and evaluation of variance in iliac bone. *Calcif Tissue Int* 1982;34: 449–455.
25. Meunier P, Courpron P, Edouard C, et al: Physiological senile involution and pathological rarefaction of bone. Quantitative and comparative histological data. *Clin Endocrinol Metab (Oxford)* 1973;2: 239–256.
26. Delling G: Age-related bone changes. *Curr Top Pathol* 1973;58:117–147.
27. Meunier PJ, Courpron P, Edouard C, et al: Bone histomorphometry in osteoporotic states, in Barzel US (ed): *Osteoporosis II.* New York, Grune & Stratton, 1979, pp 27–47.
28. Lips P, Courpron P, Meunier PJ: Mean wall thickness of trabecular bone packets in the human iliac crest: Changes with age. *Calcif Tiss Res* 1978;26:13–17.
29. Boyce BF, Courpron P, Meunier PJ: Amount of bone in osteoporosis and physiological senile osteopenia. Comparison of two histomorphometric parameters. *Metab Bone Dis Relat Res* 1978;1:35–38.
30. Meunier P, Courpron P, Giroux JM, et al: Osteoporosis. Newer methods for quantitation. *Calc Tissue Res* 1976; 21(suppl):254–360.
31. Follis RH: The inorganic composition of the human rib with and without marrow elements. *J Biol Chem* 1952;194: 223–226.
32. Vogt JH, Tonsager A: Investigations on the bone chemistry of man. Phosphatase, calcium, phosphorus and nitrogen in substantia spongiosa crista ilea. *Acta Med Scand* 1949;135:231–244.
33. Strandh J, Norlen H: Distribution per volume bone tissue of calcium, phosphorus and nitrogen from individuals of varying ages as compared with distribution per unit weight. *Acta Orthop Scand* 1965;35:257–263.
34. Casuccio C: An introduction to the study of osteoporosis. Biochemical and biophysical research in bone ageing. *Proc R Soc Med* 1962;55:663–668.

35. Rogers HJ, Weidmann SM, Parkinson A: Studies on the skeletal tissues. 2. The collagen content of bones from rabbits, oxen and humans. *Biochem J* 1952;50: 537–542.
36. Eastoe JE: The organic matrix of bone, in Bourne (ed): *Biochemistry and Physiology of Bone.* New York, Academic Press, 1956, pp 81–105.
37. Dequeker J, Merlevide W: Collagen content and collagen extractability pattern of adult human trabecular bone according to age, sex and amount of bone mass. *Biochim Biophys Acta* 1971;244:410–420.
38. Smith R: Osteomalacia, in Apley AG (ed): *Biochemical Disorders of the Skeleton.* London, Butterworth, Scientific Publishers, 1979, pp 95–132.
39. Gallagher JC, Riggs BL, Jerpbak CM, et al: The effect of age on serum immunoreactive parathyroid hormone in normal and osteoporotic women. *J Lab Clin Med* 1980;95:373–385.
40. Berlyne GM, Ben-Ari J, Kushelevsky A, et al: The aetiology of senile osteoporosis: Secondary hyperparathyroidism due to renal failure. *Q J Med* 1975;44:505–521.
41. Samaan NA, Anderson G, Adam- Mayne M: Immunoreactive calcitonin in the mother, neonate, child and adult. *Am J Obstet Gynecol* 1975;121:622–625.
42. Deftos LJ, Weisman MH, Williams GW, et al: Influence of age and sex on plasma calcitonin in human beings. *N Engl J Med* 1980;302:1351–1353.
43. Heath H, Sizemore GW: Plasma calcitonin in normal man. Differences between men and women. *J Clin Invest* 1970;60: 1135–1140.
44. Gallagher JC, Riggs BL, Eisman J, et al: Intestinal calcium absorption and serum vitamin D metabolites in normal subjects and osteoporotic patients. *J Clin Invest* 1979;64:729–736.
45. Epstein S, Bryce G, Hui S, et al: Age, sex and bone mineral metabolism, abstracted. *American Society for Bone and Mineral Research,* San Antonio, Texas, June 1983.
46. Avioli LV, McDonald JE, Lee SW: Influence of age in the intestinal absorption of ^{47}Ca absorption in women and its relation to ^{47}Ca absorption in postmenopausal osteoporosis. *J Clin Invest* 1965;44:1960–1967.
47. Montgomery RD, Haeney MR, Ross I, et al: The ageing gut: A study of intestinal absorption in relation to nutrition in the elderly. *Q J Med* 1978;47:197–211.
48. Heaney RP, Recker RR, Saville PD: Menopausal changes in bone remodelling. *J Lab Clin Med* 1978;92:964–970.
49. Riggs BL: Postmenopausal and senile osteoporosis: Current concepts of etiology and treatment. *Endocrinol Jpn* 1979;1: 31–41.
50. Gallagher J, Riggs BL, Eisman J, et al: Impaired production of 1,25 dihydroxyvitamin D in postmenopausal osteoporosis. *Clin Res* 1976;24:580A.
51. Judd HL, Korenman SG: Effects of aging on reproductive function in women, in Korenman SG (ed): *Endocrine Aspects of Aging.* New York, Elsevier Biomedical, 1982, pp 163–197.
52. Judd HL: Hormonal dynamics associated with the menopause. *Clin Obstet Gynecol* 1976;19:775–788.
53. Young, M Nordin BEC: Effects of natural and artificial menopause on plasma and urinary calcium and phosphorus. *Lancet* 1967;2:118–120.
54. Heaney RP, Recker RR, Saville PD: Menopausal changes in calcium balance performance. *J Lab Clin Med* 1978;92: 953–963.
55. Heaney RP: Calcium metabolic changes at menopause. Their possible relationship to post-menopausal osteoporosis, in Barzel US (ed): *Osteoporosis II.* New York, Grune & Stratton, 1979, pp 101–109.
56. Catherwood BD, Marcus R, Madvig P, et al: Plasma bone Gla protein in healthy aging subjects: Correlation with renal function, not with age, abstracted. *American Society for Bone and Mineral Research,* San Antonio, Texas, June 1983.
57. Gruber HE, Baylink DJ: The diagnosis of osteoporosis. *J Am Geriatr Soc* 1981; 29:490–497.
58. Turek SL: *Orthopaedics. Principles and Their Application.* Philadelphia, JB Lippincott Co, 1977.
59. Benson DR: The back: thoracic and lumbar spine, in D'Ambrosia R (ed): *Musculoskeletal Disorders–Regional Examination and Differential Diagnosis.* Philadelphia, JB Lippincott Co, 1977, p 245.

60. Siegelman SS: The radiology of osteoporosis, in Barzel U (ed): *Osteoporosis.* New York, Grune & Stratton, 1979, p 68.
61. Albright F, Reifenstein E: *The Parathyroid Glands and Metabolic Bone Disease. Select Studies.* Baltimore, Williams & Wilkins Co, 1948.
62. Avioli LV, Baran DT, Whyte MP, et al: The biochemical and skeletal heterogeneity of "post-menopausal osteoporosis," in Barzel U (ed): *Osteoporosis.* New York, Grune & Stratton, 1979, pp 49–64.
63. Whyte MP, Bergfield MA, Murphy WA, et al: Postmenopausal osteoporosis. A heterogeneous disorder as assessed by histomorphometric analysis of iliac crest bone from untreated patients. *Am J Med* 1982;72:193–202.
64. Gruber HE, Gutteridge D, Baylink D: Osteoporosis associated with pregnancy and lactation: Bone biopsy and skeletal features in three patients. *Metab Bone Dis Relat Res* 1984;5:159–165.
65. Darby AJ, Meunier PJ: Mean wall thickness and formation periods of trabecular bone packets in idiopathic osteoporosis. *Calcif Tissue Int* 1981;33: 199–204.
66. Gruber H, Ivey J, Thompson E, et al: Osteoblast and osteoclast cell number and cell activity in postmenopausal osteoporotics. *Calcif Tissue Int* 1982;34:S31.
67. Johnston CC Jr, Epstein S: The endocrinology of osteoporosis, in Parsons JA (ed): *Endocrinology of Calcium Metabolism.* New York, Raven Press, 1982, pp 467–484.
68. Riggs BL, Arnaud C, Jowsey J, et al: Parathyroid function in primary osteoporosis. *J Clin Invest* 1973;52:181–184.
69. Riggs BL: Hormonal factors in the pathogenesis of postmenopausal osteoporosis, in Barzel US (ed): *Osteoporosis II.* New York, Grune & Stratton, 1979, pp 111–121.
70. Roof BS, Piel CF, Hanson J, et al: Serum parathyroid hormone levels and serum calcium levels from birth to senescence. *Mechanisms of Ageing and Development.* 1976;5:289–304.
71. Bouillon R, Geusens P, Dequeker J, et al: Parathyroid function in primary osteoporosis. *Clin Sci* 1979;57:167–171.
72. Teitelbaum SL, Rosenberg EM, Richardson CA, et al: Histological studies of bone from normocalcemic postmenopausal osteoporotic patients with increased circulating parathyroid hormone. *J Clin Endocrinol Metab* 1976;42:537–543.
73. Taggart H, Chesnut CH III, Ivey JL, et al: Deficient calcitonin response to calcium stimulation in postmenopausal osteoporosis? *Lancet* 1982;1:8270:475–478.
74. Shamonki I, Frumar A, Tataryn I, et al: Age related changes of calcitonin secretion in females. *J Clin Endocrinol Metab* 1980;50:437–439.
75. Lore F, DiCairano G, Signorini A, et al: Serum levels of 25-hydroxyvitamin D in postmenopausal osteoporosis. *Calcif Tissue Internat* 1981;33:467–470.
76. Lund B, Sorenson OH, Lund B: Clinical applications of the 1,25-$(OH)_2D$ assay, in Norman AW, Schaefer K, Herrath D, et al (eds): *Vitamin D. Basic Research and Its Clinical Application.* Berlin, W deGruyter, 1979, pp 991–997.
77. Morita R, Yamamoto I, Fukunaga M, et al: Changes in sex hormones and calcium regulating hormones with reference to bone mass associated with aging. *Endocrinol Jpn* 1979;1:15–22.
78. Haussler M, Drezner MK, Pike W, et al: Assay of 1,25-dihydroxyvitamin D and other active vitamin D metabolites in serum: Application to animals and humans, in Norman AW, Schaefer K, Herrath D, et al (eds): *Vitamin D. Basic Research and Its Clinical Application.* Berlin, W deGruyter, 1979, pp 189–196.
79. Slovik DM, Adams JS, Neer RM, et al: Deficient production of 1,25-dihydroxyvitamin D in elderly osteoporotic patients. *N Engl J Med* 1981;305:372–374.
80. Price PA, Parthemore JG, Deftos LJ, et al: New biochemical marker for bone resorption. Measurement by radioimmunoassay of bone gla protein in the plasma of normal subjects and patients with bone disease. *J Clin Invest* 1980;66:878–883.
81. Gundberg C, Lian J, Steinberg J, et al: Carboxyglutamic acid excretion as a marker for metabolic bone disease, in DeLuca HF, Frost HM, Jee WS, et al (ed): *Osteoporosis: Recent Advances in Pathogenesis and Treatment.* Baltimore, University Park Press, 1981, p 473.

82. Ivey JL, Baylink DJ: Postmenopausal osteoporosis: proposed roles of defective coupling and estrogen deficiency. *Metab Bone Dis Relat Res* 1981;3:3–7.
83. Baylink DJ, Liu C-C: The regulation of endosteal bone volume. *J Peridontol* (special issue) 1979;50:43–49.
84. Harris WH, Heaney RP: Skeletal renewal and metabolic bone disease. *N Engl J Med* (special issue)1969;281:253–259.
85. Birkenhager-Frenkel DH: Onderzoek van biopsien uit de crista iliaca bij patienten mit osteoporosis senilis, in Orloff S (ed): *L'ostéoporose, journée de travail sur l'ostéoporose.* Brussels, Sandoz, 1966, p 16.
86. Birkenhager-Fernkel DH: Assessment of porosity in bone specimens; differences in chemical composition between normal bone and bone from patients with senile osteoporosis, in Gaillard PJ (ed): *Fourth European Symposium on Calcified Tissues.* Amsterdam, Excerpta Medica, 1966, pp 8–9.
87. Birkenhager-Frenkel DH, Birkenhager JC: Chemical analysis of bone-degree of mineralization and mineral composition, in Courvoisier B, Donath A (eds): *Symposium CEMO.* Geneva, Editions Medicine et Hygiene, Geneva, pp 165–172.
88. Manicourt DH, Orloff S, Brauman J, et al: Bone mineral content of the radius. Good correlations with physio-chemical determinations in iliac crest trabecular bone of normal and osteoporotic subjects. *Metabolism* 1981;30:57–61.
89. Henneman DH, Pak CY, Bartter FC: The solubility and synthetic rate of bone collagen in idiopathic osteoporosis. *Clin Orthop* 1982;88:275–282.
90. Burnell JM, Baylink DJ, Chesnut CH III, et al: Bone matrix and mineral abnormalities in postmenopausal osteoporosis. *Metabolism* 1982;31:1113–1120.
91. Baylink DJ, Smith L, Howard G: Osteoporosis, in Conn HF (ed): *Current Therapy 1980.* Philadelphia, WB Saunders Co, 1980, pp 455–458.
92. Manzke E, Rawley R, Vose G, et al: Effect of fluoride therapy on nondialyzable urinary hydroxyproline, serum alkaline phosphatase, parathyroid hormone, and 25-hydroxyvitamin D. *Metabolism* 1977;26:1005–1010.
93. Seeman E, Riggs BL: The treatment of postmenopausal and senile osteoporosis, in Heath D (ed): *Calcium Disorders. Clinical Endocrinology.* Cornwall, Butterworth Scientific Publications, 1982, Vol 2, pp 69–91.
94. Gordon GS: Disputanda. Dead wrong: Estrogens, osteoporosis, cancer and public policy. *J Med* 1980;11:203–222.
95. Heaney RP: Estrogens and postmenopausal osteoporosis. *Clin Obstet Gynecol* 1976;19:791–803.
96. Chesnut CH III, Gruber HE: Osteoporosis, in Conn HR (ed): *Current Therapy 1981.* Philadelphia, WB Saunders Co, 1981, pp 485–488.
97. Lindsay R, Aitken JM, Anderson JB, et al: Long-term prevention of postmenopausal osteoporosis by estrogen. *Lancet* 1976;1:1038–1041.
98. Gallagher JC, Nordin BEC: Effects of oestrogen and progestogen therapy on calcium metabolism in postmenopausal women. *Front Hormone Res* 1975;3: 150–176.
99. Recker RR, Saville PD, Heaney RP: Effect of estrogens and calcium carbonate on bone loss in postmenopausal women. *Ann Intern Med* 1977;87:649–655.
100. Horsman A, Gallagher JC, Simpson M, et al: Prospective trial of oestrogen and calcium in postmenopausal women. *Br Med J* 1977;2:789–792.
101. Gallagher JC, Riggs BL, Hamstra A, et al: Effect of estrogen therapy on calcium absorption and vitamin D metabolism in postmenopausal osteoporosis. *Clin Res* 1978;26:415A.
102. Lindsay R, McK Hart D, Kraszewski A: Prospective double-blind trial of synthetic steroid (Org OD 14) for preventing postmenopausal osteoporosis. *Br Med J* 1980;280:1207–1209.
103. Thalassinos NC, Gutteridge DH, Joplin GF, et al: Calcium balance in osteoporotic patients on long-term oral calcium therapy with and without sex hormones. *Clin Sci* 1982;62:221–226.
104. Dalen N, Furuhjilm M, Jacobson B, et al: Changes in bone mineral content in women with natural menopause during treatment with female sex hormones. *Acta Obstet Gynecol Scand* 1978;57:435–437.
105. Lindsay R, Fogelman I, Hart D: Prevention of postmenopausal bone loss using sex

steroids, in DeLuca HF, Frost H, Jee WS, Johnston CC Jr, Parfitt AM, (ed): *Osteoporosis. Recent Advances in Pathogenesis and Treatment.* Baltimore, University Park Press, 1981, pp 399–406.

106. Marshall DH, Gallagher JC, Guha P, et al: The effect of 1-alpha-hydroxycholecalciferol and hormone therapy on the calcium balance of postmenopausal osteoporosis. *Calcif Tissue Res* 1977;22 (suppl):78–84.
107. Marshall DH, Nordin BEC: The effect of 1-hydroxyvitamin D with and without oestrogens on calcium balance in postmenopausal women. *Clin Endocrinol* 1977;7(suppl):1595–1695.
108. Nordin BEC: What is the therapeutic role of sex hormones and anabolic hormones? in: *International Symposium on Osteoporosis. Virgin Islands, 1978.* New York, Biomedical Information Corp, 1979, p 50.
109. Milhaud G, Talbon J: Calcitonin treatment of post-menopausal osteoporosis. Evaluation of efficacy by principal components analysis. *Biomedicine* 1975;23: 223–232.
110. Rasmussen H, Bordier P, Marie P, et al: Effect of combined therapy with phosphate and calcitonin on bone volume in osteoporosis. *Metab Bone Dis Relat Res* 1980;2:107–111.
111. Agrawal R, Wallach S, Cohn S, et al: Calcitonin treatment of osteoporosis, in Pecile A (ed): *Calcitonin: Chemistry, Physiology, Pharmacology and Clinical Aspects.* Amsterdam, Excerpta Medica, 1981, pp 237–246.
112. Gruber HE, Ivey JL, Baylink DJ, et al: Long-term calcitonin therapy in postmenopausal osteoporosis. *Metabolism* 1984;33:295–303.
113. Lafferty FW, Spencer GE, Pearson OH: Effects of androgens, estrogens, and high calcium intakes on bone formation and resorption in osteoporosis. *Am J Med* 1964;36:514–528.
114. Riggs BL, Jowsey J, Goldsmith RS, et al: Short and long-term effects of estrogen and synthetic anabolic hormone in postmenopausal osteoporosis. *J Clin Invest* 1972;51:2659–2663.
115. Harrison JE, Hitchman AJW, Finley JM, et al: Effect of treatment on calcium kinetics in metabolic bone disease. *Metabolism* 1971;20:1107–1118.
116. Chesnut CH III, Nelp WB Baylink DJ, et al: Effect of methandrostenolone on postmenopausal bone wasting as assessed by changes in total bone mineral mass. *Metabolism* 1977;26:267–277.
117. Alioa JF, Kapoor A, Vaswani A, et al: Changes in body composition following treatment of osteoporosis with methandrostenolone. *Metabolism* 1981;30: 1076–1079.
118. Chesnut CH III, Ivey JL, Gruber HE, et al: Stanozolol in postmenopausal osteoporosis. *Metabolism* 1983;32: 571–580.
119. Baylink DJ, Bernstein DS: The effects of fluoride therapy on metabolic bone disease. A histologic study. *Clin Orthop* 1967;55:51–85.
120. Schenk RK, Merz WA, Reutter FW: Fluoride in osteoporosis: Quantitative histological studies on bone structure and bone remodelling in serial biopsies of the iliac crest, in Vischer TL (ed): *Fluoride in Medicine.* Bern, Switzerland, Huber Verlag, 1970, pp 153–167.
121. Jowsey J, Riggs BL, Kelly P, et al: Effect of combined therapy with sodium fluoride, vitamin D and calcium in osteoporosis. *Am J Med* 1972;53:43–49.
122. Reutter FW, Olah AJ: Bone biopsy findings and clinical observations in longterm treatment of osteoporosis with sodium fluoride and vitamin D_3, in Courvoisier B, Donath A (eds): *Fluoride and Bone.* Bern, Switzerland, Huber Verlag, 1978, pp 249–255.
123. Jowsey J: The long-term treatment of osteoporosis with fluoride, calcium and vitamin D, in Barzel US (ed): *Osteoporosis II.* New York, Grune & Stratton, 1979, pp 123–134.
124. Farley SM, Smith L, Baylink DJ: Characterization of the skeletal response to sodium fluoride in osteoporosis. *Clin Res* 1983;31:55A.
125. Meunier PJ, Bressot C, Vignon E, et al: Radiological and histological evolution of post-menopausal osteoporosis treated with sodium fluoride-vitamin D-calcium. Preliminary results, in Courvoisier B, Donath A, Baud C (eds): *Fluoride and Bone.* Geneva, Huber Verlag, 1978, pp 263–276.
126. Whyte MP, Teitelbaum SL Bergfeld M,

et al: Histomorphometric analysis of iliac crest bone from osteoporotic subjects following alternate sodium fluoride and calcium-vitamin D therapy. *Clin Res* 1978;26:776A.

127. Van Kesteren RG, Duursma SA, Visser WJ, et al: Fluoride in serum and bone during treatment of osteoporosis with sodium fluoride, calcium and vitamin D. *Metab Bone Dis Relat Res* 1982;4:31–37.
128. Farley JR, Wergedal JE, Baylink DJ: Fluoride acts directly on bone cells *in vitro* and interacts with a putative human skeletal coupling factor, abstracted in *Transactions of 29th Annual Meeting Orthopaedic Research Society* 1983, vol 8, p 48.
129. Riggs BL: What is the therapeutic role of sodium fluoride and should it be used routinely?, in: *International Symposium on Osteoporosis. Virgin Islands.* New York, Biomedical Information Corp, 1978, pp 52–54.
130. Christiansen C, Christensen M, Transbol I: Prophylaxis of early postmenopausal bone loss. A controlled study with oestrogen/gestagen and $1{,}25(OH)_2D_3$, in DeLuca HF, Frost HM, Jee WS, et al (eds): *Osteoporosis. Recent Advances in Pathogenesis and Treatment.* Baltimore, University Park Press, 1981, p 489.
131. Gallagher JC, Riggs BL, DeLuca HF: Effects of calcitriol in osteoporosis, in DeLuca HF, Frost HM, Jee WS, et al (eds): *Osteoporosis. Recent Advances in Pathogenesis and Treatment.* Baltimore, University Park Press, 1981, pp 419–423.
132. Gallagher JC, Riggs BL, DeLuca HF: Effect of long-term treatment with synthetic 1,25-dihydroxyvitamin D_3 in postmenopausal osteoporosis. *Clin Res* 1980; 28:777A.
133. Nordin BEC, Horsman A, Crilly RG, et al: Treatment of spinal osteoporosis in postmenopausal women. *Br Med J* 1980; 280:451–455.
134. Riggs BL, Seeman E, Hodgson SF, et al: Effect of the fluoride/calcium regimen on vertebral fracture occurrence in postmenopausal osteoporosis. *N Engl J Med* 1982;306:446–450.
135. Lund B, Jorth H, Kjaer I, et al: Treatment of osteoporosis of ageing with 1α-hydroxycholecalciferol. *Lancet* 1975;2: 1168–1171.
136. Sorenson OH, Anderson RB, Christensen MS, et al: Treatment of senile osteoporosis with 1α-Hydroxyvitamin D_3. *Clin Endocrinol (Oxf)*1977;7(suppl):1695–1755.
137. Christiansen C, Christensen MS, McNair P, et al: Prevention of early postmenopausal bone loss: controlled 2-year study in 315 normal females. *Eur J Clin Invest* 1980;10:273–279.
138. Aloia JF, Zanzi I, Vaswani A, et al: Combination therapy for osteoporosis with estrogen, fluoride, and calcium. *J Am Geriatr Soc* 1982;30:13–17.
139. Harrison JE, McNeill K, Sturtridge W, et al: Three-year changes in bone mineral mass of postmenopausal osteoporotic patients based on neutron activation analysis of the central third of the skeleton. *J Clin Endocrinol Metab* 1981;52:751–758.
140. Fleisch H, Felix R: Diphosphonates. *Calcif Tissue Internat* 1979;27:91–94.
141. Jowsey J, Riggs BL, Kelly P, et al: The treatment of osteoporosis with disodium ethane-1-hydroxy-1,1-diphosphonate. *J Lab Clin Med* 1971;78:574–584.
142. Heaney RP, Saville PD: Etidronate disodium in postmenopausal osteoporosis. *Clin Pharmacol Ther* 1976;20:593–604.
143. Saville PD, Heaney R: Treatment of osteoporosis with diphosphonates. *Semin Drug Treat* 1972;2:47–50.
144. Reeve J, Hesp R, Wooton R, et al: Clinical trial of hPTH(1-34), in "idiopathic" osteoporosis. An interim report, in Copp DH, Talmage RV (eds): *Endocrinology of Calcium Metabolism.* Amsterdam, Excerpta Medica, 1978, pp 71–74.
145. Parsons JA, Meunier PJ, Neer RM, et al: Effects of synthetic human parathyroid hormone fragment (hPTH1-34) on bone mass and bone mineral metabolism, in DeLuca HF, Frost HM, Jee WS, et al (eds): *Osteoporosis. Recent Advances in Pathogenesis and Treatment.* Baltimore, University Park Press, 1981, pp 457–465.
146. Heaney RP: Calcium intake requirement and bone mass in the elderly. *J Lab Clin Med* 1982;100:309–312.
147. Marcus R: The relationship of dietary calcium to the maintenance of skeletal integrity in man – an interface of endocrinology and nutrition. *Metabolism* 1982;31:93–101.

148. Shenk RK, Olah AJ: What is osteomalacia?, in Massry S, Ritz E, Jahn H (eds): *Phosphate and Minerals in Health and Disease.* New York, Plenum Press, 1980, pp 549–562.
149. Frame B: Concepts of osteomalacia in 1979. *Endocrinol Jpn S.R. No.* 1979;1: 101–106.
150. Frame B, Parfitt MB: Osteomalacia: current concepts. *Ann Intern Med* 1978; 89:966–982.
151. Baylink DJ: Disorders of bone and bone mineral metabolism, in Andres R, Bierman E, Hazzard W, (eds): *Principles in Geriatric Medicine.* New York, McGraw Hill, 1982.
152. Corry DB, Lee DBN: Disorders of calcium, magnesium and phosphorus homeostasis, in Gonick HC (ed): *Current Nephrology.* New York, John Wiley & Sons, 1982, vol 6, pp 187–223.
153. Gruber HE, Stauffer ME, Thompson ER, et al: Diagnosis of bone disease by core biopsies. *Semin Hematol* 1981;18: 258–278.
154. Dent CE, Stamp TCB: Vitamin D, rickets and osteomalacia, in Avioli LV, Krane SM (eds): *Metabolic Bone Disease.* New York, Academic Press, vol 1, 1977, pp 237–305.
155. Norman AW: Vitamin D metabolism and calcium absorption. *Am J Med* 1979;67 :989–998.
156. Preece MA, Tomlinson S, Ribot C, et al: Studies of vitamin D deficiency in man. *Q J Med* 1975;44:575–589.
157. Barzel US: Common metabolic disorders of the skeleton in aging, in Reichel W (ed): *Clinical Aspects of Aging.* Baltimore, Williams & Wilkins Co, 1978, pp 277–287.
158. Brautbar N, Lee DBN, Kleeman CR: The divalent ions. Calcium, phosphorus, and magnesium and vitamin D, in Frienker NF (ed): *Contemporary Metabolism*, New York, Plenum Publishing, 1982, vol 2, pp 441–526.
159. Avioli L: Management of osteomalacia. *Hosp Pract* 1979;14:109–114.
160. Singer FR, Schiller AL, Pyle EB, et al: Paget's disease of bone, in Avioli LV, Krane SM (eds): *Metabolic Bone Disease*, New York, Academic Press, 1978, Vol 2, pp 489–575.
161. Krane SM: Paget's disease of bone, in Wintrobe M, Thorn G, Adams R, et al (eds): *Harrison's Principles of Internal Medicine,* ed 7. New York, McGraw Hill Book Co, 1974, pp 1974–1976.
162. Zanzi I: Hereditary Factors, in Wallace S (ed): *Paget's Disease of Bone.* Chicago, Professional Communications Associates, 1979, pp 22–25.
163. Walpin LA, Singer FR: Reversal of severe paraparesis using calcitonin. *Spine* 1979;4:213–219.
164. Krane SM: Paget's disease of bone. *Clin Orthop Relat Res* 1977;127:24–35
165. Singer FR: Diagnosis, in Wallach S (ed): *Paget's Disease of Bone.* Chicago, Professional Communications Associates, 1977, pp 32–36.
166. Smith R: Paget's disease of bone, in Smith R (ed): *Biochemical Disorders of the Skeleton.* London, Butterworth Scientific Publications, 1979, pp 133–159.
167. Woodhouse NJY: Paget's disease of bone. *Clin Endocrinol Metab* 1972;1:125–141.
168. Canfield R, Rosner W, Skinner J, et al: Diphosphonate therapy of Paget's disease of bone. *J Clin Endocrinol Metab* 1977; 44:96–100.
169. Cherny S: Neoplasia masquerading as Paget's Disease, in Wallach S (ed): *Paget's Disease of Bone.* Chicago, Professional Communications Associates, 1977, pp 41–45.
170. Wootton R, Tellez M, Green JR, et al: Skeletal blood flow in Paget's disease of bone. *Metabol Bone Dis Relat Res* 1981; 4–5:263–270.
171. Henley JW, Croxson RS, Ibbertson HK: The cardiovascular system in Paget's disease of bone and the response to therapy with calcitonin and diphosphonate. *Aust NZ J Med* 1979;9:390–397.
172. Russell RGG, Beard DJ, Cameron EC, et al: Biochemical markers of bone turnover in Paget's disease. *Metab Bone Dis Relat Res* 1982;4–5:255–262.
173. Deftos LJ, Parthemore JG, Price PA: Changes in plasma bone Gla protein during treatment of bone disease. *Calcif Tissue Internat* 1982;34:121–124.
174. Chapuy M-C, Zucchelli P, Meunier PJ: Parathyroid function in Paget's disease of bone. *Mineral Electrolyte Metab* 1981;6: 112–118.
175. Krane SM, Kantrowitz FG, Byrne M, et al: Urinary excretion of hydroxylysine and

its glycosides as an index of collagen degradation. *J Clin Invest* 1977;59: 819–827.
176. Misra DP: Crosslink in bone collagen in Paget's disease. *J Clin Pathol* 1975;28: 305–308.
177. Milgram JW: Radiographical and pathological assessment of the activity of Paget's disease of bone. *Clin Orthop* 1977; 127:43–54.
178. Meunier PJ, Coindre JM, Edouard CM, et al: Bone histomorphometry in Paget's disease. Quantitative and dynamic analysis of pagetic and nonpagetic bone tissue. *Arthritis Rheum* 1980;23:1095–1103.
179. Rebel A, Malkani K, Basle M: Anomalies nucléaires des ostéoclastes de la maladie de Paget. *Nouv Presse Med* 1974;18: 1299–1301.
180. Mills B, Singer FR: Nuclear inclusions in Paget's disease of bone. *Science* 1976; 194:201–202.
181. Gheradi G, Cascio V, Bonucci E: Fine structure of nuclei and cytoplasm of osteoclasts in Paget's disease of bone. *Histopathology* 1980;4:63–74.
182. Rebel A, Basle M, Pouplard A, et al: Bone tissue in Paget's disease of the bone. Ultrastructure and immunocytology. *Arthritis Rheum* 1980;23:2204–2214.
183. Rebel A, Basle M, Pouplard A, et al: Towards a viral etiology for Paget's disease of bone. *Metab Bone Dis Relat Res* 1981;4–5:235–238.
184. Mills BG, Singer FR, Weiner LP, et al: Cell cultures from bone affected by Paget's disease. *Arthritis Rheum* 1980;23:1115–1120.
185. Mills BG: Comparison of the ultrastructure of a malignant tumor of the mandible containing giant cells with Paget's disease of bone. *J Oral Pathol* 1981;10:203–215.
186. Chambers TJ: Osteoblasts release osteoclasts from calcitonin-induced quiescence. *J Cell Sci* 1982;57:247–260.
187. Avramides A: Calcitonin in treatment of Paget's disease, in Wallach S (ed): *Paget's Disease of Bone.* Chicago, Professional Communications Associates, 1979, pp 69–74.
188. Doyle FH, Pennock J, Greenberg PB, et al: Radiological evidence of a dose- related response to long-term treatment of Paget's disease with human calcitonin. *Br J Radiol* 1974;47:1–8.
189. Wallach S, Avramides A, Flores A, et al: Skeletal turnover and total body elemental composition during extended calcitonin therapy of Paget's disease. *Metabolism* 1975;24:745–753.
190. Singer FR: Recent developments in the therapeutics of disorders of bone metabolism. *Ann Rep Med Chem* 1982;17: 261–269.
191. Singer FR, Fredericks RS, Minkin C: Salmon calcitonin therapy for Paget's disease of the bone. The problem of acquired resistance. *Arthritis Rheum* 1980; 23:1148–1154.
192. Hosking DJ, Huddlestone LB, Clark AJ, et al: Resistance to calcitonin during treatment of Paget's disease. *Metab Bone Dis Relat Res* 1981;2:315–320.
193. Rojanasathit S, Rosenberg E, Haddad JG Jr: Paget's bone disease: Response to human calcitonin in patients resistant to salmon calcitonin. *Lancet* 1974;2:1412–1415.
194. Wallach S: Treatment of Paget's disease. *Adv Intern Med* 1982;27:1–43.
195. Fromm GA, Schajowicz F, Casco C, et al: The treatment of Paget's bone disease with sodium etidronate. *Am J Med Sci* 1979;277:29–37.
196. Walton RJ, Russel RGG, Smith R: Changes in the renal and extrarenal handling of phosphate induced by disodium etidronate (EHDP) in man. *Clin Sci Molec Med* 1975;49:45–56.
197. Hosking DJ: Calcitonin and diphosphonate in the treatment of Paget's disease of bone. *Metab Bone Dis Relat Res* 1981;4–5:317–326.
198. Douglas DL, Russell RG, Preston CJ, et al: Effect of dichloromethylene diphosphonate in Paget's disease of bone and in hypercalcemia due to primary hyperparathyroidism or malignant disease. *Lancet* 1980;1:1043–1047.
199. Meunier PJ, Alexandre C, Edouard C: Effects of disodium dichloromethylene diphosphonate on Paget's disease of bone. *Lancet* 1979;2:489–492.
200. Arlot ME, Meunier PJ: Effects of two diphosphonates (EHDP and Cl_2MDP) on serum uric acid on pagetic patients. *Calcif Tissue Internat* 1981;33:195–198.

201. Frijlink WB, Bijvoet OL, te Velde J, et al: Treatment of Paget's disease with (3-amino-1-hydroxypropylidene)-1,1-bisphosphonate (A.P.D.) *Lancet* 1979;1: 799–803.
202. Adami S, Frijlink WB, Bijvoet O, et al: Regulation of calcium absorption by 1,25,dihydroxy-vitamin D -studies of the effects of a biphosphonate treatment. *Calcif Tissue Internat* 1982;34:317–320.
203. Riggs BL, Jowsey J: Treatment of Paget's disease with fluoride. *Semin Drug Treat* 1972;2:65–68.
204. Russell AS, Chalmer IM, Percy JS, et al: Long term effectiveness of low dose mithramycin for Paget's disease of bone. *Arthritis Rheum* 1979;22:215–218.

CHAPTER 12 Pharmacodynamics and Pharmacokinetics of Drugs in the Elderly

Kenneth L. Duchin

As we age, physiologic changes occur that may influence the pharmacokinetics of a drug and ultimately lead to alterations in the pharmacology and/or toxicity of a given agent. This review will focus on the mechanisms responsible for altered pharmacokinetics in the elderly and the changes in the pharmacodynamics of drugs in this patient population. These are important issues that physicians, pharmacists, and nurses, should be aware of since the use of drugs in the elderly will continue to expand, primarily because the proportion of the population in the Western world over 65 years old will grow from 11% to 15% by the year 2040.[1] In addition, it is well known that older individuals have more illnesses and hospitalizations than do younger people, and their periods of acute care are longer.

Several studies have established that the frequency of adverse reactions to drugs in the elderly is higher than in younger patients. In a study of over 700 patients at the Johns Hopkins Hospital, it was found that 24% of patients over the age of 80 years had adverse drug reactions, compared to 11.8% of patients 41 to 50 years old.[2] In a series of 1160 consecutive patients, the incidence of adverse reactions was 15.4% in patients over 60 years old and rose to 20.3% in those over 70.[3] In another study, 177 out of 6063 consecutive admissions to the University of Florida Hospital were a consequence of drug-induced illnesses.[4] Seventy-three or 41% of these patients were over the age of 60.

Normally, the intensity and duration of drug action is determined mainly by the concentration of free drug at the site of action. In old age, two mechanisms are responsible for altered drug effects. One is a change in the pharmacodynamics of the drug in the patient, secondary to changes in receptor sensitivity, impaired homeostasis, and disease. The second and the one that has been most widely studied is the age-related change in drug pharmacokinetics, which includes drug absorption, distribution, and disposition.

PHARMACODYNAMICS

Changes in pharmacodynamics with age are difficult to study in vivo, but there is some evidence suggesting that tissue or receptor sensitivity is altered in the elderly. Several examples of age-related changes in pharmacodynamics are presented.

β-Adrenoceptor Blockers

Evidence exists that there may be fundamental age differences in the physiology of the autonomic nervous system. Some,[5,6] but not all studies,[7] indicate that there is a positive correlation between plasma norepinephrine levels and age. As suggested by Rowe and Troen,[8] this may be related to the selection of subjects and various definitions of the basal state. The number of β-adrenoceptors in the membrane fractions of lymphocytes have been found to correlate negatively with age, without any changes in the affinity for the receptor.[9] This is consistent with the lower products of AMP in membrane preparations of lymphocytes from elderly subjects compared to young subjects after β-adrenergic stimulation.[10] This may explain the reduced chronotropic response to isoproterenol as age increases.[11] Furthermore, Feely and Stevenson[12] have reported a reduced effect of propranolol in the elderly.

Antihypertensives

An impaired baroreceptor response[13] and a reduction in peripheral venous tone[14] contribute to the postural hypotension in the elderly. Older patients have also been reported to be very sensitive to the antihypertensive and CNS effects of methyldopa and other centrally acting antihypertensives.[15] These factors, therefore, must be considered in the selection of the proper dose of antihypertensive medications in this patient population.

Anticoagulants

Studies have shown that older patients are more sensitive to the effects of both heparin[16] and warfarin.[17] The increased risk of hemorrhagic complications may, in part, be due to a diminished mechanical hemostatic response in the presence of degenerative vascular disease.[18] Elevated sensitivity to warfarin in the elderly was not found by all investigators.[19,20] One group reported inhibition of the synthesis of vitamin K-dependent clotting factors in the elderly without any changes in the rate of clotting factor degradation.[20] This may be related to a deficiency of vitamin K, secondary to reduced dietary intake, decreased absorption, or altered pharmacokinetics of the vitamin itself.[20]

Sedative and Anxiolytic Agents

Castleden et al[21] have reported a greater impairment of psychomotor performance in the elderly than in young subjects following a 10-mg oral dose of nitrazepam. However, there were no significant pharmacokinetic differences between the two groups. Others have also found that there is greater depression of the CNS with diazepam at any given plasma drug concentration in the elderly than in the young.[22,23] The elderly are also more susceptible to the toxic effects of flurazepam and therefore a lower initial dose is used compared to younger patients.[24] At equivalent blood concentrations of ethanol, older subjects have been reported to have greater impairment of reaction time, memory, and hearing than their younger counterparts.[25] Elderly patients are very sensitive to barbiturates as the reaction to this class of drugs ranges from mild restlessness to frank psychosis.[26] For this reason, barbiturates are rarely used in geriatric medicine.

PHARMACOKINETICS

The principal factors that govern the amount of free drug at its site of action are represented schematically in Figure 12-1 and the probable changes in these interrelated pharmacokinetic processes that occur with aging are indicated.

Absorption

Normally, drug absorption is usually a passive, saturable diffusion process that does not require energy expenditure. It proceeds proportionally to the concentration gradient and to the lipid-water partition coefficient of the drug. Several changes may occur in the gastrointestinal (GI) tract of elderly people that could, at least in part, contribute to altered drug absorption. First, there may be reduced gastric-parietal cell function, leading to impaired acid secretion and an elevation in gastric pH.[27] This will lead to a slower rate, but not extent, of absorption in the elderly for drugs whose absorption is pH-dependent (eg, digoxin, phenobarbital).[28] Increases in stomach pH are also accompanied by delayed gastric emptying and movement of the drug from the stomach to the small intestine, where most of the absorption occurs. Mesenteric blood flow has been reported to be 40% to 50% lower in the elderly compared to younger patients.[28] Other possible reasons for reduced absorption of drugs in the elderly include decreased GI motility, atrophy of macro- and microvilli, and increased connective tissue.[29] Furthermore, dietary patterns shift as we age and, in general, geriatric patients consume less food than younger patients, leading to decreases in gastric emptying. Decreased mastication, secondary to the loss of teeth, may also affect absorption of a drug when taken with food. Because polypharmacy is widespread in

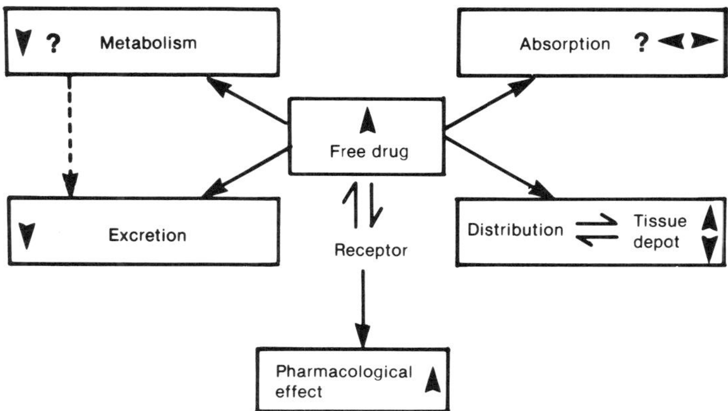

Figure 12-1 A schematic representation of pharmacokinetic changes (heavy arrows) in the elderly which may influence pharmacological activity. (Reproduced with permission from O'Malley K, Judge TG, Crooks J: Geriatric clinical pharmacology and therapeutics, in Avery G (ed): *Drug Treatment.* Newtown, Pa, ADIS Press, 1980, p 160.)

this patient population, there may be specific drug interactions within the GI tract that may alter drug absorption. Although the aforementioned factors may indirectly influence drug absorption, there is little evidence to suggest that oral absorption of a drug is markedly impaired in old age, although not every drug has been studied. Presumably, surface area and blood flow are sufficient to allow adequate absorption. Well-controlled studies suggest that the rate and extent of absorption of acetaminophen and lorazepam are not impaired in elderly subjects.[10]

Turning to drugs that are administered intramuscularly or topically, absorption may be reduced since tissue perfusion may be impaired, and skin hydration may be lower and keratinization increased in the elderly compared to their younger counterparts. These physiologic changes could conceivably reduce permeability to the drug and the concentration gradient.

Distribution

The movement of a drug from the central (blood) compartment into the tissues is dependent upon the mass of the tissue, its degree of perfusion, and the partition characteristics of the drug between blood and tissue, which is dependent on membrane permeability, intra- and extracellular pH, tissue, and plasma protein binding. The term describing drug distribution is known as the volume of distribution (V_d) which is estimated from the ratio of the amount of drug in the body to the blood or plasma concentration of unbound or total drug factored for body weight. This value, however, can only be determined with accuracy when the drug is administered intravenously. The use of V_d may represent the initial space into which the drug immediately distributes following rapid intravenous (IV) administration (V_c), the volume that is found when the drug reaches steady state (V_{dss}), and during distribution equilibrium ($V_{d\beta}$). In general, V_{dss} and $V_{d\beta}$ are nearly equivalent. However, when larger differences are present, V_{dss} is a better indicator of the factors determining distribution and $V_{d\beta}$ is useful in calculating dosage regimens.[30]

It is well known that body composition changes with age, and there are important differences between young and old adults. Total body water, both in absolute terms and as a percentage of body weight, decreases by 10% to 15% between the ages of 20 and 90 years.[31] By definition, this leads to a smaller V_d for water-soluble drugs, and a higher concentration of drug per unit volume, if the dosage is not adjusted. For instance, ethanol and antipyrine, which are both confined to total body water, have a smaller V_{dss} in elderly than in younger subjects. Furthermore, the ratio of lean body weight to fatty tissue changes, even without any changes in overall body weight. Generally, between the second and ninth decades of life, body fat increases from about 18% to 36% in men and in women from 33% to 45% of body weight.[32] Lean body mass, which is composed primarily of muscles, liver, brain, and kidney decrease by 20% to 30% with the decline starting in the fifth decade.[32] Thus, V_d for lipid-soluble drugs will increase and blood levels will decrease as one ages. The most classical example of a change in V_d with respect to age is that of diazepam. Both V_c and V_{dss} have been shown to increase linearly over a fourfold range from 20 to 80 years of age.[33,34] Similar findings have been reported for chlordiazepoxide.[35,36] In contrast, other benzodiazepines, oxazepam[36] and lorazepam[37] do not appear to exhibit any age-related changes in V_d. The weaker lipophilicity of the latter two benzodiazepines probably contribute to the failure of these drugs to increase their distribution in the elderly.

The V_d for a given drug may change in the elderly secondary to other physiological mechanisms. Bender[38] found that there is a 1% per year decline in cardiac output from the second to the eighth decade of life, although brain, liver, and kidney have smaller reductions in blood flow. This may lead to alterations in V_c and $V_{d\beta}$ since both are dependent on delivery of drug to the tissues.[39] For instance, following IV administration of lidocaine, 20 to 40 minutes may be required to reach $V_{d\beta}$ in the young, whereas 90 to 200 minutes may be required to reach this state in the elderly.[40]

An important factor governing the distribution of a drug is the degree of binding to biological macromolecules. Tissue binding and its possible age-related alterations have received little attention, even though it may be extremely important in drug distribution and pharmacokinetics. Many drugs circulate in the blood as reversible complexes with albumin and other macromolecules such as α_1-acid glycoprotein (AAG), and lipoproteins. This binding restricts the distribution of drug out of the vasculature and the V_d is related to the proportion of unbound drug.[31] Plasma albumin concentration decreases with age,[40] thus more free drug would be expected to be available for distribution. The decrease in albumin is probably secondary to reduced albumin synthesis, increased albumin catabolism, and undernutrition. The extent of a change in the proportion of a drug that is bound to plasma protein depends on the extent to which the drug is normally bound. If only a small proportion of the drug is bound, a significant alteration in percent binding (eg, 20% to 50%) will not markedly affect the disposition of the drug. On the other hand, if a drug is highly protein bound (eg, 98%), a 10% reduction in the proportion bound will result in more drug available for redistribution into tissues and perhaps the clearance of the agent might increase, depending on how it is eliminated.

Protein binding of phenytoin has been shown to be decreased in the elderly as there is an age-related increase in the proportion of drug unbound in plasma from 9.9% at 17 years to 12.7% at 53 years.[41] The increase in free drug was clearly related to the decline in albumin levels. Hayes et al[42] also showed a similar decline in warfarin binding as age increased that was correlated to the concentrations of plasma albumin. Protein binding of diazepam has also been reported to decline in the elderly.[35] However, not all studies have clearly demonstrated that there are age-related changes in plasma protein binding of phenytoin,[43] warfarin,[42] and diazepam.[34] The differences in protein binding could be due to varying technics for determining protein binding and with the variety of study populations, each composed of a small number of subjects.

Basic drugs may also bind to membrane phospholipids and AAG. The latter has been shown to be elevated in the elderly and in many unrelated inflammatory diseases such as arthritis, cancer, and myocardial infarction.[44] A variety of drugs such as lidocaine, chlorpromazine, the tricyclic antidepressants, and propranolol hydrochloride have been shown to bind to AAG.[45]

Medication given concomitantly may also result in competitive displacement of drugs from their binding sites in plasma. This may be exaggerated in the older population. For instance, significantly higher free fractions of both salicylates and sulfadiazine in plasma were found in older subjects compared to younger ones even though they both received the same doses.[46]

Changes in drug distribution in the elderly, secondary to alterations in protein binding, body composition, and tissue perfusion, may lead to alterations in drug concentration at the receptors, and also in drug elimination. The former has not been well studied, whereas the latter has been, especially regarding elimination half-life (t½) of the drug, as shown in the following equation:

$$t\tfrac{1}{2} = \frac{\ln 2\ (V_d)}{Cl_B} \quad (1)$$

where Cl_B = body clearance, defined as the overall efficiency of drug removed from the body and includes hepatic and extrahepatic metabolism plus renal and biliary excretion. Because V_d can change in older patients, using half-life as an index of drug elimination can be misleading when considering disappearance of a drug. The higher half-life values in the elderly for diazepam, chloradizepoxide, and lidocaine are due primarily to the age-related increase in V_d. Body clearance is considered to be the most appropriate parameter for elimination of drug from the body. The one situation where half-life alone is helpful is in predicting the time it takes to achieve maximum steady-state levels. Multiplying the half-life by five will give a reasonable estimate of the time required to achieve maximum therapeutic effect or the end of the acute drug toxicity risk period.

Although the distribution of drugs in the elderly can be different compared to younger subjects, there is no consistent pattern that might aid in the prediction of either the mechanisms or the magnitude of the alterations. This type of information must be developed on an individual drug basis and the clinical significance of any differences between drug distribution in young and old patients must be evaluated.

Drug Metabolism

The biotransformation of a drug into another compound with or without pharmacologic activity occurs primarily in the liver. Two types of biotransformation reactions occur. Phase I reactions include the oxidations (hydroxylation, N-dealkylation, sulfoxidation), the reductions, and the hydrolyses. These reactions yield a more polar (water-soluble) product that may retain a portion of the pharmacologic activity of the parent drug. The second major type of reaction is the phase II reaction and involves conjugation or attachment of the drug to a larger substituent, usually glucuronic acid, sulphate, glycine, or another group. The resulting conjugates, with little or no pharmacologic activity are more polar than the parent drug and are excreted in the urine. Some drugs may pass through both phase I and II reactions before being eliminated, whereas others only pass through either phase I or phase II. Although liver function tests in healthy elderly adults may be within normal limits, these tests do not estimate the capacity of the drug-metabolizing enzymes, the ones responsible for the phase I and II reactions. Undernutrition, a decline in liver mass, and the number of hepatocytes may contribute to a decrease in drug-metabolizing enzymes in the elderly. Pirttiaho et al[47] found a correlation between cytochrome P-450, an enzyme involved in phase I reactions, and liver weight in a population ranging from 20 to 60 years of age. In another study, though, there was no correlation between cytochrome P-450 activity and age.[48] Nevertheless, based on indirect methods, (ie, clearance of drugs extensively metabolized in the liver and total amounts of metabolites eliminated in the urine), there is evidence to suggest the elderly may have a reduced ability to metabolize a number of drugs. This would lead to reduced total drug clearance and higher steady-state levels during chronic dosing. On the other hand, optimal liver function is required for the conversion of an inactive drug to one or more metabolites (eg, tricyclic antidepressants) than for maintenance of effective drug levels of the parent drug.

Table 12-1 summarizes metabolized drugs whose clearance may be altered with respect to age. In the absence of clearance data, one cannot simply rely on plasma half-life, since there may have been age-related changes in V_d. Most of the drugs with a reduced plasma clearance in the elderly are oxidized (primarily hydroxylation or demethylation). Reductions in drug oxidation are not universal in the elderly, since clearances comparable to those in young subjects have been found for warfarin, lidocaine, and nitrazepam. Clearance of phenytoin increases with age. Hayes et al[43] found that the kinetics of this drug

Table 12-1
Studies of the Relation of Age to the Clearance of Drugs Cleared by Hepatic Biotransformation

Drug or Metabolite	Initial Pathway of Biotransformation
Evidence suggesting age-related reduction in clearance	
Antipyrine	Oxidation(OH,DA)
Diazepam	Oxidation(DA)
Chlordiazepoxide	Oxidation(DA)
Desmethyldiazepam	Oxidation(OH)
Desalkylflurazepam	Oxidation(OH)
Clobazam	Oxidation(DA)
Alprazolam	Oxidation(OH)
Quinidine	Oxidation(OH)
Theophylline	Oxidation
Propranolol	Oxidation(OH)
Nortriptyline hydrochloride	Oxidation(OH)
Small or negligible age-related change in clearance	
Oxazepam	Glucuronidation
Lorazepam	Glucuronidation
Temazepam	Glucuronidation
Warfarin	Oxidation(OH)
Lidocaine	Oxidation(DA)
Nitrazepam	Nitroreduction
Flunitrazepam	Oxidation(DA),nitroreduction
Isoniazid	Acetylation
Ethanol	Oxidation(alcoholol dehydrogenase)
Metoprolol	Oxidation
Digitoxin	Oxidation
Prazosin hydrochloride	Oxidation
Data conflicting or not definitive	
Meperidine hydrochloride	Oxidation(DA)
Phenylbutazone	Oxidation(OH)
Phenytoin	Oxidation(OH)
Imipramine hydrochloride	Oxidation(OH,DA)
Amitriptyline hydrochloride	Oxidation(OH,DA)
Acetaminophen	Glucuronidation,sulfation
Amobarbital	Oxidation(OH)

*OH denotes hydroxylation and DA dealkylation. (Reprinted with permission from Greenblatt et al.[1])

are complex, being dose-dependent and influenced by plasma albumin concentration and affinity for the drug. To date, there is no evidence that the biotransformation of drugs that undergo reduction or hydroxylation are affected by the aging process.

There have not been any age-related differences in metabolism of drugs undergoing phase II reactions such as isoniazid (acetylation), indomethacin (glucuronide and sulfate conjugation), and oxazepam and lorazepam (glucuronidation).

Hepatic blood flow, rather than the drug-metabolizing enzymes, is the major determinant of plasma clearance for a number of drugs.[49] A 40% to 45% reduction in total liver blood flow, secondary to the decline in cardiac output, may be observed in the elderly.[27] Drugs that are highly extracted by the liver have reduced clearances in older patients after oral and IV administration compared with young adults. The systemic clearance of propranolol and indocyanine green correlated with each other and are depressed in the elderly.[50] For reasons that are unclear, the clearance of lidocaine, another drug that is rapidly extracted by the liver, did not correlate with age.[40]

In evaluating the changes with age in the drug-metabolizing enzymes, one must also consider the environmental stimulants, such as smoking, atmospheric pollutants, and the presence of other drugs that may inhibit or stimulate the activity of these enzymes.[51] Smoking, for instance, has clearly been shown to induce the activity of the drug-metabolizing enzymes and increases total metabolic clearance for a number of drugs including theophylline, phenacetin, propoxyphene, and propranolol. Using the clearance of antipyrine, the activities of these enzymes increased to a greater extent in the young than in the elderly.[50] In addition, early mortality tends to select against heavy smokers in the geriatric population.[1] Furthermore, marijuana smoking appears to have greater inducing effect than cigarette smoking.[52] Further studies are needed to determine why the inducibility of the drug-metabolizing enzymes decreases with age.

Based on the comprehensive studies of Vestal and Wood,[50] old age is associated with two distinct processes that may effect drug elimination: decreases in liver blood flow, secondary to the reduction in cardiac output; and an age-related reduction in the effect of cigarette smoking on intrinsic clearance, which reflects hepatic drug metabolism. The effects of age on drug elimination will therefore depend on whether the drug has a high or low extraction, and on the route of drug administration (oral or IV). For example, when a poorly extracted drug is administered orally or IV, any age-related decrease would be expected to occur mainly in the smokers, because the oral (intrinsic) and IV (systemic) clearances are almost equivalent and are not importantly affected by liver blood flow. On the other hand, a highly extracted drug when given orally has a decreased clearance secondary to the age-related decline in liver blood flow whereas clearance need not necessarily decline following IV administration of the same drug.

The ingestion of large amounts of ethanol, in the absence of severe liver disease, increases the clearance of many drugs, probably by induction of the drug-metabolizing enzymes.[1] On the other hand, acute alcohol ingestion inhibits the oxidative, but not the phase II type of reactions. However, there are no studies of the effects of alcohol ingestion on metabolism of drugs in the elderly. It is presumed though that the use of alcohol is lower in the elderly than in the young, and like smoking, the inducibility of these enzymes is greater in the younger adult.[1]

Salem et al[53] have demonstrated that chronic (2 weeks) administration of the hypnotic drug dichloralphenazone to young and old subjects was associated with an increase in the elimination of quinidine and antipyrine. However, the pharmacokinetic alterations of these drugs was much greater in the younger subjects.

Cimetidine is widely used as an antiulcer agent. It has been shown to bind to cytochrome P-450,[54] and, in addition, to reduce hepatic blood flow.[55] Several studies[56,57] have shown higher propranolol blood levels during chronic cimetidine therapy.

Since aging is a dynamic and individual process, it is difficult, if not impossible, to obtain a representative population to study the biotransformation of drugs with respect to age. One must consider many factors when selecting a population to study such as smoking habits, genetics, life style, and concomitant disease. Because polypharmacy is so common in the elderly, any one of the drugs may interact with the agent that is being evaluated. Furthermore, the clinical investigator should have sensitive analytical methods for the assay of the metabolities in both blood and urine, particularly for the major ones in quantity and the pharmacologically active ones. In the future, it might be possible to relate the metabolism of the given agent to the metabolism of a model compound that has been well studied, such as antipyrine.

The data available to date suggests, often by indirect means, that there is a decrease in the metabolic activity and of the adaptive capacity of the biotransformation enzymes with age in man. For some drugs, the decreased elimination rates of a series of oxidized drugs support diminished biotransformation in the elderly. For other oxidized drugs, there is no decrease in metabolism with age. Hydrolysis, reductions, and phase II reactions do not appear to have any age-related differences with respect to rate and biotransformation of drugs. While pharmacokinetic comparisons following single doses of drug given to elderly and young subjects are interesting, the steady-state concentrations of drug following the same dose to the same two groups are of much greater clinical relevance. In a limited number of studies, the increases in steady-state levels secondary to reduced biotransformation, of some drugs, but not all, correlated with advancing age.[58] Obviously, further work is needed to determine to what extent age alters drug metabolism for the major drugs used in geriatric medicine.

Drug Elimination

The total body clearance of a drug represents a hypothetical volume of blood from which the drug is completely cleared per unit of time. Total clearance is the best indicator for quantitating the removal or elimination of a drug. Most drugs are cleared by one or more organs, usually the kidneys or liver, and total clearance cannot exceed blood flow to the organ or organs responsible for clearance.

The following equation summarizes the relationship between the steady-state blood level (C_{ss}), dose, and clearance (Cl_B):

$$C_{ss} = \frac{\text{dose per unit time}}{Cl_B} \qquad (2)$$

Clearance is a major factor in the extent of drug accumulation during multiple dosing. Thus, for any given dose, as Cl_B declines, C_{ss} will increase. Assuming clinical efficacy and toxicity are related to C_{ss}, then effects are readily diminished or enhanced when Cl_B rises or falls, respectively. If Cl_B is known to be lower in one setting than another, it would be appropriate to modify the dosage schedule to compensate for the reduction in Cl_B. As mentioned earlier, there is a progressive decline in liver blood flow as we age. Similarly, the kidney's ability to remove a drug diminishes with time. Glomerular filtration rate (GFR) decreases by 30% to 45% over the age range of 30 to 90 years, with an acceleration of the decline after the middle of the sixth decade.[59] Renal blood flow also falls by about 10% per decade beginning at about age 40.[39]

The decline in renal function dictates an alteration in the dosage regimen of certain drugs in the elderly, analogous to the situation in chronic renal failure. For drugs that are primarily excreted by the kidneys ($>60\%$ of the dose), the total clearance will predictably decline approximately in proportion to the reduced GFR. Without an alteration in the dose, higher blood levels of the drug and their renally excreted metabolites in the elderly will be observed, and there is an increased risk of enhanced pharmacologic actions and drug toxicity. Leikola and Vartia[60] were the first to demonstrate a correlation between age and excretion of penicillin. Not unexpectedly they found higher serum levels in the elderly compared to younger patients. Similar findings were made for a variety of other drugs, including tetracyclines, procainamide, hypoglycemic agents, and lithium.[61]

The age-dependent kinetics of two aminoglycosides, kanamycin sulfate and gentamicin sulfate, were studied by Lumholtz et al.[62] The half-lives of both drugs were higher in older patients; kanamycin from 107 ± 27 to 330 ± 154 minutes and gentamicin from 93 ± 26 to 216 ± 60 minutes. Serum creatinine in these patients ranged from 0.7 to 1.3 mg/dL. The extreme variability in plasma half-lives, without the clearance data, suggests that dose regimens based solely upon serum creatinine cannot be satisfactorily applied in all age groups.[63] Decreased renal function in the elderly may also result in inadequate concentrations of antibiotics used to treat urinary tract infections (eg, nitrofurantoin, chloramphenicol, and amdinocillin[61]).

For drugs that are extensively excreted unchanged in the urine and have a narrow therapeutic index, a reduction in the dose in the elderly must be considered in any treatment plan. Table 12-2 lists drugs whose dosages are usually reduced in the elderly. In general, changes in GFR, estimated by creatinine clearance, relate well to changes in the renal clearance of drugs. Although many drugs are excreted by tubular secretion, as well as being filtered by the glomerulus, it appears that total renal clearance parallels glomerular filtration even when tubular secretion is the main route of excretion. There is, however, evidence which suggests that the tubular secretion of basic drugs declines more rapidly than glomerular filtration.[64] Therefore, individualization of the dosage regimen based on GFR must be done for each patient. Knowledge of the patient's serum creatinine concentration may not be accurate because of the decline of muscle mass and lean body mass relative to total body weight in old age. Furthermore, since serum creatinine levels depend on creatinine turnover as well as renal creatinine clearance, the true decrease in renal function may not elevate the serum creatinine. Therefore, reliance on this parameter as the sole index of renal function in this patient population may not be accurate. Creatinine clearance, based on a 24-hour urinary excretion of creatinine and a 12-hour serum creatinine concentration, taken in the absence of a protein-rich meal,[65] is a much better indicator of renal function. When a complete urine collection is not possible, creatinine clearance can be estimated from serum creatinine on the basis of an equation[66] or nomograms[67] that utilize age, sex, and body weight as described elsewhere in this volume.

A modified dosage schedule would allow the concentration of drug in the blood in the elderly to be equivalent to that in the young patient with normal renal function. This may be accomplished by (1) decreasing the dose but maintaining the usual dosage interval, (2) administering the usual dose but at less frequent intervals, or (3) a combination of both approaches. In general, loading doses do not have to be modified in the presence of decreased renal function; however, maintenance doses do require adjustment. It should be stressed that no dosage regimen can produce a concentration/time profile in a patient with impaired renal function identical to that in the normal patient. Depending on the drug, its pharmacokinetics, and the indication for which it is intended, one must select a dosage regimen that will provide a similar peak, trough, or average blood level during the dosage interval compared to normal subjects, assuming there are no

Table 12-2
Examples of Drugs Usually Given in Reduced Dosage in the Elderly

Carbamazepine	Metoclopramide hydrochloride
Clomethiazole	Nitrazepam
Chlorpropamide	Meperidine hydrochloride
Digoxin	Sulthiame
Flurazepam hydrochloride	Thioridazine
Furosemide	Thyroxine
Haloperidol	Vitamine D
Levodopa	Warfarin

significant age-related changes in distribution and metabolism.

The use of a decreased dose, given at the conventional dosage interval to elderly patients with impaired renal function, will provide similar blood steady-state concentration as patients with normal renal function, except that the peak and trough levels will be lower and higher, respectively. This will prevent drug accumulation and its associated toxicity, and avoid large fluctuations between peak and trough levels. For drugs with short elimination half-lives, relative to the dosing interval, and whose efficacy relates more closely to peak rather than steady-state blood levels (eg, aminoglycoside antibiotics), a dosage regimen that includes the usual dose, but at prolonged dosage interval, may be more appropriate.

The maintenance dose that is to be administered at the usual frequency in the elderly patient with impaired renal function may be estimated as a fraction of the dose usually administered to a patient with normal renal function. This fraction may be calculated from the ratio of the whole body clearance of the drug in renal dysfunction to that in the young patient with normal renal function, using the known relationship of the drug's clearance to creatinine clearance. This is based on the mean steady-state blood concentration (C_{ss}) following drug administration which is given by

$$C_{ss} = F \cdot D/Cl \cdot \tau$$

where F = the bioavailability of the drug following oral or intramuscular administration, (F = 1 after IV administration), D = dose administered, Cl = whole body clearance, and τ = dosage interval. Assuming the same C_{ss} is required for therapeutic effect in patients with normal (N) and decreased renal function (U) then

$$\frac{F_N \cdot D_N}{Cl_N \cdot \tau_N} = \frac{F_U \cdot D_U}{Cl_U \cdot \tau_U}$$

and if F and τ are not altered by poor renal function, then the dose in the uremic patient (D_U) would be

$$D_U = \frac{Cl_U \cdot D_N}{Cl_N}$$

where Cl_U/Cl_N is the dose reduction factor. The value for Cl_U originates from the equation of the regression line of clearance of the drug plotted against creatinine clearance. Cl_N is generally obtained from studies in normal volunteers.

Conversely, the usual dose may be administered at prolonged dosage intervals as

$$\tau_U = \frac{Cl_N \neq \tau_U}{Cl_U}$$

where τ_U and τ_N are dosage intervals for uremic and normal patients, respectively.

Alternatively, a simple and easy-to-use nomogram for some drugs is available.[68] If no information about the clearance of the drug is known, a conservative approximation may be made by simply expressing the creatinine clearance in the elderly patient as a fraction of the normal value (120mL/min).

In summary, the reduction in renal function and the associated impairment of urinary excretion of drugs and their metabolites in the elderly is well established. In the absence of any age-independent renal disease, the magnitude of the functional decrease in this organ is no greater than about 50%. It is extremely important to modify the dosage regimen for those drugs that are excreted primarily in the urine (>60% of the dose) and which have a relatively small difference between the concentration of drug producing the therapeutic effect and that causing unacceptable adverse reactions. Due to interpatient variability, these modifications are only a first approximation that may need further refinement based on plasma drug levels achieved and clinical assessment.

CONCLUSION

Over the next several decades, there will be an increase in the developed countries in the number and proportion of the population constituted by the elderly. These patients consume a disproportionate share of both prescribed and over-the-counter medications and suffer from an increased incidence of side effects. It must be recognized that aging is not a uniform process and interpatient variability increases with age. Because the responsiveness and disposition of some drugs are altered in the elderly, clinical trials of drugs that are to be used in geriatric medicine should be performed for investigational and marketed drugs. Obviously, this is more important with drugs that have a narrow therapeutic index. In all cases, the physician must individualize therapy and keep in mind that the pharmacodynamics and pharmacokinetics of drugs may be clearly different in the older population.

REFERENCES

1. Greenblatt DJ, Sellers EM, Shader RI: Drug disposition in old age. *N Engl J Med* 1982;306:1081–1088.
2. Seidl LG, Thornton GF, Smith JW, et al: Studies on the epidemiology of adverse drug reactions. III. Reactions in patients on a general medical service. *Bull Johns Hopkins Hosp* 1966;119:299–315.
3. Hurwitz N: Predisposing factors in adverse reactions to drugs. *Br Med J* 1969;1: 536–539.
4. Caranasos CJ, Stewart RB, Cluff LE: Drug induced illness leading to hospitalization. *JAMA* 1974;228:713–717.
5. Lake CR, Ziegler MG, Coleman MD, Kopin IJ: Age-related plasma norepinephrine levels are similar in normotensive and hypertensive subjects. *N Engl J Med* 1977;296:208–209.
6. Sever PS, Osikowska B, Birch M, et al: Plasma noradrenaline in essential hypertension. *Lancet* 1977;1:1078–1081.
7. deChamplain J, Eowsineau D: Lack of correlation between age and circulating catecholamines in hypertensive patients. *N Engl J Med* 1977;297:672.
8. Rowe JW, Troen BR: Sympathetic nervous system and aging. *Endocr Rev* 1980; 1:167–179.
9. Schocken D, Ruth G; Reduced beta-adrenergic receptor concentrations in aging man. *Nature* 1977;267:856–858.
10. Dillon N, Chung S, Kelly J, et al: Age and beta adrenoceptor-mediated function. *Clin Pharmacol Ther* 1980;27:769–772.
11. London GM, Sarfar ME, Weiss YA, et al: Isoproterenol sensitivity and total body clearance of propranolol in hypertensive patients. *J Clin Pharmacol* 1976;16:174–182.
12. Feely J, Stevenson IH: The influence of aging on propranolol concentration, binding and efficacy in hyperthyroid patients. *J Clin Exp Gerontol* 1979;1:173–184.
13. Gribbon G, Pickering TG, Sleight P, et al: Effect of age and high blood pressure on baroreflex sensitivity in man. *Circ Res* 1971;29:424–431.
14. Caird FI, Andrews GR, Kennedy RD: Effect of posture on blood pressure in the elderly. *Br Heart J* 1973;35:527–530.
15. Dollery CT, Harrington J: Methyldopa in hypertension. Clinical and pharmacological studies. *Lancet* 1962;1:759–763.
16. Jick H, Stone K, Borda IT, et al: Efficacy and toxicity of heparin in relation to age and sex. *N Engl J Med* 1968;279:284–286.
17. O'Malley K, Stevenson IH, Ward CA, et al: Determinants of anticoagulant control in patients receiving warfarin. *Br J Clin Pharmacol* 1977;4:309–314.
18. Crooks J: Aging and drug disposition–pharmacodynamics. *J Chronic Dis* 1983; 36:85–90.
19. Jones BR, Baran H, Reidenberg MM: Evaluating patients' warfarin requirements. *J Am Geriatr Soc* 1980;28:10–12.
20. Shephard AMM, Herrick DS, Moreland TA, et al: Age as a determinant of sensitivity of warfarin. *Br J Clin Pharmacol* 1977;4:315–320.
21. Castelden CM, George CF, Marcer D, et al: Increased sensitivity to nitrazepam in old age. *Br Med J* 1977;1:10–12.
22. Reidenberg MM, Levy M, Warner H, et al: Relationship between diazepam dose, plasma level, age and central nervous system depression. *Clin Pharmacol Ther* 1978;23:371–374.

23. Giles HG, MacLeod SM, Wright JR, et al: Influence of age and previous use on diazepam dosage required for endoscopy. *Can Med Assoc J* 1978;118:513–514.
24. Greenblatt DJ, Allen MD, Shader RI: Toxicity of high dose flurazepam in the elderly. *Clin Pharmacol Ther* 1977;21:355–361.
25. Roberstontchabo EA, Arenberg D, Vestal RE: Age differences in memory performance following ethanol infusion, in *Proceedings of the 10th International Congress on Gerontology* (Jerusalem, Israel) 1975; 2:62(abstract 455).
26. Bender AD: Pharmacologic aspects of aging. A survey of the effect of age on drug activity in adults. *J Am Geriatr Soc* 1964; 12:114–134.
27. Geokas MC, Haverback BJ: The aging gastrointestinal tract. *Am J Surg* 1969; 117:881–892.
28. Lamy PP: Comparative pharmacokinetic changes and drug therapy in an older population. *J Am Geriatr Soc* 1982;30: 511–519.
29. Prescott LF, Nimmo WS (eds): *Drug Absorption. Proceedings of the Edinburgh International Conference.* Lancaster, England, MTP Press 1981.
30. Tozer TN: Concepts basic to pharmacokinetics. *Pharmacol Ther* 1981;12:109–131.
31. Vestal RE, Norris AH, Tobin JD, et al: Antipyrine metabolism in man: influence of age, alcohol, caffeine, and smoking. *Clin Pharmacol Ther* 1975;18:425–432.
32. Novak LP: Aging, total body potassium, fat free mass, and cell mass in males and females between ages 18 and 85 years. *J Gerontol* 1972;27:438–443.
33. Klotz U, Avant GR, Hoyampa A, et al: The effects of age and liver disease on the disposition and elimination of diazepam in adult man. *J Clin Invest* 1975;55:347–359.
34. Greenblatt DJ, Allen MD, Hermatz JS, et al: Diazepam disposition determinants. *Clin Pharmacol Ther* 1980;27:301–312.
35. Shader RI, Greenblatt DJ, Harmatz JS, et al: Absorption and disposition of chlordiazepoxide in young and elderly male volunteers. *J Clin Pharmacol* 1977;17: 709–718.
36. Greenblatt DJ, Diroll M, Harmatz JS, et al: Oxazepam kinetics: Effects of age and sex. *J Pharmacol Exp Ther* 1980;215:86–91.
37. Greenblatt DJ, Allen MD, Locniskar A, et al: Lorazepam kinetics in the elderly. *Clin Pharmacol Ther* 1979;26:103–113.
38. Bender AD: The effect of increasing age on the distribution of peripheral blood flow in man. *J Am Geriatr Soc* 1965;13:192–198.
39. Riegelman S, Loo JCK, Rowland M: Shortcomings in pharmacokinetic analysis by conceiving the body to exhibit properties of a single compartment. *J Pharm Sci* 1968; 57:117–123.
40. Woodford-Williams E, Alvarez D, Webster B, et al: Serum protein patterns in normal and pathological aging. *Gerontologia* 1964;10:86–99.
41. Hooper WD, Bochner F, Eodie MJ, et al: Plasma protein binding of diphenylhydantoin: effects of sex hormones, renal and hepatic disease. *Clin Pharmacol Ther* 1974;15:276–282.
42. Hayes MJ, Langman MJS, Short AH: Changes in drug metabolism with increasing age. 1. Warfarin binding and plasma proteins. *Br J Clin Pharmacol* 1975;2: 69–72.
43. Hayes MJ, Langman MJS, Short AH: Changes in drug metabolism with increasing age. 2. Phenytoin clearance and protein binding. *Br J Clin Pharmacol* 1975; 2:73–79.
44. Piafsfy KM, Borga O, Odar-Cederloff I, et al: Increased plasma protein binding of propranolol and chlorpromazine mediated by disease-induced elevations of α_1-acid glycoprotein. *N Engl J Med* 1978;299:1435–1439.
45. Shand DG: Biological determinants of altered pharmacokinetics in the elderly. *Gerontology* 1982;28:(suppl 1):8–17.
46. Wallace S, Whiting B, Runcie J: Factors affecting drug binding in plasma of elderly patients. *Br J Clin Pharmacol* 1976;3: 327–330.
47. Pirttiaho HI, Sotaniemi EA, Ahlquist J, et al: Liver size and indices of drug metabolism in alcoholics. *Eur J Clin Pharmacol* 1978;13:61–67.
48. Kremers P, Beaune P, Cresteil T, et al: Cytochrome P-450 monoxygenase activities in human and rat liver microsomes. *Eur J Biochem* 1981;118:599–606.
49. Wilkinson GR, Shand DG: A physiological approach to hepatic drug clearance. *Clin Pharmacol Ther* 1975;18:377–390.

50. Vestal RE, Wood AJ: Influence of age and smoking on drug kinetics in man. *Clin Pharmacokinet* 1980;5:309–319.
51. Sjoqvist F, Alvan G: Aging and drug disposition metabolism. *J Chronic Dis* 1983; 36:31–37.
52. Jusko WJ, Gardner MJ, Mangione A, et al: Factors affecting theophylline clearance: age, tobacco, marijuana, cirrhosis, congestive heart failure, obesity, oral contraceptive, benzodiazepines, barbiturates, and ethanol. *J Pharm Sci* 1979;68: 1358–1366.
53. Salem SAM, Rajiayabun P, Shepherd AMM, et al: Reduced induction of drug metabolism in the elderly. *Age Ageing* 1978;7:68–73.
54. Pelkonen O, Puurunen J: The effect of cimetidine on *in vitro* and *in vivo* microsomal drug metabolism in the rat. *Biochem Pharmacol* 1980;29:3075–3080.
55. Brogden RN, Heel RC, Speight TM, et al: Cimetidine: A review of its pharmacological properties and therapeutic efficacy in peptic ulcer disease. *Drugs* 1978;15:93–131.
56. Feely J, Wilkinson GR, Wood AJJ: Reduction of liver blood flow and propranolol metabolism by cimetidine. *N Engl J Med* 1981;304:692–695.
57. Reimann IW, Klotz U, Siems B, et al: Cimetidine increases steady-state plasma levels of propranolol. *Br J Clin Pharmacol* 1981;12:785–790.
58. Stevenson IH, Salem SAM, Shepherd AMM: Studies on drug absorption and metabolism in the elderly, in Crooks J, Stevenson IH (eds): *Drugs and the Elderly.* Baltimore, University Park Press, 1979, pp 51–63.
59. Rowe JW, Andres R, Tobin JD, et al: The effect of age on creatinine clearance in men: a cross-sectional and longitudinal study. *J Gerontol* 1976;31:155–163.
60. Leikola E, Vartia KO: On penicillin levels in young and geriatric subjects. *J Gerontol* 1957;12:48–52.
61. Wilkinson GR: Drug distribution and renal excretion in the elderly. *J Chronic Dis* 1983;36:91–102.
62. Lumholtz B, Kampmann J, Siersbaek-Nielsen K, et al: Dose-regimen of kanamycin and gentamicin. *Acta Med Scand* 1974;190:521–524.
63. Cutler RE, Orne BM: Correlation of serum creatinine concentration and kanamycin half-life. *JAMA* 1969;208:539–543.
64. Reidenberg MM, Camacho M, Kluger J, et al: Aging and renal clearance of procainamide and acetylprocainamide. *Clin Pharmacol Ther* 1980;28:732–735.
65. Mayersohn M, Conrad KA, Achari R: Effect of a cooked meal on estimates of creatinine clearance. *Clin Pharmacol Ther* 1983;33:264.
66. Cockcroft DW, Gault MW: Predictions of creatinine clearance from serum creatinine. *Nephron* 1976;16:31–41.
67. Chennavasin P, Brater DC: Nomograms for drug use in renal disease. *Clin Pharmacokinet* 1981;6:193–214.
68. Dettli L: Elimination kinetics and dosage adjustment of drugs in patients with kidney disease. *Prog Pharmacol* 1977;1:1–34.

CHAPTER 13

Dialysis of the Elderly Patient

William Stacy
Domenic Sica

Dialysis and kidney transplantation were first employed as substitution therapy for end-stage renal disease (ESRD) in the early 1960s. During the first decade of development and implementation of both modes of therapy, the scarcity of treatment facilities resulted in the exclusion of "high risk" patients from most programs. Those excluded included patients with disease of other systems; those who were considered unable to cooperate; and those at the extremes of age. Many centers rather arbitrarily set the upper limits of age for dialysis at 45 to 50 years.[1] By the mid-1960s, however, a few centers had begun accepting older patients and could demonstrate that age per se was not a contraindication to substitution therapy for ESRD.[2–4] Age remained, however, a significant factor in patient selection criteria in many units primarily because of limited availability of funds.[5]

In 1973 Congress authorized funding of the End-Stage Renal Disease Program. The Social Security Act was amended to provide payment for at least 80% of all costs incurred for kidney substitution therapy. These benefits are applicable to all who are eligible for social security benefits regardless of their ability to pay. This subsequently resulted in a dramatic increase in treatment facilities so that therapy should now be available in the United States to all who can be expected to benefit, regardless of age. The rate of acceptance for treatment of new patients in the older age ranges has steadily increased in the United States and most industrialized nations.[6] A notable exception is the situation in the United Kingdom where the acceptance rate for patients over age 50 lags considerably behind other European nations and the United States because of rationing of facilities.[7–10]

END-STAGE RENAL DISEASE

End-stage renal disease (ESRD) may be defined as that level of renal function at which conservative measures alone are no longer adequate for the maintenance of an asymptomatic and prolonged existence. It is easy to determine when intervention with substitution therapy is required if the patient is overtly uremic. The relatively asymptomatic patient whose course of renal failure is insidious presents a more difficult problem. There is no uniformity of opinion as to when it is best to start dialysis in such a patient. For example, Bonomini et al advocate initiation of dialysis when the endogenous creatinine clearance has diminished to a level between 10 and 21 mL/min.[11,12] Alternatively, Berlyne and Giovannetti feel that with conservative management many patients will do well until the creatinine clearance reaches 5 mL/min.[13]

Creatinine clearance is the most common clinically employed measure for evaluation of progressive renal insufficiency. It is important to realize that with age the serum creatinine ceases to be an accurate indicator of the level of renal function. Kampmann et al[14] have shown that there is a substantial decline in urinary creatinine excretion with age. Between the ages of 20 and 90 creatinine excretion falls from 23.8 mg/kg/d to 9.4 mg/kg/d.[14] This change in rate of excretion is not reflected by a rise in serum creatinine because there is a parallel decrease in creatinine production by muscle. Therefore, with progressive aging renal function may be continuously declining despite maintenance of the same serum creatinine value.

Our tendency is to adopt a "middle of the road" approach between these extremes. In our experience most adult patients gain the greatest benefits from dialytic intervention at or just below a glomerular filtration rate (GFR) of 10 mL/min. This level of function usually results in a BUN of 100 mg/dL or greater or a serum creatinine of 10 mg/dL. BUN is a function of protein intake which may be quite deficient in the elderly; thus, the BUN on occasion will not reach values of 100 mg/dL prior to the need for dialytic intervention.

Some patients do quite well with a GFR of less than 10 mL/min, particularly if high urine volumes and adequate sodium excretion can be maintained. These patients must be followed very closely, however, lest they suddenly become overtly uremic. Only a rare patient will thrive with a GFR of 5 mL/min or less. Some patients may require dialysis despite a GFR greater than 10 mL/min. This is particularly true of the patient who exhibits marked degrees of sodium retention and/or intractable heart failure. In our experience it is unusual for a patient not to respond to conservative measures when the GFR exceeds 15 mL/min.

It is unwise to forestall dialysis until the patient, particularly an elderly one, has overt manifestations of uremia. Such uremic findings would include pericarditis, encephalopathy, severe gastrointestinal (GI) disturbances, general debility, or life-threatening disturbances in electrolyte or acid-base balance. An elderly patient with one or more of these manifestations of the uremic syndrome usually requires hospitalization, and if recovery is successful it is necessarily prolonged. It is far better to anticipate these more catastrophic events and begin dialysis a short time before it is absolutely required. Frequently, the early manifestations of the uremic syndrome are subtle and not easily detected by patient or physician. The patient may experience a change in life style brought about by fatigue in the early afternoon, or perhaps a loss of appetite and occasional vomiting after meals may be the earliest symptoms. The family sometimes notices a decrease in attentiveness and mental sharpness not obvious to the physician. These subtle changes are difficult to detect in the elderly patient or they may even be attributed to intercurrent events. When the elderly patient with severely compromised renal function fails to thrive, it may become necessary to begin dialysis as a therapeutic trial. If the uremic syndrome is present, unequivocal improvement can be expected within a week or so of adequate dialysis.

MAGNITUDE OF THE PROBLEM

The prevalence of treatable ESRD in the United States is currently unknown. The total number of patients on dialysis has steadily increased each year with no sign that an equilibrium in the ESRD population has been reached. According to the ESRD Annual Report to Congress for 1981 the total dialysis population registered with the Medicare program increased by more than 6900 patients (15.4%) during 1980.[15] Since there is little evidence that the incidence of terminal renal failure is increasing or that the mortality rate of dialysis patients has been greatly improved, this steady increase most likely reflects a general liberalization of inclusion criteria for patients into ESRD programs and an increasing availability of treatment facilities.

The liberalization of admission criteria for dialysis clearly includes an increasing tendency to provide treatment for many elderly patients who at one time would have been excluded. The proportion of dialysis patients in the United States aged 55 years and older has increased from 7% in 1967 to near 54% by 1979.[16,17] The greatest increase in incidence of treated ESRD patients in recent years has been in the older age groups (Table 13-1).[6] The trend toward acceptance of older patients for ESRD replacement therapy is also occurring in Europe except, perhaps, in Great Britain (see above).[18]

The incidence of treatable ESRD (as estimated by the number of dialysis patients) varies widely within the United States. In 1979 the number of dialysis patients of all ages was estimated to range from 983 per million population in the District of Columbia to only 20 per million population in Wyoming. The mean value for the entire nation was 204.7 per million. Rates for other developed nations are also quite variable but, in general, are lower.[19]

From the foregoing, it can be seen that an accurate determination of the magnitude of the ESRD problem in the elderly is not yet possible. It will depend in large part on the availability of resources for commitment to this population group. The experience of the Kaiser Foundation Health Plan of Northern California regarding the incidence of referral for treatment of ESRD may be one of the better sources of incidence data now available for the United States. These data are derived from a closely scrutinized membership of over 1 million whose age and sex distribution differ little from the total population in the area of coverage. In their experience the mean age-adjusted annual incidence rate was 44.9 per million total population per year. Rates climbed steeply with increasing age going to 99.1 per million for the 60- to 69-year-old age group and 154.3 per million for those 70 years of age and older.[20] Other surveys in Connecticut[21] and the Delaware Valley[22] have also demonstrated rising incidence rates with age.

Several surveys have confirmed that incidence rates are considerably higher for blacks than for whites in all age groups studied.[20,23,24] Data recently reported from

Table 13-1
Medical ESRD Program Incidence Rates per Million Population, by Age, Sex, and Race, 1978–1980

	1978	1979	1980	% Change 1978–1980
Total	71	78	82	15
Age				
0–14	6	6	7	17
15–24	26	26	24	−8
25–34	53	54	58	9
35–44	85	84	86	1
45–54	120	135	136	13
55–64	173	193	204	18
65–74	208	230	241	16
75+	96	134	153	59

Adapted from Eggers et al.[6]

Jefferson County, Alabama indicate that the rate of ESRD treatment of blacks over the age of 50 is approximately four times that of whites. The greatest rate disparity, however, was in the 30- to 39-year-old age group,[24] where the rate of ESRD for blacks was 9.02 times that for whites.

The above data suggest that in the United States we may expect an annual ESRD acquisition rate in our older population to be at least 100 per million population per year. The rate for any given area will be both age- and race-dependent, and as of yet the equilibration point in the population has not been reached.

The ESRD program is very costly. The Health Care Financing Administration estimates that the total ESRD program, including all dialysis and transplant patients, will cost 1.8 billion in 1982 and 2.8 billion by 1986.[15] It is likely that management of ESRD in the population over age 50 years will account for more than one half of these funds.

The treatment options for the patient with ESRD are listed in Table 13-2. It is our view that patients and families should be well informed regarding such treatment options and be offered any that might carry a reasonable chance for success. Patients should also be allowed to change treatment programs when they feel it is in their best interest as long as their choices remain both rational and technically feasible.

The transplant option in the elderly is well covered in another chapter of this text and will not be addressed here. It should be stated, however, that the risks attendant to the transplantation process in older patients are greater than the risks of hemodialysis.[25]

Table 13-2
Treatment Options in End-Stage Renal Disease Management

Conservative measures alone
Protein restriction
Electrolyte restriction
Control fluid volume
Control acid-base balance
Phosphate binders
Dialysis
Hemodialysis
Peritoneal dialysis
Transplantation
Cadaver donor
Living related donor

Conservative Management

It is neither reasonable nor desirable that every patient with severe kidney failure should receive substitution therapy. Many patients, particularly the very old, may have severe CNS disease that precludes any meaningful existence. A few patients will have neoplasms, infections, or cardiovascular disease that renders substitution therapy of any type ineffective if not frankly dangerous. Finally, there will be some individuals who, with a clear understanding of the problems at hand, will elect not to accept either dialysis or transplantation. For these patients conservative measures are mandated to prevent the unnecessary discomfort that accompanies protracted nausea and vomiting or pulmonary edema.

For many patients severe salt and water restriction and the use of very large doses of diuretics are necessary to prevent fluid overload, although this is not universally required. A few patients, despite endogenous creatinine clearances less than 5 mL/min, are still capable of adequate if not excessive excretion of salt and water. This is most commonly seen in chronic obstructive uropathy, as seen in the spinal cord injury patient with persistent bladder dysfunction (stones, infection, obstruction). Restriction of salt and water in such patients will result in hypotension, cramps, fatigue or anorexia.

Dietary potassium restriction is seldom necessary as long as urine volume remains high (greater than 1 L/24 h). In those patients who do tend to retain potassium, diuretics such as the long-acting thiazide-like drugs including metolazone,[26] with or without a loop diuretic, can induce sufficient potassium excretion to prevent hyperkalemia. An occasional patient may require the mineralocorticoid-like substance, fludrocortisone, in small amounts coupled with a diuretic. Oral exchange resins such as sodium polystyrene sulfonate are poorly tolerated in most patients and are best avoided if required for long periods. Severe dietary potassium restriction is rarely needed and if instituted is often poorly tolerated.

An additional concern in the predialytic management of the elderly patient approaching ESRD is the application of sound principles of drug and diet therapy. As the creatinine clearance decreases below 30 mL/min, drug-dosing regimens commonly used in the elderly must be altered. Careful attention must be given to the dosages for a variety of agents in common use, such as digoxin,[27] cimetidine,[28] aminoglycoside antibiotics,[29] and antihypertensives.[30] In addition, the commonly employed class of drugs termed the nonsteroidal anti-inflammatory agents (NSAID) are capable of altering renal function by impairing blood flow to the kidney.[31] A number of factors augment this deleterious response including age and/or preexistent dehydration.[32] Though the dosage adjustment for NSAID in the elderly is not known, careful attention must be paid to the circumstances in which they are utilized.

For several decades the principle of restricting protein intake and optimizing the biologic quality of protein has been employed in the management of progressive renal failure. This serves several purposes. One of the most important is to delay the time when dialysis will eventually be needed since chronic renal failure (CRF) usually progresses inexorably. This progression of CRF may occur because of a hyperfiltration phenomenon in the remaining undamaged nephrons with resultant glomerulosclerosis[33] or as the result of disturbances in calcium and phosphorus homeostasis.[34] Such calcium and phosphorus disturbances commonly present as hypocalcemia and hyperphosphatemia and lead to the potential for an elevation in the (calcium × phosphorus) product. This in turn lends itself to a tendency for deposition of these minerals in soft tissues.[34]

Dietary restriction of protein serves several purposes including restricting the ingested quantities of potassium, phosphorus, sulfur, and both protein and nonprotein nitrogen. This restriction diminishes the requirement for excretion of potassium, phosphorus, sulfate, urea, and uric acid by the already compromised kidney. The patient's tendency to develop hyperkalemia, hyperphosphatemia, acidosis, and/or azotemia is then diminished. Such a diet serves to slow the rate at which a CRF patient approaches dialysis. This is particularly germane to the elderly patient in whom substantial risk exists once ESRD management has been initiated. If such a diet is used, it must be carefully tailored to avoid malnutrition and muscle wasting due to progressive negative nitrogen balance, and it must be sufficiently palatable to ensure patient compliance.

Hemodialysis

Approximately 80% of the ESRD population in the United States is managed by hemodialysis. Most of these patients receive in-center care assisted by training staff with less than 15% performing home dialysis.[15] Because of the high incidence of cardiovascular disease in the elderly, it was assumed by many in the early 1960s that older patients could not be managed successfully with hemodialysis. It was felt that vascular access would be difficult to establish and that tolerance of extracorporeal circulation would be limited because of circulatory insufficiency. Certainly, severe cardiovascular disease makes successful dialysis difficult, but it has not proved to be a problem of sufficient magnitude to prevent the widespread use of hemodialysis in older patients.

A number of centers have demonstrated a reasonable rate of success with chronic hemodialysis in older patients. Among the first large groups reported were 29 patients over age 50 (mean age 55) from Minneapolis.[3] All of these patients were managed by in-center hemodialysis as were 93 younger patients (mean age 35) with whom comparisons were made. A number of parameters were studied including cannula survival, transfusion requirements, hospitalization, surgical procedures, and rehabilitation, and in all instances the older group did at least as well as the younger patients.

Ghantous et al concluded from their experience with dialysis and transplantation of 60 patients aged from 50 to 80 years that both a reasonable and pleasant experience was possible in older patients with ESRD,[35] though they noted several problems felt to be unique to elderly patients. Cardiovascular complications were more common in the older patients; this required maintenance of a high hematocrit in these patients and therefore a greater number of transfusions. Ghantous et al also felt that systemic infections were poorly tolerated in the older patients. Half of the patients studied were successfully managed with home hemodialysis, clearly indicating their tolerance of the procedure and an ability to adapt to a complicated treatment program.

One of the oldest populations of patients reported is that of Chester et al from Georgetown University.[36] They described their results with hemodialysis of 45 patients who started maintenance hemodialysis after age 70 (mean age 75), nine of whom were over age 80. The older patients were compared to a younger group of 70 patients (mean age 42). The older patients had more medical problems upon entrance into the ESRD program (5.0 ± 0.3 *v* 2.5 ± 0.2) and a higher overall mortality rate. In general these older patients did well, and the authors did not find that chronological age, per se, was a contraindication to hemodialysis and that indeed they could not identify any criteria to assist the clinician in deciding who would and who would not respond well to hemodialysis.

One of the largest series of older hemodialysis patients reported to date is that of Walker et al,[37] who described their experience with 154 patients over 50 years of age treated by hemodialysis. These patients were part of a group of 576 patients with ESRD treated in the Nashville area from July 1965 to June 1975. Their older patients had a survival rate of 92% at 1 year. The 3-year survival rates in those over the age of 50 were similar to those of their patients under 50 years. From the fourth year on, however, the older patients had significantly lower survival rates. The older patients received fewer transfusions and had fewer hospital days than the younger patients. These differences appear, at least in part, related to the greater number of younger patients who were subjected to bilateral nephrectomy. The general well-being and rehabilitation status was felt to be comparable between the two groups and compliance appeared better in older patients. This group also found that home hemodialysis was a feasible alternative for many older patients.

There have been no studies, to our knowledge, that have specifically addressed the issue of problems peculiar to older patients who are supported by chronic hemodialysis. It is clear from our own experience and that anecdotally described by others that there are some problems unique to the elderly hemodialysis patient.

Table 13-3 lists complications that may be associated with the hemodialysis procedure. There is no reason to believe that the older patient is subject to more iatrogenic complications such as equipment malfunction. These, then, will not be discussed.

It seems logical that establishment of vascular access would be a major problem in the older patient because of the greater degree of peripheral vascular disease expected in this group. Although this may in fact be a serious problem in select patients, most authors have not reported it to be of a magnitude great enough to limit the applicability of hemodialysis in the elderly.

Table 13-3
Complications of Hemodialysis

Vascular access–related
  Infection
  Increased cardiac output
  Vascular insufficiency distal to access
  Repeated access thrombosis
  Inadequate flow
  Carpal tunnel syndrome

Hypotension

Encephalopathies
  Dialysis dementia
  Disequilibrium
  Subdural hematoma

Dialysis-induced hypoxia

Membrane-induced leukopenia

Iatrogenic complications
  Blood line rupture
  Improper bath composition or temperature
  Contamination of dialysate
    Chemical
    Bacterial
    Pyrogens

Bleeding from anticoagulation

Muscle cramps

In fact, in some series the experiences with access in older patients was no worse than with younger patients.[35,38] Preliminary data obtained during the first year of a prospective study of vascular access complications by the Medical Review Board of the ESRD Network Coordinating Council of the Virginias suggest that age does influence the decision regarding the type of vascular access initially attempted. A subcutaneous arteriovenous (A-V) fistula was the first choice for access in 65 of 87 (75%) nondiabetic patients under age 50 years, but was the first choice in only 92 of 195 (49%) nondiabetic patients 50 years or older. The remaining patients in both age groups had creation of an A-V communication via a synthetic graft. These data suggest that the surgeons selected the synthetic A-V graft for first access attempt in the older patients more often, either because they anticipated A-V fistula failure due to the presence of overt vascular disease or because of their previous poor experience with older patients. Additional data from this audit suggest that short-term survival (<1 year) of a first access was the same in young and older patients (Westervelt FB, Turner MS: Medical Review Board, ESRD Network of the Virginias, personal communication, 1984). It is very likely that vascular insufficiency distal to an A-V access of any type would be more common in older patients than in younger, but to date this has not been documented.

Cardiac failure because of excess shunting of blood through an A-V fistula is rare. It has been empirically observed that if the fistula size is limited to 8 mm, heart failure related to the A-V communication almost never occurs.[39] It is unlikely that this represents a problem unique to elderly patients.

Membrane-induced leukopenia is a phenomenon unique to extracorporeal circulation procedures and was first described in association with hemodialysis by Kaplow and Goffinet.[40] A few minutes after the initiation of dialysis, the majority of the circulating polymorphonuclear leukocytes are sequestered within capillaries, particularly in the lung, resulting in a sudden drop in the total circulating leukocyte count. These sequestered neuotrophils return to the circulation within two to three hours despite continuation of dialysis. The pathophysiology of this phenomenon is not understood but clearly requires contact of the neutrophils with the dialysis tubing and membrane with the subsequent activation of complement.[41] The short- and long-term consequences of this phenomenon remain unknown. It can be reduced to some degree by the use of dialysis membranes that are more biocompatible such as those made of polyacrylonitrile.[42] We know of no evidence that membrane-induced leukopenia is more or less severe or of more or less consequence in older patients.

Dialysis-induced hypoxemia is another unique and poorly understood phenomenon associated with hemodialysis. A few minutes after the start of dialysis the arterial oxygen tension of most patients drops by 10 to 15 mmHg and usually remains down for the duration of dialysis. Mechanisms that may be involved include: plugging of pulmonary capillaries with sequestered neutrophils (see above),[41] loss of CO_2 via the dialyzer thereby reducing respiratory drive,[43] and increased oxygen consumption during dialysis.[44] This phenomenon does not appear to be influenced by age. Although the magnitude of reduction in oxygen tension is not particularly significant in an otherwise normal individual, it may well be an important factor in that patient who begins dialysis with impaired pulmonary function and abnormal oxygenation. The degree of reduction in O_2 tension may be reduced by the use of bicarbonate bath.[45] We frequently administer oxygen to those patients who begin dialysis with poor oxygenation in an attempt to lessen the degree of dialysis-induced hypoxia. We have been concerned, but unable to prove, that dialysis-induced hypoxia has been a contributing factor to the development of hypotension and ventricular irritability in patients with preexisting cardiopulmonary disease as may be seen in the elderly.

Hypotension is one of the most common complications of hemodialysis. Walker et al[37] noted that during dialysis some of their older patients suddenly become profoundly hypotensive with loss of consciousness. Frequently this occurred without typical prodromal signs such as sweating, apprehension, or tachycardia. They also noted that this cardiovascular collapse was more difficult to reverse than that seen in younger patients. We have frequently observed this same reaction in our older patients even though extracellular fluid (ECF) volume losses have been minimal during the dialysis session. We believe that this phenomenon is primarily due to impaired cardiovascular responsiveness that is clinically inapparent until one or more of the factors peculiar to the hemodialysis procedure are brought into play. This, in our experience, is the most frightening and serious complication unique to the elderly patient.

The multiple factors that may contribute to hypotension during dialysis are listed in Table 13-4. A decrease in ECF volume is a consequence of every dialysis procedure unless extraordinary care is exercised to prevent it. From 100 to 200 mL of blood is needed to fill the dialyzer and tubing. As urea and other solutes are rapidly removed from the ECF compartment, osmolality drops faster in the extracellular compartment than in the intracellular (ICF) compartment and some ECF shifts into the ICF compartment at the expense of blood pressure.[46] As additional ECF is removed by the dialyzer, blood pressure control may become increasingly difficult. With this continuous reduction in ECF, blood pressure can only be maintained if there is an appropriate increase in cardiac output and/or reduction in the ECF by vasoconstriction.

The response of the cardiovascular system may be impaired by a number of factors. The moderate reduction in oxygen tension observed in most patients shortly after the start of dialysis (see above) may result in impaired cardiovascular responsiveness.[47–49] Additional problems peculiar to the individual patient include primary cardiovascular disease,[50] autonomic neuropathy,[51] antihypertensive agents, and poor response to catecholamines.[52] It is not unreasonable then to assume that, on average, older patients are more likely

Table 13-4
Hypotension of Hemodialysis

Reduction in extracellular volume
Priming of dialyzer
Fluid removal by ultrafiltration alone
Intracellular shifts of fluid
Impaired cardiovascular responsiveness
Primary disease of heart and vessels
Autonomic neuropathy
Impaired response to catecholamines
Acetate accumulation
Hypoxemia
Antihypertensive agents

to have one or more of the above factors operative than younger patients.

Strategies aimed at reducing the occurrence and severity of hypotension during hemodialysis are directed toward limiting the rate and magnitude of ECF volume reduction and when possible eliminating those factors that may impair cardiovascular responsiveness (Table 13-4). The patient must be encouraged to restrict salt and fluid intake. This eliminates the necessity for removal of large volumes of fluid during dialysis and control of interdialytic hypertension can be achieved with little or no antihypertensive medication. If it is necessary to remove a large volume of fluid, the use of "sequential dialysis" may prove helpful.[53,54] This is a procedure in which the rapid removal of fluid (ultrafiltration) and dialysis of solutes (diffusion) are separated. Fluid is removed rapidly, usually during the first part of the procedure, without flow of dialysate (or bath) so that the fluid removed is essentially isotonic and little or no change in ECF osmolality occurs. This avoids the intracellular fluid shifts and other problems related to dialysis-induced changes in ECF osmotic pressure. When sufficient fluid has been removed, dialysate flow is started, and dialysis continues in the usual fashion without the need for significant additional fluid removal. We have found sequential dialysis to be quite helpful in the management of some of our older, more unstable patients though it should not be used as a substitute for patient education and compliance.

The dialysis procedure contains factors capable of reducing cardiac performance. Modification of these factors is possible but entails additional cost to both the patient and the provider of the service. Dialysis may be conducted in a less vigorous fashion using a dialyzer with small priming volume and less efficiency though a longer period of dialysis will be required to achieve adequate waste removal. The use of a bath with bicarbonate as the source of base eliminates the potential cardiovascular depressant effects of acetate and may decrease the degree of dialysis-induced hypoxemia. It should be noted, though, that Mehta was unable to demonstrate a difference in left ventricular performance when isovolemic acetate dialysis and bicarbonate dialysis were compared in seven patients with initially depressed cardiac function.[55] While a dialysate containing bicarbonate may sometimes be preferable to one containing acetate, its use remains limited because most existing dialysis equipment would have to be modified or replaced at a considerable expense to allow the use of bicarbonate as a dialysate buffer. At present it seems prudent to recommend bicarbonate dialysate only for those patients in whom a definite benefit can be demonstrated.

The hemodialysis procedure as usually performed efficiently removes osmotically active solutes of low molecular weight such as urea from the ECF resulting in a rapid drop in ECF osmolality. The shift of urea and perhaps other solutes from the ICF is somewhat slower than their removal from the ECF. The result is relative hypertonicity in the ICF compartment with a shift of fluid from the ECF to the ICF. This fluid shift has several consequences including an increase in spinal fluid pressure. This increased intracerebral pressure has been suggested to be the etiology of the dialysis disequilibrium syndrome.[56-58] In the patient who is just starting dialysis this syndrome may be quite severe, particularly if the first few dialysis sessions are of usual efficiency and duration. The patient may have severe headache, restlessness, agitation, nausea, and vomiting, and in the more severe cases, seizures, coma, or psychotic behavior. This problem can be minimized by starting the new dialysis patient slowly with a few short dialysis sessions using a small, less efficient dialyzer. Some patients exhibit symptoms of disequilibrium even after having been on dialysis for years. They complain of headache, somnolence, nausea, and fatigue toward the end of the dialysis procedure and sometimes for 12 to 24 hours afterwards. This can prove quite distressing to some patients, limiting their performance in the immediate postdialysis period. Various measures may be used to alleviate this problem. A less vigorous but longer dialysis will help some, while others have fewer symptoms when a bath of higher osmolality (higher sodium concentration) is used.[59] The use of bicarbonate bath may also be of value.[60] We do not believe that disequilibrium is more significant in the elderly patient.

Muscle cramps are a very distressing complication for some patients during or after hemodialysis. They appear related, at least in some patients, to the rapidity with which solute and fluid are removed. They are largely prevented by better patient compliance so that less fluid need be removed at each dialysis session and by less efficient (and therefore longer) dialysis. If this does not prove possible the administration of mannitol, normal saline, or hypertonic sodium chloride solution is frequently beneficial.[61] These substances act by mitigating the reduction in ECF osmotic pressure due to the rapid removal of urea and other solutes. Muscle cramps are neither more nor less severe nor more frequent in the older population of hemodialysis patients.

Other than the complications related to the dialysis procedure itself, a number of problems may exist which relate to the persistence of the uremic condition (Table 13-5). A number of encephalopathic disturbances can occur in the chronic dialysis patient.[62] In the elderly patient these must be carefully separated from the entity of atherosclerotic cerebral vascular disease, which is rarely reversible. Uremic encephalopathy, though common to far-advanced renal insufficiency, may still be seen in inadequately dialyzed patients. When faced with an undiagnosed encephalopathy a not unreasonable approach might be an increase in the intensity of dialysis. A severe encephalopathy termed "dialysis dementia" is characterized by dementia, speech impairment, myoclonus, and seizures.[63,64] It is felt by some to be related to the excessive deposition of aluminum in brain gray matter.[65] A major source of excessive aluminum has been secondary to the transference of aluminum across the dialyzer from contaminated water used to prepare dialysate.[66] An additional source of aluminum is from its GI absorption, particularly when aluminum-containing phosphate binders are ingested.[67] Finally, unexplained neurologic findings or dementia should suggest the possibility of a subdural hematoma.[68] This is of particular concern for the elderly patient who may on occasion fall and incur head trauma.

Despite major emphasis on the control of secondary hyperparathyroidism in the dialysis patient, it continues to be a problem. Therapy includes control of the serum phosphorus with phosphate-binding antacids, dietary restriction of phosphate,[69] normalization of the serum calcium with exogenous calcium supplementation,[70] raising the dialysate calcium concentration,[71] and utilizing vitamin D analogues when indicated.[72–74] If this proves unsuccessful, the end result may include pathologic bone fractures and bone pain. Pre-existing metabolic bone disease such as osteoporosis would only compound the pathologic alterations in bone. Additional complications of secondary hyperparathyroidism include

Table 13-5
Persistent Uremic Problems

A. Encephalopathies
   1. Subdural hematoma
   2. Uremic encephalopathy
   3. Dialysis dementia
   4. Atherosclerotic cerebrovascular disease
B. Secondary hyperparathyroidism
   1. Metabolic bone disease
   2. Vascular calcification
   3. Visceral calcification
C. Arteriosclerotic cardiovascular disease
D. Anemia
E. Nonaccess-related infection
F. Gastrointestinal effects
   1. Bleeding
   2. Constipation
   3. Perforation
G. Dermatologic effects
H. Articular disease

both vascular[75] and visceral calcification. The latter sometimes culminates in cardiac rhythm disturbances[76] or oxygen diffusion abnormalities in the lung.[77]

A leading cause of death in ESRD patients is from myocardial infarction. It is for this reason that it has been asserted that the rate of development of atherosclerosis is accelerated in hemodialysis patients.[78,79] The data in support of this are few. In fact, if one examines the risk for an ischemic event in individuals on hemodialysis who entered into dialysis *without* established ischemic heart disease, the risk appears no greater than that found in a nondialysis population with comparable risk factors.[80,81] Metabolic and hemodynamic alterations induced by hemodialysis may unmask pre-existing ischemic heart disease. Additionally, several factors intrinsic to the dialysis population may influence coronary risk. These include the demographic characteristics of the population, in that the number of patients being dialyzed over the age of 50 has increased dramatically in the last decade. Recent studies by Rostand[82] have demonstrated that there exists an age-related rise in risk for the development of symptomatic ischemic heart disease. This was found to be most prominent in whites and women. Of additional importance is the fact that hypertension has accounted for a large portion of all renal failure in the United States, and studies[82,83] have shown hypertension to be an important risk factor in the acceleration of atherosclerosis in a hemodialysis population. Diabetics are entering the dialysis population at increasing rates and this also may contribute to the coronary risk in a hemodialysis population.

Though a number of uremia-associated metabolic disturbances occur, that which is most commonly implicated as being atherogenic is the hyperlipidemia observed in dialysis patients. This occurs in about 30% of the hemodialysis population[84] and results in isolated elevation in the triglyceride values of blood. In particular, there is a decrease in high-density lipoproteins and an increase in low-density lipoproteins in this population.[85] This abnormality is important since in a nondialysis population it has been shown to be a sensitive indicator of coronary risk.[86]

The use of glucose and acetate in the dialysate bath may promote hyperlipidemia but this is of uncertain clinical significance.[87] The major deleterious effects of hemodialysis are the result of hemodynamic stresses to the coronary vasculature resulting from the dialysis procedure. When hemodynamic stress is coupled with anemia, the risk of dialysis-associated angina is real with or without existing coronary artery stenosis.[88]

Anemia is the most common hematologic problem encountered in an elderly population. The degree of anemia is mild and insignificant in comparison to that seen in most hemodialysis patients (6 to 8 g/dL) including elderly ones. The causes of anemia in a nondialytic elderly population are related to GI blood loss and to nutritional deficiency conditions such as folate deficiency.[89] The causes of anemia in an elderly dialysis population are somewhat different and explain to some extent its severity in this population. First, the incidence of blood loss is greater in the dialysis population. Loss of some blood remaining in the dialyzer at the end of each treatment is inevitable and may vary between 5 and 50 mL per dialysis session.[90] Periodic laboratory examinations are necessary and are another source of blood loss. Heparinization is required during hemodialysis, and this coupled to existing organ pathology and/or inevitable trauma may lead to a number of bleeding complications including subdural hematomas,[68] hemopericardium,[91] retroperitoneal hematomas,[92] hemorrhagic pleural effusions,[93] and, most importantly, GI bleeding.[94,95] Folic acid is easily dialyzed so that its levels diminish during hemodialysis.[96] A diet consisting of 69 to 80 g protein is sufficient to supply the necessary amount of lost folate.[97] If, as occurs in the elderly, dietary habits preclude this, then oral folate supplementation becomes mandatory. Finally, and most importantly, there exists decreased erythropoietin production[98] as well as inhibitors of heme synthesis and erythroid proliferation in the uremic state.[99] These latter two mechanisms explain the relative severity of anemia in a dialysis population. The observation that hematocrits are comparably higher in chronic ambulatory peritoneal dialysis (CAPD) patients who were previously on hemodialysis may relate to the ability of the more porous peritoneal membrane to remove large molecular weight erythropoietic inhibitors.[100]

The effects of this severe anemia (6 to 8 g/dL) when untreated may be of particular concern in the elderly. Its presence is probably the cause of the common symptoms of fatigue and lethargy. In addition, the anemia alters cardiac function in hemodialysis patients. Systemic vascular resistance decreases, cardiac output increases, and mean arterial pressure remains constant. As a result of these changes left ventricular work load increases.[101] When the anemia is coupled with hypervolemia the likelihood of development of heart failure is great, particularly if the patient is elderly and has pre-existing cardiac disease.

Treatment of anemia is quite critical in the elderly. For those who are symptomatic, blood transfusions sufficient to maintain a hemoglobin of 10 g/dL should be employed. If iron deficiency exists, oral iron supplementation should be used. In this instance, it is important to realize that serum iron levels are unreliable in dialysis patients[102] and that serum ferritin levels should be measured if a noninvasive means of diagnosing iron deficiency is sought.[103] A final therapy that may be used is the administration of androgens. Use of androgens, in most instances, will increase hematocrit by about 5%. It appears that intramuscular nandrolone decanoate is particularly effective in this regard.[104] These agents probably act to stimulate remnant erythropoietin production and secondarily to directly stimulate the marrow.[105] The incidence of side effects from injectable androgens is on the order of 25% and their use should be reserved for patients with hemoglobin values less than 8 g/dL or for those with symptomatic anemia.[104] A particular side effect of androgens germane to the elderly is the masculinization that occurs with their use. This may, among other things, cause an increase in muscle mass and an increase in creatinine thereby raising the possibility of inadequate dialysis. Also, androgens may lead to prostatic growth and cause symptomatic urinary retention in those elderly males who continue with good urine output despite dialysis.

It is well known that the effectiveness of the immune system decreases with age. Both cell-mediated immunity and the humoral response to foreign antigens diminish, at least in part due to thymic involution and an imbalance of regulatory T-lymphocytes.[106,107] These changes are modest and are not the sole answer for the increased susceptibility of older patients to infection. When the effect of senescence on the immune system is combined with that of uremia there may exist a situation capable of leading to life-threatening infection. Uremia causes a number of alterations in the effector limbs of immunity. Granulocytes demonstrate subnormal locomotion[108] and variable defects in phagocytosis and intracellular killing.[109] A moderate lymphopenia is also encountered due to a decrease in both T- and B-lymphocytes.[110] Decreased lymphocyte transformation[111] as well as cutaneous anergy may be seen.[112]

Both access-related[113] and nonaccess-related[114,115] infections are common in dialysis patients. These infections are most often caused by common bacterial pathogens. Ghantous et al[35] have noted that frequent infectious complications occurred in their older dialysis and transplant patients. Septicemia if present was generally fatal accounting for 45% of all fatalities.[35] Keane and Rau[116] have also described a higher incidence of death due to infections in older patients compared to their younger counterparts. Their nondiabetic patients over age 60 had 7.8 infection-related deaths/1000 treatment months as compared to 1.4 infection-related deaths/1000 treatment months in the younger patients. Interestingly, Keane and Rau felt that the higher incidence of death in the older patients was not due to the inability to mount a response to an individual infection but rather to the increased number of infections occurring in this group.

Most authors do not mention GI bleeding as a major or common complication in the elderly dialysis population though Chester et al[36] noted that elderly patients had a higher incidence of GI bleeding (22% *v* 7% in the control group) requiring more transfusions (6.9 U/yr compared to 3.4 U/yr). It would not be surprising to observe a higher incidence of acute and chronic GI blood loss in this population. The elderly dialysis patient has a high incidence of diverticula,[117] angiodysplasia,[118] and carcinoma[119] in addition to the other usual causes of GI bleeding seen in nonuremic patients such as peptic ulcer disease or reflux esophagitis. In addition, any bleeding site is likely to become evident because of the intermittent heparinization that is required for hemodialysis. The treatment of GI bleeding when present is straightforward and entails similar treatment strategies as in the nonuremic population.

It is well known that the incidence of colonic diverticula increases with increasing age. Perhaps 50% of the population over 60 will have one or more colonic diverticula.[120,121] Complications of colonic diverticulosis, particularly perforation, have recently been recognized as a significant cause of morbidity and mortality in the older ESRD population,[122,123] and may relate to the significant constipating effects of the commonly employed phosphate binders.[124,125]

In our experience, perforation of the colon in the older ESRD patient is a very insidious illness. Patients frequently have vague abdominal pain and low-grade fever for several days before the illness becomes so pronounced as to warrant hospital admission and evaluation. Frequently patients do not exhibit signs of acute peritonitis until very late in the course of the illness. Our experience with four cases of colonic perforation has led us to be very aggressive in the older patient who presents with abdominal complaints. If low-grade fever is present, we generally admit these patients and aggressively pursue the diagnosis of perforated colon.

Dermatologic complaints are common in the dialysis population regardless of age.[126] They usually consist of xerosis and pruritus and may in part relate to the extent of secondary hyperparathyroidism.[127] A number of treatment modalities have been employed for pruritus including symptomatic management with antihistamines, cholestyramine resin,[128] ultraviolet phototherapy,[129] oral charcoal,[130] and intravenous lidocaine.[131] In certain instances pruritus responds dramatically to subtotal parathyroidectomy.

A final consideration is that of wound healing in the elderly. Wounds generally heal slowly demonstrating decreased tensile strength and an increased risk of disruption.[132] This is an important consideration in an elderly dialysis population that is one frequently operated upon.

Hemodialysis patients are prone to a number of joint and tendon abnormalities. For this reason the elderly dialysis patient should be assessed carefully when they voice musculoskeletal complaints. Spontaneous tendon ruptures occur and may be associated with the extent of secondary hyperparathyroidism.[133] Carpal tunnel syndrome is also being reported with increasing frequency in dialysis patients.[134] A number of crystal-induced diseases can occur including gout, pseudogout,[135] and calcium oxalate microcrystalline deposition.[136] These crystal-induced diseases are sometimes difficult to differentiate from the periarticular inflammatory episodes associated with soft tissue calcification. A final consideration is that of septic arthritis. This is more common in the dialysis population than in a general population.[137] It tends to be multiarticular and most commonly the result of a staphylococcal species which has entered the systemic circulation via the vascular access. Though crystal-induced disease occurs in this population, if other systemic complaints coexist with a syndrome of joint disease the diagnosis of septic arthritis should be carefully considered.

Table 13-6
Advantages of Peritoneal Dialysis

No anticoagulation
Slower rate of solute removal
Slower rate of fluid removal
Simple technic and safe equipment
Excellent potential for home use
Avoids dialysis-induced leukopenia and hypoxemia

PERITONEAL DIALYSIS

Table 13-6 lists some of the advantages of peritoneal dialysis. It is clear that some of these advantages are particularly germane to the elderly. The longer, slower dialysis effected avoids many of the complications of hemodialysis, particularly sudden hypotension and disequilibrium. The technics are easy to learn and can be performed at home without assistance.

The first trials of peritoneal dialysis for the management of chronic renal failure were conducted in the early 1960s. It appears that the first ESRD patient managed by repeated peritoneal dialysis in the United States was a patient treated by Doolan and Ruben[138] followed shortly by four patients reported by Merrill et al.[139] These early attempts were not particularly successful primarily because of difficulties with long-term access to the peritoneal cavity. Peritoneal dialysis remained an impractical method of long-term management of the ESRD patient until the introduction of an acceptable chronic indwelling peritoneal catheter by Tenchkhoff and Schecter in 1968.[140] Subsequent modifications of this catheter have made it the most widely used peritoneal access device.

Several variations of peritoneal dialysis are currently available. The first technic employed was intermittent (or periodic) peritoneal dialysis (IPD). With this method the patient receives a series of rapid exchanges of peritoneal dialysate. This occurs over a period of 12 to 24 hours, one or more times per week, for a total time on dialysis of about 40 hours per week. For many patients this long period of dialysis proves inconvenient, and an alternative is to perform unattended overnight IPD several nights per week with an automated cycling device. This technic has been used by only a small portion of the dialysis population. It is a reasonable alternative for many older patients, especially those who have someone at home who can help them with the necessary tubing connections and the operation of the cycling device.

Wider acceptance of peritoneal dialysis as an alternative for the ESRD patient has come with the introduction of continuous ambulatory peritoneal dialysis (CAPD) as originally described by Popovich et al.[141] This is a closed system peritoneal dialysis technic using an indwelling peritoneal access device (Tenckhoff catheter), a connecting tubing set, and a collapsible plastic bag that contains dialysate. Fresh dialyzing fluid is gravity-fed into the peritoneal cavity from the plastic bag as rapidly as possible. The bag remains attached to the tubing, and when empty both are rolled up and carried in a convenient pocket. After several hours the fluid is drained back into the bag. The spent bag of fluid is then discarded, and a fresh bag of solution is connected by sterile technic to the system and infused. The average patient makes three to five exchanges per day leaving the last exchange of the day in overnight. The inefficiency of this technic does not limit its effectiveness because it provides a means of continuous solute exchange. Surprisingly good control of BUN levels, acid-base, and fluid and electrolyte balance can be achieved.[142] A variation of CAPD called cyclical peritoneal dialysis (CCPD) allows three to five exchanges to take place overnight with the aid of an automatic cycler, with the last exchange being allowed to remain in the abdomen during the day.[143]

In the early stages of CAPD, the elderly were not felt to be good candidates for this procedure. This arose from the feeling that they were incapable of making the necessary aseptic tubing changes because of failing vision and declining motor skills. Despite the initial concerns, subsequent experience has shown that age alone is not a criterion for exclusion of patients from a CAPD program. In fact, the recent development of mechanical aids that facilitate tubing connections may make this procedure available to patients with severe visual and motor impairment, and therefore increase the number of elderly patients in which this procedure may be used.

Kay et al[143] have reported favorable results in a small series of CAPD patients over 65 years of age. In their population of 44 patients successfully trained for CAPD, the 18 patients who were over 65 years old (mean age 73.7 ± 5.1) did just as well as the 26 patients under 65 years old (mean age 48 ± 13.7 years). There was no difference in biochemical values, complication rate, or frequency of episodes of peritonitis. The mortality was the same in both groups, but the length of follow-up (average 14.5 months under 65 years and 17.6 months over 65) was not long enough to conclude that mortality rates would not be subsequently greater in the older age group. Similar results have been described by Nicholls et al.[144] In their unit, 38 patients over age 60 with ESRD were treated with CAPD for up to 3 years. Patient survival at 1 and 2 years was 72% and 61% respectively which compared favorably to European data for survival of hemodialysis patients in the over 55-year-old age group.

Table 13-7 displays the experience of the National Institutes of Health (NIH) National CAPD Patient Registry from January 1, 1981 through June 30, 1984.[145] The fact that approximately 30% of registered patients are over age 60 suggests that, at least early in the history of this procedure, physicians are finding older patients suitable candidates for CAPD. The rate at which patients transfer off CAPD to another type of dialysis is shown in Table 13-8, in which data, again from the National CAPD Registry, indicate that the rate of transference off CAPD is virtually the same for all ages (Table 13-8). The Toronto group has, however, found that increasing age is a risk factor for failure of CAPD, but not for the development of peritonitis.[146] These data suggest that while old age may imply some increased risk of early failure of CAPD, it is by no means an overwhelming risk factor. Several problems common to the CAPD population are likely to be more prevalent in the older patient. These include exacerbation of pre-existing peripheral vascular

Table 13-7
Age Distribution of Patients Registered with the National CAPD Registry

Age Group (yr)	Total No.	Patients (%)
0–10	115	(1.8)
11–20	214	(3.4)
21–30	568	(8.9)
31–40	1000	(15.7)
41–50	982	(15.4)
51–60	1505	(23.7)
61–70	1419	(22.3)
71–80	537	(8.4)
81–90	21	(0.3)
	6361	(100)

Adapted from Steinberg et al.[145]

Table 13-8
Cumulative Probability of Transferring off CAPD–National CAPD Registry Patients

Months from Placement onto CAPD	Age 20–59 Years (%)	Age ≥60 Years (%)
0	0	0
3	2.6	2.6
6	7.1	6.4
9	12.8	13.7
12	18.4	20.9
15	24.0	25.3
18	28.7	27.7

Adapted from Steinberg et al.[145]

disease by hypotension, abdominal hernias, and low back pain.

CAPD frequently results in good blood pressure control in the previously hypertensive patient.[142] This lowering of blood pressure may, however, exacerbate the effects of peripheral vascular disease. Brown et al[146] recently described five patients with severe pre-existing peripheral vascular disease involving the lower extremities who had exacerbation of the effects of their peripheral vascular disease following a drop in systemic pressure associated with starting CAPD; amputations were required in four. The fifth had improvement in claudication following an increase in blood pressure after switching from CAPD to IPD. Despite significant lowering of the blood pressure, their patients demonstrated no CNS symptoms of hypotension. Peritoneal dialysis, in and of itself, probably does not cause or enhance peripheral vascular disease. Rather the lowering of blood pressure with the peritoneal dialysis may lower perfusion pressure to an already compromised vascular bed resulting in symptoms of ischemia. Wehling et al[147] have recently described a 63-year-old male CAPD patient who developed nonocclusive ischemic colitis due to hypotension when on CAPD. The colitis resolved following an increase in blood pressure even though CAPD was continued.

Low back pain associated with constantly carrying the 2 L of peritoneal fluid is a well-recognized cause of CAPD failure. Aging is associated with degenerative changes in the spine, poor posture, and poor muscle tone, all of which predispose the patient to back problems. It seems reasonable to refer patients who have back problems to a physical therapist who might then instruct them in an exercise program and the proper means of back protection.[148]

The increased intra-abdominal pressure appears to predispose CAPD patients to abdominal hernias. Digenis et al[149] have recently described 22 patients from the Toronto Western Hospital CAPD population of 192 patients who developed abdominal hernias. The mean age of their hernia patients was significantly greater than their total CAPD population. Rubin et al,[150] however, did not find age to be a predisposing factor in their small series of 12 patients. It appears appropriate to carefully search for and repair pre-existing abdominal hernias before starting chronic peritoneal dialysis. Patients may resume CAPD after successful repair.

In summary, we feel that peritoneal dialysis is an excellent alternative for the older ESRD patient, being particularly applicable to the home dialysis of older patients. The risk of a sudden catastrophe, inherent to hemodialysis, is avoided. The simplicity and flexibility of the technic permits adaptation to varied life styles.

MORTALITY

Data from several large dialysis registries[151] and the United States Department of Health and Human Resources[6] clearly indicate that the mortality rate of dialysis patients increases with increasing age. Several large series of patients recently reported from large centers and small geographical areas also support the conclusion that age at onset of end-stage disease is a major determinant of survival among ESRD patients.[152–154]

This difference in survival does not mean that elderly ESRD patients universally have a poor prognosis. Eggers et al[6] have pointed out that much of the increase in mortality in older age groups can be attributed to underlying age mortality irrespective of renal disease. When compared to the mortality rate of the total population in their own age group, survival of ESRD patients in younger age groups is much worse. The mortality rate for the younger ESRD patients may be 60 to 80 times that for all persons of the same age, whereas older ESRD patients may experience less than a tenfold increase in mortality over the general population of the same age (Table 13-9). When viewed in this perspective, the survival of older patients is not

Table 13-9
Five-Year Mortality Rates for US Population and Medical ESRD Dialysis Patients by Age, 1973–1979

Age Group	Five-Year Mortality (%) *Total Population*	*ESRD*	Ratio (ESRD/Total Population)
0–14	0.5	40	80
15–24	0.6	36	60
25–34	0.7	44	63
35–44	1.3	47	36
45–54	3.1	54	17
55–64	7.2	59	8
65–74	14.8	70	5
75+	31.1	78	3

Adapted from Eggers et al.[6]

nearly as grim as the mortality data might suggest. In fact, several groups have found survival of older dialysis patients over the short term to be comparable to their younger population. Cohen et al[3] found a slightly better survival rate over a 4-year period for a group of 29 dialysis patients over age 50 when compared to their larger population of patients under age 50. Another early study of 302 patients, most of whom had been followed for less than 3 years, reported by Lewis et al,[155] revealed a small increase in mortality in dialysis patients over 45 years of age that proved not to be statistically significant. Bailey et al[156] also found only a slight increase in mortality in their group of chronic hemodialysis patients who started dialysis between the age of 50 and 80 years. Chester et al[36] also described an acceptable survival in a review of 45 patients over age 70. Two-year survival was 42% in the older group and 58% in younger controls. Undoubtedly patient selection has led, in part, to the relatively good survival of the older patients in these earlier series since it was more difficult to deny therapy to a younger patient with multiple risk factors than to an older patient with similar problems.

It is obvious that age is not the only major factor that affects the survival of the ESRD dialysis population. Other significant risk factors include diabetes mellitus, coronary artery disease, cerebrovascular accidents, chronic obstructive pulmonary disease, nonskin malignancy, left ventricular failure, and severe hypertension.[153,157] The occurrence of one or more of these risk factors in the younger population of ESRD patients tends to reduce their survival rate so that it approximates the rate seen in uncomplicated older patients.[157] From the foregoing, we believe that one can conclude that the survival of older patients treated for ESRD by dialysis is acceptable and with careful patient selection can approximate that of young patients over the short term.

SUMMARY

The elderly ESRD patient can be successfully managed by dialysis. Virtually every dialysis technic has been used effectively in appropriately selected patients. Mortality rates, degree of rehabilitation, and quality of life currently achieved in older dialysis patients is acceptable. Age alone should not be a criterion for selection of patients for dialysis.

REFERENCES

1. Hegstrom RM, Murray JP, Pendrac JS, et al: Hemodialysis in the treatment of chronic uremia. *Trans Am Soc Artif Intern Organs* 1961;7:136–149.

2. Johnson WJ, in *Proceedings of the Conference on Dialysis as a "Practical Workshop."* New York, National Dialysis Committee, June 24–26, 1966, p 5.
3. Cohen SL, Comty CM, Shapiro FL: The effect of age on the results of regular hemodialysis treatment. *Proc Eur Dial Transplant Assoc* 1970;7:254–272.
4. Figueroa JE: Dialysis in older patients. *Postgrad Med J* 1969;45:205–210.
5. Abram HS, Wadlington W: Selection of patients for artificial and transplanted organs. *Ann Intern Med* 1968;69:615–620.
6. Eggers PW, Connerton R, McMullan M: The medical experience with end-stage renal disease. *Health Care Financial Rev*, in press, 1984.
7. Wing AJ: Why don't the British treat more patients with kidney failure? *Br Med J* [*Clin Res*] 1983;287:1157–1158.
8. Brynger H, Brunner FP, Chantler C, et al: Combined report on regular dialysis and transplantation in Europe. *Proc Eur Dial Transplant Assoc* 1979;17:4–86.
9. Taube DH, Winder EA, Ogg CS, et al: Successful treatment of middle aged and elderly patients with end-stage renal disease. *Br Med J* [*Clin Res*] 1983;286: 2018–2020.
10. Berlyne CM: Over 50 and uremic – death. The failure of the British National Health Service to provide adequate dialysis facilities. *Nephron* 1982;31:188–190.
11. Bonomini V, Albertazzi A, Bortolotti GC, et al: When to start dialysis and transplantation, in Giovannetti S, Bonomini V, D'Amico G (eds): *Proceedings of the Sixth International Congress of Nephrology.* Basel, S Karger, 1975, pp 680–691.
12. Bonomini V, Albertazzi A, Vangelista A, et al: Residual renal function and effective rehabilitation in chronic dialysis. *Nephron* 1976;16:89–99.
13. Berlyne GM, Giovannetti S: When would entry into a regular hemodialysis occur? *Nephron* 1976;16:81–82.
14. Kampmann J, Siersbak-Nielsen K, Kristensin M, et al: Rapid evaluation of creatinine clearance. *Acta Med Scand* 1974; 196:517–520.
15. *End-Stage Renal Disease Annual Report to Congress.* Health Care Financing Administration, document No. HCFA 82-02144, 1981, p 3.
16. Evans RW, Blagg CR, Bryan FA Jr: Implications for health care policy: a social and demographic profile of hemodialysis patients in the United States. *JAMA* 1981;245:487–491.
17. Becker EL: Finite resources and medical triage. *Am J Med* 1979;66:549–550.
18. Broyer M, Brunner FP, Brynger H, et al: Combined report on regular dialysis and transplantation in Europe, XII, 1981. *Proc Eur Dial Transplant Assoc* 1982;19:2–86.
19. Relman AS, Rennie D: Treatment of end-stage renal disease: Free but not equal. *N Engl J Med* 1980;303:996–998.
20. Hiatt RA, Friedman GD: Characteristics of patients referred for treatment of end-stage renal disease in a defined population. *Am J Public Health* 1982;72:829–833.
21. Pearson DA, Stranova TJ, Thompson JD: Characteristics of Connecticut patients receiving services for end-stage uremia. *Public Health Rep* 1975;90:440–448.
22. Mausner JS, Clark JK, Coles BI, et al: An area-wide survey of treated end-stage renal disease. *Am J Public Health* 1978;68:166–169.
23. Easterling RE: Racial factors in the incidence and causation of end-stage renal disease. *Trans Am Soc Artif Intern Organs* 1977;23:28–33.
24. Rostand SG, Kirk KA, Rutsky EA, et al: Racial differences in the incidence of treatment for end-stage renal disease. *N Engl J Med* 1982;306:1276–1279.
25. Sommer BG, Ferguson RM, Davin TD, et al: Renal transplantation in patients over 50 years of age. *Transplant Proc* 1981;13: 33–35.
26. Epstein M, Lepp RA, Hoffman DS, et al: Potentiation of furosemide by metolazone in refractory edema. *Curr Ther Res* 1977; 21:656–667.
27. Ewy GA, Kapadia GG, Yao L, et al: Digoxin metabolism in the elderly. *Circulation* 1969;39:449–453.
28. Somogyi A, Rohner HG, Gugler R: Pharmacokinetics and bioavailability of cimetidine in gastric and duodenal ulcer patients. *Clin Pharmacokinet* 1980;5:84–94.
29. Cronin RE: Aminoglycoside nephrotoxicity: pathogenesis and prevention. *Clin Nephrol* 1979;11:251–256.
30. Stenbaëk Ø, Myhre E, Broadwall EK, et al: Hypotensive effect of methyldopa in

renal failure asociated with hypertension. *Acta Med Scand* 1972;191:333–337.

31. Dunn MJ, Zambraski EJ: Renal effects of drugs that inhibit prostaglandin synthesis. *Kidney Int* 1980;18:609–622.
32. Blackshear JL, Davidman M, Stillman T: Identification of risk for renal insufficiency from non-steroidal antiinflammatory drugs. *Arch Intern Med* 1983;143:1130–1134.
33. Brenner BM, Meyer TW, Hostetter TH: Dietary protein intake and the progressive nature of kidney disease: the role of hemodynamically mediated glomerular injury in the pathogenesis of progressive glomerular sclerosis in aging, renal ablation, and intrinsic renal disease. *N Engl J Med* 1982;307:652–659.
34. Ibels LS, Alfrey A, Haut AL, et al: Preservation of function in experimental renal disease by dietary restriction of phosphate. *N Engl J Med* 1978;298:122–126.
35. Ghantous WN, Bailey GL, Zschaeck D, et al: Long-term hemodialysis in the elderly. *Trans Am Soc Artif Intern Organs* 1971; 17:125–128.
36. Chester AC, Rakowski TA, Argy WP, et al: Hemodialysis in the eighth and ninth decades of life. *Arch Intern Med* 1979;139: 1001–1005.
37. Walker PJ, Ginn HE, Johnson HK, et al: Long-term hemodialysis for patients over 50. *Geriatrics* 1976;31:55–61.
38. Rathaus M, Bernheim JL: Are your elderly patients good candidates for dialysis? *Geriatrics* 1978;33:56–66.
39. Ahern DM, Maher JF: Heart failure as a complication of hemodialysis: arteriovenous fistula. *Ann Intern Med* 1972;77:201–204.
40. Kaplow LS, Goffinet JA: Profound neutropenia during the early phase of hemodialysis. *JAMA* 1968;203:1135–1137.
41. Craddock PR, Fehr J, Brigham KL, et al: Complement and leukocyte mediated pulmonary dysfunction in hemodialysis. *N Engl J Med* 1977;296:769–774.
42. Shin J, Matsua M, Shinko S, et al: A study on hemodialysis leukopenia using various dialyzers. *J Dial* 1980;4:51–62.
43. Aurigemma N, Feldman N, Gottlieb M, et al: Arterial oxygenation during hemodialysis. *N Engl J Med* 1977;287:871–873.
44. Patterson RW, Nissenson AR, Miller J, et al: Hypoxemia and pulmonary gas exchange during hemodialysis. *J Appl Physiol* 1981;50:259–264.
45. Nissenson AR: Prevention of dialysis-induced hypoxemia by bicarbonate dialysis. *Trans Am Soc Artif Intern Organs* 1980;26:339–342.
46. Rodrigo F, Shideman J, McHugh R, et al: Osmolality changes during hemodialysis: Natural history, clinical correlations and influence of dialysate, glucose, and IV mannitol. *Ann Intern Med* 1977;86:554–561.
47. Novello A, Kelsch RC, Easterling RE: Acetate intolerance during hemodialysis. *Clin Nephrol* 1976;5:29–32.
48. Aizawa Y, Ohmori T, Imai K, et al: Depressant action of acetate upon the human cardiovascular system. *Clin Nephrol* 1977;8: 477–480.
49. Graffe U, Multinovich J, Follette C, et al: Less dialysis induced morbidity and vascular instability with bicarbonate in dialysate. *Ann Intern Med* 1978;88:332–336.
50. Lazarus JM, Lowrie EG, Hampers CL, et al: Cardiovascular disease in uremic patients on hemodialysis. *Kidney Int* 1975; (suppl 2):S167–S175.
51. Kersh ES, Kronfield SJ, Unger A, et al: Autonomic insufficiency in uremia as a cause of hemodialysis-induced hypotension. *N Engl J Med* 1974;290:650–653.
52. Ulmann A, Drueke T, Zingraff J, et al: The response of heart rate to isoproterenol in hemodialyzed patients before and after parathyroidectomy. *Clin Nephrol* 1977;7: 58–60.
53. Bergstrom J, Asaba H, Furst P, et al: Dialysis, ultrafiltration, and blood pressure. *Proc Eur Dial Transplant Assoc* 1976;13:293–300.
54. Rouby JJ, Rottembourg J, Duronde JP, et al: Hemodynamic changes induced by regular hemodialysis and sequential ultrafiltration hemodialysis: A comparative study. *Kidney Int* 1980;17:801–810.
55. Falls WF, Stacy WK, Bear ES, et al: Dialysis-induced change of extracellular fluid volume in man. *Proc Dial Transplant Forum* 1972;2:155–160.
56. Wakim KG: The pathophysiology of the dialysis disequilibrium syndrome. *Mayo Clinic Proc* 1969;44:406–429.

57. Arieff AI, Guisado R, Massry SG, et al: Central nervous system pH in uremia and the effects of hemodialysis. *J Clin Invest* 1976;58:306–311.
58. Arieff AI, Massry SG, Barrientos A, et al: Brain water and electrolyte metabolism in uremia: Effects of slow and rapid hemodialysis. *Kidney Int* 1973;4:177–187.
59. Port FK, Johnson WJ, Klass DW: Prevention of dialysis disequilibrium syndrome by use of high sodium concentration in the dialysate. *Kidney Int* 1973;3:327–333.
60. Graefe U, Milutinovich J, Follette WC, et al: Less dialysis-induced morbidity and vascular instability with bicarbonate in dialysate. *Ann Intern Med* 1978;88:332–336.
61. Wilkinson R, Barber SG, Robson V: Cramps, thirst and hypertension in hemodialysis patients–the influence of dialyzate sodium concentration. *Clin Nephrol* 1977;7:101–105.
62. Tyler HR: Neurologic disorders in renal failure. *Am J Med* 1968;44:734–748.
63. Alfrey AC, Mishell JM, Burks J, et al: Syndrome of dyspraxia and multifocal seizures associated with chronic hemodialysis. *Trans Am Soc Artif Intern Organs* 1972; 18:257–261.
64. Pierides AM, Edwards WG, Cullum UX, et al: Hemodialysis encephalopathy with osteomalacic fractures and muscle weakness. *Kidney Int* 1980;18:115–124.
65. Arieff AI, Cooper JD, Armstrong D, et al: Dementia, renal failure and brain aluminum. *Ann Intern Med* 1979;90:741–747.
66. Flendrig JA, Kruis H, Das HA: Aluminum intoxication: The cause of dialysis dementia. *Proc Eur Dial Transplant Assoc* 1976;13:355–363.
67. Kovarik J, Graf H, Meisinger V, et al: Influence of phosphate binders on serum aluminum levels in patients on chronic hemodialysis. *Mineral Electrolyte Metab* 1979;2:242.
68. Leonard A, Shapiro FL: Subdural hematoma in regularly hemodialyzed patients. *Ann Intern Med* 1975;82:650–658.
69. Goldsmith RS, Furszyfer J, Johnson WJ, et al: Control of secondary hyperparathyroidism during long-term hemodialysis. *Am J Med* 1971;50:692–699.
70. Meyrier A, Marsac J, Richet G: The influence of a high calcium carbonate intake on bone disease in patients undergoing hemodialysis. *Kidney Int* 1973;4:146–153.
71. Malluche HH, Ritz E, Lange HP, et al: Changes of bone histology during maintenance hemodialysis at various levels of dialysate calcium concentration. *Clin Nephrol* 1976;6:440–447.
72. Teitelbaum SL, Bone JM, Stein PM, et al: Calciferol in renal insufficiency. *JAMA* 1967;235:164–167.
73. Chan JCM, Oldhom SB, Holick MF, et al: 1-alpha-hydroxyvitamin D_3 in chronic renal failure. A potent analogue of the kidney hormone, 1,25 dihydroxycholecalciferol. *JAMA* 1975;234:47–52.
74. Pierides M, Ward MK, Alvarez-Ude F, et al: Long-term therapy with $1,25(OH)_2D_3$ in dialysis bone disease. *Proc Eur Dial Transplant Assoc* 1976;12:237–244.
75. Meema HE, Oreopoulos DG, Deueber GA: Arterial calcifications in severe chronic renal disease and their relationship to dialysis treatment, renal transplant and parathyroidectomy. *Radiology* 1976;121: 315–321.
76. Schwartz KV: Heart block in renal failure and hypercalcemia. *JAMA* 1976;235:1550.
77. Conger JD, Hammond WS, Alfrey AC, et al: Pulmonary calcification in chronic dialysis patients. Clinical and pathologic studies. *Ann Intern Med* 1975;83:330–336.
78. Lindner A, Charra B, Sherrard DJ, et al: Accelerated atherosclerosis in prolonged maintenance hemodialysis. *N Engl J Med* 1974;290:697–701.
79. Lazarus JM, Lowrie EG, Hampers CL, et al: Cardiovascular disease in patients on hemodialysis. *Kidney Int* 1975;7(suppl 2): S167–S175.
80. Rostand SG, Gretes JC, Kirk KA, et al: Ischemic heart disease in patients with uremia undergoing maintenance hemodialysis. *Kidney Int* 1979;16:600–611.
81. Nicholls AJ, Edwards N, Catto GRD, et al: Accelerated atherosclerosis in long-term dialysis and renal-transplant patients. Fact or fiction? *Lancet* 1980;1:276–278.
82. Rostand SG, Kirk KA, Rutsky EA: Relationship of coronary risk factors to hemodialysis-associated ischemic heart disease. *Kidney Int* 1982;22:304–308.
83. Vincenti F, Amend WJ, Abele J, et al: The role of hypertension in hemodialysis-associated atherosclerosis. *Am J Med* 1980;68:363–369.

84. Bagdade JD, Casaretto A, Albers JJ: Effect of chronic uremia, hemodialysis and renal transplantation on plasma lipids and lipoproteins in man. *J Lab Clin Med* 1976;87:37–48.
85. Bagdade JD, Albers JJ: Plasma high density lipoprotein concentrations in chronic hemodialysis and renal transplant patients. *N Engl J Med* 1977;296:1436–1439.
86. Castelli WP, Doyle JT, Gordon T, et al: HDL cholesterol and other lipids in coronary heart disease. The cooperative lipoprotein phenotyping study. *Circulation* 1977;55:767–772.
87. Morris RJ, Srikantaiah MV, Davidson WD: Effect of uremia on incorporation of acetate into rat plasma and tissue lipids. *Metabolism* 1980;29:311–316.
88. Rutsky EA, Rostand SG: Cardiac performance and coronary risk in chronic hemodialysis patients. *The Kidney* 1983;16:1–8.
89. Seligman PA: Hematologic and oncologic problems in the elderly, in Schrier R (ed): *Clinical Internal Medicine in the Aged.* Philadelphia, WB Saunders Co, 1982, pp 280–295.
90. Lindsay RM, Burton JA, King P, et al: Dialyzer blood loss. *Clin Nephrol* 1973;1: 24–28.
91. Alfrey AC, Goss JE, Ogden DA, et al: Uremic hemopericardium. *Am J Med* 1968;45:391–400.
92. Milutinovich J, Follette WC, Scribner BN: Spontaneous retroperitoneal bleeding in patients on chronic hemodialysis. *Ann Intern Med* 1977;86:189–192.
93. Galen MA, Steinberg SM, Lowrie EG, et al: Hemorrhage pleural effusion in patients undergoing chronic hemodialysis. *Ann Intern Med* 1975;82:359–361.
94. Stewart JH, Tuckwell LA, Sinnett PF: Peritoneal and haemodialysis: a comparison of their morbidity and of the mortality suffered by dialyzed patients. *Q J Med* 1965;35:407–420.
95. Eschbach JW: Hematologic problems of dialysis patients, in Drukker W, Parsons FM, Maher JF (eds): *Replacement of Renal Function by Dialysis.* Boston, M Nijoff, 1983, pp 630–645.
96. Whitehead VM, Comty CH, Posen GA, et al: Homeostasis of folic acid in patients undergoing maintenance hemodialysis. *N Engl J Med* 1968;279:970–974.
97. Hemmeloff AKE: Folic acid status of patients with chronic renal failure maintained by dialysis. *Clin Nephrol* 1977;8: 510–513.
98. Caro J, Brown S, Miller O, et al: Erythropoietin levels in uremic nephric and anephric patients. *J Lab Clin Med* 1979; 93:449–458.
99. Fisher JW: Mechanism of the anemia of chronic renal failure. *Nephron* 1980;25: 106–111.
100. Zappacosta AR, Caro J, Erslev A: Normalization of hematocrit in patients with end-stage renal disease in continuous ambulatory peritoneal dialysis. *Am J Med* 1982;72:53–57.
101. Duke M, Abelmann WH: The hemodynamic response to chronic anemia. *Circulation* 1969;39:503–515.
102. Bell JD, Kincaid WR, Morgan RG, et al: Serum ferritin assay and bone marrow iron stores in patients on maintenance hemodialysis. *Kidney Int* 1980;17:237–241.
103. Gokal R, Millard PR, Weatherall DJ, et al: Iron metabolism in hemodialysis patients. *Q J Med* 1979;48:369–391.
104. Neff MS, Goldberg J, Slifkin RF, et al: A comparison of androgens for anemia in patients on hemodialysis. *N Engl J Med* 1981;304:871–875.
105. Singer JW, Adamson JW: Steroids and hematopoiesis. II. The effect of steroids on in vitro erythroid colony growth: Evidence for different target cells for different classes of steroids. *J Cell Physiol* 1976;88:135–144.
106. Walton WK: The failing immune system. *J Chronic Dis* 1983;36:129–135.
107. Weksler ME: Senescence of the immune system. *Med Clin North Am* 1983;67:263–271.
108. Sinwatratananonta P, Sinsakul V, Stern K, et al: Defective chemotaxis in uremia. *J Lab Clin Med* 1978;92:402–407.
109. Goldblum SE, Reed WP: Host defenses and immunologic alterations associated with chronic hemodialysis. *Ann Intern Med* 1980;93:597–613.
110. Kauffman CA, Manzler AD, Phair JP: Cell-mediated immunity in patients on long-term hemodialysis. *Clin Exp Immunol* 1975;22:54–61.
111. Touraine JL, Touraine F, Revillard JP, et al: T-lymphocytes and serum inhibitors of

cell-mediated immunity in renal insufficiency. *Nephron* 1975;14:195–208.
112. Sengar D, Rashid A, Harris J: In vitro cellular immunity and in vivo delayed hypersensitivity in uremic patients maintained on hemodialysis. *Int Arch Allergy Appl Immunol* 1974;47:829–838.
113. Dobkin JE, Miller MW, Steighegel NH: Septicemia in patients on chronic hemodialysis. *Ann Intern Med* 1978;88:28–33.
114. Nsouli KA, Lazarus MJ, Schoenbaum SC, et al: Bacteremic infection in hemodialysis. *Arch Intern Med* 1979;139: 1255–1258.
115. Keane WF, Shapiro FL, Raji L: Incidence and type of infections occurring in 445 chronic hemodialysis patients. *Trans Am Soc Artif Intern Organs* 1977;23;41–47.
116. Keane WF, Rau LR: Host defenses and infectious complications in maintenance hemodialysis patients, in Drukker W, Parsons FM, Maher JF (eds): *Replacement of Renal Function by Dialysis.* Boston, M Nijhoff, 1983, pp 646–658.
117. Bailey GL, Griffiths H, Lock JP, et al: Gastrointestinal abnormalities in uremia, abstract in *5th Annual Meeting American Society of Nephrology.* Washington, DC, 1971, p 5.
118. Cunningham JT: Gastric telangiectasias in chronic hemodialysis patients: A report of six cases. *Gastroenterology* 1981;81: 1131–1133.
119. Jacobs C, Reach I, DeGoulet P: Cancer in patients on hemodialysis. *N Engl J Med* 1979;300:1279–1280.
120. Marousos ON, Truelove SC, Lumsden K: Transit times of food in patients with diverticulosis or irritable colon syndrome and normal subjects. *Br Med J* 1967;3: 760–762.
121. Parks TG: Natural history of diverticular disease of the colon. *Clin Gastroenterol* 1975;4:53–69.
122. Adams PL, Rutsky EA, Rostand SG, et al: Lower gastrointestinal tract dysfunction in patients receiving long-term hemodialysis. *Arch Intern Med* 1982;142:303–306.
123. Lipschutz DE, Easterling RE: Spontaneous perforation of the colon in chronic renal failure. *Arch Intern Med* 1973;132: 758–759.
124. Johnson WJ, O'Brien PC: Effectiveness of intestinal phosphate binders in patients maintained by hemodialysis. *Nephron* 1978;21:123–130.
125. Welch JP, Schweizer RT, Bartus SA: Management of antacid impactions in hemodialysis and renal transplant patients. *Am J Surg* 1980;139:561–568.
126. Young AW Jr, Sweeney EW, David DS, et al: Dermatologic evaluation of pruritus in patients on hemodialysis. *NY State J Med* 1973;73:2670–2674.
127. Hampers CL, Katz AI, Wilson RE, et al: Disappearance of "uremic" itching after subtotal parathyroidectomy. *N Engl J Med* 1968;279:695–697.
128. Silverberg DS, Iaina A, Reisin E, et al: Cholestyramine in uraemic pruritus. *Br Med J* 1977;1:752–753.
129. Gilchrest BA, Rowe JW, Brown RS, et al: Relief of uremic pruritus with ultraviolet phototherapy. *N Engl J Med* 1977;297: 136–138.
130. Pederson JA, Matter BJ, Czerwinski AW, et al: Relief of idiopathic generalized pruritus in dialysis patients treated with activated oral charcoal. *Ann Intern Med* 1980;93:446–448.
131. Tapia L, Cheigh JS, David DS, et al: Pruritus in dialysis patients treated with parenteral lidocaine. *N Engl J Med* 1977; 296:261–262.
132. Mendoza CB Jr, Postlethwait RW, Johnson WD: Incidence of wound disruption following operation. *Arch Surg* 1970;101: 396–398.
133. Morein G, Goldschmidt Z, Pauker M, et al: Spontaneous tendon ruptures in patients treated by chronic hemodialysis. *Clin Orthop* 1977;124:209–213.
134. Jain VK, Cestero RVM, Baum J: Carpal tunnel syndrome in patients undergoing hemodialysis. *JAMA* 1979;242:2868–2869.
135. Ellman MH, Brown NL, Katzenberg CA: Acute pseudogout in chronic renal failure. *Arch Intern Med* 1979;139:795–796.
136. Hoffman GS, Schumacher R, Paul H, et al: Calcium oxalate microcrystalline-associated arthritis in end-stage renal disease. *Ann Intern Med* 1982;97:36–42.
137. Mathews M, Shen FH, Lindner A, et al: Septic arthritis in hemodialyzed patients. *Nephron* 1980;25:87–91.
138. Drukker W: Peritoneal dialysis: A historical review, in Drukker W, Parsons FM, Maher J (eds): *Replacement of Renal*

Function by Dialysis. Boston, M Nijhoff, 1983, pp 410–439.
139. Merrill JP, Sabbaga E, Henderson L, et al: The use of an indwelling plastic conduit for chronic peritoneal irrigation. *Trans Am Soc Artif Intern Organs* 1962;8:252–255.
140. Tenckhoff H, Schechter W: A bacteriologically safe peritoneal access device. *Trans Am Soc Artif Intern Organs* 1968;14:181–186.
141. Popovich RP, Moncrief JW, Decherd JB, et al: The definition of a novel portable/wearable equilibrium peritoneal dialysis technique, abstracted. *Am Soc Artif Intern Organs* 1976;5:64.
142. Popovich RP, Moncrief JW, Nolph KD, et al: Continuous ambulatory peritoneal dialysis. *Ann Intern Med* 1978;88:449–456.
143. Kaye M, Pajel PA, Somerville JP: Four years experience with continuous ambulatory peritoneal dialysis (CAPD) in the elderly. *Perit Dial Bull* 1983;3:17–19.
144. Nicholls AJ, Waldek S, Platts MM, et al: Impact of continuous ambulatory peritoneal dialysis on treatment of renal failure in patients aged over 60. *Br Med J [Clin Res]* 1984;288:18–19.
145. Steinberg SM, Cutler SJ, Novak JW, et al: Characteristics of participants and selected outcome measures for the period January 1, 1981 through June 30, 1983, in *Report of the National CAPD Registry of the National Institutes of Health*, Bethesda, Maryland, 1984.
146. Brown PM, Johnston KW, Fenton SS, et al: Symptomatic exacerbation of peripheral vascular disease with chronic ambulatory peritoneal dialysis. *Clin Nephrol* 1981;16:258–261.
147. Wehling M, Jenni R, Steurer J, et al: Ischemic colitis in a patient undergoing CAPD. *Perit Dial Bull* 1982;2:123–124.
148. Hamodraka-Mailis A: Pathogenesis and treatment of back pain in peritoneal dialysis patients. *Perit Dial Bull* 1983;3(suppl):S41–43.
149. Digenis GE, Khanna R, Mathews R, et al: Abdominal hernias in patients undergoing continuous ambulatory peritoneal dialysis. *Perit Dial Bull* 1982;2:115–117.
150. Rubin J, Raji S, Teal N, et al: Abdominal hernia in patients undergoing continuous ambulatory peritoneal dialysis. *Arch Intern Med* 1982;142:1453–1455.
151. Disney AP, Correll RL: Report of the Australian and New Zealand combined dialysis and transplant registry. *Med J Aust* 1981;1:117–122.
152. Roberts JL: Analysis and outcome of 1063 patients trained for home hemodialysis. *Kidney Int* 1976;9:363–374.
153. Hutchinson TA, Thomas DC, MacGibbon B: Predicting survival with end-stage renal disease: an age-equivalence index. *Ann Intern Med* 1982;96:417–423.
154. Weller JM, Port FK, Swartz RD, et al: Analysis of survival of end-stage renal disease patients. *Kidney Int* 1982;21:78–83.
155. Lewis EJ, Foster DM, De La Puente J, et al: Survival data for patients undergoing chronic intermittent hemodialysis. *Ann Intern Med* 1969;70:311–315.
156. Bailey GL, Mocelin AJ, Griffiths HJL, et al: Hemodialysis and renal transplantation in patients of the 50–80 age group. *J Am Geriatr Soc* 1972;20:421–428.
157. Shapiro FL, Umer A: Risk factors in hemodialysis patient survival. *Am Soc Artif Intern Organs* 1983;6:176–184.

CHAPTER 14 Renal Transplantation in the Elderly

Ashley Baquero
Mitchell H. Goldman

The elderly population has steadily increased in numbers since the beginning of this century.[1] Advances in chronic hemodialysis and peritoneal dialysis, as well as more sophisticated technics in vascular and peritoneal access surgery, have made long-term maintenance dialysis a routine treatment for patients with end-stage renal disease. Historically, most patients who are considered ideal transplant candidates have no complicating disease and are between the age of 16 and 45 years. Ironically, many of the patients who die of kidney disease are over the age of 50.[2] The number of transplants performed on patients over 50 years is increasing, but this population represents at present a minority of transplant recipients. In the ESRD Network 30 (Virginia and West Virginia), of 458 renal allografts done from 1977 to 1980, only 83 were performed in patients over 50 years of age.[3] Of this group, 82 were cadaver transplants and one was a living related donor transplant from a sibling. Of 403 patients who received cadaver allografts, 180 (45%) were alive and had good renal function 1 year after transplant. An additional 28 patients (7%) died with good renal function. In the subgroup of 82 patients over 50 years of age, 38 patients (46%) were alive and had good renal function 1 year after transplant. Additionally, 10 patients (12%) died with good renal function. Thus, both groups had similar 1-year graft survival, but the mortality rate was higher in the older group and was similar to that encountered in the same age group treated with chronic hemodialysis.[4]

In general, cadaver renal transplantation carries lower graft and patient survival when compared to living related donor allografts. The availability of living related donors for patients over 50 years of age is limited. Parents are no longer living and siblings are apt to be old or have complicating diseases which eliminate them as potential donors. Consideration of a young child for organ donation to an aged parent represents a special ethical problem in our society. With the application of the donor-specific blood transfusion (DST) protocol introduced by Salvatierra,[5] the number of living related donors may be expected to increase. However, the great majority of those recipients of advanced age will still depend on cadaver donors for transplantation. In the general transplant population, chronic glomerulonephritis and chronic tubulo-interstitial nephritis constitute the two most common causes of ESRD. Among the older age group there is also a preponderance of polycystic degeneration and atherosclerotic and hypertensive nephrosclerosis.

SELECTION OF TRANSPLANT CANDIDATES

The criteria for selection of transplant candidates among patients over 50 years of age do not necessarily differ from the general criteria for selection in younger groups. A biologically well-maintained patient without major pulmonary disease who is free of uncontrolled malignancy or infection should be considered for transplantation. It is a fact that older patients with ESRD are a high-risk group regardless of the modality of treatment used. This poor prognosis is related to the numerous associated diseases seen in patients over 50 years of age. In addition, there is some evidence that atherosclerosis is accelerated in the dialysis population, perhaps because of abnormalities in blood lipoprotein constituents.[6]

Prior to transplantation all transplant candidates undergo a series of laboratory evaluations which are similar to the preoperative workup for major surgery (Table 14-1). In addition, the routine pretransplant evaluation involves specific immunologic studies including red cell ABO and Lewis typing and tissue-typing of the HLA-A, -B, -C, and -D loci using peripheral lymphocytes. Serial circulating lymphocytotoxic antibody determinations are also performed by testing the recipient's serum against a panel of known lymphocyte donors. Sera are collected for donor-specific crossmatching. When a potential living related donor is evaluated, a mixed lymphocyte culture (MLC) is carried out and patients in whom the stimulation index is high are considered for donor-specific transfusion. When donor-specific transfusion is utilized, pretreatment with azathioprine should be considered to decrease the possibility of sensitization.[7]

All patients undergo a urologic evaluation. A voiding cystourethrogram is performed to: (*a*) delineate the anatomy of the bladder and urethra, (*b*) measure the capacity of the bladder, (*c*) evaluate for the presence of ureterovesical reflux, (*d*) evaluate the emptying mechanism, and (*e*) identify potential urosepsis. Any anatomical obstruction to urinary outflow should be repaired prior to transplantation. If significant ureteral reflux is present, nephrectomy and total ureterectomy are indicated. When an adequate emptying mechanism is absent, an ileal conduit or repeated bladder catheterization by the patient may be entertained, but both methods are associated with an increased risk of infection. Small bladders are usually enlarged after transplantation. A urine culture is obtained from a catheterization specimen at the time of the cystourethrogram.

The upper gastrointestinal (GI) tract is evaluated for the presence of peptic ulcer disease. If ulcer, obstruction, or heavy scarring is found or if the patient has a strong history of peptic ulcer disease, highly selective vagotomy is performed prior to transplantation.

Table 14-1
Pretransplant Evaluation

Routine Preoperative Laboratory Workup
- CBC
- Blood type
- Electrolytes
- Blood sugar
- Urinalysis
- Chest X-ray film
- ECG
- Coagulation studies

General Pretransplant Workup
- Tissue typing
- Monthly cytotoxic antibody levels
- MLC with living related donor
- Voiding cystourethrogram
- Upper GI series
- Urine culture
- Bilateral nephrectomy and/or splenectomy
- Blood transfusions

Considerations in Older Patients
- Urological: prostate examination, cystoscopy
- GI: barium enema
- Cardiovascular: stress test, MUGA scan, angiography
- Cerebrovascular: carotid artery Doppler evaluation
- Peripheral vascular disease: noninvasive vascular laboratory studies
- Pulmonary: sputum cultures, pulmonary function tests
- Infections: PPD skin test
- Endocrine: glucose tolerance test

CBC = complete blood cell count, MLC = mixed lymphocyte culture, MUGA scan = multiple gated blood pool scintigraphy

In the past, bilateral nephrectomy and splenectomy were part of the pretransplant preparation. Now, bilateral nephrectomy is performed only in patients with ureteral reflux, polycystic kidneys with documented urinary tract infection or bleeding, recurrent pyelonephritis, and in selected patients with intractable hypertension. The beneficial effect of pretransplant splenectomy is controversial. In some patients who are leukopenic prior to transplantation, splenectomy may be considered. While the salutary effect of pretransplant blood transfusions is now widely accepted, the number and timing of blood transfusions remain unclear. Most centers recommend three to five transfusions during the year prior to transplantation. Some authors believe that a blood transfusion given at the time of surgery has the same beneficial effect without the risk of sensitization. There are several considerations specific to the elderly candidates which should be noted in the pretransplant workup.

Urologic complications Obstructive benign prostatic hypertrophy (BPH) is commonly seen after 50 years of age and should be surgically corrected prior to transplantation. Hematuria in this age group should lead to a workup for malignancy. Transitional cell carcinoma of the bladder is usually a contraindication to transplantation because it may be multifocal and may recur. Localized renal cell carcinoma, treated by total excision, does not contraindicate transplantation.

Gastrointestinal complications Unlike younger patients, ulcer disease is not usually a problem in the elderly. However, since it has catastrophic sequelae, its presence should be sought in the elderly. In addition, many patients over 50 years of age who are on hemodialysis have diverticulosis. Colon perforation is an almost uniformly fatal complication in renal allograft recipients. In selected cases with severe localized diverticulosis, a segmental colectomy should be considered before transplantation. All attempts must be made to prevent constipation after transplantation because cecal perforation is catastrophic. Careful attention should be paid to the constipating characteristics of certain antacids, and a stool softener used.

Cardiovascular complications Septic and cardiovascular complications are the most common causes of death in the posttransplant period. An exhaustive evaluation of the patient's cardiac status is imperative. A history of chest pain, which would suggest the presence of coronary artery disease, is of great value and warrants further evaluation such as a stress test, nuclear medicine scans, ejection fraction determination, and coronary angiography. Many patients have received renal allografts after successful coronary artery bypass surgery. Congestive heart failure must be controlled before transplantation.

Peripheral vascular disease The incidence of occlusive disease of the hypogastric artery in a general population of renal transplant recipients as reported by Starzl et al[8] is approximately 20% though higher incidence values have been observed by others in patients aged 40 or over. The use of the common iliac or external iliac artery for arterial inflow may be necessary. With the availability of noninvasive vascular laboratories, a pretransplant vascular evaluation could help discover severe iliofemoral disease needing surgical correction prior to transplantation. In the case of mild to moderate arteriosclerotic iliac disease, a pretransplant Doppler ultrasound evaluation would be useful in selecting the best iliac artery for use at the time of transplantation.

Five transplant recipients in our series had posttransplant cerebrovascular accidents. Four of these occurred during the first year after transplant. All of them resulted in the death of the patient. Carotid artery disease should never be overlooked and if symptomatic disease or severe flow-limiting lesions are present, endarterectomy of the involved artery is indicated before transplantation.

Pulmonary evaluation Those individuals with a history of heavy smoking and chronic cough, sputum production, and exertional dyspnea should undergo pulmonary function tests. Although pulmonary insufficiency is almost never severe enough to contraindicate surgery, pulmonary function tests are useful in selecting patients who will be at high risk for postoperative pulmonary complications. The patient with chronic bronchopulmonary infection presents a problem when given immunosuppressive therapy for transplantation. Many elderly patients have a long history of smoking and have excessive perioperative secretions with subsequent atelectasis and pneumonitis. Preoperatively, sputum culture and sensitivity is mandatory since it will facilitate subsequent control of pulmonary infection. Sputum stain and cultures for acid-fast bacilli are also performed. A PPD skin test is applied, if indicated. Any suspicious abnormality in the chest film must be diagnosed and treated appropriately before transplantation. Tuberculosis is treated for at least 6 months to 1 year before transplantation is considered. Postoperative incentive spirometry and physiotherapy are mandatory.

DONOR AGE

Controversy exists regarding the functional quality of the aging kidney. Although the glomerular filtration rate (GFR) and creatinine clearance decrease with age,[9,10] the serum creatinine level remains normal, probably because of changes in lean body mass. Friedman et al[11] have shown that radioisotope scanning of the kidney is commonly abnormal in elderly patients. It is difficult to explain these changes, especially in the absence of proteinuria or reduced kidney size. One explanation for the functional defects in the aging kidney involves intrarenal vascular changes.[12] Several clinical studies differ concerning the use of kidneys from different donor age groups. This difference may be because of lack of controls in the recipient age group. When both donor and recipient ages are controlled, the difference disappears. Donor age does not seem to have a deleterious effect on the outcome of kidney transplantation using cadaver donors or living donors.[13,14]

OPERATIVE CONSIDERATIONS

The operative technic of renal transplantation has been described by many authors and is uniformly accepted. Classically, the renal artery is sutured end-to-end to the hypogastric artery and the renal vein is sutured end-to-side to the iliac vein. A ureteroneocystostomy completes the operation. Careful ligation of recipient lymphatics helps to prevent postoperative lymphocele. Since over 40% of renal transplant recipients over the age of 40 years have hypogastric artery occlusive disease, alternatives to using the hypogastric artery must be entertained. The common iliac artery or the external iliac artery can be used as the host site for an end-to-side arterial anastomosis. The discrepancy in the wall thickness between these two arteries makes the anastomosis difficult, but this may be overcome by using a Carrel patch of donor aorta (Figure 14-1). On occasion, the common iliac artery and the external iliac artery are also involved in the disease process and the use of vein patch, donor aortic patch, or prosthetic graft may be necessary.

Endarterectomy of the hypogastric artery may also be performed. Occasionally, opening of the common iliac artery through a longitudinal arteriotomy is indicated to be sure that the endarterectomy has been carried out completely and that no loose plaque remains in the common iliac or the external iliac arteries. Pseudoaneurysm after endarterectomy has not been a problem. However, because of the lack of compliance of the endarterectomized vessel, it is wise to free the hypogastric artery over its full length in order to have a long, gentle curve rather than a kink at the area of the anastomosis. The use of heparin is not necessary in either the end-to-end or end-to-side anastomosis. Every means to provide a good arterial inflow should be attempted prior to the arterial anastomosis. If a poor inflow is discovered after completion of the arterial anastomosis, the allograft must be flushed with cold solution to prevent additional warm ischemia and other sites for arterial anastomosis quickly chosen.[15] Care is taken to avoid damaging the intima of the arteries and to avoid kinking of the anastomosis because these may be causes of postoperative renal artery stenosis.

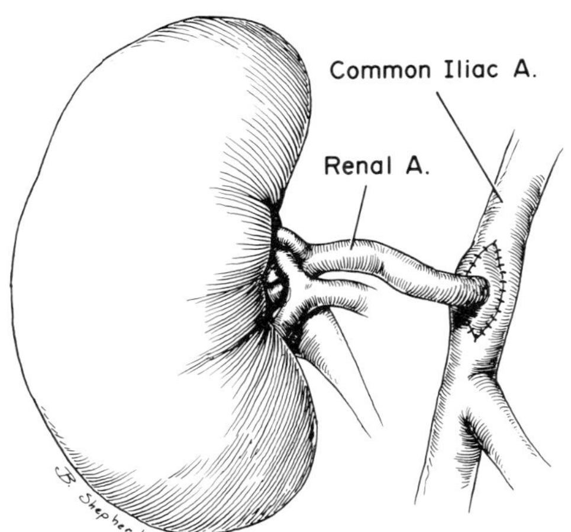

Figure 14-1 Ordinarily the renal artery is anastomosed to the hypogastric artery in an end-to-end fashion. However, when there are multiple renal arteries or when the hypogastric artery has extensive atherosclerosis, an end-to-side anastomosis using a Carrel patch of donor aorta may be performed with the recipient's common iliac artery.

Several technics have been described for the ureteroneocystostomy. The Politano-Leadbetter[16] technic is probably the most widely used. In recent years, more transplant surgeons have been using the Lich technic.[17] Briefly, the Politano-Leadbetter technic consists of an internal ureteroneocystostomy in which the distal ureter is tunneled through the submucosa of the bladder wall in the inferolateral aspect of the bladder. An anterior cystotomy is required for this procedure. The Lich technic is an external ureteroneocystostomy in which the distal end of the ureter is anastomosed to the mucosa of the bladder wall in the anterolateral position and then is covered with the seromuscular layers of the bladder wall. Another technic advocated by some authors[18] is the pyeloureterostomy using the recipient's own ureter. Each method has its advantages and disadvantages and every transplant surgeon should be familiar with them (Figure 14-2).

After flow is re-established to the allograft, a renal biopsy is performed. In addition, a capsulotomy is performed to prevent renal allograft rupture. While the use of postoperative drains is somewhat controversial, a suction catheter may be useful in the immediate postoperative period to eliminate hematomas and subsequent wound infection.[19]

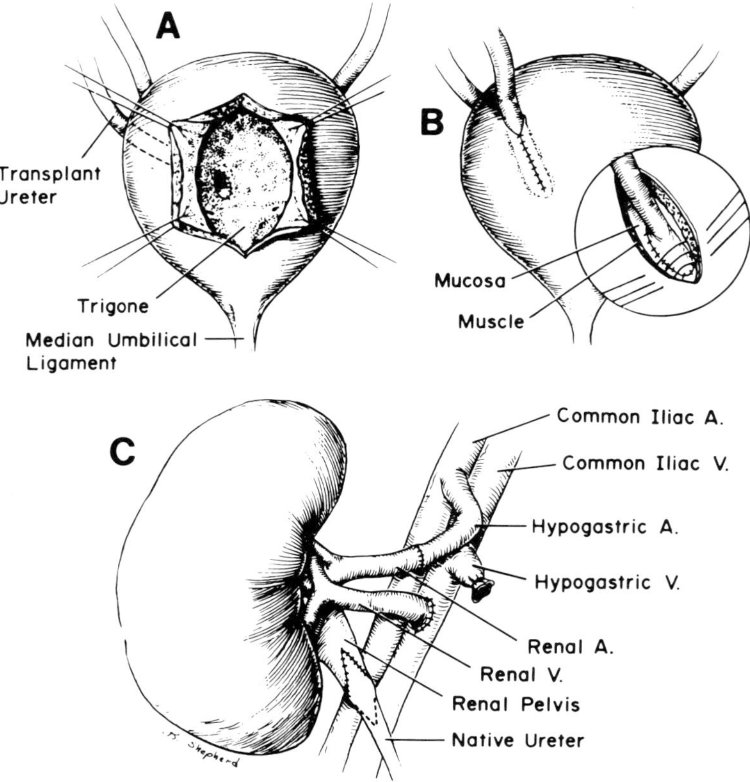

Figure 14-2 Three methods of establishing continuity of the urinary tract in transplantation of the kidney: Politano-Leadbetter technic of submucosal tunnel through a cystotomy (A); submucosal tunnel of Lich using a ureteral-mucosal anastomosis (B); and pyeloureterostomy (C).

POSTOPERATIVE CARE

The majority of transplant recipients usually do not require special care. The surgery itself is done retroperitoneally and unless complications arise, it should not cause much discomfort to the patients. Most transplant centers have their own unit to which patients return from the recovery room. In centers where a transplant unit is not available, it is wise to send patients to the intensive care unit for at least 24 hours. Care is taken to prevent contact with contagious diseases and strict aseptic technic is used. After the transplant, fluid management is of utmost importance, especially in cadaver donors, where some delay in function of the allograft is frequently encountered. The central venous pressure must be monitored and in patients with compromised cardiopulmonary function, a Swan-Ganz catheter is indicated. Intravascular volume must be maintained to ensure adequate renal blood flow.[20] When acute tubular necrosis (ATN) occurs, a high dose of diuretics should be considered since it has been observed that this occasionally induces a high output renal failure which is considerably easier to manage. Often the patient will not require postoperative dialysis. When immediate function is obtained, the postoperative course should be smooth and recovery fast.

Anti-embolic stockings are used routinely and passive exercises in bed with early ambulation is encouraged. Oral intake is started as early as the evening of or the day after surgery. The Foley catheter is removed two to five days after surgery, depending on the type of ureteroneocystostomy used.

Immunosuppressive Therapy

Human immunocompetence decreases with age.[21] Whether the aging process is responsible for the decrease in immunocompetence or the loss of normal immune response plays a role in the aging process is still controversial. Nevertheless, all renal allograft recipients beyond the pediatric age group are given similar immunosuppressive therapy. Azathioprine and steroids remain the most widely used immunosuppressive agents following transplantation. Local radiation, lymphoplasmapheresis, thoracic duct drainage, total lymphoid irradiation, and antithymocyte globulin (ATG)[22–24] may be part of different protocols around the world. In the near future, more specific and sophisticated immunologic monitoring and more specific and less toxic immunosuppressive agents will be available for practical use.[25]

Recent reports with cyclosporine are encouraging.[26,27] Lower doses of steroids are needed when used in combination with cyclosporine; thus steroid-related complications are decreased. This is of great value, especially in diabetic patients. Also, evidence is available that cyclosporine may permit better patient and graft survival in the elderly group as reported by Ringden et al.[28] However, complications related to the use of cyclosporine have been described. Hirsutism, nausea, vomiting, tremor, nephrotoxicity, hepatotoxicity, hypertension, and lymphoma are among the complications seen with cyclosporine therapy. The application of monoclonal antibodies to the manipulation of the immune system is promising. Whatever immunosuppressive regimen is used, the tendency is to reduce the prednisone dose given to elderly patients in many transplant centers.[29,30]

REJECTION

The classic picture of rejection is characterized by oliguria, enlargement and tenderness of the graft, malaise, fever, leukocytosis, hypertension, weight gain, and peripheral edema. However, the clinical manifestations of allograft rejection are not always fully expressed. The most reliable clinical signs of ongoing rejection are weight gain and decrease in urinary output associated with elevation of the serum creatinine and BUN. Serial radionuclide scans are also useful in establishing the diagnosis of rejection. A slight delay in the vascular phase and a decreased excretory rate are seen in association with rejection.[31] Other methods of evaluating the disturbance in renal blood flow which occurs during transplant rejection have been described.[32,33] Renal biopsy is an excellent diagnostic tool, but is not always necessary. Fine needle aspiration biopsy may be helpful in differentiating rejection from other causes of a poorly functioning kidney.[34] Urinary tract infection, obstruction by lymphocele or hematoma, urinary leak, and vascular complications must all be ruled out. The diagnosis of rejection is made even more difficult when cyclosporine is used as the primary immunosuppressive agent. The nephrotoxicity of cyclosporine may be confused with rejection. Assays for cyclosporine blood levels and renal biopsy will help in differentiating rejection from cyclosporine nephrotoxicity. Also, there is some indication that cytomegalovirus may produce a glomerulonephritis which may clinically mimic rejection.[35] In this situation, treatment with increased doses of corticosteroids is contraindicated. Creatinine clearance, fractional sodium clearance, urinary and serum β-2-microglobulins, and urinary thromboxane-B_2 have also been used in diagnosing rejection.[36,37] It is especially important in the elderly population to make a clear-cut diagnosis of rejection in order to avoid the complications of steroid toxicity. When the diagnosis of rejection has been made, methylprednisolone, antithymocyte globulin (ATG), plasmaleukopheresis, local irradiation, and monoclonal antibodies have been used to treat the rejection episode. Cyclosporine may also have a role in the treatment of rejection. Second and third episodes of rejection may be treated; however, the treatment of multiple rejection episodes has to be weighed against the prognosis for ultimate graft function and the increase in complications associated with higher quantitative doses of immunosuppressive drugs.

At the Medical College of Virginia and the McGuire Veterans Administration Medical Center, of the 48 grafts lost in the first year, the cause in 21 (44%) was death. Rejection was the second leading cause of graft loss, involving 13 patients (27%) who rejected their allografts. Primary nonfunction allografts were seen mainly during the early years of the transplant programs and accounted for nine grafts lost (19%). In addition, urinary complications were the cause of graft loss in four patients (8%). One graft loss (2%) was due to discontinued immunosuppression, and in one (2%) the cause of loss was undetermined. Thus in the elderly renal transplant recipient, death from complications of transplantation occurs more often than rejection. This would suggest that lowering the immunosuppressive dose coupled with less vigorous antirejection therapy, and acceptance of graft failure in some instances, might improve the long-term results of transplantation in this group. Also, it is expected that the introduction of new immunosuppressive drugs such as cyclosporine will contribute to a better graft and patient survival.

COMPLICATIONS

Most clinical complications of transplantation occur in the first year after transplantation. Postoperative complications include arterial occlusion or leakage, venous thrombosis, urinary leakage, lymphocele, hematoma, and wound infection.[19,38,39] Vascular problems in the elderly may be related to the advanced atherosclerosis seen in this population.[40] Wound infection may be treated with postoperative antibiotics. Other complications are closely related to the type and quantity of immunosuppression, especially in patients over 45 who seem to be at a higher risk.

The most common complications seen in the first year after transplantation in the elderly are sepsis, myocardial infarction, and cerebrovascular accidents. Urosepsis from bladder catheterization or from urinary retention caused by prostatic hypertrophy is common.[41] Pulmonary infections are also common and must be diagnosed and treated aggressively. Sputum cultures, tracheal aspiration, bronchoscopy, and open or closed pulmonary biopsy are used expeditiously to diagnose accurately the nature of a pulmonary infiltrate so that appropriate therapy may be instituted. Because of the higher incidence of diverticula in the elderly, diverticulitis is more often seen both in the dialysis and in the transplant population. Perforation or abscess in association with diverticulitis has up to an 80% mortality and should be diagnosed aggressively. Often the immunosuppressed patient will not manifest the usual signs of abdominal catastrophe. There may be vague or diffuse abdominal pain without peritoneal signs. Fever or leukocytosis may be absent. Pancreatitis, mesenteric ischemia, appendicitis, and perforated peptic ulcer may be considered in the differential diagnosis and should be quickly evaluated. However, surgical exploration on the basis of a suspicion of an abdominal catastrophic event may be the only means of making the diagnosis and may be life-saving. Exteriorization or resection of the diseased colon with diversion should be performed. Appropriate antibiotics should be given and the immunosuppression regimen reduced when possible.

Malignancy is also seen frequently in the immunosuppressed population. This is also true for the elderly population and the coexistence of immunosuppression and an older age group of patients may result in an increased occurrence of malignancy.

Squamous cell carcinomas of the skin, Kaposi's sarcoma, lymphomas, and cervical carcinoma are all seen in a higher incidence in the immunosuppressed population. In addition, cyclosporine has been associated with an increased incidence of both polyclonal and monoclonal lymphomas. Surprisingly, the malignancies commonly associated with the older age group, such as colon, prostatic, and pulmonary cancer, have not been reported to be increased after transplantation. This is perhaps due to the relatively recent extension of transplantation to the geriatric population, the resultant small numbers of recipients, and the shorter follow-up of this group. As graft survival becomes longer and as more elderly patients receive allografts, more intensive surveillance for these malignancies will be warranted. Other complications seen in the elderly transplant population are easily bruised and friable skin, diabetes mellitus, musculoskeletal disturbances, hypertension, cataracts, polycythemia, Cushing's syndrome, and renal artery stenosis.[42]

In the Medical College of Virginia–McGuire Veterans Administration Medical Center series, 74 patients over 50 years of age received 85 allografts. The 1- and 2-year actuarial graft survival was 43% and 37%, respectively (Figure 14-3). Of the 74 patients, 22 (30%) died during the first year after transplantation. Of the 22 deaths during the first year, 11 patients (50%) died of septic complications; four (19%) of cerebrovascular accidents; three of myocardial infarction, one of whom was on dialysis; one of lymphoma; one of liver failure complicated by sepsis; one of pulmonary insufficiency complicated by sepsis; and one was a surgical mortality following repair of renal artery stenosis. Of the 11 patients who died from primary septic complications, six patients (54%) never had a rejection episode. It seems from this experience and from information reported in other series that lowering the immunosuppressive dose in the elderly patient may result in better patient survival without changing the actual graft survival. Long-term complications of transplantation were related mostly to cardiovascular problems. Of the 40 patients in the Medical College of Virginia–McGuire VA Medical Center series who were followed from 1 to 4 years after transplantation, only two died, one from myocardial infarction and the other from cerebrovascular accident. Other complications of peripheral vascular disease were seen in this population which necessitated treatment in a fashion similar to the nontransplant population.

SUMMARY

The practice of surgery in the geriatric age group is a challenge. Renal transplantation as an alternative for the elderly patient with end-stage renal disease can be successful if careful attention is paid to the assessment of associated diseases and the correct application of immunosuppressive regimens. The early mortality rate associated with transplantation may be lowered by reducing the septic and vascular complications with lower doses of immunosuppression. If a low complication and mortality rate can be maintained, the rehabilitation

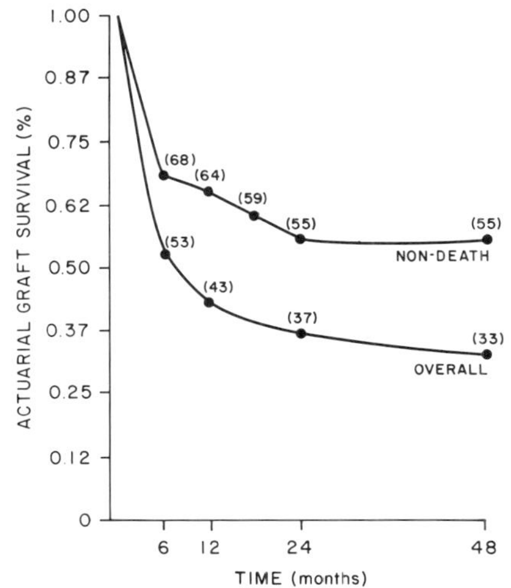

Figure 14-3 Cadaver graft survival in recipients over the age of 50 years old using conventional immunosuppression. The "non-death" group represents graft survival in patients who did not die of early complications such as sepsis and cardiovascular disease.

and independence achieved with a successful transplant make renal transplantation in elderly patients with chronic renal failure a reasonable option.[43–45]

REFERENCES

1. Rowe JW: Influence of age on renal function. *Residents Staff Physicians* 1978; 24:49–55.
2. *Vital Statistics of the United States 1980 Mortality.* US Dept of Health, Education and Welfare, Public Health Service, National Vital Statistics Division, 1963, vol 2, part A.
3. End Stage Renal Disease Network 30. Transplantation Outcome Survey, 1980.
4. Krakauer H, Grauman JS, McMullun MR, et al: The recent US experience in the treatment of end-stage renal disease by dialysis and transplantation. *N Engl J Med* 1983; 308:1558–1563.
5. Cochrum KC, Hanes D, Potter D, et al: Donor specific blood transfusions in HLA-O-disparate one haplotype-related allografts. *Transplant Proc* 1979;11:1903–1907.
6. Goldberg AP, Harter HR, Patsch W, et al: Racial differences in plasma high-density lipoproteins in patients receiving hemodialysis. *N Engl J Med* 1983;308:1245–1252.
7. Anderson CB, Sicard GH, Etheridge E: Pretreatment of renal allograft recipients with azathioprine and donor-specific blood products. *Surgery* 1982;92:315–321.
8. Starzl TE, Porter KA, Husberg BS, et al: Renal homotransplantation – Part II. *Curr Probl Surg* 1974;5:1–54.
9. Davies DF, Shock NW: Age changes in glomerular filtration rate, effective renal plasma flow, and tubular excretory capacity in adult males. *J Clin Invest* 1950;29: 496–507.
10. Lewis WH, Alving AS: Changes with age in the renal function of adult men. *Am J Physiol* 1938;123:505–515.
11. Friedman SA, Raizner AE, Rosen H, et al: Functional defects in the aging kidney. *Ann Intern Med* 1972;76:41–45.
12. Takazakura E, Sawabu N, Handa A, et al: Intrarenal vascular changes with age and disease. *Kidney Int* 1972;2:224–230.
13. Speybroeck JV, Feduska N, Amend W, et al: The influence of donor age on graft survival. *Am J Surg* 1979;137:374–377.
14. Matas AJ, Simmons RL, Kjellstrand CM, et al: Transplantation of the aging kidney. *Transplantation* 1976;21:160–161.
15. Geis PW, Giacchino JL, Jacobi RJ, et al: Technical considerations in elderly renal allograft recipients. *Am J Surg* 1976; 132:332–335.
16. Politano VA, Leadbetter WF: An operative technique for correction of vesicoureteral reflux. *J Urol* 1958;79:932–941.
17. McDonald JC, Rohr MS, Frentz BD: External ureteroneocystostomy and ureteroureterostomy in renal transplantation. *Ann Surg* 1979;190:663–667.
18. Jaffers GJ, Cosimi BA, Delmonico FL, et al: Experience with pyeloureterostomy in renal transplantation. *Ann Surg* 1982;196: 588–593.
19. Muakkassa WF, Goldman MH, Mendez-Picon G, et al: Wound infection in renal transplant patients. *J Urol* 1983;130:17–19.
20. Carlier M, Squifflet JP, Dirson Y, et al: Maximal hydration during anesthesia increases pulmonary arterial pressures and improves early function of human renal transplants. *Transplantation* 1982;34: 201–204.
21. Weigle WO, Parks DE: Effect of aging on immune and tolerant states. *Fed Proc* 1978;37:1253–1257.
22. Thomas F, Mendez-Picon G, Peace K, et al: Effect of antilymphocyte-globulin potency on suvival of cadaver renal transplants. *Lancet* 1977;2:671–674.
23. Pilepich MV, Sicard GA, Breaux SR, et al: Renal graft irradiation in acute rejection. *Transplantation* 1983;35:208–211.
24. Allen NH, Dyer P, Geoghegan T, et al: Plasma exchange in acute renal allograft rejection: A controlled trial. *Transplantation* 1983;35:425–428.
25. Ellis TM, Berry CR, Mendez-Picon G, et al: Immunological monitoring of renal allograft recipients using monoclonal antibodies to human T-lymphocyte subpopulations. *Transplantation* 1982;33:317–319.
26. Starzl TE, Klintmalm GBG, Weil R, et al: Cyclosporin A and steroid therapy in sixty-six cadaver kidney recipients. *Surg Gynecol Obstet* 1981;153:486–494.
27. Halloran PF, Lein J, Aprile M, et al: Preliminary results of a randomized comparison of cyclosporine and Minnesota anti-

lymphoblast globulin. *Transplant Proc* 1982;14:627–630.
28. Rinden O, Ost L, Klintmalm C: Improved outcome in renal transplant recipient above 55 years of age treated with cyclosporine A and low doses of steroids. *Transplant Proc* 1983;15(4):2507–2512.
29. Ost L, Groth CG, Lindholm B, et al: Cadaveric renal transplantation in patients of 60 years and above. *Transplantation* 1980;30:339–340.
30. Lundgren G, Fehrman I, Gunnarsson R, et al: Cadaveric renal transplantation in patients over 55 years of age with special emphasis on immunosuppressive therapy. *Transplant Proc* 1982;14:601–604.
31. Salvatierra O, Powel MR, Price DC, et al: The advantages of I^{131}-orthoiodohippurate scintiphotography in the management of patients after renal transplantation. *Ann Surg* 1974;180:336–342.
32. Arima M, Ishibash M, Usami M, et al: Analysis of the arterial blood flow patterns of normal and allografted kidneys by the directional ultrasonic Doppler technique. *J Urol* 1979;122:587–591.
33. Berland LL, Lawson TL, Adams M, et al: Evaluation of renal transplants with pulsed Doppler duplex sonography. *J Ultrasound Med* 1982;1:215–222.
34. Hayry P, von Willebrand E: Transplant aspiration cytology in diagnostic evaluation of renal allografts. *Transplant Proc* 1981;13:1575–1578.
35. Richardson WP, Colvin RB, Cheeseman SH, et al: Glomerulopathy associated with cytomegalovirus viremia in renal allografts. *N Engl J Med* 1981;305:57–63.
36. Schweizer RT, Moore R, Bartus SA, et al: Beta 2 microglobulin monitoring after renal transplantation. *Transplant Proc* 1981;13:1620–1623.
37. Foegh ML, Zmudka M, Cooley C, et al: Urine I-TxB_2 in renal allograft rejection. *Lancet* 1981;2:431–434.
38. Goldman MH, Burleson RL, Tilney NL, et al: Calyceal cutaneous fistulae in renal transplant patients. *Ann Surg* 1976;184: 679–681.
39. Goldman MH, Leapman SB, Handy RD, et al: Renal allograft rupture with iliofemoral thrombophlebitis. *Arch Surg* 1978;113: 204–205.
40. Goldman MH, Tilney NL, Vineyard GC, et al: A twenty-year survey of arterial complications of renal transplantation. *Surg Gynecol Obstet* 1975;141:758–760.
41. Belitsky P, Lannon SG, MacDonald AS, et al: Urinary tract infections (UTI) after kidney transplantation. *Transplant Proc* 1982;14:696–699.
42. Reinitz ER, Goldman MH, Sais J, et al: Evaluation of transplant renal artery blood flow by Doppler sound-spectrum analysis. *Arch Surg* 1983;118:415–419.
43. Sommer BG, Ferguson RM, Davin TD, et al: Renal transplantation in patients over 50 years of age. *Transplant Proc* 1981;13: 33–35.
44. Abele R, Novick AC, Braun WE, et al: Long term results of renal transplantation in recipients with a functioning graft for 2 years. *Transplantation* 1982;34:264–267.
45. Vollmer WM, Wahl PW, Blagg CR: Survival with dialysis and transplantation in patients with end-stage renal disease. *N Engl J Med* 1983;308:1553–1558.

CHAPTER 15 Hypertension in the Aged

James R. Sowers
Edward T. Zawada, Jr.

The geriatric population (generally defined as 65 years of age or older) is a rapidly growing segment of our society. There are now over 25 million Americans 65 years of age or older, and it is projected that by 1990 there will be approximately 29 million. Cardiovascular disease and stroke account for the majority of deaths in this group and considerable morbidity in individuals over 65 years of age. There is accumulating evidence that increased cardiovascular morbidity and mortality in the geriatric population are associated with systolic-diastolic or isolated systolic hypertension. Although the benefits of correcting combined systolic-diastolic hypertension in the elderly are now clear, treatment of isolated systolic hypertension remains controversial. In this chapter we will examine the prevalence and risks of geriatric hypertension. We will address possible unique pathogenetic mechanisms involved in hypertension in the elderly. Finally, we will discuss the evaluation and approach to treatment of hypertension in elderly patients.

PREVALENCE AND RISK

In the United States approximately 40% of whites and more than 50% of blacks aged 65 to 74 years have systolic-diastolic hypertension (defined as systolic >160 mmHg and diastolic >95 mmHg) or isolated systolic hypertension (systolic blood pressure 160 mmHg and diastolic pressure <95 mmHg), and 30% have borderline hypertension (systolic pressure 140 to 159 mmHg and diastolic pressure 90 to 94 mmHg.[1] Diastolic blood pressure tends to peak at 50 to 60 years of age while systolic pressure continues to rise with age.[1] It appears that the majority of patients with systolic-diastolic hypertension developed elevated blood pressures in middle age which persisted into later years. A rise in systolic pressure results from a loss of elasticity within the major arteries, which get progressively thicker and more rigid secondary to the atherosclerotic process. Mean systolic blood pressure rises 20 to 40 mmHg from age 60 to 89 years, is higher for women than men at all ages, and affects as many as a third of all people over age 65. It is likely that the above figures are overestimations of the true prevalence of hypertension, particularly systolic hypertension in the elderly, because they are generally based on single blood pressure determinations. The variability of systolic blood pressure has been found to be greater in older persons.[2] It has been suggested that perhaps one third of elderly patients diagnosed as having systolic hypertension on the basis of a single measurement would prove not to have elevated pressures on subsequent determinations.[3]

Data collected from the Framingham Study have provided considerable prospective evidence of the risk of hypertension in the elderly.[4–8] From the initial cohort to 5127 persons, aged 20 to 62 years followed for 26 years with biennial examinations, it was observed that the major risk factors for cardiovascular disease including hypertension are operative throughout life. In this study borderline hypertension was defined as systolic/diastolic blood pressure levels of 140/90 to 160/95 mmHg and definite hypertension as blood pressure levels greater than 160/95 mmHg. Borderline as well as definite hypertension both were associated with an increase in mortality from coronary artery disease and stroke for men and women when compared with those with normal blood pressures. The differences became more prominent with advancing age, particularly for women. This observation clearly refuted the long-held fallacy that hypertension in elderly women is a relatively benign condition. The risk of higher blood pressure in older women appeared greatest for coronary heart disease, the risk for stroke ranging from equal to slightly greater for hypertensive elderly women as compared with men. In the Veterans Administration study,[9] age was an important factor determining morbidity and mortality. Though only 20% of all patients in that study were older than 60 years, half the morbidity was in the elderly, congestive heart failure and stroke being the most common morbid complications.

That systolic hypertension is a significant risk factor for cardiovascular morbidity and mortality is clear from the results of a number of studies. The Build and Blood Pressure Study[10] conducted by the Society of Actuaries demonstrated that, even in the face of normal diastolic blood pressures, mortality was increased by a moderate elevation of systolic blood pressure (158 to 176 mmHg). This was true for individuals below and over 60 years of age. In a study involving the follow-up of 72 residents of a California retirement community for 6 years[11] cardiovascular mortality was seven times as great in patients with systolic hypertension than in a matched control group whose blood pressures were below 140/90 mmHg. Myocardial infarction occurred twice as often in those with elevated systolic blood pressure, and angina and strokes were almost three times as frequent. The Framingham Study demonstrated that both men and women with elevated systolic but normal diastolic blood pressures are at increased risk for cardiovascular complications.[8–12] One group of investigators examined the incidence of stroke in 3400 individuals aged 65 to 74 years.[13] Hypertension occurred in 43% of the cohort, and the hypertensive subjects had twice the frequency of stroke of normotensives. Systolic hypertension was a stronger determinant of stroke than diastolic blood pressure elevation, although both were associated with increased risk. In the Chicago stroke study[14] the mortality due to coronary artery disease was increased 1.7 times, and the mortality due to all types of cardiovascular-renal causes was increased twofold in men and women aged 65 to 74 years who had systolic hypertension. Additionally, the incidence of all types of stroke as well as nonembolic brain infarction was 2.5 times greater in patients with isolated systolic hypertension.

From the above data it is clear that isolated systolic hypertension is associated with increased morbidity and mortality. However, it is not clear whether these complications are directly caused by the systolic hypertension or whether underlying atherosclerosis is responsible for the complications as well as the systolic hypertension. A major unanswered question is whether systolic hypertension accelerates development of atherosclerosis.

PATHOPHYSIOLOGY

Although the prevalence of hypertension increases with age in the United States this is not true for some of the primitive societies in Africa[15] and the Pacific islands.[16] Whereas in our society advancing age is associated with an increased incidence of obesity,[17] this trend is not observed in those primitive societies. Obesity appears to be associated with an increased incidence of hypertension,[18] which could explain the observation of age-related increases in hypertension in the United States but not in some primitive societies. In the primitive societies without age-related increases in hypertension there is a tendency to ingest much smaller amounts of sodium than is consumed in the United States. Indeed, there is evidence that age-related increases in blood pressure in this country may be related to decreased ability to excrete a sodium load with increasing age. Luft et al[19] reported that normal subjects older than 40 years of age excrete a saline load more slowly than matched controls under 40 years of age. These investigators suggested that the delayed natriuretic response after volume expansion can be attributed to decreasing glomerular filtration rate (GFR) associated with aging. In another investigation[20] an inverse correlation was observed between age and ability to excrete a saline load in the relatives of essential hypertensives but not in controls. These observations have been interpreted as suggesting that genetically determined aberrancies in the handling of sodium associated with increasing age may play a role in the increasing incidence of hypertension in individuals consuming diets high in sodium which is common in our industrialized society. There is also evidence that elderly individuals consume proportionately more sodium which is perhaps related to decreased salt taste acuity with aging.[21] Although genetic factors may predispose to high blood pressure, they may not be a critical determinant of age-related increases in blood pressure. Hamilton et al[22] found that relatives of hypertensive and normotensive propositi have identical positive regression lines for age and blood pressure. Although the regression line was higher in relatives of propositi with hypertension, the slope of regression was identical in both groups. These observations suggest that what is inherited in the relatives of hypertensives is a tendency to have higher blood pressures at any age and not a tendency for blood pressure to rise excessively with increasing age.

Other factors that have been implicated in the rising incidence of hypertension with advancing age include the loss of vascular elasticity, and impairment of baroreceptor and renal function. An age-related increase in systolic pressure is related to the loss of distensibility of the aorta and other large arteries which become progressively thicker and more rigid from atherosclerosis. As the aorta becomes more rigid, blood is forced into a confined restricted vessel. Thus, the systolic pressure rises at a steeper slope as a result of a loss of arterial compliance.[3] Increasing atherosclerosis of the carotid and aortic vessel walls also leads to impairment of baroreceptor function with advancing age.[23] Baroreceptor reflexes act primarily as an inhibitory control over medullary vasomotor centers to decrease sympathetic activity. Increased central afferent nerve traffic induced by increases in intra-arterial pressure inhibits sympathetic outflow from the vasomotor center, resulting in a decrease in cardiac rate and peripheral vasodilatation that buffers the initial blood pressure increase. A decline in baroreceptor sensitivity with aging in man has been demonstrated by showing decreased cardiovascular response rates to drugs that reduce blood pressure and diminished bradycardia in response to a pressor injection of phenylephrine.[23] Sluggish baroreceptor function in the elderly may play a role in the development of hypertension and the increased variability of blood pressure with advancing age.[2] Impaired baroreceptor function probably also plays a role in the high incidence of orthostatic hypotension, particularly with antihypertensive therapy, that elderly patients experience.

Age-related changes in renal functions may have important implications regarding both the pathogenesis and treatment of hypertension in the elderly. Beginning in the fourth decade there are decreases in renal cortical mass, renal cortical blood flow, and GFR.[24] With aging there is a general reduction in the nephron population, with diminished glomerular and tubular surface area in the surviving nephrons.[25] As a result of these changes the aged kidney lacks the ability to maximally concentrate and dilute urine in the presence of different solute loads. As previously discussed, decreased ability to excrete a sodium load could result in sodium retention. This retention of sodium could then contribute to the development of hypertension and renin suppression in the elderly.[26] Elderly hypertensive patients placed on sodium restriction and diuretics may lose larger amounts of sodium with accompanying greater degrees of volume depletion, resulting in orthostatic hypotension.

With advancing age there are changes in endocrine systems which play a role in blood pressure regulation. Sympathetic nervous system activity is a well-established determinant of blood pressure maintenance especially in response to postural changes, intravascular volume depletion, and stress.[27–29] Plasma norepinephrine levels in the circulation reflect principally the activity of the peripheral sympathetic nervous system.[30] Plasma levels of norepinephrine increase with advancing age reflecting an age-related increase in sympathetic nervous activity.[26,28,31–33] This age-related elevation in plasma norepinephrine has been reported to be greater with assumption of an upright posture[31–33] than in the supine position in the morning. These age-related increases in supine and upright plasma norepinephrine levels are independent of increases in obesity occurring in aging (Figure 15-1).[33] There is an age-related decrease in clearance of norepinephrine with the greatest decreases occurring from the third to the fifth decades but with little alteration in

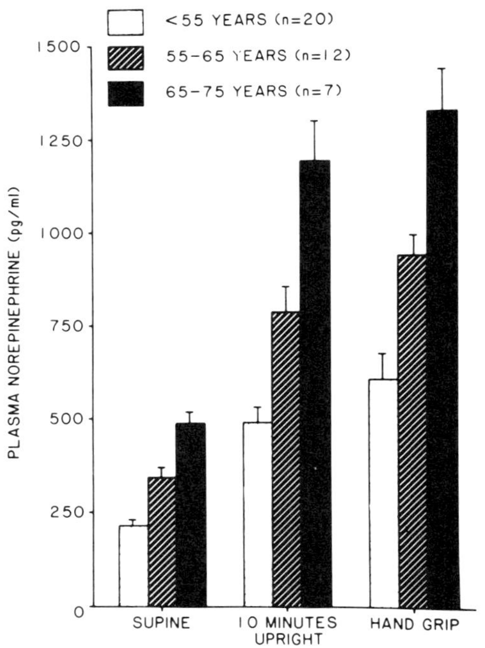

Figure 15-1 Mean (±SEM) plasma NE responses to 10 minute upright posture and 5 minute isometric handgrip exercise in three age groups of men.

clearance thereafter.[34] Recent observations that plasma norepinephrine levels continue to increase in subjects 65 to 75 years of age[33] suggest that increases in norepinephrine secretion rather than decreases in clearance are responsible for age-related increases in plasma norepinephrine. Consistent with this concept is the observation that plasma levels of dopamine-beta-hydroxylase, the enzyme involved in converting dopamine to norepinephrine, increases progressively with age.[35] This enzyme is secreted in stoichiometrically equal amounts with norepinephrine during sympathetic nerve stimulation.[36]

Older subjects have been found to have consistently higher plasma levels of norepinephrine throughout a 24-hour sampling period.[27] Age-related differences were greater at night when plasma levels in older subjects (60 to 80 years old) exceeded those in younger subjects (20 to 30 years old) by 75%. The older individuals had considerably less stage 4 sleep, less rapid eye movement (REM) sleep, and much more wakefulness.[37] There was a relationship between increased nocturnal norepinephrine levels and nighttime wakefulness. These results may suggest that heightened sympathetic activity in the elderly interferes with REM and stage 4 sleep. Alternatively, increased nighttime wakefulness in the elderly could result in heightened sympathetic activity and greater nighttime secretion of norepinephrine. These observations may be particularly relevant in light of observations of an increased incidence of hypertension in people with sleep disorders.[38]

In contrast to levels of norepinephrine, plasma epinephrine[26,27] and dopamine[39] have not been found to increase with aging. Elevated levels of norepinephrine in the presence of normal levels of dopamine with aging may have significance with respect to altered sodium homeostasis and an increased incidence of hypertension with aging. Stimulation of renal sympathetic nerves and renal arterial infusion of norepinephrine result in sodium retention.[40] In contrast, dopamine acts as a natriuretic hormone directly inhibiting proximal renal tubular reabsorption of sodium.[41] Thus in the elderly hypertensive patient who inappropriately retains sodium with a high salt intake there may be an imbalance within the sympathetic nervous system in which there is a relative deficiency of dopamine to oppose the sodium-retaining properties of increased plasma norepinephrine. This concept of an age-related dopamine deficiency takes on an added significance in light of the vasodepressor effects of dopamine and dopamine agonists in essential hypertension.[42]

The imbalance in the sympathetic nervous system with aging may also be reflected in the counterregulatory effects of the β- and α-adrenergic systems. When tissues are chronically exposed to high levels of catecholamines they undergo a process of desensitization with a fall in functional β-adrenergic receptor activity.[43] No such down-regulation of α-adrenergic receptors has been demonstrated. Increasing levels of plasma norepinephrine with aging and accompanying diminished β-adrenergic activity, particularly in respect to β-adrenergic induced vasodilation, could then allow unopposed α-adrenergic activity and result in vasoconstriction.

There is considerable evidence that both basal plasma renin activity (PRA) and its response to various stimuli decrease with age, particularly in elderly hypertensive patients.[26,44–46] An inverse relationship between levels of diastolic blood pressure and PRA was noted in one of these studies.[44] In another study[26] the slopes for the renin-age relationships were similar in normotensive and mild hypertensive subjects but steeper in those with moderate to severe hypertension. These observations suggest an independent effect of elevated blood pressure to decrease PRA levels, particularly in elderly hypertensives. Increases in total body sodium and extracellular fluid volume are rarely found in the elderly and thus do not explain the suppression of the renin angiotensin axis with aging. One regulator of renal renin release is the sympathetic nervous system. Most evidence suggests that β-adrenergic receptors are involved in mediating renal renin release in response to renal nerve stimulation and circulating catecholamines.[47] Thus, one factor which may play a role in the decreased renin responses with aging is decreased β-adrenergic activity mediating renal renin release. A decrease in renal mass and alterations in the renal vasculature, particularly in elderly hypertensives, could account for lesser renal secretion of renin.

Plasma levels of aldosterone usually parallel those of PRA and it would be expected that an age-related decrease in aldosterone would accompany that of PRA. An age-associated decrease in plasma aldosterone as well as urinary aldosterone excretion have been described.[45,48–51] In a recent study[51] decreases in urinary excretion and plasma concentration of aldosterone were interpreted as being secondary to decreases in aldosterone secretion, since the metabolic clearance of aldosterone was not altered with aging. However, in this study neither plasma aldosterone concentration nor PRA decreased with age when these measurements were made in blood samples from recumbent subjects on an unrestricted sodium diet. Weidmann et al[26] observed no significant correlation between upright plasma aldosterone concentration and age in normotensive and essential hypertensive subjects. Supine plasma aldosterone and both supine and upright PRA were observed to decline significantly with increasing age in both study groups. These observations suggest an inappropriately elevated aldosterone response to upright posture despite decreased PRA responses with increasing age. Other investigators[52] have reported less binding of aldosterone to an aldosterone-binding globulin with increasing age in normal controls and to a lesser extent in essential hypertensive patients. In these studies the metabolic clearance rate of aldosterone was lower in hypertensive patients, but did not correlate with age. These investigators proposed that biologically active (free) aldosterone levels did not decrease with age in hypertensives, and in fact may be etiologically related to the development of hypertension in elderly patients. Elevated levels of 18-hydroxydeoxycorticosterone have been observed in some patients with low renin essential hypertension but no association with advancing age has been noted.[53,54] That volume expansion may occur in the elderly is suggested by the observation that there is a decrease in the sensitivity to angiotensin II of the adrenal zona glomerulosa in older subjects.[55] Thus, the role of mineralocorticoids in volume expansion and the development of hypertension with aging remains to be elucidated.

In recent years, investigations have demonstrated that renal prostaglandin E_2 (PGE_2) synthesis can affect renal blood flow,[56] GFR,[57] free water excretion,[58] renin production,[59,60] and urinary sodium excretion.[61] Therefore, interest has developed in determining whether PGE_2 may contribute to or mediate the volume-vasoconstriction events in essential hypertension. Since PGE_2 is a vasodilator[56] and increases sodium excretion,[61] it is hypothesized that a relative deficiency of PGE_2 could contribute to the pathogenesis of essential hypertension.[62,63] This hypothesis has been supported by data showing that patients with essential hypertension have a decreased excretion of PGE_2, which reflects decreased intrarenal production.[64–66] We undertook a study to confirm and extend these observations to include the effect of age on PGE_2 excretion in humans with and without essential hypertension.[67]

Four groups of human subjects were studied. Group 1 consisted of seven normal young male volunteers with a mean age of 28 ± 1 years (range 23 to 33 years). Group 2 consisted of 11 young male essential hypertensives with a mean age of 32 ± 1 years (range 24 to 39 years). Group 3 consisted of eight older normotensive men with a mean age of 56 ± 1 years (range 49 to 63 years). Group 4 consisted of 25 older men with essential hypertension whose mean age was 55 ± 2 years (range 41 to 71 years). All subjects had normal renal function as defined by serum creatinine less than 1.3 mg/dL. All patients were on ad lib normal diets. Twenty-four-hour urinary sodium excretion measurements revealed greater than 2 g salt intake in all cases. All medications were discontinued for 1 week prior to obtaining the measurements of urinary prostaglandin excretion ($UPGE_2v$). Twenty-four-hour urine collections were obtained from all four groups. Urine was collected without preservatives and aliquots were frozen until assayed. Urinary PGE_2 excretion was measured by radioimmunoassay using the Dray antibody.[68] All results are expressed as mean ± SEM. Statistical analysis was done using the Student paired t-test. This antibody has been shown to be specific for PGE_2.

The results are summarized in Figures 15-2–15-5. In Figure 15-2 it can be seen that the young male controls (group 1), had a urinary PGE_2 excretion ($UPGE_2v$) of 865.6 ± 128.3 ng/d.

The young hypertensives in group 2 had $UPGE_2v$ of 588.0 ± 171.0 ng/d. There was no statistical difference between the two groups. Also, it can be seen in Figure 15-2 that group 3, the older male controls, had a $UPGE_2v$ of 993.9 ± 302.6 ng/d while group 4, the older male patients with essential hypertension, had $UPGE_2v$ of 195.0 ± 42.6 ng/d. These two groups were significantly different ($P<.001$).

Figure 15-3 compares the normotensive subjects, groups 1 and 3, to the hypertensive patients, groups 2 and 4. The $UPGE_2v$ was 888.2 ± 172.4 ng/d for the normotensive population and 315.3 ± 66 ng/d for the hypertensive population

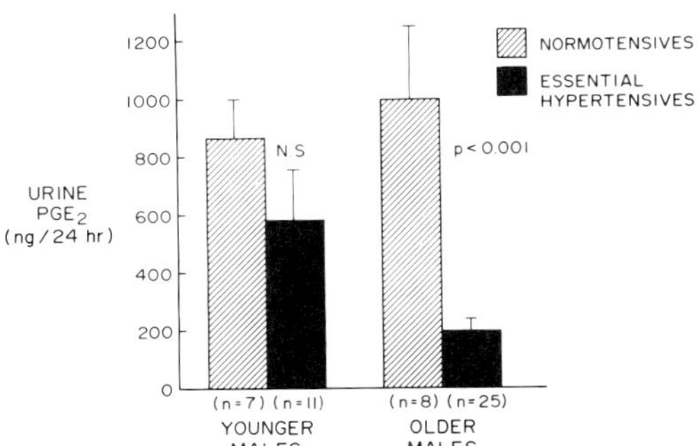

Figure 15-2 Urinary prostaglandin E_2 excretion in four groups of human subjects: normal young men (group 1); young hypertensive men (group 2); nonhypertensive older men (group 3); hypertensive older men (group 4).

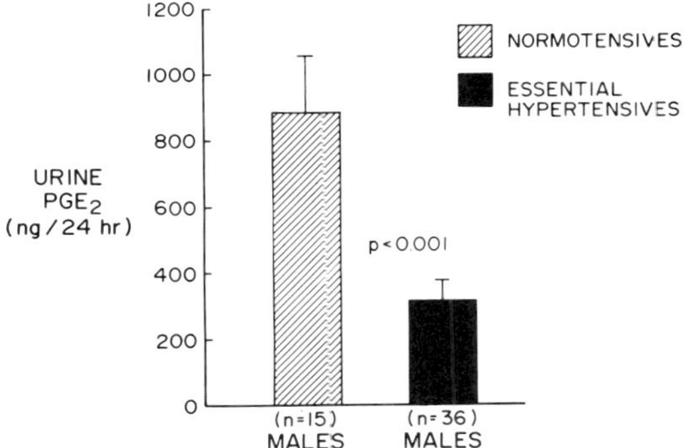

Figure 15-3 Urinary prostaglandin E_2 excretion in all hypertensives *v* all normal controls.

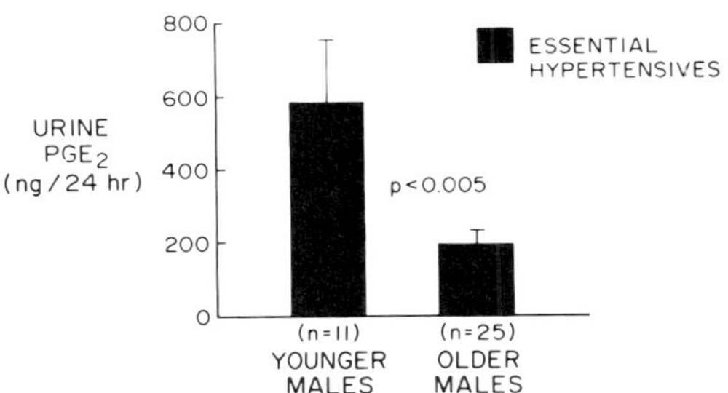

Figure 15-4 Urinary prostaglandin E_2 excretion in hypertensives: older *v* younger men.

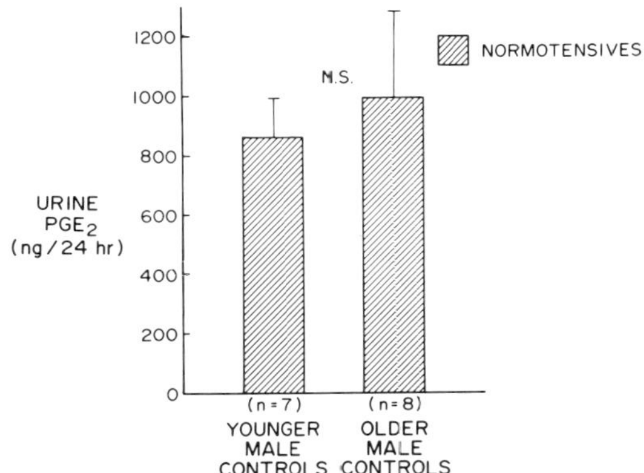

Figure 15-5 Urinary prostaglandin E_2 excretion in normal controls: older *v* younger men.

($P<.001$). Figure 15-4 compares the subpopulations of hypertensive subjects separated by age (ie, group 2, younger hypertensives; and group 4, older hypertensives). There was a statistically significant lower $UPGE_2v$ in older compared with younger hypertensive patients ($P<.005$). In Figure 15-5 it can be seen that comparison of the two control normotensive groups, 1 and 3, revealed no significant difference between these control groups.

Several authors have demonstrated that urinary PGE_2 excretion is decreased in patients with essential hypertension.[65-67] Tan et al also have investigated PGE_2 urinary excretion in patients with renovascular hypertension and primary aldosteronism.[69] Patients from both groups had urinary PGE_2 excretion not significantly different from controls. This finding led the authors to the conclusion that decreased PGE_2 excretion is not caused by increased blood pressure alone and that renin may not be an important determinant in PGE_2 excretion since the patients with high renin states (renovascular hypertension) and low renin states (primary aldosteronism) had similar PGE_2 excretion. This second conclusion is substantiated by the lack of statistical correlation of PRA and PGE_2 excretion in patients with essential hypertension in their study and the study of Weber et al.[66]

Our data confirm the finding that PGE_2 urinary excretion is decreased in patients with essential hypertension. However, we also examined the effect of age on urinary excretion of PGE_2 in normals compared with hypertensives. Our findings indicate that age alone will not decrease PGE_2 excretion. Our controls all had similar urinary levels regardless of age. However, we did find a statistical difference in excretion of PGE_2 between younger hypertensives and older hypertensives. It should be noted that the degree of blood pressure elevation was similar in both groups of hypertensive patients. Also, all renin levels measured in these hypertensives were in the low normal range.

There are at least two possible explanations for the differences in excretion of PGE_2 between the two groups of hypertensive patients. First, one could postulate that prolonged essential hypertension may eventually cause enough kidney dysfunction, not evident by elevated serum creatinine levels, to decrease PGE_2 excretion. In our hypertensive patients creatinine clearances were measured in all cases. There was a significant inverse correlation between $UPGE_2v$ and creatinine clearance, $r=.47$, $P<.01$, in these hypertensive patients. The second explanation for our findings could be that essential hypertension in the young and in the elderly have a different pathophysiology, similar to differences in the role of the renin-angiotensin system in the hypertension seen in these two age groups. One could postulate that a disordered prostaglandin synthetic pathway plays a greater role in hypertension in the elderly. Evaluation of this postulate will require a longitudinal study of younger hypertensive patients with normal PGE_2 excretion to see if their PGE_2 excretion decreases with age.

In summary, our study confirmed the finding that PGE_2 excretion is decreased in patients with essential hypertension, especially elderly patients with essential hypertension. Aging, itself, is not accompanied by changes in PGE_2 excretion. The decreased $UPGE_2v$ may reflect end-organ damage due to prolonged hypertension or may contribute to the pathophysiology of hypertension in the elderly hypertensives. Impaired renal prostaglandin synthesis in these patients may be responsible for impaired sodium excretion which in turn could produce hypertension in these patients.

TREATMENT OF GERIATRIC HYPERTENSION

The value of treating diastolic hypertension in the elderly is well established. In the VA cooperative study[9] 81 of the patients were over age 60 at randomization, and when this elderly group was analyzed separately the incidence of morbid events over a mean duration of 3.3 years was very high. There was a striking reduction in morbidity following antihypertensive therapy in those with diastolic pressures in the range of 90 to 104 mmHg. Furthermore, patients who had a major complication of hypertension before treatment benefited most. In the Hypertensive Detection and Follow-up Program (HDFP)[70,71] the therapeutic goal was a diastolic blood pressure <90 mmHg for those with an entry diastolic blood pressure >100mmHg and a 10 mmHg decrease for those with a lower diastolic blood pressure. In the elderly (aged 60 to 69 years) this therapeutic goal was achieved in 75% of those receiving stepped care and 55% of those receiving routine referred care, a better result than in younger patients in this study. Furthermore, blood pressure control in patients over 60 was associated with a 16.4% reduction in mortality over those referred to their routine source of medical care. Both the HDFP and the European Working Party on High Blood Pressure in the Elderly (EWPHE)[72] have demonstrated that elderly patients do tolerate antihypertensive drugs well. The HDFP study used chlorthalidone in step 1 and either reserpine or methyldopa in step 2. The EWPHE study is a larger European evaluation of treatment of diastolic hypertension in patients over 60 which is currently in progress, but data already available indicate that elderly patients can be safely treated with as much or more benefit than younger patients. The EWPHE study is employing hydrochlorothiazide with triamterene in step 1 and methyldopa in step 2.

Treatment of isolated systolic hypertension in the elderly remains controversial. There are no data from a prospective, well-controlled clinical study designed to determine if control of isolated systolic hypertension improves prognosis. A cooperative trial on the treatment of predominantly systolic hypertension has been undertaken by the National Heart, Lung, and Blood Institute and the Institute on Aging, but it will likely be 1990 before the final data are available.

Since cardiovascular complications, kidney damage, and hemorrhagic and thrombotic strokes are more closely linked to systolic than to diastolic blood pressure, it is probably appropriate to treat systolic hypertension aiming for a very gradual reduction in blood pressure. One prominent investigator has suggested that he aims for a gradual initial reduction in systolic pressure to the 140- to 160-mmHg range.[3]

In treating the elderly hypertensive patient, other factors must be taken into consideration. The presence of end-organ damage with hypertension greatly increases the risk of additional complications. Diabetes and hypercholesterolemia coexisting with hypertension considerably increase the risk of myocardial infarction and sudden death. Therefore, it appears important to aggressively treat almost all elderly patients with target organ damage for other concomitant risk factors.[73] The value of antihypertensive therapy following strokes in preventing recurrences of strokes has been evaluated in two studies. In one study the overall occurrence of strokes appeared to be decreased by therapy in patients above 70 years of age.[74] In another study beneficial effects were not seen in patients over 65.[75]

Antihypertensive therapy must be administered even more cautiously in elderly patients who have suffered strokes as the poor cerebral autoregulatory ability in the elderly may be even further impaired in the presence of cerebral vascular disease.[76] The rate of complications from hypertension is at least twice as great in blacks, and the mortality ratio two times higher for hypertensive men than for women.[77] Therefore treatment should probably be initiated at lower blood pressures in males and blacks than in females and whites up to age 75. For both men and women older than 75 years, antihypertensive therapy should be reserved for control of hypertensive heart failure and progressive retinal or renal damage.[76]

Multiple blood pressure measurements should be made before deciding to treat a geriatric patient with antihypertensive therapy, because systolic blood pressures fluctuate widely in elderly patients with rigid, poorly compliant aortas. One investigator recommends obtaining three measurements on each of at least three office visits over a period of weeks before deciding to initiate therapy.[3] Once the diagnosis of hypertension has been made, an evaluation for secondary causes of hypertension is seldom necessary in elderly hypertensives. If the blood pressure is found to be very high in an elderly patient previously normotensive, the possibility of atherosclerotic renovascular hypertension must be considered.

It is generally agreed that antihypertensive therapy in the elderly should be initiated with reduction in salt and caloric intake, especially if the patient is a heavy salt user and is obese. However, lifetime dietary patterns are often difficult to change in the elderly and drug therapy is often necessary. Although the concern over decreased compliance in the elderly hypertensive has been voiced by many, the HDFP[70,71] study demonstrated that compliance with antihypertensive therapy in the elderly may be better than that in younger age groups. A slow careful explanation with written reinforcement is often quite helpful in prescribing antihypertensive medications to the elderly who are often on numerous other drugs. A careful search for medications which may be exacerbating the hypertensive state in the elderly should also be made. Compliance, particularly in elderly patients, is often improved by maintaining a simple regimen (once or twice daily) that has a low incidence of side effects.[77] Other practical factors that may make successful treatment in the elderly more difficult include poor hearing or eyesight, difficulty in opening safety caps on bottles, limited income, and the consumption of processed foods which are high in sodium and very low in potassium.

Elderly patients are particularly prone to side effects of antihypertensive medication because of physiologic changes that occur with aging. A common adverse effect of antihypertensive drugs in the elderly is related to decreased ability to maintain cerebral blood flow following decreases in cerebral perfusion pressure. Autoregulatory mechanisms normally maintain cerebral blood flow constant despite considerable fluctuations in blood pressure. In elderly hypertensives, particularly those with occlusive cerebrovascular diseases, the lower limit of autoregulation rises, and reductions in blood pressure are often associated with reduced cerebral perfusion. Clinical manifestations include dizziness, orthostatic falls, and even transient ischemic episodes or strokes.[78,79] Reductions in baroreceptor sensitivity in the elderly may allow very large orthostatic drops in blood pressure to occur after initiating antihypertensive therapy. This may result in episodes of dizziness, fainting, and falls when the elderly patient receiving antihypertensive therapy rises from a supine or sitting position. Hypovolemia, a frequent occurrence in elderly patients with predominantly systolic hypertension increases the propensity for severe orthostatic hypotension in elderly patients with sluggish baroreceptor function. The propensity for orthostatic hypotension is further increased by the limited compensatory cardiovascular responses in the elderly with large falls in blood pressure.

Alterations in the absorption, distribution volume, and metabolism of drugs must also be considered in prescribing antihypertensive drugs for the geriatric population. Delays in gastric emptying and decreased gastric acid production can decrease absorption of drugs in the small intestine. Aging may affect drug distribution in a number of ways. Decreases in skeletal muscle mass along with increases in adipose tissue could alter the distribution of certain drugs that partition into certain tissues, ie, fat *v* water-soluble characteristics. Reductions in cardiac output associated with aging could decrease the rate of delivery of drugs to tissues responsible for their clearance, ie, kidney and liver. Renal excretion of drugs is often reduced because of the reduction in glomerular and tubular function with aging. Age-associated changes in hepatic function may also affect drug elimination. Liver blood flow declines with aging, probably reflecting the reduction in cardiac output. Propranolol is a commonly prescribed antihypertensive drug which is metabolized by the liver following absorption into the portal circulation. When metabolism of propranolol was compared in aged and younger subjects, plasma levels were high in the elderly suggesting reduced hepatic metabolism.[80] However, higher levels of propranolol in the elderly do not result in excessive pharmacologic effects because of the marked decrease in β-adrenergic function with advancing age.[43]

A stepped care approach would appear to be appropriate in the treatment of elderly hypertensive patients as it is in younger hypertensives. Diuretics employed in the VA cooperative study,[9] the HDFP studies,[70,71] and the ongoing EWPHE studies[72] generally are well accepted by patients and are the most commonly used first-step therapy for aged hypertensives. Both hydrochlorothiazide and chlorthalidone have been used successfully as the step-1 treatment regimen in elderly hypertensives. An appropriate initial regimen would be a small dose of a diuretic of intermediate duration of action such as 12.5 or 25 mg hydrochlorothiazide each morning. The patient should be evaluated in 1 week, and if the hypertension has not been corrected, then the thiazide can be given twice daily. Because of poor dietary intake of potassium, elderly patients are more likely to develop hypokalemia while taking thiazides. Thus potassium chloride supplements may be needed, even while taking low doses of thiazides. Potassium-containing salt substitutes are a relatively inexpensive means of replacing potassium in these patients. The EWPHE[72] is employing a combination of triameterene with hydrochlorothiazide to reduce potassium loss. Thiazides are also more likely to cause either chemical or clinical diabetes mellitus in the elderly.[81] The onset of elevated glucose is usually gradual but may occur within the first weeks of therapy. It is generally mild, although hyperosmolar nonketotic diabetic coma is more likely to occur with thiazide therapy in the elderly hypertensive with decreased renal function. Hyperuricemia may occur, and serum uric acid levels should be obtained before and at 1 or 2 months after initiation of thiazide therapy. Additionally, thiazides may adversely affect serum lipoproteins.[82] A recent prospective study[83] of elderly male hypertensive patients in Australia showed a higher mortality in patients with vascular disease treated with diuretics alone compared with controls and those treated with propranolol. This report, as well as the observation that there was no reduction in deaths from myocardial infarction in the elderly in the VA cooperative study,[9] suggest that diuretics may not represent optimal therapy in elderly hypertensive patients with significant vascular or ischemic heart disease. Thiazides should be used with considerable caution in elderly patients with impaired renal or hepatic function. With decreased renal function thiazides may accumulate and cause renal function to deteriorate further. In patients with impaired hepatic function, thiazides may precipitate hepatic coma. Thus, thiazide diuretics, although generally accepted as the first line of drug therapy in elderly hypertensives, must be used with considerable caution in these patients.

If hypertension is not adequately controlled with thiazides, the second line of therapy could be with methyldopa, clonidine hydrochloride, β-blockers, calcium antagonists, or possibly reserpine. Central-acting sympathetic inhibitors such as methyldopa, clonidine, and reserpine are effective antihypertensives in the elderly but can be associated with certain side effects that are more commonly manifested in the elderly. These include orthostatic hypotension, decreased mental acuity, depression, sexual dysfunction, nasal stuffiness, and dry mouth. Clonidine is probably associated with less orthostatic hypotension and fluid retention than the other two medications. Although daytime somnolence is a relatively common problem with clonidine therapy, this side effect can be minimized by administering the drug as a single evening dose.[84] In the elderly hypertensive patient, therapy should be begun with 0.1 mg PM and doses increased slowly, at 2- to 3-week intervals. Methyldopa has some advantages in the elderly patient in that it only minimally compromises cardiac output and renal blood flow. However, methyldopa may produce a drug fever, hepatitis, a positive Coombs test, and occasionally hemolytic anemia. Patients with prior liver disease and the elderly are especially at risk of developing hepatitis. Mental depression, nightmares, and insomnia are less common side effects which usually occur with daily doses greater than 500 mg. Methyldopa is excreted primarily via the kidneys, and patients with impaired renal function may require lower doses. The elderly patient with impaired hepatic and renal function is especially susceptible to decreased metabolism.

Some have advocated β-adrenergic blocking agents as the first-line therapy for elderly patients with hypertension.[85,86] β-blocking agents generally cause fewer CNS side effects such as sedation and less problems with postural hypotension. However, there is evidence of decreased responsiveness to β-adrenergic blocking agents in elderly patients.[43] There is also an increased incidence of adverse side effects associated with propranolol therapy in the elderly.[87] Water-soluble β-blockers such as atenolol are primarily cleared by the kidney and may accumulate in the elderly with impaired renal function. Lipid soluble β-blockers such as propranolol are largely metabolized by the liver, and the rate of this metabolism decreases with age.[80] All β-blockers should be carefully used in the elderly since they have been demonstrated to decrease renal blood flow and GFR.[88] Although selective β_1-blockers such as atenolol may prove to be safer antihypertensive agents in the elderly, the use of any β-blocker in older patients with evidence of left ventricular failure or bronchoconstrictor disease should be avoided. Propranolol has been shown to blunt the insulin response to glucose, and propranolol-induced hyperosmolar nonketotic coma has been reported.[89] β-blockers can also mask the symptoms of hypoglycemia. Vasoconstriction, even to the extent of producing Raynaud's phenomenon, has been observed in patients receiving propranolol. Obviously this is a significant consideration in treating elderly patients with compromised peripheral blood flow.

Calcium antagonists such as nifedipine, verapamil, and diltiazem hydrochloride may prove to be safe and effective antihypertensive agents in elderly patients. Calcium antagonists, or slow channel blocking agents, by blocking calcium-mediated electromechanical coupling in contractile vascular smooth muscle, produce arterial dilatation in peripheral vessels as well as the coronary vascular bed.[90,91] Verapamil and nifedipine block the entry of calcium into the cell, and diltiazem increases the exit of calcium from the cell. The calcium antagonists are commonly used as step-2 and even step-1 drugs in the management of hypertension in other countries.[92,93] Arteriolar dilation produced by the calcium antagonists would be expected to trigger a reflexive increase in β-adrenergic-mediated reflex tachycardia.[94] However, reflex tachycardia is probably minimal in elderly patients with sluggish baroreceptor function. Calcium antagonists do exert negative inotropic and chronotropic effects on the heart and must be used carefully in the elderly patient who may have borderline left ventricular function and possible conduction disturbances.[90] Other direct-acting vasodilators such as hydralazine hydrochloride may be useful as second- or third-line drugs for treating hypertension in the elderly. Vasodilators such as hydralazine and prazosin hydrochloride are contraindicated in patients with dissecting aneurysm and should be used with extreme caution in patients with left ventricular dysfunction.[95] Other side effects of both hydralazine and prazosin are sodium and water retention and peripheral edema, which are problems more likely to occur in the elderly hypertensive patient.

In treating elderly hypertensive patients one should attempt to keep the number of medications and number of daily doses to a minimum in that the elderly may have more difficulty in following complicated dosage schedules, reading the labels, and opening safety-proof caps. Careful follow-up with reinforcement of the importance of taking antihypertensive medication is particularly important in elderly patients. One must be aware of other drugs which the patient may be placed on which may interact with, or interfere with the action of antihypertensives. This is particularly important in those elderly patients who are taking many drugs.

Finally, from our studies on prostaglandin physiology in elderly hypertensives,[67] another important therapeutic consideration arises. Care should be used in the use of prostaglandin-inhibitory drugs in elderly hypertensive patients. Such drugs as aspirin and nonsteroidal anti-inflammatory drugs, which are frequently used in the elderly, may aggravate the pathophysiology of the renal prostaglandin synthetic pathways, which may play a role in the hypertension seen in these patients. Since at present there is no way to enhance renal prostaglandin synthesis, at least avoidance of further impairment of renal prostaglandin synthesis by limitations of frequency and total dose of aspirin and nonsteroidal anti-inflammatory drugs in elderly hypertensives is suggested.

ACKNOWLEDGMENT

Figures 15-2–15-5 are reprinted by permission of S Karger, Basel, from Zawada ET, MacKenzie TA, Johnson M: The importance of age on prostaglandin E_2 excretion in normal and hypertensive men. *Nephron* 1984;38:178–182.

REFERENCES

1. *National Health Examination Survey-United States 1960–1962.* US Dept of Health, Education, and Welfare, 1964, series II.
2. Drayer JIM, Weber MA, DeYoung JL, et al: Circadian blood pressure patterns in ambulatory hypertensive patients. Effects of age. *Am J Med* 1982;73:493–499.
3. Gifford RW: Isolated systolic hypertension in the elderly. *JAMA* 1982;247:781–785.
4. Kannel WB, Wolf PA, Verter J, et al: Epidemiologic assessment of the role of blood pressure in stroke: The Framingham Study. *JAMA* 1970;214:301–304.
5. Kannel WB, Castelli WP, McNamara PM, et al: Role of blood pressure in the development of congestive heart failure. *N Engl J Med* 1972;287:78–81.
6. Kannel WB: Role of blood pressure in cardiovascular disease: The Framingham Study. *Angiology* 1975;26:1–14.
7. Shurtleff D, Secton EO: *Some Characteristics Related to the Incidence of Cardiovascular Disease and Death: The Framingham Study, 18-Year Follow-up.* US Dept of Health, Education and Welfare, publication no. (NIH) 74-599, 1974.
8. Kannell WB, Wolf PA, McGee DL: Systolic blood pressure, arterial rigidity, and risks of stroke: The Framingham Study. *JAMA* 1981;245:1225–1229.
9. Veterans Administration Cooperative Study Group on Antihypertensive Agents: Effects of treatment on morbidity in hypertension. III. Influence of age, diastolic pressure, and prior cardiovascular disease, further analysis of side effects. *Circulation* 1972; 45:991–1004.
10. Morton PA: Ordinary insurance: The Build and Blood Pressure Study. *Trans Soc Actuaries* 1959;11:987–997.
11. Colandrea MA, Friedman GD, Nichaman

MZ, et al: Systolic hypertension in the elderly: An epidemiologic assessment. *Circulation* 1970;41:239–245.

12. Kannel WB, Gordon T, Schwartz MJ: Systolic versus diastolic blood pressure and the risks of coronary heart disease: The Framingham Study. *Am J Cardiol* 1971; 77:335–346.
13. Shekelle RB, Ostfeld AM, Klawans HL: Hypertension and risks of stroke in an elderly population. *Stroke* 1974;5:71–75.
14. Dyer AR, Stamler, J, Shekelle RB, et al: Hypertension in the elderly. *Med Clin North Am* 1977;61:513–529.
15. Shaper AG: Blood pressure studies in East Africa, in Stamler J, Stamler R, Pullman TN (eds): *The Epidemiology of Hypertension*, New York, Grune & Stratton, 1967, pp 139–145.
16. Lovell RRH: Race and blood pressure with special reference to Oceania, in Stamler J, Stamler R, Pullman TN (eds): *The Epidemiology of Hypertension*, New York, Grune & Stratton, 1967, pp 122–129.
17. Durnin JVGA, Womerskley J: Body fat assessed from total body density and its estimation from skinfold thickness: measurements on 481 men and women aged from 16 to 72 years. *Br J Nutr* 1974;32: 77–97.
18. Sowers JR, Whitfield L, Catania R, et al: Role of the sympathetic nervous system in blood pressure maintenance in obesity. *J Clin Endocrinol Metab* 1982;54:1181–1186.
19. Luft FC, Grim CE, Fineberg N, et al: Effects of volume expansion and contraction in normotensive whites, blacks, and subjects of different ages. *Circulation* 1979;59:643–650.
20. Grim CE, Luft FC, Miller JZ, et al: Effects of sodium loading and depletion in normotensive first degree relatives of essential hypertensives. *J Lab Clin Med* 1979;94:764–770.
21. Grzegorczyk PB, Jones SW, Mistretta CM: Age-related differences in salt taste acuity. *J Gerontol* 1979;34:834–840.
22. Hamilton MG, Pickering GW, Roberts AF, et al: The aetiology of essential hypertension: The role of inheritance. *Clin Sci* 1954;13:273–282.
23. Gribbin B, Pickering TG, Sleight P, et al: Effect of age and high blood pressure on baroreflex sensitivity in man. *Circ Res* 1971;29:424–429.
24. Hollenberg NK, Adams DF, Solomon HS, et al: Senescence and the renal vasculature in normal man. *Circ Res* 1974;34:309–316.
25. Papper S: The effects of age in reducing renal function. *Geriatrics* 1973;28:83–87.
26. Weidmann P, Beretta-Piccoli C, Ziegler WH, et al: Age versus urinary sodium for judging renin, aldosterone, and catecholamine levels: Studies in normal subjects and patients with essential hypertension. *Kidney Int* 1978;14:619–628.
27. Stene M, Panagiotis N, Tuck ML, et al: Plasma norepinephrine levels are influenced by sodium intake, glucocorticoid administration, and circadian changes in normal man. *J Clin Endocrinol Metab* 1980;51:1340–1345.
28. Henry DP, Luft FC, Weinberger MH, et al: Norepinephrine in urine and plasma following provocative maneuvers in normal and hypertensive subjects. *Hypertension* 1980; 2:20–28.
29. Whitfield L, Sowers JR, Tuck ML, et al: Dopaminergic control of plasma catecholamine and aldosterone responses to acute stimuli in normal man. *J Clin Endocrinol Metab* 1980;51:724–729.
30. Wallin G, Sundloff G, Eriksson BM, et al: Plasma noradrenaline correlates to sympathetic muscle nerve activity in normotensive man. *Acta Physiol Scand* 1981;111: 69–73.
31. Lake CR, Ziegler MG, Coleman MD, et al: Age-adjusted plasma norepinephrine levels are similar in normotensive and hypertensive subjects. *N Engl J Med* 1977;296:208–209.
32. Young JB, Rowe JW, Pallotta JA, et al: Enhanced plasma norepinephrine response to upright posture and oral glucose administration in elderly human subjects. *Metabolism* 1980;29:532–539.
33. Sowers JR, Rubenstein LZ, Stern N: Plasma norepinephrine responses to posture and isometric exercise increase with age in the absence of obesity. *J Gerontol* 1983;38:315–317.
34. Esler M, Skems H, Leonard P, et al: Age-dependence of noradrenaline kinetics in normal subjects. *Clin Sci* 1981;60:217–219.
35. Friedman LS, Ohuchi T, Goldstein M, et al: Changes in human serum dopamine-B-hydroxylase with age. *Nature* 1972;236: 310–311.
36. Weinshilbonm RM, Thoa NB, Johnson DB,

et al: Proportional release of norepinephrine and dopamine hydroxylase from sympathetic nerves. *Science* 1971;174:1349–1351.

37. Printz PN, Halter J, Benedetti C, et al: Circadian variation of plasma catecholamines in young and old men: Relation to rapid eye movements and slow wave sleep. *J Clin Endocrinol Metab* 1979;49:300–304.
38. Stern N, Beahm E, Sowers JR, et al: The effect of age on circadian rhythm of blood pressure, catecholamines, plasma renin activity, prolactin and corticosteroids in essential hypertension. Read before Endocrine Society 65th Annual Meeting, San Antonio, Texas 1983, No. 772.
39. Franco-Morselli R, Elghozi JL, Joly E, et al: Increased plasma adrenalin in benign essential hypertension. *Br Med J [Clin Res]* 1977;2:1251–1254.
40. Besarb A, Silva P, Landsberg L: Effects of catecholamines on tubular function in the isolated perfused rat kidney. *Am J Physiol* 1977;233:F39–F44.
41. Bello-Reuss E, Higashi Y, Kaneda Y: Dopamine decrease fluid reabsorption in straight portions of rabbit proximal tubule. *Am J Physiol* 1982;242:F634–F640.
42. Sowers JR, Golub MS, Berger ME, et al: Dopaminergic modulation of pressor and hormonal responses in essential hypertension. *Hypertension* 1982;4:424–429.
43. Vestal RE, Wood AJJ, Shand DG: Reduced beta-adrenoreceptor sensitivity in the elderly. *Clin Pharmacol Ther* 1979;26:181–186.
44. Tuck ML, Williams GH, Can JP: Relation of age, diastolic pressure and known duration of hypertension to presence of low renin essential hypertension. *Am J Cardiol* 1973;32:632–637.
45. Crane MG, Harris JJ: Effect of aging on renin activity and aldosterone excretion. *J Lab Clin Med* 1976;87:949–959.
46. Noth RH, Lassman MN, Tan SY, et al: Age and renin-aldosterone system. *Arch Intern Med* 1977;137:1414–1417.
47. Osborne JL, DiBona GF, Thames MD: Beta-1 receptor mediation of renin secretion elicited by low frequency renal nerve stimulation. *J Pharmacol Exp Ther* 1981;216:265.
48. Salvetti A, Pedrinelli R, Poli L, et al: The relationship of plasma and urinary aldosterone with sodium balance, plasma renin activity and age in normal subjects. *J Nucl Med Allied Sci* 1977;21:7–17.
49. Weidman P, DeMyttenaere-Buroztein S, Maxwell MH, et al: Effect of aging on plasma renin and aldosterone in normal man. *Kidney Int* 1975;8:325–333.
50. Zadik Z, Kowarski AA: Normal integrated concentration of aldosterone and plasma renin activity: Effect of age. *J Clin Endocrinol Metab* 1980;50:867–869.
51. Hegstad R, Brown RD, Jiang N, et al: Aging and aldosterone. *Am J Med* 1983;74: 442–448.
52. Nowaczynski W, Genest J, Kuchel O, et al: Age- and posture-related changes in plasma protein binding and metabolism of aldosterone in essential and secondary hypertension. *J Lab Clin Med* 1977;90:475–489.
53. Melby JC, Dale SL: Adrenal steroidogenesis in "low renin" or hyporeninemic hypertension. *J Steroid Biochem* 1975;6:761–766.
54. Messerli FH, Kuchel O, Nowaczynski W, et al: Mineralocorticoid secretion in essential hypertension with normal and low renin activity. *Circulation* 1976;53:406–410.
55. Takeda R, Morimoto S, Uchida K, et al: Effect of age on plasma aldosterone response to exogenous angiotensin II in normotensive subjects. *Acta Endocrinol* 1980;94: 553–558.
56. Tannenbaum J, Splawinski JA, Oates JA, et al: Enhanced renal prostaglandin production in the dog. I. Effects on renal function. *Circ Res* 1975;36:197–203.
57. Schnermann J, Briggs JP: Participation of renal cortical prostaglandins in the regulation of glomerular filtration rate. *Kidney Int* 1981;19:802–815.
58. Anderson RJ, Berl T, McDonald KM, et al: Evidence for an in vivo antagonism between vasopressin and prostaglandin in the mammalian kidney. *J Clin Invest* 1975;56: 420–426.
59. Bolger PM, Eisner GM, Ramwell PW, et al: Effect of prostaglandin synthesis on renal function and renin in the dog. *Nature* 1976;259:244–245.
60. Freeman RN, Davis JO, Dietz JR, Renal prostaglandins and the control of renin release. *Hypertension* 1982;4(suppl 2): 106–112.
61. Kirschenbaum MA, Stein JH: The effect of inhibition of prostaglandin synthesis on urinary sodium excretion in the conscious dog. *J Clin Invest* 1976;57:517–521.

62. McGiff JC, Vane JR: Prostaglandins and the regulation of blood pressure. *Kidney Int* 1975;8:S262–S270.
63. Lee JB, Patak RV, Mookerjee BK: Renal prostaglandins and the regulation of blood pressure and sodium and water homeostasis. *Am J Med* 1976;60:798–816.
64. Tan SY, Sweet P, Mulrow PJ: Impaired renal production of prostaglandin E_2: A newly identified lesion in human essential hypertension. *Prostaglandins* 1978;15:139–150.
65. Abe K, Seino M, Yasujima M, et al: Studies on renomedullary prostaglandin and renal kallikrein-kinin system in hypertension. *Jpn Circ J* 1977;41:873–880.
66. Weber PC, Siess W, Scherer B: Possible significance of renal prostaglandins in essential hypertension. *Clin Exp Hypertens* 1980;2(3–4):741–760.
67. MacKenzie TA, Zawada ET, Johnson M: The effect of age on urinary prostaglandin excretion in normal and hypertensive men. *Nephron* 1984;38:178–182.
68. Dray R, Charvonnel B, Maclouf J: Radioimmunoassay of prostaglandins R, E, and E_2 in human plasma. *Eur J Clin Invest* 1975;5:311–318.
69. Tan SY, Bravo E, Mulrow PJ: Impaired renal prostaglandin E_2 biosynthesis in human hypertensive states. *Prostaglandins Med* 1978;1:76–85.
70. Hypertension Detection and Follow-up Program Cooperative Group: Five-year findings of the Hypertension Detection Follow-up Program I. Reduction in mortality of persons with high blood pressure, including mild hypertension. *JAMA* 1979;242: 2562–2571.
71. Hypertension Detection and Follow-up Program Cooperative Group: Five-year findings of the Hypertension Detection and Follow-up Program II. Mortality by race, sex, and age. *JAMA* 1979;242:2572–2577.
72. Amery A, Berthaux P, Birkenhager W: Antihypertensive therapy in patients above 60 years: Fourth interim report of the European Working Party on High Blood Pressure in Elderly. *Clin Sci Mol Med* 1978;55:263–270.
73. Truett J, Cornfield J, Kannel WB: A multivariant analysis of the risk of coronary heart disease in Framingham. *J Chronic Dis* 1967;20:511–524.
74. Hypertension-Stroke Cooperative Study Group: Effect of antihypertensive treatment in stroke recurrence. *JAMA* 1974; 229:409–418.
75. Carter AB: Hypotensive therapy in stroke survivors. *Lancet* 1978;1:485–489.
76. Heller RF, Rose G: Current management of hypertension in general practice. *Br Med J* 1977;1:1441–1444.
77. Stamler R, Stamler J, Civinelli J, et al: Adherance and blood pressure response to hypertensive treatment. *Lancet* 1976;2: 1317–1318.
78. Jackson G, Pierscianowski TA, Mahon W, et al: Inappropriate antihypertensive therapy in the elderly. *Lancet* 1976;2: 1317–1318.
79. Graham OI: Ischemic brain damage of central perfusion type after treatment of severe hypertension. *Br Med J* 1975;4:739–743.
80. Castleden CM, Kaye CM, Parsons RL: The effect of age on plasma levels of propranolol and practolol in man. *Br J Clin Pharmacol* 1975;2:303–306.
81. Amery A, Berthaux P, Aulpitt C: Glucose intolerance during diuretic therapy. *Lancet* 1978;1:681–683.
82. Gluck Z, Baumgartner G, Wadmann P: Increased ratio between serum B- and lipoproteins during diuretic therapy: an adverse effect. *Clin Sci Mol Med* 1978;55:325–328.
83. Morgan T, Adam W, Carney S: Treatment of mild hypertension in elderly males. *Clin Sci* 1979;57:355–357.
84. Putzeyz MR, Hoobler SW: Comparison of clonidine and methyldopa on blood pressure and side effects in hypertensive patients. *Am Heart J* 1972;83:464–468.
85. Eisulo A, Huno A, Munter J: The effect of alprenolol in elderly patients with raised blood pressure. *Acta Med Scand [Suppl]* 1974;554–523.
86. O'Malley K, O'Brien MR: Management of hypertension in the elderly. *N Engl J Med* 1980;302:1397–1401.
87. Greenblatt DJ, Koch-Weser J: Adverse reactions to propranolol in hospitalized medical patients: a report from the Boston Collaborative Drug Surveillance Program. *Am Heart J* 1973;86:478–484.
88. Bauer JH, Brooks CS: The long term effect of propranolol therapy on renal function. *Am J Med* 1979;66:406–410.
89. Podolsky S, Pattarina CG: Hyperosmolar

nonketotic diabetic coma–A complication of propranolol therapy. *Metab Clin Exp* 1973;22:685–693.

90. Flickenstein A: Specific pharmacology of calcium in myocardium cardiac pacemakers and vascular smooth muscle. *Annu Rev Pharmacol Toxicol* 1977;17:149–166.
91. Thorens S, Hacusler J: Effects of some vasodilators on calcium translocation in intact and fractionated vascular smooth muscle. *Eur J Pharmacol* 1979;54:79–91.
92. Olivari M, Bartocelli C, Polese A, et al: Treatment of hypertension with nifedipine, a calcium antagonist agent. *Circulation* 1979;59:1056–1062.
93. Karvajima I, Veda K, Kamata C, et al: A study on the effects of nifedipine in hypertensive crisis and severe hypertension. *Jpn Heart J* 1978;19:455–467.
94. Amelie JP, Landmark K: The effect of nifedipine on the sinus and atrioventricular node of the dog after β-adrenergic receptor blockade. *Acta Pharmacol Toxicol (Cophenh)* 1978;42:287–291.
95. Koch-Weser J: Vasodilator drugs in treatment of hypertension. *Arch Intern Med* 1974;133:1017–1027.

CHAPTER 16 Renovascular Hypertensive Disease in the Elderly

C. Scott Norris
Mitchell H. Goldman

Blood pressure is a physiologic parameter which changes with age. In population studies, it is a strong predictor of morbidity and mortality when pathologically elevated.[1] Epidemiologic evidence suggests that approximately 10% of the population of the United States is hypertensive with a diastolic blood pressure greater than 90 mmHg. However, upon reaching the sixth decade of life, the incidence of high blood pressure (systolic pressure greater than 160 mmHg, or diastolic pressure greater than 95 mmHg) rises to 33%.[2] Reversible causes of hypertension occur in 2% to 10% of hypertensive patients with renal arterial occlusive disease being the most common lesion encountered.[3] Atherosclerosis is responsible for the majority of renovascular lesions in the elderly. Although the prevalence of atherosclerotic renovascular disease varies between 25% and 80% in different series, the actual frequency is dependent upon the prevailing age and race of the patients seen by any institution. Because of sampling bias and the lack of simple and precise screening technics, an accurate estimate of this disease in the geriatric population is unavailable.

Recent advances in diagnostic and interventional technics have significantly expanded the options available to the practicing clinician. Application of these newly developed methods in the high-risk elderly population has substantially reduced the morbidity and mortality associated with the diagnosis and treatment of renovascular disease. Thus, a reemphasis on seeking this curable cause of hypertension has arisen.

PATHOPHYSIOLOGY

Information about experimental renovascular hypertension has been provided through the efforts of many investigators. Goldblatt established the canine model which has been used by most investigators as a model of renovascular hypertension.[4] In subsequent work kidney extracts containing renin were isolated, and they were found to be capable of producing hypertension experimentally.[5] The chemical configuration,[6] cellular origin within the juxtaglomerular apparatus,[7] and enzymatic sequences of interactions leading from renin synthesis to angiotensin generation and finally to aldosterone secretion[8] have further contributed to our understanding of the pathophysiology of renovascular hypertension. Other factors such as age, sex, race, diurnal variation in secretion, and drug interactions are all known to be capable of influencing plasma renin activity, and therefore, of playing a role in the diagnosis and therapy of hypertension related to excess activity of the renin-angiotensin-aldosterone axis.[9]

Many processes are known to regulate renin secretion (Figure 16-1). Decreased perfusion pressure to the kidney can activate intrinsic vascular receptors and these in turn stimulate renin secretion.[10] Alterations in the sodium or chloride content of tubular fluid, when detected at the macula densa, can stimulate tubuloglomerular feedback and then renin release.[11] Extrinsic autonomic modulation,[12] central nervous system (CNS) activity through the renal nerves,[13] as well as humoral mech-

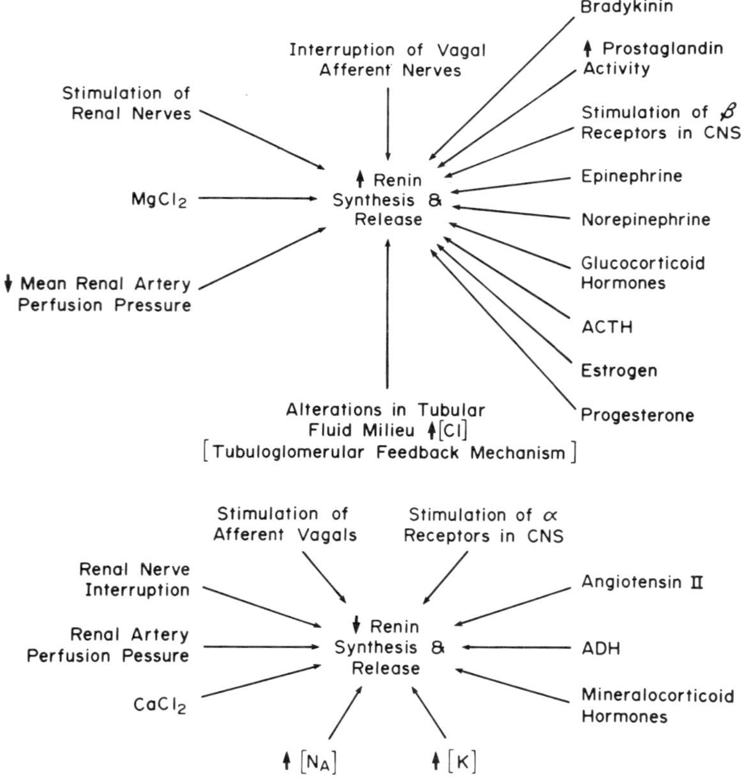

Figure 16-1 Circulating factors which may influence renin synthesis and release.

anisms are also capable of contributing to the complex regulation of renin synthesis and secretion.

The relationship between renal artery stenosis and hypertension is further complicated by the not uncommon finding of renal artery stenosis in nonhypertensive patients.[14] Retrospective autopsy findings have revealed that in 50% of all patients with a renal arterial lesion reducing vessel diameter by 50%, that clinical hypertension was absent.[15] Moreover, many cases of renal artery stenosis that cause hypertension are not associated with pathologic renin secretion.[16] Finally, the saralasin test, which utilizes an intact angiotensin antagonist, is reported to be negative in 22% of patients with subsequent surgical cure of hypertension.[17] This confusing picture is partially resolved by examining microvascular changes in "two kidney" animal models of renovascular hypertension; these models demonstrate contralateral microvascular arteriolar changes and persistence of hypertension even when arterial continuity has been re-established. Thus, experimental work as well as clinical evidence suggest that underlying contralateral and ipsilateral arteriolar nephrosclerosis may be an important cause of the elevated blood pressure associated with renovascular hypertension (Figure 16-2).

PATHOLOGY

Hypertensive nephropathy is associated with consistent morphologic changes regardless of a primary or secondary etiology of the disease (Figure 16-3). Arterioles initially undergo hyaline degeneration and later, with more malignant forms of disease, fibrinoid necrosis.[18] In certain instances, degeneration is seen to extend into the glomerular tuft. Intralobular and

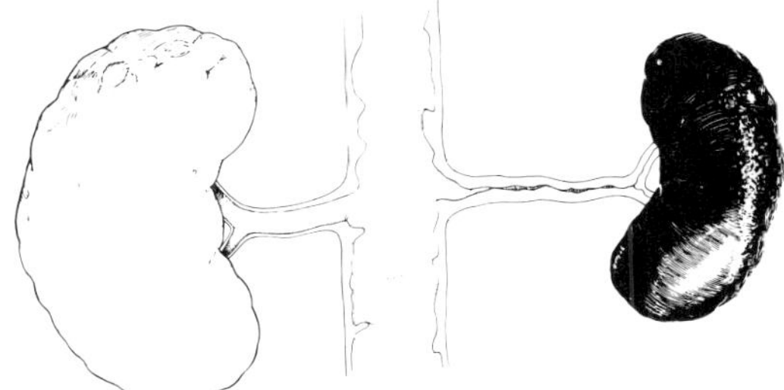

Figure 16-2 Underlying nephrosclerosis distal and contralateral to main renal artery occlusive lesion may explain failure to cure hypertension following reinstatement of adequate perfusion.

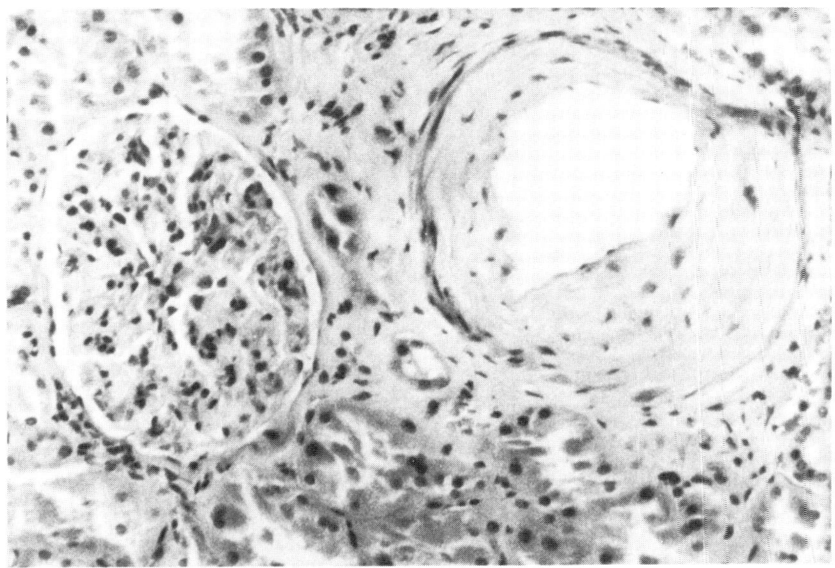

Figure 16-3 Photomicrograph demonstrating hypertensive nephropathy. (H & E stain × 400).

arcurate arteries demonstrate intimal proliferation and medial hypertrophy. A broad spectrum of glomerular involvement is seen, depending upon the severity and duration of hypertension. The natural history of this advancing disease process is comprised of varying degrees of necrosis with extension of fibrinous debris from the afferent arteriole into the glomerular tuft and finally by the development of complete sclerosis. The tubules and collecting ducts may reveal focal atrophy and interstitial fibrosis with a variable chronic inflammatory infiltrate. With optimal control of hypertension, subintimal fibroplasia in the large and medium-sized arteries may be the only finding in the absence of thrombonecrotic changes in arterioles and glomeruli.

Many forms of flow-restricting lesions of the main renal artery and its primary and secondary branches have been reported. Primary atherosclerotic disease[19] and aneurysm of the renal artery[20] may both be associated with thrombosis and subsequent hypertension. Atheromatous or mycotic emboli,[21] external compression,[22] adrenal and renal neoplasia or cysts,[23] congenital bands,[24] retroperitoneal fibrosis,[25] and arteritis[26] have all been implicated as causes of hypertension. Aortitis,[27] postirradiation stenosis,[28] transplant stenosis,[29] primary fibromuscular disease,[30] coarctation of the aorta,[31] and arteriovenous fistulae[32] may also lead to renovascular form of hypertension. In the elderly patient atherosclerotic disease of the aorta and the proximal 2 cm of the renal artery is the most likely etiology causing renovascular hypertension.

CLINICAL PRESENTATION

The reported incidence of renovascular hypertension is variable, depending upon the race and patient age being sampled. Blacks infrequently suffer from renovascular disease, yet when it is present, especially in later decades, it is most likely to be of atherosclerotic origin. The elderly patient may present with an abrupt acceleration of long-standing essential hypertension with evidence of extrarenal peripheral vascular disease or azotemia being present.[33] Medical control of preexisting hypertension may become increasingly difficult with a requirement for multiple drug therapy. Chemical evidence of renal failure if present may be disproportionate to that expected for the patient's age. Physical findings are remarkable for absent or attenuated carotid, subclavian, radial, aortic, femoral, or distal lower extremity pulsation, which may in turn be associated with bruits. An inordinately prominent aortic pulse indicates the presence of aneurysmal disease. Careful examination of the legs and feet may reveal either a unilateral cool extremity, atrophic skin changes, and ischemic ulcers or gangrene about the heel, malleolus, or toes. Painful bluish discoloration of the toes or fingers may be the result of a proximal embolic shower. Fundoscopy is remarkable for the changes of hypertensive retinopathy, including arteriovenous nicking, copper wire arteriolar changes, flame-shaped hemorrhages, and soft and hard exudates. One third of the patients will have a detectable flank bruit, and one third will demonstrate aortic calcification on plain abdominal film.[34] The mean age of the atherosclerotic group in most series ranges from 50 to 54 years. Ten percent of these same patients will have an associated abdominal aortic aneurysm. Symptomatic peripheral atherosclerotic disease will be present in 10% to 15%, and an additional 10% to 15% of these patients will experience transient ischemic attacks or stroke prior to contemplated surgery. Twenty percent of this patient population will have associated symptomatic coronary artery disease.[35] Many individuals are incidentally discovered to harbor minor renal (nonflow-reducing, less than 50% diameter reduction) lesions on aortography for nonrenal atherosclerotic disease. Forty percent of this occult disease so observed will progress over time into significant lesions.[36]

RADIOLOGY

Radiologic tests for imaging the kidney and its vasculature include intravenous (IV) urography, isotope renal flow studies, both of which require excretory function, and intra-arterial and IV (digital subtraction) arteriography. Rapid sequence urography, can be performed following injection of contrast, but requires an intact glomerular apparatus. The nephrogram phase of this study normally reveals the left kidney to be 0.5 cm longer than the right, and a discrepancy of greater than 1.5 cm is suggestive of the presence of renal artery stenosis. Delay in the nephrogram is suggestive of either ischemic atrophy or reduction in flow within the kidney. There will be visualization of the pelvocalyceal system because of an intact glomerular filtration process, but it is delayed along with the nephrogram phase. Also, notching of the renal pelvis or proximal ureter can sometimes be noted and is due to extrinsic collateral circulation. This test is associated with a sensitivity and specificity rate of 78% and 87% respectively.[37]

Intra-arterial selective angiography is universally accepted as the diagnostic standard for arterial lesions and should routinely include oblique views in order to adequately assess the majority of lesions. Most disease of secondary renal branches requires arteriography to adequately visualize the lesions. This invasive procedure is associated with 1% incidence of morbidity and a 0.1% mortality.[38] It should be cautioned, though, that the mere demonstration of renal arterial occlusive disease by arteriography does not insure remission of hypertension following revascularization. Recent advances in computerized arteriography and digital subtraction angiography have shown promising results in the hands of a limited number of investigators with an accuracy rate of 80% to 87%.[39] This procedure has a 1% to 2% incidence of contrast reactions and a less than 0.01% mortality, the former being most acceptable for a diagnostic test.[40]

SCREENING TECHNICS AND PREOPERATIVE ASSESSMENT

The insensitivity and nonspecificity of present mass screening technics have led many physicians to rely on medical therapy in the majority of patients with hypertension. Studies of peripheral plasma renin activity as a screening technic have yielded a 26% sensitivity and a 95% specificity in contrast to saralasin infusion which has a reported 52% sensitivity and 85% specificity.[41] These values are improved somewhat when standardized conditions are utilized prior to plasma renin determination, yet the results remain less than optimal. Standard conditions entail discontinuing all antihypertensive medications 2 weeks prior to testing, several days of a sodium-restricted diet, maintaining a supine posture for several hours, and diuretics given orally or parenterally prior to renin determinations. Despite employing these standard conditions, it is important to realize that the ultimate utility of peripheral plasma renin activity is limited by the fact that 16% of patients with essential hypertension will have increased values.[42]

Duplex-echo-Doppler technology has been applied in recent years to the noninvasive evaluation of renal artery stenosis. Early reports have documented the feasibility of interrogation of both renal artery and vein hemodynamics transcutaneously. Our laboratory has investigated duplex technology from an experimental and clinical perspective and has found this device to be reliable for the detection of renal artery stenosis of greater than or equal to 60% diameter reduction and for the prediction of increased renovascular resistance.[43] The parameters used to assess renal artery stenosis include a localized increase in systolic frequency, spectral broadening at the point of stenosis, and a fall in systolic Doppler shift at points distal to the stenosis (Figure 16-4). There may also be a filling in of the systolic window

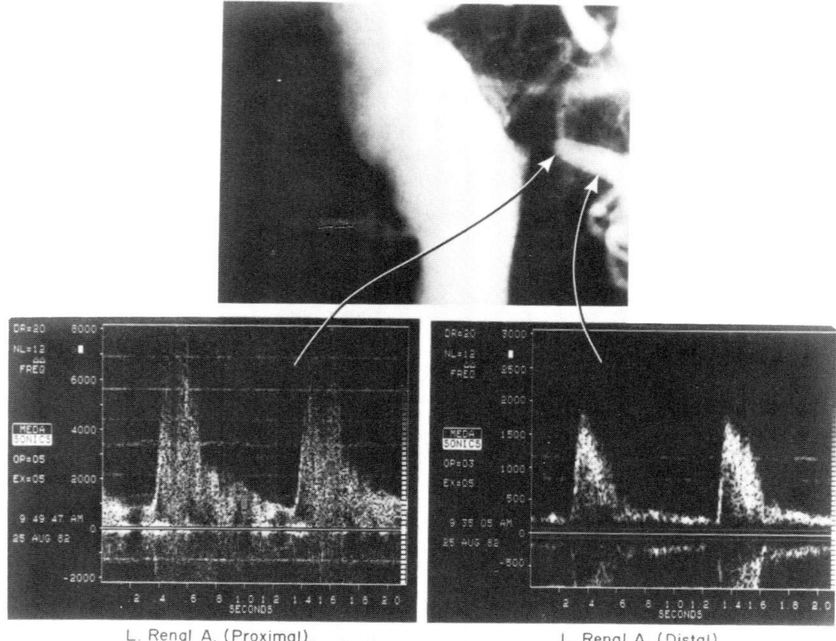

Figure 16-4 Spectral analysis from duplex interrogation of proximal stenotic and distal normal renal artery (× 400).

and an associated wall bruit. Using a 3 mHz probe, the peak systolic frequency exceeds 4 kHz in all vessels with greater than 60% diameter reduction, while only 5% of normal vessels are accompanied by this frequency response. Patients having satisfactory B-mode images, yet undetectable renal artery velocity signals, have been subsequently demonstrated as having an atrophic kidney or a totally occluded renal artery. A total of 120 patients have been studied and hemodynamic profiles were successfully measured throughout the course of the renal arteries bilaterally in 113 (94%) of them. Forty-three of the patients subsequently underwent contrast arteriography which validated renal artery morphology and documented sensitivity and specificity rates of 83% and 97%, respectively. Diastolic/systolic frequency ratios, in an organ normally characterized by high diastolic flow, were capable of differentiating age-matched hypertensive and symptomatic atherosclerotic patients from controls (Figure 16-5). These clinical studies of renal artery velocity disturbances using duplex-echo-Doppler scanning demonstrate noninvasive detection of renal artery stenosis and estimation of parenchymal renovascular resistance. Factors precluding satisfactory scanning, such as patient obesity, aneurysm, operation, or recent oral intake, may be overcome in the future by improvements in technic and instruments.

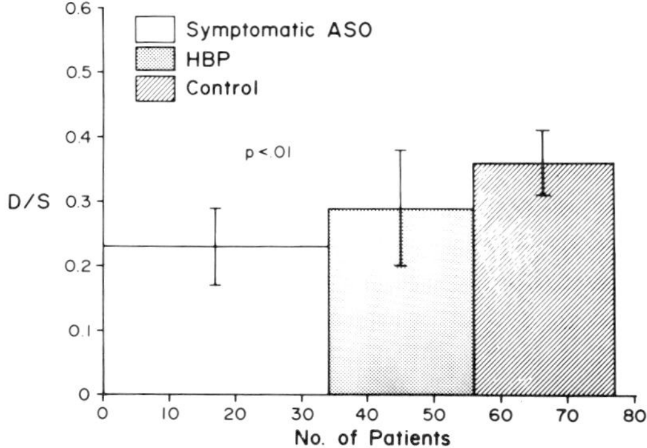

Figure 16-5 Duplex noninvasive measure (index of diastolic/systolic frequency) of microvascular resistance from age-matched normal, hypertensives (two-drug × 10 years), and patients with symptomatic peripheral vascular disease.

Following identification of a critical renal artery stenosis in a hypertensive patient, most authors support physiologic evaluation to substantiate renin dependency of the hypertension. Patients should be restricted to a 2-g sodium intake for two consecutive days, and should receive 40 mg furosemide daily prior to renal vein sampling for plasma renin activity. In addition, ideally, all antihypertensive medication should be discontinued for several weeks, and patients should be instructed to maintain a supine posture for several hours before testing.[44] To ensure accurate and effective sampling renin sampling should be performed before or a considerable period after angiography. The administration of a provocative agent such as hydralazine hydrochloride or captopril increases renin secretion and further improves diagnostic accuracy. Studies adhering to these strict conditions have correctly predicted the results of surgical treatment in 98% of patients when renal vein renin ratios were greater than 1.5.[45] Some investigators have emphasized that a renal/systemic renin index which exceeds 0.48 is the result of suppression of renin secretion in the contralateral kidney.[46]

Despite the obvious renin dependency of most forms of renovascular hypertension, many reports have documented surgically cured renovascular hypertension that has not been associated with preoperative renin dependence. Furthermore, patients with essential hypertension have shown a 20% to 25% incidence of lateralizing renin values. The functional significance of renal ischemia can be further investigated by bilateral ureteral catheterization and split function testing. A 25% to 60% reduction in urine volume, 15% reduction in urine sodium concentration, and 25% to 50% difference in urine creatinine concentration implies unilateral ischemia on the affected side. Following IV administration of para-aminohippurate (PAH), a substance used to measure renal blood flow, a 25% reduction of its clearance on the affected side is a further indication of functional significance. These studies have identified 97% of significant lesions.[44] There are many disadvantages to split renal function studies including technical dissatisfaction in 10% to 20% of the cases and 20% false-positive and 48% false-negative results.[47]

SURGICAL INTERVENTION VERSUS MEDICAL THERAPY

Once a flow-restricting renal artery stenotic lesion has been identified and the ipsilateral kidney is proved to secrete abnormal levels of renin, the decision regarding medical *v* surgical therapy must be resolved (Figure 16-6). Trials comparing medical and surgical therapy, though poorly controlled and not randomized, suggest a prolonged longevity with surgical intervention.[48] Instituting a prolonged course of medical therapy for hypertension is often made difficult because of poor compliance, undesirable side effects, and not infrequently inadequate control of the hypertension.[49] Moreover, effective control of the blood pressure existing proximal to a stenotic lesion may result in lowering perfusion pressure to the involved kidney with the result being ischemia and atrophy of that kidney. When selecting a course of therapy, the physician must be aware that renal arterial lesions are often both progressive and recurrent and in certain

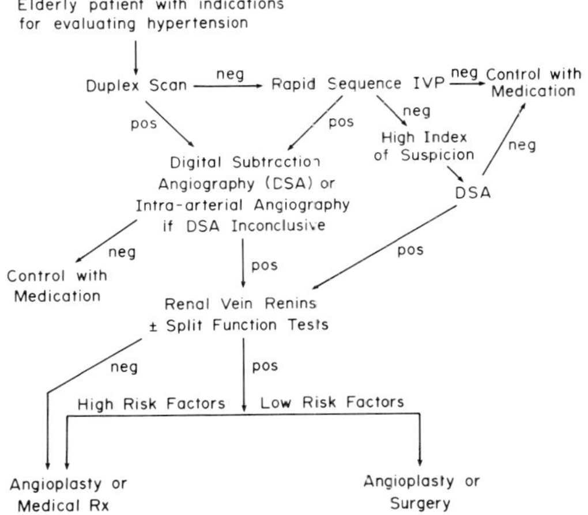

Figure 16-6 Systematic approach to evaluating the hypertensive elderly patient.

instances multiple or bilateral lesions exist. Poor selection of surgical measures for management of this disease may be associated with a 10% to 20% incidence of failure within 3 months thereby leading to nephrectomy in 10% of cases.[46] Patients with bilateral renal artery stenosis or evidence of diffuse atherosclerotic disease have a 3% to 15% perioperative mortality rate[50] in contrast to a 2% to 3% mortality rate for fibromuscular dysplasia.[51] The potential for recovery of renal function following revascularization is dependent upon the extent of underlying nephrosclerosis that has occurred as the result of the ischemic insult. Other criteria that support attempts at revascularization include evidence of collateral circulation, viable glomeruli on biopsy, and a patent distal renal artery as demonstrated by arteriography or operative exploration.[52]

Percutaneous transluminal angioplasty (PTA) has had excellent results in the correction of stenotic lesions with a 90% primary success rate and 3% technical failures. Calcification of the renal artery wall and severe tortuosity with an acutely angled takeoff from the aorta are situations that present technical difficulties which may preclude angioplasty.[53] Atherosclerosis of the aorta, iliac, and femoral vessels and the presence of aneurysmal disease may also interfere with successful dilation.[54] Cure or improvement in hypertension has been observed with successful PTA despite occasional nonlateralizing renal vein renin determinations. This procedure has also been successful in transplant renal artery stenosis with improvement in renal function subsequent to the reinstatement of adequate perfusion. The long-term patency rate of the renal artery following PTA is presently not established, and difficulties from re-stenosis have been reported. Complications include acute renal failure, distal emboli and infarction, renal artery perforation, thigh hematoma, intimal tears, distal extremity gangrene, and balloon segment rupture.

PREOPERATIVE PREPARATION

Preoperative assessment of the elderly patient who is selected for operative intervention must include an in-depth evaluation and screening for occult cerebrovascular and cardiovascular disease (Figure 16-7). The technic of carotid Doppler interrogation utilized for cerebrovascular testing has provided a sensitive and specific means of identifying carotid occlusive disease.[55] Additionally, echocardiographic evaluation of the left ventricle during resting and stressed conditions has provided objective criteria useful in identifying occult coronary artery disease as manifested by a reduced ejection fraction and dyskinetic segmental wall motion.[56] Individuals with significant coexisting disease should initially undergo repair of these lesions in hopes of minimizing this

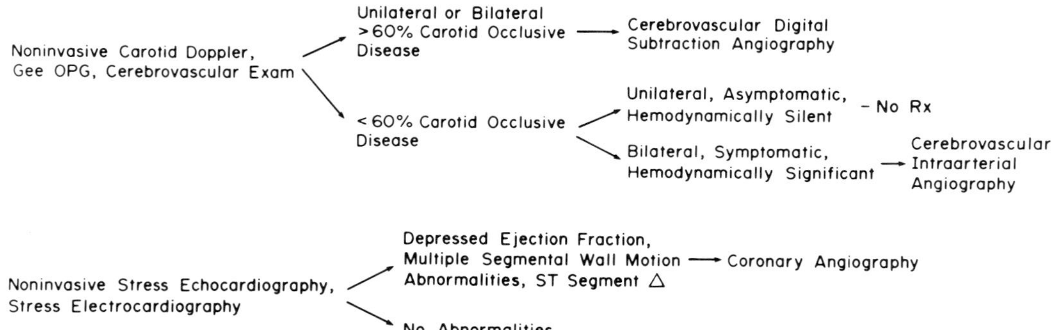

Figure 16-7 Noninvasive evaluation of cerebrovascular and cardiovascular systems in high-risk patients.

as a source of perioperative morbidity and mortality. Long-acting antihypertensive agents should be discontinued 2 weeks prior to surgery and electrolyte abnormalities, if present, appropriately managed. Short-acting agents may be employed for the temporary control of blood pressure. Preoperative pulmonary artery catheterization and pressure monitoring may be useful for optimal hydration prior to and during surgery.

OPERATIVE TECHNIC

Though approaches and technics for surgical repair of renal artery stenosis vary, there are standard measures which are usually taken intraoperatively. Patient positioning on the operating table must be carefully designed to coincide with the preoperative assessment and subsequent operative plan. Bilateral exploration of the renal arteries may be performed through a midline incision once the patient has been placed in a supine position with arms at the sides. Optimal exposure for a unilateral repair may be best achieved through a retroperitoneal exploration following positioning on a kidney rest with moderate dorsiflexion and rotation of the patient. Skin preparation and draping should include the chest, abdomen, and both legs to allow easy procurement of a saphenous vein. Renal ischemic time is best kept under 60 minutes. To preserve renal function, mannitol and furosemide are given 20 minutes prior to interruption of renal blood flow, and fluids are administered in volumes adequate to maintain physiologic central pressure. Intraoperative anticoagulation with heparin is also routinely used.

Midline Approach for Unilateral Disease

Once the abdomen has been entered, a general exploration is undertaken. The small bowel is retracted to the contralateral side of the repair and packed. When exposure of the right kidney is the primary objective, the right colon is mobilized by dividing the lateral peritoneal reflection from the hepatic flexure to beyond the cecum and retracting the second and third portions of the duodenum cephalad and medially allowing access to the right renal vein and inferior vena cava (Figure 16-8). Further exposure of the vena cava can be achieved by division of the posterior lumbar and right gonadal veins. Once the vena cava and left renal vein can be retracted, the origin of the right renal artery may be appreciated. The renal artery and aorta are dissected from the surrounding neural and lymphatic elements. Control of the aorta is obtained between the celiac and superior mesenteric artery, and the entire length of the renal artery from its origin to the first major division is exposed. Intravenous heparin, 3000 to 5000 units, is given three minutes prior to the interruption of blood flow, and the aorta is partially occluded around the orifice of the renal artery. Local endarterectomy of the renal artery is performed with a renal arteriotomy which is extended onto the aorta. This approach provides poor exposure for the aortic portion of the endarterectomy where disease often originates, yet may be appropriate for focal mid- to distal one third renal artery lesions. Care must

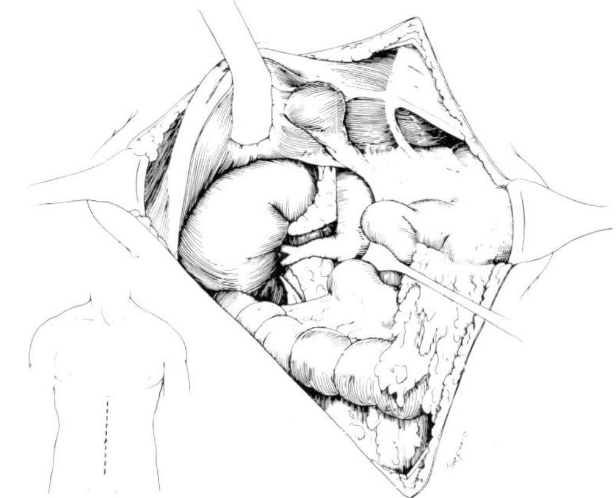

Figure 16-8 Schematic illustration of midline approach to exposure of the right kidney and vascular pedicle.

be taken to establish the proper plane for endarterectomy. With the use of a blunt instrument, the endarterectomy is advanced in a circumferential manner proximally and distally until the occlusive segment can be retracted from the wound margins. The end point of dissection must be closely inspected for smooth margins, and tacking sutures may be required to reduce the likelihood of future dissection. Following endarterectomy, the renal artery is often thin-walled and may require vein patch angioplasty.

Exposure of the left kidney is achieved by mobilizing the left descending colon, splenic flexure, and distal half of the transverse colon. The gastrocolic ligament and splenocolic attachments are divided while retracting the colon inferiorly and medially. The adrenal, gonadal, and posterior lumbar veins may be ligated and divided to allow further mobilization of the inferior vena cava and left renal vein. This will in turn yield an access plane for dissection of the left renal artery.

With extensive atherosclerotic involvement of the aorta and orifices of the renal arteries, a transaortic approach for endarterectomy should be considered. Complete mobilization of the aorta to a point above the superior mesenteric artery (SMA) and below the iliac bifurcation is warranted. The lower lumbar arteries are divided to gain aortic mobility. Following heparinization, clamps or tourniquets are placed on the proximal SMA and distal renal arteries to avoid back bleeding. The aorta is occluded either between the celiac and SMA or just distal to the SMA. A vertical anterior aortotomy is made, and the endarterectomy is performed as previously described with fixation of the raw plane of intima with mattress sutures. Dissection is continued to the ostia of the renal arteries where the plane is carefully extended into the renal artery until a normal intima appears (Figure 16-9). Occasionally, the plaque may be "milked" out of the renal artery. The contralateral side is operated on in a similar fashion, and the dissection is extended cephalad to the superior mesenteric artery. Once completed, the aortotomy is flushed with dilute heparin and the clamps are released to free loose plaques or thrombi. The intima of the renal artery is inspected through the orifice for loose flaps, and the aortotomy is then closed. Occasionally, additional incisions are made in the renal arteries to ensure an adequate endarterectomy. Disadvantages of this method include the necessity for aortic cross clamping since the ensuing bilateral renal ischemia is associated with significant morbidity and mortality.

Bypass grafting for occlusive disease is yet another alternative. This may include resection of short diseased segments and placement of interposition grafts. Aortorenal bypass grafts are associated with favorable short- and long-term results.[57] This procedure avoids the extensive aortic dissection required with endarterectomy

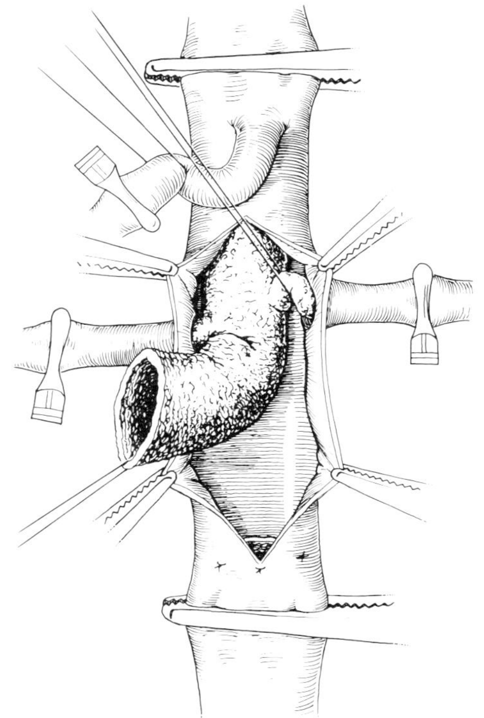

Figure 16-9 Aortorenal endarterectomy is useful from an anterior transaortic approach in the presence of severe coexisting aortic disease.

and can be adapted to multisegmental fibrous lesions or disease of the secondary vessels. Autogenous hypogastric artery,[58] splenic artery,[59] and saphenous vein have all been used as the grafting vessel. Dacron, although associated with a high rate of early thrombosis, may be an alternative interconnecting substance.[60] Meticulous technic must be employed with saphenous vein procurement, selecting a vessel of 4 to 6 mm in diameter with careful ligation of its tributaries. The vein is left in situ until the vessel is ready for anastomosis, and then it is dilated with autologous heparinized blood. The patient is heparinized prior to interrupting flow to the kidney, and the bypass graft is positioned in a fashion to ensure a comfortable orientation. An end-to-side or end-to-end renal anastomosis is performed with tapering of the saphenous vein as necessary. The aortic anastomosis is performed between the renal artery and the inferior mesenteric artery. Following mobilization of the aorta and identification of a suitable location free of atherosclerotic plaque, a Satinsky clamp is placed on the anterolateral portion of the infrarenal aorta in a tangential fashion. A 12- to 15-mm aortotomy is performed, and the vein graft is oriented in a comfortable position anterior to the renal veins and vena cava. The proximal anastomosis is performed following tapering of the saphenous vein utilizing a similar technic as was employed distally (Figure 16-10). When an end-to-end anastomosis is planned, the graft is sewn to the aorta prior to performing the distal anastomosis. An alternative to bypass grafts to the left renal artery in the face of severe atherosclerosis involving the aorta may include mobilizing the splenic artery proximal to its division within the hilum of the spleen and using this vessel as a conduit. Contraindications to this procedure may include splenic artery occlusive disease, pancreatitis, and pseudocyst.[61] Additional potential sources for inflow to the right kidney are the hepatic, gastroduodenal, superior mesenteric or iliac arteries. Though these arteries are readily available for use, their mobility and anatomic location require a more extensive dissection in order to achieve adequate length for grafting.

Ablative Surgery

The surgeon is occasionally left with the performance of a total nephrectomy as the only therapeutic alternative. Failure of partial nephrectomy, unilateral total renal infarction, severe nephrosclerosis, or poor flow through a previous repair with preexisting elevated renin secretion may necessitate total nephrectomy. In the past, the totally occluded renal artery with a nonfunctioning kidney inevitably resulted in nephrectomy though more recently successful attempts at revascularization have been reported. This decision should be preceded by selective arteriography that demonstrates peripheral collaterals or retrograde filling of the distal renal artery by collaterals. Evidence of back bleeding, at the time of surgery, distal to the occluded segment and intraoperative histology demonstrating viable glomeruli may also support the decision to attempt revascularization rather than to proceed with nephrectomy.

Partial nephrectomy may be indicated for a localized disease process in the hopes of preserving some remaining function

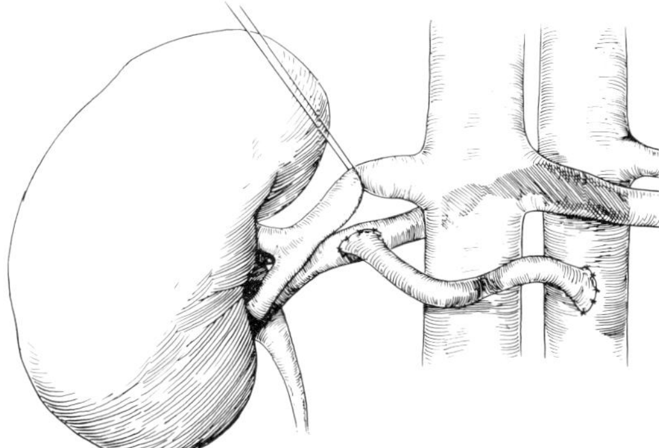

Figure 16-10 Schematic illustration of aortorenal bypass grafting with tapering of graft at anastomosis.

(Figure 16-11), or for segmental ischemia from branch lesions that are technically inadequate for grafting or dilation. Polar nephrectomy is performed by exposing the renal pedicle and then selectively isolating the proximal diseased secondary branch vessels. Vital dyes (indigo carmine, methylene blue) are infused within the diseased branch vessels to identify the poorly perfused tissue. The capsule is then divided and retracted toward the pedicle while hemostasis is improved by applying gentle pressure across the renal parenchyma while holding the kidney between the thumb and fingers. After resection of the diseased parenchyma, shallow figure-of-eight sutures are placed over the exposed transected vessels (Figure 16-12). The collecting system is closed separately following which the renal pelvis is injected with dilute methylene blue to verify that the system is watertight. The capsular flaps are retracted over the raw parenchymal surface and sutured with horizontal mattress sutures. Mannitol is infused following partial nephrectomy to prevent obstruction of the collecting system by clot formation.

Segmental lesions affecting branches of the anterior division of the renal artery that are inaccessible to bypass or dilatation are best managed by midsegmental resection. Selective angiography is necessary to precisely define the occlusive lesions. The hilum of the kidney is identified and the secondary branch vessels are carefully isolated. Traction sutures are placed around arterial branches supplying the vascular segment. These vessels are injected with methylene blue thereby delineating the ischemic parenchyma, which is then compared to the corresponding arteriogram. The arteries and veins supplying this segment are ligated and divided. The calyceal portion of the devitalized parenchyma is transected and closed. The cap-

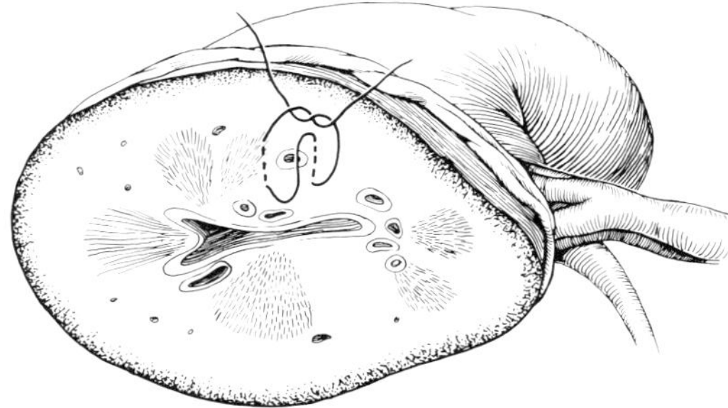

Figure 16-12 Operative technic to gain hemostasis when performing polar nephrectomy.

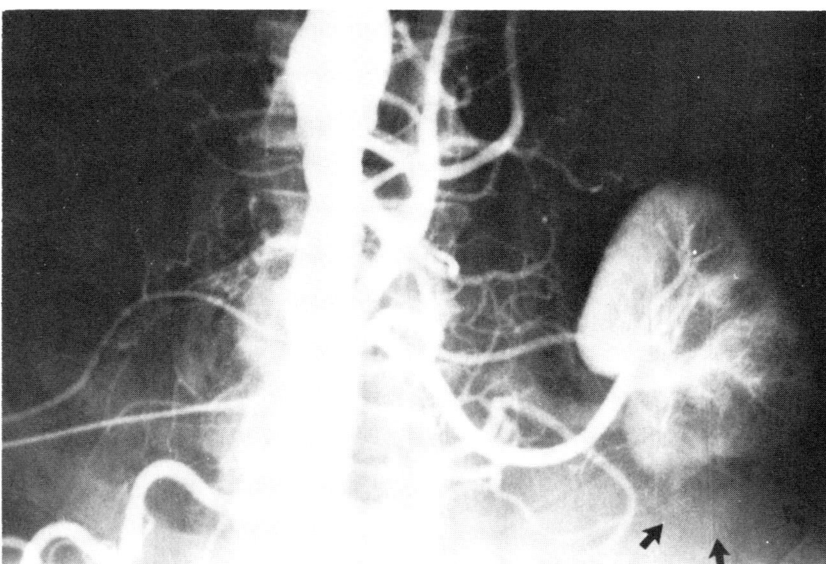

Figure 16-11 Isolated infarcted segment of the kidney may be responsible for persistent hypertension.

sule is divided in a coronal direction exposing the wedge of demarcated tissue. Mannitol and heparin are administered prior to clamping the main renal artery at which time the central wedge of tissue is excised. Residual bleeders are ligated on the cut surface of parenchyma, and the calyceal system is inspected to ensure a tight closure. Clamps are removed from the main renal artery, and further inspection is performed to ensure adequate hemostasis. The collecting system may be infused with dye to document a closure that is hydrostatically complete. The capsule overlying the two poles is approximated with horizontal mattress sutures, and Gerota's capsule is closed leaving drains juxtaposed to the kidney.

Autotransplantation – Ex Vivo Renal Surgery

In the presence of extensive atheromatous aortic disease precluding an aortic anastomosis and when other sources of inflow (splenic artery, superior mesenteric artery, hepatic artery) are judged to be poor alternatives, autotransplantation may be an option.[62] The kidney is explanted utilizing similar technics as with an allograft, and the ureter is left in a comfortable position, not requiring division. During the harvesting procedure, care must be taken to ensure that a maximum length of renal vessel and ureter, if necessary, are preserved. Ex vivo renal surgery has allowed access to secondary branch vessels previously inaccessible to microvascular repair or dilatation.

Combined Aortoiliac and Renal Artery Disease

Combining aortofemoral bypass grafting or aneurysmectomy with renal revascularization is associated with a higher perioperative and late mortality, 6% and 25% respectively, because of complications from generalized atherosclerosis. The 53% incidence of cure or improvement in patients with combined disease is less satisfactory than the 87% cure rate associated with focal renovascular involvement alone.[52] Assessment of these patients necessitates comparing the morbidity and mortality for each problem with the estimated longevity of the patient and the expected results from surgery. Most patients selected for aortic surgery should be capable of tolerating the additional stress of concomitant renal revascularization. In the event of unforeseen technical difficulties, the surgeon may select intraoperative balloon dilatation or PTA following successful postoperative recovery.

RESULTS

Surgical intervention is associated with a wide spectrum of complications that varies with the center, operative technic, and patient population. Thrombosis and hemorrhage are the most frequently experienced difficulties and may be attributed to errors in surgical technic. False aneurysm and aortoenteric fistula are additional complications which may be late occurrences.[63] Aortic thrombosis and distal extremity embolization from plaque dislodgement may occur during or subsequent to the initial angiography procedure or following surgical manipulation. Late aneurysmal graft dilatation with autogenous saphenous vein and iliac artery have also been reported.[64] Postoperative hypertension despite a functioning bypass graft is another disappointing result the surgeon must be prepared to face and usually results from intraparenchymal disease. Preoperative technics that allow assessment of the microvascular status of a kidney may supplement existing physiologic studies and result in an improved patient selection. Experimental models of graded microvascular resistance have been sensitive and accurate in categorizing existing methods of flow velocity analysis. Significantly increased levels of resistance[43] are demonstrated when transcutaneous application of this technic is applied to patient populations recognized to harbor microvascular disease.

Elderly patients with renovascular hypertension experience the poorest results from surgical intervention. An aggressive preoperative assessment to identify and eradicate potential sources of operative morbidity has significantly improved perioperative results and has made operative intervention a more viable alternative in otherwise high-risk individuals.[65] The natural history of renal function in this population is that of a steady deterioration with the passage of years. Therefore, the coexistence of renovascular disease would presumably influence the management decision favoring maximal attempts at salvage of a still functioning kidney.

Within the elderly patient population, those patients at lowest risk who are most likely to benefit from normalization in renal perfusion as measured by preoperative evaluation (angiography, differential renal vein renin, microvascular resistance) should be advised to select surgical therapy at an experienced institution. Poor-risk patients with a less definitive preoperative assessment or evidence of generalized atherosclerosis may best be managed with PTA. Although this technic has not been shown to have a longevity equivalent to that of surgery, there will still be at least short-term benefits in renal function and blood pressure. With the improved screening and imaging technics now available, these patients can be closely followed and scheduled for repeat dilatation procedures as necessary.

REFERENCES

1. Five-year Findings of the Hypertension Detection and Follow-up Program. *JAMA* 1979;242(23):2562–2571.
2. Kannel WB, Gordon T, Sorlie P, et al: Physical activity and coronary vulnerability. The Framingham Study. *Cardiovas Dig* 1971;6:28–40.
3. Foster JH: Recognition and management of renovascular hypertension. *Hosp Pract* 1975;10(10):61–70.
4. Goldblatt H: Experimental renal hypertension. *Am J Med* 1948;4:401–402.
5. Pickering GW, Prinzmetal M, Kelsall AR: Assay of renin in rabbits with experimental renal hypertension. *Clin Sci* 1942;4:401–402.
6. Skeggs LT, Marsh WH, Kahn JR, et al: The purification of hypertension. *J Exp Med* 1954;100:363–370.
7. Edelman R, Hartroft PM: Localization of renin in juxtaglomerular cells of rabbit and dog through the use of the fluorescent-antibody technique. *Circ Res* 1961;9:1069–1077.
8. Ganong WF, Mulrow PJ: Evidence of secretion of an aldosterone-stimulating substance by the kidney. *Nature* 1961;190:115–116.
9. Laragh JH: Peptide hormones, in Berson SA, Yalow RS (eds): *Methods of Investigative and Diagnostic Endocrinology.* New York, American Elsevier, 1973, vol 2B, pp 1168–1174.
10. Abe Y, Okahara T, Kishimoto T, et al: Relationship between intrarenal distribution of blood flow and renin secretion. *Am J Phsyiol* 1973;225:319–323.
11. Thurau K: Renal hemodynamics. *Am J Med* 1964;36:698–719.
12. Ganong WF, Reid IA: Sympathetic nervous system and central alpha- and beta-adrenergic receptors in the regulation of renin secretion, in Onesti G, Fernandes M, Kim KE (eds): *Regulation of Blood Pressure by the Central Nervous System. Fourth Hahnemann International Symposium on Hypertension.* New York, Grune & Stratton, 1976, p 201.
13. Ueda H, Yasuda H, Takabatake Y: Increased renin release evoked by mesencephalic stimulation in the dog. *Jpn Heart J* 1967;8:498–506.
14. Holley KE, Hunt JC, Brown AL, et al: Renal artery stenosis: A clinical-pathologic study in normotensive and hypertensive patients. *Am J Med* 1964;37:14–22.
15. Dustan HP, Humphries AW, de Wolfe VG, et al: Normal arterial pressure in patients with renal arterial stenosis. *JAMA* 1964;187:1028–1029.
16. Amsterdam EA, Couch NP, Christlieb AR, et al: Renal vein renin activity in the prog-

nosis of surgery for renovascular hypertension. *Am J Med* 1969;47:860–868.
17. Tucker RM: Renal arterial hypertension: diagnosis and management. *Cardiovasc Clin* 1978;9:165–181.
18. Heptinstall RH: Renal biopsies in hypertension. *Br Heart J* 1954;16:133–141.
19. McCormack LJ, Dustan HP, Gifford RW, et al: Pathology of renal artery disease. *Postgrad Med* 1966;40:348–354.
20. Popowniak KL, Gifford RW, Straffon RA, et al: Aneurysms of the renal artery: an analysis of 51 cases. *Postgrad Med* 1966; 40:255–262.
21. Lessman RK, Johnson SF, Coburn JW, et al: Renal artery embolism: clinical features and long-term follow-up of 17 cases. *Ann Intern Med* 1978;89:477–482.
22. Halpern M, Currarino G: Vascular lesions causing hypertension in neurofibromatosis. *N Engl J Med* 1965;273:248–252.
23. Weidmann P, Siegenthaler W, Ziegler WH, et al: Hypertension associated tumors adjacent to renal arteries. *Am J Med* 1969; 47:528–533.
24. D'Abreu F, Strickland B: Developmental renal artery stenosis. *Lancet* 1962;2:517–521.
25. Rinke Von W, Kalkowski H, Wedler B, et al: Doppelseitige Nierenarterienstenose bei retroperitonealer Fibrose (Morbus Ormond). *Zentralbl Chir* 1978;103:242–245.
26. Heptinstall RH: Polyarteritis (periarteritis) nodosa and rheumatoid arthritis, in Heptinstall RH (ed): *Pathology of the Kidney.* Boston, Little, Brown and Co, 1974, vol 2, pp 601–638.
27. Prince RK, Skelton R: Hypertension due to syphilitic occlusion of main renal arteries. *Br Heart J* 1948;10:29–33.
28. Lawson JD, Boerth R, Foster JH, et al: Diagnosis and management of renovascular hypertension in children. *Arch Surg* 1977; 112:1307–1316.
29. Doyle TH, McGregor WR, Fox PS, et al: Homotransplant renal artery stenosis. *Surgery* 1975;77:53–60.
30. Harrison EG, McCormack LJ: Pathologic classification of renal artery disease in renovascular hypertension. *Mayo Clin Proc* 1971;46:161–167.
31. Alpert BS, Bain HH, Balfe JW, et al: Role of the renin-angiotensin-aldosterone system in hypertensive children with coarctation of the aorta. *Am J Cardiol* 1979;43: 828–834.
32. McAlhany JC Jr, Black HC Jr, Hanback LD Jr, et al: Renal arteriovenous fistula as a cause of hypertension. *Am J Surg* 1971; 122:117–120.
33. Perloff D, Sokolow M, Wylie EJ, et al: Hypertension secondary to renal artery occlusive disease. *Circulation* 1961;24:1286–1304.
34. Swinton NW: Clinical presentation and natural history of renovascular hypertension, in Breslin DJ, Swinton NW, Livertino JA, et al (eds): *Renovascular Hypertension.* Baltimore, Williams & Wilkins, 1982, pp 73–77.
35. Wollenweber J, Sheps SG, Davis GD: Clinical course of atherosclerotic renovascular disease. *Am J Cardiol* 1968;21: 60–71.
36. Meaney TF, Dustan HP, McCormack LJ: Natural history of renal arterial disease. *Radiology* 1968;91:881–887.
37. Thornbury JR, Stanley JC, Fryback DG: Hypertensive urogram: A nondiscriminatory test for renovascular hypertension. *Am J Roentgenol* 1982;138:43–49.
38. Sigstedt B, Lunderquist A: Complications of angiographic examinations. *Am J Roentgenol* 1978;130:455–460.
39. Smith CW, Winfield AC, Price RR, et al: Evaluation of digital venous angiography for the diagnosis of renovascular hypertension. *Radiology* 1982;144:51–54.
40. Coleman WP, Ochsner SF, Watson BE: Allergic reactions in 10,000 consecutive intravenous urographies. *South Med J* 1964; 54:1401–1404.
41. Grim CE, Luft FC, Weinberger MH, et al: Sensitivity and specificity of screening tests for renal vascular hypertension. *Ann Intern Med* 1979;91:617–622.
42. Maxwell MH, Marks LS, Varady PD, et al: Renal vein renin in essential hypertension. *J Lab Clin Med* 1975;86:901–909.
43. Norris CS, Pfeiffer JS, Rittgers SE, et al: Noninvasive evaluation of renal artery stenosis and renovascular resistance: experimental and clinical studies. *J Vasc Surg* 1984;1:192–201.
44. Dean RH, Oates JA, Wilson, JP, et al: Bilateral renal artery stenosis and renovascular hypertension. *Surgery* 1977;81:53–62.
45. Strong CG, Hunt JC, Sheps SG, et al: Renal

venous renin activity–enhancement of sensitivity of lateralization by sodium depletion. *Am J Cardiol* 1971;27:602–611.

46. Stanley JC, Fry WJ: Surgical treatment of renovascular hypertension. *Arch Surg* 1977;112:1291–1297.
47. Russell RP: Renal hypertension. *Surg Clin North Am* 1974;54:349–361.
48. Hunt JC: Renovascular hypertension, in Earley LE, Gottschalk CW (eds): *Diseases of the Kidney*. Boston, Little, Brown and Co, 1979, pp 1357–1384.
49. Genest J, Boucher R, Rojo-Ortega JM, et al: Renovascular hypertension, in Genest J, Koiw E, Kuchel O (eds): *Hypertension*. New York, McGraw-Hill Book Co, 1977, pp 815–840.
50. Ernst CB, Stanley JC, Marshall FF, Fry WJ: Renal revascularization for arteriosclerotic renovascular hypertension: Prognostic implications of focal renal arterial vs. overt generalized arteriosclerosis. *Surgery* 1973; 73:859–867.
51. Stanley JC, Fry WJ: Renovascular hypertension secondary to arterial fibrodysplasia in adults: Criteria for operation and results of surgical therapy. *Arch Surg* 1975;110: 922–928.
52. Libertino JA, Zinman L, Breslin DJ, et al: Renal artery revascularization: restoration of renal function. *JAMA* 1980;244:1340–1342.
53. Madias NE, Ball JT, Millan VG: Percutaneous transluminal renal angioplasty in the treatment of unilateral atherosclerotic renovascular hypertension. *Am J Med* 1981;70:1078–1084.
54. Schwarten DE, Yune HY, Klatte EC, et al: Clinical experience with percutaneous transluminal angioplasty (PTA) of stenotic renal arteries. *Radiology* 1980;135:601–604.
55. Blackshear WM, Phillips DJ, Thiele BL, et al: Detection of carotid occlusive disease by ultrasonic imaging and pulsed Doppler spectrum analysis. *Surgery* 1979;86:698–706.
56. Mason SJ, Weiss JL, Weisfeldt ML, et al: Exercise echocardiography: detection of wall motion abnormalities during ischemia. *Circulation* 1979;59:50–59.
57. Stanley JC, Ernst CB, Fry WJ: Fate of 100 aortorenal vein grafts: characteristics of late graft expansion, aneurysmal dilation, and stenosis. *Surgery* 1973;74:931–944.
58. Lye CR, String ST, Wylie EJ, et al: Aortorenal arterial autografts: late observations. *Arch Surg* 1975;110:1321–1326.
59. Wylie EJ: Vascular replacement with arterial autografts. *Surgery* 1965;57:14–21.
60. Kaufman JJ: Long-term results of aortorenal dacron grafts in the treatment of renal artery disease. *J Urol* 1974;111: 298–304.
61. Straffon RA, McLaughlin TC, Kiser WS, et al: The saphenous vein bypass graft in the treatment of renovascular hypertension. *Trans Am Assoc Genitourin Surg* 1970; 62:47–56.
62. Hardy JC: High ureteral injuries: Management by autotransplantation of the kidney. *JAMA* 1963;184:97–101.
63. Nerstrom B, Engell HC: Operative treatment of renovascular hypertension: a study of 60 consecutive patients with follow-up findings between 1 and 7 years postoperatively. *Ann Surg* 1972;176:590–596.
64. Foster JH, Dean RH, Pinkerton JA, et al: Ten years experience with the surgical management of renovascular hypertension. *Ann Surg* 1973;177:755–766.
65. Pechan BW, Novick AC, Stewart BH, et al: Endarterectomy and patchgraft angioplasty in treatment of atherosclerotic renovascular hypertension. *Urology* 1979;14:487–490.

CHAPTER 17 Pathology of the Aging Lower Urinary Tract

Robert H. Lippman

URINARY BLADDER

Embryology

The urogenital sinus develops from the endoderm of the cloaca. From the urogenital sinus evolves most of the urethra, urinary bladder, and in the male the prostate; in the female, the vestibule. The bladder trigone represents the incorporation of the mesonephric duct (mesoderm) into the bladder. In the male the trigone is the region between the ureters and the deferential ducts, all of which are derived from the mesonephric duct[1] (Figure 17-1).

Anatomy

The urinary bladder is a viscus with transitional epithelium covering the luminal surface and submucosa, and the detrusor muscle comprising the bulk of the bladder wall. The detrusor consists of interlacing fascicles of smooth muscle which condense at the bladder neck. The muscle bundles continue on as longitudinal fibers in the urethra. The muscle of the trigone is a continuation of the muscle fibers found in the wall of the ureter. These fibers insert in the verumontanum in the male and in the terminal urethra in the female. Smooth muscle contraction results in contraction of the bladder; this leads to a funneling effect at the bladder neck where the resultant shortening of the urethra leads to urethral closure. The urogenital diaphragm is composed of voluntary skeletal muscle (Figure 17-1). It permits short-term urethral closure and interruption of the urinary

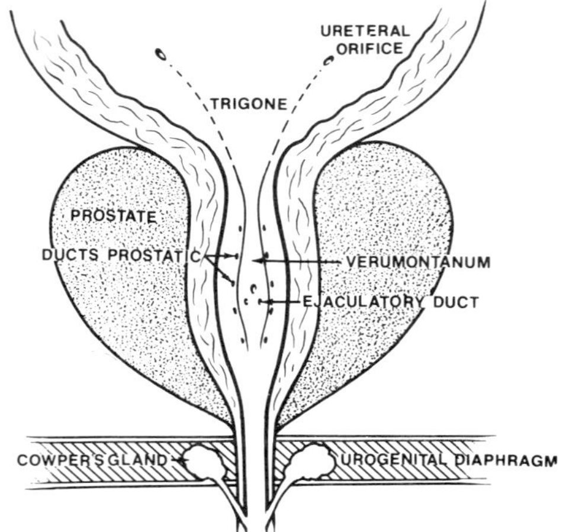

Figure 17-1 Anatomy of bladder and prostate.

stream. Urinary continence is maintained by many factors including both the radius and the length of the urethra, the muscular and elastic tissue configuration about the bladder neck, and possibly a relationship to vascular erectile tissue.[2]

Hormones

The trigone is sensitive to steroid hormones as are other derivatives of the mesonephric duct. Decreased estrogen which may follow menopause or oophorectomy characteristically leads to epithelial thinning in the lower urinary tract.[3]

AGING

There are three major categories of age-related functional changes in the urinary bladder: those changes associated with urinary outlet obstruction, urinary incontinence, and the decreased bladder capacity and increased postvoiding residual seen to occur in both men and women who demonstrate neither obstruction nor incontinence.[2,4] Vesicular outlet obstruction may be either neurogenic or anatomical in origin. Macroscopic changes in the obstructed and the incontinent urinary bladder demonstrate similar features: trabeculation and/or diverticula of the wall. The major difference between the obstructed and the incontinent bladder exists in either's capacity to effect the amount of urine retained after voiding. This is usually increased with obstruction and decreased with incontinence. In outlet obstruction the first event is dilation of the vesicle; this is then followed by detrusor muscle hypertrophy as might be seen in any muscle-lined hollow viscus operating against obstruction including the heart or gallbladder. The detrusor contracts as a unit and therefore hypertrophy occurs uniformly. The hypertrophied bundles of detrusor muscle are termed trabeculae. The trabecular prominence is increased by the dilatation of the bladder wall at sites located between these interlacing muscle bundles. Elevation of intraluminal pressure during micturition or with chronic obstruction can lead to the herniation of mucosa between these muscle bundles. The earliest types of herniation are called *cellules* or *saccules*. When the herniation projects beyond the limits of the bladder wall a pseudodiverticulum is formed (pseudo because the outpouching is devoid of a complete muscle coat). Conventionally, these outpouchings are known simply as bladder diverticula. As with any blind pouch these false diverticula are prone to the development of infection, ulceration, or calculus formation. In either the obstructed or incontinent bladder the most common location for pseudodiverticula is in a lateral location at or near the ureteral orifices or at the site of the urachus, both areas being foci of natural weaknesses in the detrusor coat.[5] Trabeculae are almost always present whereas diverticula may only develop during micturition.[6] Chronic dilation with trabeculation may ultimately destroy the ureteral valve effect seen to occur with micturition, since the ureter (or infrequently, ureters) may no longer be embedded within the detrusor muscle. Consequently, with increased intraluminal pressure urine may reflux into the ureter. Hydroureter may result, eventually leading to hydronephrosis and/or pyelonephritis. The development of trabeculation and diverticula increases in frequency with aging because of detrusor hypertrophy and the loss of supporting elastic tissue.[2] Age-associated changes in bladder collagen and elastin occur as well and are discussed below.

The major causes of urinary bladder obstruction in the elderly are benign prostatic hyperplasia in the male and urethral mucosal prolapse in the female. Andersen et al examined 17 healthy elderly males and found trabeculation in ten patients, including one with a pseudodiverticulum. Eight of the ten patients with trabeculation had slight degrees of prostatic hypertrophy without frank obstructive symptoms.[7] Dymock (cited in ref #2) identified urethroceles in 69 of 100 geriatric females. In these 69 patients, 44 demonstrated minimal mucosal protrusion, 14 prominent mucosal protrusion, and in 11 marked prolapse was present. Nine of these women also exhibited urethral caruncles. This study also revealed a positive statistical correlation for incontinence and inflammation with the observed anatomical changes but no correlation with either parity or infection. Of interest, nine patients had vaginal prolapse coexistent with urethroceles.[2] Bladder neck stenosis is felt to be a product of chronic infection and therefore is a secondary change as is trabeculation and pseudodiverticulum formation; it will, though, amplify any of the pre-existent changes.[2]

Aging produces decreased tone in voluntary smooth muscle. In the lower urinary tract this manifests as weakness in the pelvic floor[2] and as decreased tone and strength of the external urinary sphincter. The latter observation restates the similarity in this relationship to that of vaginal prolapse and urethral mucosal prolapse as was demonstrated in the work of Dymock.[2] Brocklehurst and Dillane performed cystographic studies in 47 incontinent women whose age ranged from 72 to 91 years. Fifty percent of these patients exhibited laxity of the pelvic floor.[2] Parvinen et al, also employing cystographic studies, examined 59 incontinent women. They found descended bladders in 17% of their patients; 22% and 27% of their patients exhibited pseudodiverticula and trabeculation respectively.[6] Brocklehurst and Dillane[8] found 32% of their patients to have pseudodiverticula and 60% to manifest both trabeculation and cellules.[2] Parvinen et al found ureteral reflux associated with urinary tract infection but not with either trabeculation or diverticula. However, trabeculation was most prominent when infection coexisted.[6]

Since the urinary bladder is derived from the urogenital sinus and mesonephros, it is not surprising that bladder epithelium has proved to be hormonally responsive. Squamous epithelium of the vaginal type is found in the trigone of 50% of normal adult females and in a smaller proportion of males.[9] In the female the squamous epithelium of the bladder continues as the surface lining epithelium of the urethra. In females this epithelium may exhibit cyclical changes of a cytohormonal nature as occur in the vagina. However, any cyclical changes in urinary bladder epithelium are irregular compared to the vaginal epithelium and are in general delayed.[10]

The squamous epithelium of the trigone, bladder base, and urethra is natural to these locations and is present in the absence of inflammation or other disease. Squamous epithelium can develop as a metaplastic process in other areas, particularly as a response to chronic inflammation. This squamous metaplasia is much more common in females, probably because of their shortened urethra which predisposes to a higher incidence of both inflammation and infection.

Biochemical alterations in the bladder's structure have been observed with aging. Cortivo et al[11] found minor variations in the collagen content of the bladder wall in children between the ages of 3 months and 8 years, and in adults aged 48 to 70 years. These observations were unaffected by the presence or absence of vesicular outlet obstruction in either the children or adults who were studied. Collagen content was calculated based on the known constant proportion of hydroxyproline in collagen since hydroxyproline is unique to collagen. Elastin composition, however, was altered in the presence of outlet obstruction in both groups and its alteration was dependent on the age of the individual. The compositional change of elastin consisted of an increase in its content of polar amino acids. Total elastin content of the bladder increased if the obstruction existed in either the infants or the adults but not if it was present in children. These biochemical findings were supported by comparable anatomic changes demonstrated by histologic staining for elastin. The authors attributed the lack of difference in elastin content between normal and obstructed children to a lesser degree of obstruction in this 4- to 8-year-old patient population.[11] Susset et al[12] also examined bladder collagen content as a function of either age and/or sex. They found no differences when the results were factored by age or sex up to the age of 50. However, in contrast to Cortivo et al,[11] they found significantly greater collagen content in the female relative to the male, in the areas of both the detrusor and trigone. Susset et al suggested that this difference might reflect an increase in smooth muscle in the male bladder relative to its connective tissue content; they also suggested that benign prostatic hyperplasia in the older male, by producing bladder outlet obstruction, might have led to such smooth muscle hypertrophy of the bladder wall.[12]

PROSTATE

Embryology

The prostate develops from epithelial cords which arise from the cephalad urethra (urogenital sinus derivative) at the end of the third month of gestation. In the male five glandular groups develop which eventually correspond to the five lobes of the prostate. Analogous development in the female leads to the formation of the urethral and paraurethral glands.[1] In the first postnatal week 10 to 20% of the acini, predominantly in the posterior and lateral lobes, have adult-like glands. This glandular activity is apparently induced by maternal hormones present at term since it disappears after the first month of life. Squamous metaplasia may also be present in the fetal and neonatal periurethral tissues, but regresses within the first month of life. The squamous metaplasia is also probably related to the rise in maternal estrogens occurring at term since it can be retained in young mice who are administered exogenous estrogen for a time following birth.[13] The prostate, following its early burst of postnatal activity, remains involuted until approximately the age of 10.

Anatomy

The prostate gland has two morphologic sectors. Within the urethral muscle coats lie three sets of periurethral lobes: the anterior, median, and lateral lobes. The anterior lobes drain to the roof of the urethra. The median lobes lie between the urethra and deferential canal and drain to the floor of the urethra, cephalad to the verumontanum. The two lateral lobes drain to the lateral aspects of the urethra (Figure 17-1). These periurethral lobes of the prostate in the male correspond to the urethral and paraurethral glands in the female. The two posterior prostatic lobes are situated outside the urethral muscle coats. They drain to the urethral floor cephalad to the verumontanum and have no anatomical equivalent in the female.[14]

Histology

The classic work on the maturation and involution of the prostate by R.A. Moore, published in 1936,[15] remains unchallenged to this day. This work has been extensively quoted and will serve as the basis for several subsequent statements in this chapter. Moore described the existence of five types of epithelium in the mature prostate. In the absence of pathologic change the luminal cells vary from a cuboidal to a columnar type, representing resting and apocrine states, respectively. Pseudostratified luminal epithelium when present was felt to represent hyperplastic change. Different luminal cell types can be found in the same acinus. Beneath the luminal epithelium is an irregular layer of basal cells. Transitional epithelium may be found in the major ducts near the urethra. The prostatic stroma is composed of collagen, smooth muscle, and elastin fibers.[15]

Hormones

The prostate is acted upon by hormones throughout its evolution-involution cycle. In addition to the previously noted fetal and neonatal hormonal responses of the prostate, developmental changes in the prostate with age represent clear examples of its responsiveness to testosterone. As prostatic development progresses from puberty it requires both gonadotropin and intact testes with testosterone being the actual effector of prostatic cellular development. Either hypophysectomy or castration prevents the onset of puberty, but only testosterone (androgen) replacement is necessary for prostatic maturation to occur.

Androgens stimulate the prostatic epithelium whereas estrogens primarily influence fibromuscular tissue. This is analogous to the dual effects of estrogen and progestin noted to occur in the female breasts. Estrogen also stimulates fibromuscular tissue development in the male breast, an observation which in part explains the observed gynecomastia in patients with chronic liver failure. In general, estrogens counteract the effect of androgens on the prostate. Estrogen levels in the male remain relatively constant after maturity whereas the level of androgens clearly declines after the fourth decade. With age there also occurs an increased binding capacity of testosterone-binding globulin. The net effect is a marked decrease in the circulating level of unbound or active testosterone. Animal studies further suggest that the age-related involution of the prostate results from decreased circulating hormone and not from an altered end-organ response. In the fox, prostatic involution occurs between mating seasons with functional prostatic morphology and activity recurring prior to the next mating season. Further evidence for the role of testosterone in prostatic morphologic development can be derived from the senile changes observed in animals and the atrophy of the prostate that follows hormonal ablation in man. Such atrophy is readily reversed with testosterone administration.[16]

Aging

Epithelial cell activity in the prostate begins at approximately 10 years of age, and from ages 12 to 14 acinar proliferation occurs. The period of maturation is from 13 to 45 years of age[15] with the full prostatic mass in the adult being attained during the third decade. By this time there has occurred an eightfold increase in prostatic mass relative to that present at age 10. In the absence of hypertrophy the mean prostatic mass is 11 g (range 7 to 16 g)[17] and there is no statistical difference in either prostatic volume or water content ($82 \pm 2\%$) from age 20 to 90 years.[15,17]

Prostatic involution occurs at the same time as circulating levels of testosterone decline. Physiologic atrophy of the gland involves all of its components though not in an equal manner. The presenile period (age 45 to 60 years) is a time when rapid involution occurs. The predominant characteristic of the presenile prostate is the marked variability of its cellular components, since the mature gland demonstrates a uniform histology. This marked variability in the appearance of the presenile glands can occur in a number of foci and may thus significantly change the normal morphologic appearance of the prostate. Pseudostratified epithelia becomes more common and pseudoacini develop within the luminal epithelium, a finding unique to the presenile period. Spindle metaplasia of the epithelium occurs and there is an increase in the stromal connective tissue. Periacinar connective tissue thickens from 5 to 15 μm during maturity to 20 to 50 μm in the presenile period. Two types of acinar change are described by Moore[15] to occur in the presenile period. *Simple acinar atrophy* involves only the acini without affecting the stroma. The entire lobule is usually affected, but a single acinus may be involved. The epithelium is reduced in height, becoming cuboidal or, less commonly, rectilinear in appearance. Slight thickening of the basement membrane is found. *Sclerotic atrophy* involves both stromal tissue as well as glandular structures. The early change of epithelial flattening is associated with proliferation of periacinar fibroblasts. Acinar involution usually involves the entire lobule producing small, collapsed, tightly packed acini. In the late stages of sclerotic atrophy the acini become obliterated and are replaced by hyalinized collagen with 50% of all acini destroyed by age 80 years. This process is seldom accompanied by an inflammatory response. In the female similar atrophic changes have been described in Bartholin's gland. Moore concluded that sclerotic atrophy is independent of vascular insufficiency and represents an involutional sclerosis similar to that seen in the postmenopausal uterus,[15] a structure similarly deprived of its major hormonal influence.

The period of senile prostatic involution extends from approximately 60 to 75 years of age. It is characterized by slow, virtually static atrophic changes with the corpora amylacea becoming more prominent during this period. Beyond age 75 is the advanced senile period characterized by diffuse atrophy.

Moore summarized prostatic changes with age as follows[15]:

Finding	*Age (yr)*
Slight irregularity in epithelial height	40–45
Lobular atrophy	45–50
Loss of epithelial secretory activity	50–60
Initial appearance of sclerotic atrophy	60–65
Stromal changes of smooth muscle atrophy and increased connective tissue first appear	60–70
Corpora amylacea increase in size and number	65+

Using these histologic criteria, Moore was able to estimate a patient's age within 10 years for those patients whose age was less than 74 years.

Hyperplasia Prostatic hyperplasia evolves later than senile atrophy and is primarily periurethral in location. Two types of hyperplasia have been described. Nodular or benign prostatic hyperplasia (BPH) involves both glandular structures and stroma (Figure 17-2A and B). The histologic features of BPH are those of enlarged acini, intraluminal projections of papillary epithelium (Figure 17-3B), and the absence of a capsule (a criterion for an adenoma). Benign prostatic hyperplasia is found in approximately 80% of males over the age of 40 years with the incidence increasing to 95.5% of all males by the eighth decade.[15]

Secondary hyperplasia is characterized by diffuse irregular epithelial hyperplasia in an acinus which otherwise shows involution. Epithelial folds, one feature of BPH, are not seen in secondary hyperplasia. In secondary hyperplasia there is an increase in connective tissue with no stromal reaction and it is rarely seen in the absence of senile changes. Secondary hyperplasia is not seen prior to the sixth decade and is usually observed after the seventh decade. In contrast to BPH, which is predominantly periurethral in location, secondary hyperplasia is most commonly seen in the posterior lobes of the prostate. The incidence of secondary hyperplasia is quite

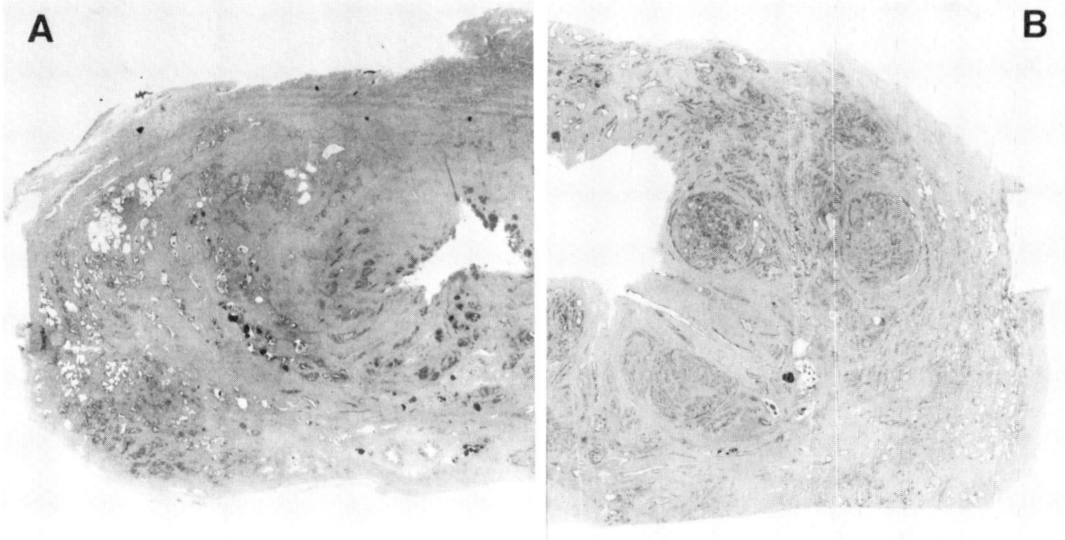

Figure 17-2 Prostate. **A.** Macroscopic view of normal prostate in a 61-year-old man. **B.** Benign (nodular) prostatic hyperplasia in a 68-year-old man.

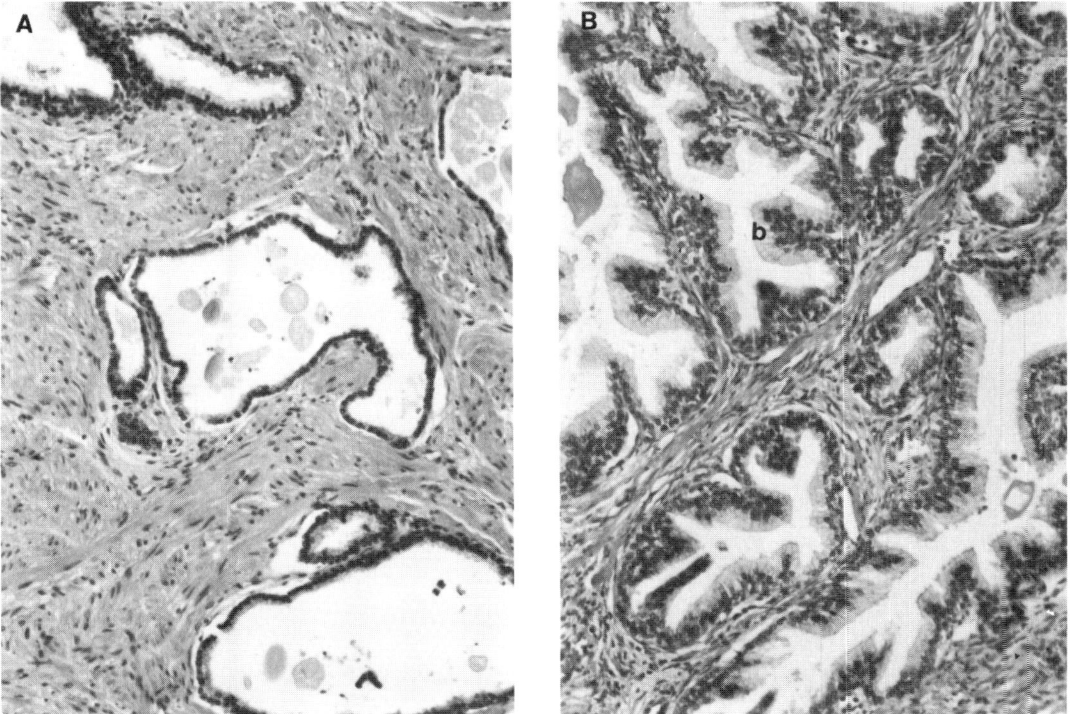

Figure 17-3 Prostatic histopathology. **A**. Pathologic involution in a 61-year-old man. Note short (involuted) glands without secretion. **B**. Nodular hyperplasia in a 68-year-old man. Note folding of hyperplastic epithelium (b-bolsters).

low; only 5% of glands with senile change will demonstrate it.[15] Similar nonuniform hyperplasia has been described in the prostates of aged dogs[13] and in response to androgen administration in castrated rats.[18] Moore felt that secondary hyperplasia might result from irregular hormonal stimulation combined with a nonuniform tissue response.[15]

Pathologic involution Age-dependent changes in the prostate must be differentiated from other more clinically significant pathologic processes. The term pathologic involution, as utilized by Moore,[15] reflects the effects of systemic illness on the involution process. It represents an acceleration of expected involutional changes; this is similar to the decreases in organ mass with age found by Harbitz for all organs in the male genital tract in patients suffering with chronic debilitating illnesses.[19-23] The histologic features of pathologic involution include diminished epithelial cell height, a low columnar or cuboidal cell type, and the absence of cellular secretion (Figure 17-3A). Both stromal change and sclerosis are conspicuously absent. The corpora amylacea have fewer laminations and lack calcification thereby supporting the concept of their accelerated evolution (ie, accelerated prostatic involution). Castration can be thought of as one cause of pathologic involution since it leads to an abrupt cessation of testicular androgen secretion as opposed to the gradual age-related decline (see below). Postcastration changes are more uniform than those that occur in senile involution; this finding supports the concept of irregular hormonal stimulation mediating the varied morphologic changes seen during the presenile period and beyond. In man, 90 days after castration there is a marked decrease in the height of epithelial cells in the prostate. During the ensuing weeks epithelial cell atrophy progresses with loss of mucosal papillations. Simultaneous stromal changes manifest as prominent periacinar stromal collars. By 120 and 150 days postcastration the histologic appearance is that of sclerotic atrophy. Administration of exogenous androgen will reverse much of the atrophy induced by castration.[15]

Metaplastic transformation is another pathologic condition which alters the prostatic epithelium. As a secondary response to various stimuli, the glandular epithelium may transform to a transitional, spindle, or squamous epithelium. In general, metaplastic epithelium is more resistant to the effects of an adverse environment than is the native glandular epithelium. Squamous or transitional metaplasia is usually associated with prostatic infarction. This is a common finding since infarction is present in approximately 25% of prostates with demonstrable BPH.[24] The blood supply to the prostate decreases with age, affecting the periurethral vessels to a greater extent than the capsular arteries.[16] Benign prostatic hyperplasia appears to cause infarcts by compression of vessels supplying hyperplastic tissue, compromising blood flow to the tissue, or by literal outgrowth of its blood supply. Trauma, including that following transurethral prostatic resection, and infection are also common inciting events for epithelial metaplasia. Hormones can also induce metaplasia; excess exogenous, or endogenous, estrogens usually produce squamous metaplasia of the prostatic epithelium. Metaplasia can also be age-dependent or be found as a spontaneous process (spindle metaplasia) in the presenile prostate. Spindle metaplasia when present is typically confined to the ducts.[24]

Carcinoma Cancer of the prostate must be considered in part as an age-related disorder. Harbitz and Haugen[19] found foci of carcinoma in 34% of a series of 200 consecutive autopsies performed on men over the age 40 years. In this series all 70 patients with foci of carcinoma were over the age 50 years. The incidence of carcinoma increased with advancing age such that 52% of the autopsied patients with carcinoma were over the age 80 years. The lesion was occult in 32.7% of the patients in the series reported by Harbitz and Haugen.[19] These same authors cite two other series in which the rate of occurrence of occult prostate carcinoma was 27.3% and 39.7% respectively.[19]

Harbitz and Haugen found that 80% of the malignancies in their series were peripheral in location.[19] Other series report values equally as high (80% to 95%) for the development of prostatic carcinoma in the periphery of the gland. The cause of prostatic cancer is unknown. Its origin within the posterior lobes of the prostate and the known involutional response of prostate cancer to estrogens implies a strong relationship with prior androgenic stimulation. Paradoxically, prostatic atrophy, hyperplasia, and malignancy all become evident during that time of life when testosterone is decreasing in concentration in the blood. One possible explanation is that prostatic carcinoma, a slowly progressive malignancy, arises early in life during a period of high testosterone levels and then remains quiescent and occult in most men. Though this hypothesis appears attractive it offers no ready explanation as to what factors might promote the further development of such a malignancy.[5,24]

Biochemical changes Age-related changes have been identified in the character of prostatic secretions. Resnick and Stubbs[25] described several protein fractions in prostatic fluid which could be separated by SDS polyacrylamide gel electrophoresis. The lowest molecular weight fraction the more commonly isolated in the older patients, but no association could be demonstrated between this protein and either benign or malignant disease.

Acid phosphatase is an antigenically distinct secretory product of prostatic epithelium. It is the only marker presently known to be of any clinical value in the evaluation of prostatic disease. Serum concentrations of acid phosphatase are elevated in those patients with prostatic carcinoma whose disease has extended beyond the capsule of the prostate. Acid phosphatase values also decline with age; in fact, the age-related changes in acid phosphatase may be nothing more than a reflection of the dependence of this enzyme on circulating testosterone levels, which also decline with age. Acid phosphatase levels also are low prior to maturity, following castration, or subsequent to estrogen administration. A lack of correlation exists between prostatic fluid acid phosphatase activity and the presence of BPH.[26] This fact lends little support to the theory that estrogen levels influence the development of BPH since a straightforward estrogen effect should lead to a decrease in acid phosphatase activity. Moore's early concept of uneven hormonal stimulation and response with aging still remains to be excluded as an important step in the development of BPH.

PENIS

Little has been written about age-related changes in the penis. Tyukov[27] has described particular vascular alterations, the first evidence of which is fibroelastosis of trabeculae in the corpus spongiosum during the fourth decade. This is then followed by progressive sclerosis of the arteries and veins. Similar sclerotic changes occur in the corpus cavernosum. Any vascular changes that occur have become generalized by the end of the sixth decade of life. Tyukov has speculated that alterations in the venous system may be important in age-associated impotence.[16,27] It is not known if similar vascular phenomena occur in the clitoris.

SEMINAL VESICLES

Anatomy and Embryology

The seminal vesicles are a pair of convoluted sacculated tubes which merge with the vas deferens to form the ejaculatory duct (Figure 17-1). The average length of each vesicle is 41 mm; the width is approximately one third the length. Each vesicle consists of a coiled main duct, of average length 100 mm, from which numerous side ducts arborize with alveolar glands arising from these ducts.[28]

The seminal vesicles bud from the deferential duct near its site of entry into the urogenital sinus during the third fetal month. There is no homologue of the seminal vesicles in the female.

Age-related Changes

Functional Secretory activity ordinarily begins at puberty. With advancing age there is both an impairment in vesicular emptying and a decreased fructose concentration in secretions.[28]

Gross morphology From childhood to puberty there is little change in the seminal vesicles, but at puberty a rapid growth phase begins. Though their mass stabilizes at maturity (age 20 years) both the length of the duct and its volume continue to increase well into the fourth decade. After maturity there occurs a gradual reduction in volume despite the mass remaining relatively constant into the ninth decade. The number of side ducts and the ratio of length to breadth of each vesicle does not vary after puberty. The ampulla of the deferential duct also enlarges rapidly at puberty, stabilizing in its growth at either age 25 or at age 50, depending on which of two conflicting reports one chooses to believe.[13,29] No association has yet been found between these seminal vesicle changes and any prostatic pathology.[28]

Microscopy The epithelium of the seminal vesicles changes with its development and maturation. Alterations are most obvious in the luminal surface cells and are unapparent in the basal and pseudostratified cells. In the fetus only a single layer of columnar cells is evident. During childhood the mucosa develops a finely reticulated appearance with a papillomatous morphology whereas in the juvenile years the epithelium assumes a villous appearance. Alveoli can be found in the mucosa for the first time at this stage of life. At puberty the surface cells demonstrate an irregular columnar appearance and the mucosa becomes highly reticulated as it develops a proliferating villous appearance. The alveoli greatly enlarge at puberty, further increasing the mucosal surface area. The adult surface epithelium is quite variable, being columnar, cuboidal, or squamous in character. Any proliferative morphology present as a juvenile eventually disappears with the epithelium assuming a villous pattern as in the juvenile. Deep alveoli first develop along the side ducts at approximately the age of 20 with their development completed by age 40 years. With advanced age the epithelium of the alveoli again becomes papillomatous as in childhood. The relative number of all alveoli in the distal (apical) vesicles starts to decrease by the fourth decade. The number of proximal alveoli declines sharply in the fifth decade. Atrophic changes are less prominent in the ampulla and ejaculatory ducts, and the relative frequency of deep alveoli in the ampulla increases with advancing age. The relationship of these age-related morphologic changes to the observed age-dependent hormonal variation is discussed in the next section.[28]

Golden yellow lipochrome pigment accumulates in the surface epithelium of the mature seminal vesicle. This degenerative product is seldom seen prior to puberty.[28] Prior to puberty the vesicular wall thickness exceeds the breadth of the lumen. At puberty, the lumen widens appreciably producing an apparent reduction in wall thickness. Postmaturity thinning of the wall occurs concurrently with mucosal atrophy.[28]

Hormonal Influences

The simple fact that seminal vesicles develop only in the male presents a compelling argument for the influence of androgenic hormones in the development of the seminal vesicle. It is of interest that a proliferative mucosal pattern never develops in the newborn. Progestational hormones, which are in high concentration at term, have androgenic effects, but obviously do not exert an effect similar to that induced by the surge in testosterone secretion at puberty. Morphologic alterations secondary to the pubertal hormone surge have been previously described. Androgenic activity (ie, testosterone) is also responsible for the onset of cellular secretion and for the glandular storage of both fat and glycogen. Androgens also produce an increase in the vascularity as well as the blood flow to the seminal vesicles of both normal and castrated rats.[13]

The symmetrical proliferative changes in the mucosa up to maturity and the atrophic changes after maturity follow in sequence; as androgenic activity rises and falls with age the morphologic phase is patterned after the prevailing androgen level. Any hormonal change that occurs will slightly precede the morphologic alterations that it has induced.

Estrogens stimulate development of fibrous, and to a lesser extent, muscular tissue, and they suppress development and maturation of the male genital tract. After puberty, estrogens depress seminal vesicle secretory function. Any estrogenic effect can only be reversed by large doses of androgen.[13]

TESTES

Embryology and Anatomy

The testes develop from the mesoderm of the genital ridge. In the fifth week of development, the primordial germ cells, migrating from the endoderm of the yolk sac, arrive at the sexually indifferent gonad. In the male these germ cells induce the differentiation of the testes. The primitive sex cords differentiate into the testes cords which in the hilar area of the testis then divide into a network which will eventually become the rete testis. The testes cords develop a horseshoe shape, the limbs of which become the tubuli recti (straight tubules) and the arch the tubuli contorti (convoluted tubules). The epithelium of the cords differentiate into the Sertoli cells, and the Leydig cells develop from the mesenchyme. The rete testis anastomose with segments of the mesonephric ducts to become the efferent ductules. The mesonephric (Wolffian) duct immediately distal to the efferent ductules develops convolutions and becomes the epididymis. The remainder of the Wolffian duct becomes the vas or ductus deferens and terminates at the prostatic utricle. The sex tubules remain solid until puberty at which time a lumen develops. The testes migrate from the abdominal cavity into the scrotum after the seventh month of intrauterine life, completing their descent in the first postnatal year.[1] At the same time Leydig cells first demonstrate a storage capacity for neutral fat.

The vascular supply to the testis originates from the aorta, inferior to the renal arteries. After these testicular arteries give branches to the ureters, cremaster muscles, and the epididymides, they continue on as the internal spermatic arteries. The arteries then divide into the testicular branches at the hilar region, ramify as interlobular arteries (Figure 17-4), and descend medially before proceeding laterally up to the apices.[30] The proximal vasculature supplies the anterior and lower portion of the testis; the distal vessels supply the posterior and upper aspects. Intertubular arteries penetrate the parenchyma ending as peritubular capillaries.[31]

Hormones

The testes are hormonally productive and responsive. They are the second largest source of androgen after the adrenal glands and also produce estrogen. The Leydig cells are the probable source of testicular sex steroids with testosterone being the major androgen produced. In utero, androgens induce the sexual orientation of the brain and the involution of the Müllerian system; they are secreted by Leydig cells which

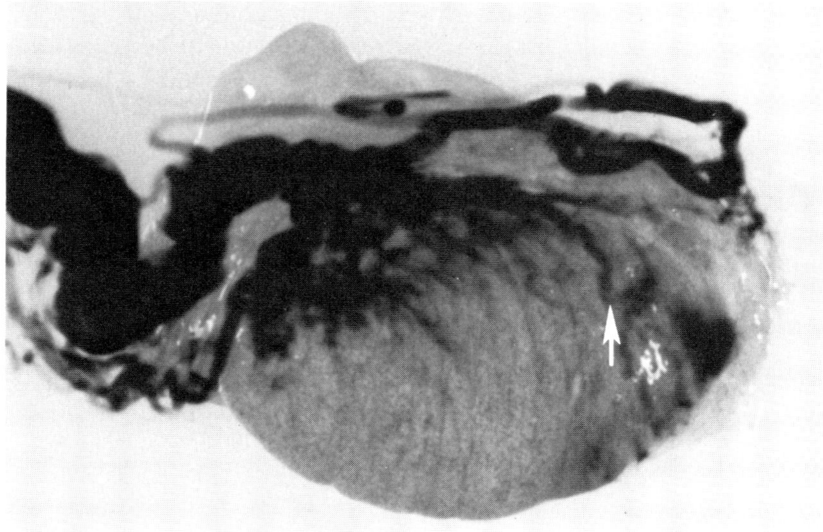

Figure 17-4 Vascular supply of the testis. Arterial and early venous angiography. Interlobular arteries arise from the internal spermatic artery. Note coiling (arrow) of the interlobular arteries in this 69-year-old male.

have been activated by chorionic gonadotropin. Postnatally, hormonal secretion by Leydig cells ceases until the surge in gonadotropin activity that occurs at puberty. During adolescence, androgens affect the secondary sexual characteristics as well as primary and secondary genital organ maturation. The metabolic effects of androgens are varied. They encompass retention of electrolytes, calcium, phosphorus, and nitrogen, osteoblast stimulation and resultant epiphyseal fusion, and increased protein anabolism including muscular development. Plasma testosterone levels slowly but steadily decline after the sixth decade. This decrease is in both plasma concentration and in the fraction which is unbound or physiologically active. Unbound testosterone falls by approximately 15% in the sixth and seventh decades and by about 30% in the ninth decade. To some extent the deterioration of the male with aging is related to this decrease in androgen levels (see below). Testicular estrogen may play a part in feedback control of gonadotropin secretion as estrogen is more effective in this feedback than is testosterone.[31,33]

Sexual activity has a demonstrable age dependency. Erection may occur from birth and ejaculation has been recorded as early as 5 months of age. Ejaculation usually begins during puberty (age 11 to 15 years) with spermatozoa first appearing at this time. Sexual activity declines gradually but steadily starting in the third decade with age being the single greatest factor affecting the frequency of orgasm. The postorgasmic refractory period prolongs rapidly beginning at age 20.[30]

Anatomic Changes with Age

Mass Harbitz found that, in men with normal prostatic histology, testicular mass increased with age ($r=0.490$, $P<0.05$). The range of testicular mass, minus epididymis, was 20 to 40 g. However, in the face of benign prostatic hyperplasia with or without carcinoma or atypical glandular hyperplasia, testicular mass decreased with age, and showed a negative regression line slope ($r=-0.446$, $P<0.001$). Patients with protracted disease demonstrated decreased testicular mass with age, in association with a decreased body mass with no specific relationship to cardiac disease or diabetes mellitus in particular. Harbitz avoided assigning any significance to the relationship of prostatic hyperplasia and diminished testicular mass.[20] However, there is a likely relationship based on the known effects of decreased effective testosterone and/or increased estrogen levels. Estrogen does induce testicular atrophy, and the paraurethral prostate (BPH) is also stimulated by estrogen.

Seminiferous tubules Harbitz also examined seminiferous tubular mass.[21] He found similar changes as noted in testicular mass, including the relationships to prostatic histology. He also noted a marked reduction in mass following estrogen therapy. He found a general preservation of tubular mass in patients with prostatic carcinoma, and suggested that prostatic hyperplasia and neoplasia reflected predominant estrogenic and androgenic influences, respectively, thereby suggesting that testicular mass, and hence function, as seen in these groups, was a concurrent effect of sex steroids. Honore, however, felt that no definitive conclusions could be drawn based on this relationship.[21,30]

Spermatogenesis is initiated at puberty and follows as the result of a rise in gonadotropin secretion as well as Leydig cell, germ cell, and Sertoli cell maturation. It peaks in activity during the fourth decade with 90% of the tubules being active. In the fifth through seventh decades spermatogenesis falls with only 50% of the tubules being active. There follows a slow and steady decline after age 70 such that approximately 10% of tubules are active in the ninth decade.[30,33]

Classical reports dealing with age-related changes in the tubules have noted shortening of the epithelium and both tubular narrowing and angling of what were previously round tubules.[30,34] Honore found dilation of the rete testes, usually associated with dilation of both the vas deferens and epididymis, and noted sperm stasis.[33] The most prominent age-related change in the testis is seminiferous tubule sclerosis (Figure 17-5A and B). Honore observed a general correlation between the level of sclerosis and advancing age. He defined tubular sclerosis as a progressive fibrosis of the tunica propria leading to complete tubular hyalinization.[33] Differing from the classical descriptions of Sasano and Ichijo, who found basement membrane thickening beginning abruptly in the fourth and fifth decades,[30] Honore found no evidence of basement membrane thickening.[33] Like Harbitz[23] he observed a milder degree of sclerosis in association with prostatic carcinoma.[35] Honore divided tubular sclerosis into two patterns. In one pattern the predominant features were those of interstitial fibrosis and severe sclerosis of small arteries and arterioles, a pattern not associated with any Leydig cell changes (Figure 17-5D). In the second pattern there existed a correlation between Leydig cell hyperplasia and the degree of severity of tubular sclerosis (Figure 17-5C). This Leydig cell hyperplasia was concurrent with degenerative changes in the Leydig cells such as cytoplasmic vacuolization, nuclear pyknosis, and crystals of Reinke. Honore also described a patchy peritubular and perivascular chronic inflammatory infiltrate composed of both small and large lymphocytes as well as plasma cells and was associated with severe tubular sclerosis.[33] These findings are similar to those previously reported by Suoranta.[34]

Sasano and Ichijo[30] found that hernialike protrusions in the tubular walls abruptly increased in frequency in the sixth and seventh decades with a steady decline thereafter. These outpouchings were more common in tubules undergoing active spermatogenesis. These authors agreed with Hatakeyama et al[32] that such herniations represented regenerative attempts by tubules.[30] Additional work by Suoranta showed that in normal testes these herniations had no relationship to the vasculature.[34]

Leydig cells As stated above, Leydig cell

hyperplasia (Figure 17-5C) may be found with tubular sclerosis and degenerative cellular changes such as cytoplasmic vacuolization or nuclear pyknosis. An additional degenerative change is the accumulation of lipofuscin pigment within cellular cytoplasm. Harbitz found that a statistically significant negative correlation existed between Leydig cell mass and age in men with BPH ($r = -0.413$, $P < 0.001$) and in men with BPH and prostatic cancer ($r = -0.343$, $P < 0.05$).[22]

Sertoli cells Harbitz found an insignificant correlation between decreasing Sertoli cell mass and advancing age and observed no change in the Sertoli cell mass with advancing age in patients whose prostatic morphology was normal. Virtually no Sertoli cells were present in patients who had received 12 or more months of estrogen therapy.[23]

Theories Three major theories have emerged on the pathogenesis of age-related testicular atrophy. The least prominent hypothesis suggests autoimmune destruction of the tubules. This theory is supported by the presence of inflammatory infiltrates in the testes as described by Honore[33] as well as by the observed lack of any inflammatory change in genetic conditions associated with sterility (eg, Klinefelter's syndrome). In general, inflammatory infiltrates are only found in those testes undergoing active spermatogenesis. This theory is unlikely but cannot be completely refuted, though does not bear up under the

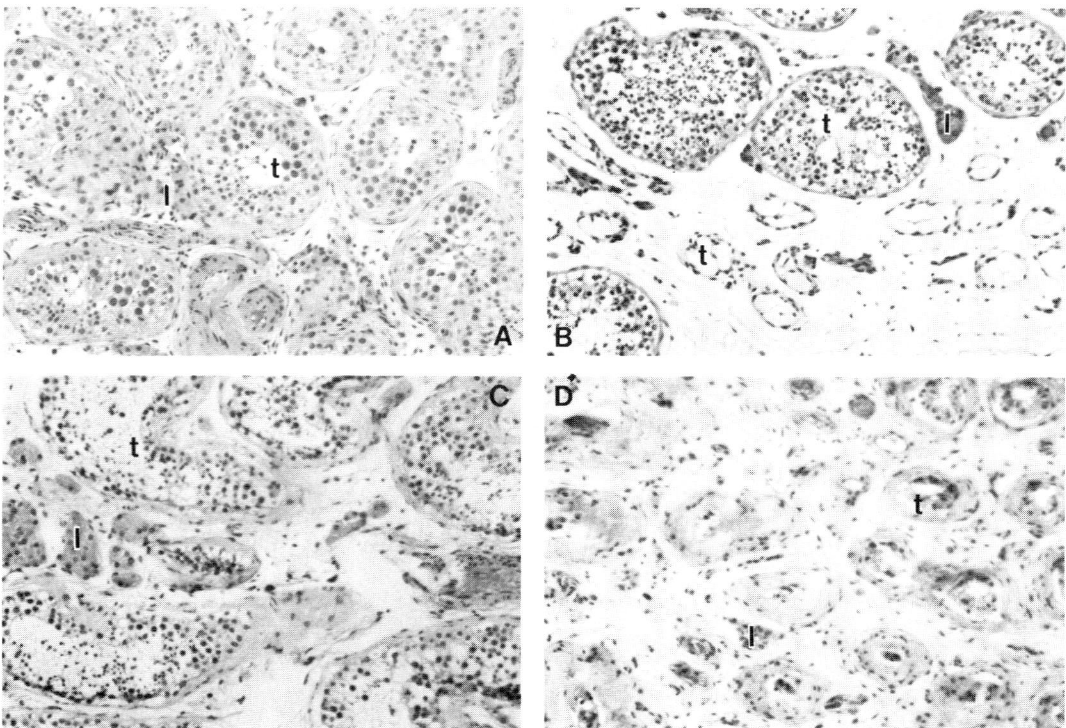

Figure 17-5 Testicular tubular changes with age. **A.** Seminiferous tubules of a 64-year-old man, relatively normal for age except for mild peritubular fibrosis and reduced spermatid production (t = seminiferous tubules, l = Leydig cells). **B.** Seminiferous tubules of an 85-year-old man, within normal limits for age. Note admixture of well-preserved and severely atrophied tubules. **C.** Seminiferous tubules of a 66-year-old man with prostatic carcinoma. No diethylstilbesterol therapy. There is decreased tubular mass, peritubular fibrosis, and Leydig cell hyperplasia. **D.** Seminiferous tubules of a 61-year-old man who died of liver failure. There is virutally complete tubular sclerosis. Leydig cells are not hyperplastic.

weight of subsequent concepts. It is probable though that none of these theories are mutually exclusive and that all of them contribute to some degree to senescent changes in the testes. Honore's description of patterns of tubular sclerosis appear to be the result of two separate processes: ischemia, and ineffective production of testosterone. Honore implied that the hyperplasia of degenerative Leydig cells may be a trophic response to increased gonadotropin secretion secondary to decreased feedback by falling testosterone levels.[33]

Vascular changes It is clear that the extreme of vascular change–frank ischemia–produces degenerative changes in the testes. Both spermatogenesis and androgen production decrease after a few minutes of ischemia.[34] In general, vascular insults produce more severe changes in the tubules than in the interstitium. Sasano and Ichijo found that senile changes were most prominent in the terminal arborizations of the testicular vessels.[30] Takizawa and Hatakeyama[29] noted regions at the very periphery of the vascular supply which were subject to focal tubular atrophy and/or hyalinization with no apparent relationship to age. These foci are in limited areas including tissue adjacent to the rete testis, the neighboring portion to the connective tissue septa, and the subcapsular area.[29] This suggests that poor or decreasing vascular supply may accelerate the development of senile changes. In areas where a marginal blood supply exists, tissue atrophy is inevitable, occurring well before any change expected from advancing age.

Studies of testicular microvasculature have shown age-related changes at all levels of the vascular tree. In young males up to the age of 35 years, the interlobular arteries are straight; any coiling present is well organized and the peritubular vascular plexus is undisturbed. Beginning in the fifth decade the vascular coiling becomes increasingly disorganized and the interlobular arteries become more erratic in their course through the testes, these changes becoming more prominent with age (Figure 17-4).[29] Takizawa and Hatakeyama found that vascular coiling was secondary to involutional change and the degree of vascular alteration proportional to the decrease in testicular mass.[29] They felt that coiling did, itself, promote testicular atrophy (see below) which was contrary to the conclusions drawn by Suoranta.[34] Joffre and Kormano[34] showed identical arterial coiling in the fox testis which proved to be reversible. During the nonbreeding season male fox testes involute with a reduction in connective tissue and total collagen; also, the larger arteries of the testis passively coil as the organ shrinks. Vessels which supply only the tunica albuginea do not coil. As the testis regains mass with the approach of the breeding season, the arterial coiling lessens. Coiling is totally absent during the breeding season. Testicular capillary blood flow increases with increasing testicular mass and is probably under hormonal control. All vascular changes remain reversible as long as there are no degenerative changes in the vessels themselves.[36] Arterial degeneration is well documented in humans: Takizawa and co-workers have shown that testicular arteriolar hyalinization begins at puberty, and progresses increasingly until it peaks in the third decade. The hyaline vascular change progresses to scarring and becomes more prominent with aging.[29]

Age-dependent testicular capillary changes have also been described. Tubular herniations as well as age-related changes may distort peritubular capillaries. Intrinsic capillary alterations also occur, and during the third and fourth decades peritubular capillary anastomoses form annular structures of a uniformly fine caliber. In the fifth and sixth decades an early age-related change–capillary transfiguration or distortion–develops. In advanced disease there is extensive loss of the fine meshwork and annular structure of the capillaries and a decrease in their absolute number, these changes now being irreversible.[27]

Age-dependent change is less prominent in testicular veins than in arteries. With aging, veins demonstrate various degrees of distortion and irregularity in their luminal diameter.[29]

Based on the foregoing events Takizawa and Hatakeyama[29] concluded that there exists age-dependent changes in the testicular microvasculature which may produce or promote testicular atrophy. They felt that the breakdown of the peritubular capillary network is of major importance in the loss of testicular parenchyma. They attributed much of the capillary destruction to reduced capillary blood flow secondary to sclerosis of the main testicular artery, coiling and distortion of the interlobular arteries, and possibly the decreased cardiac output resulting from age. Peritubular capillary distortion by tubular herniations was also felt to play a role in the capillary destruction. Takizawa and Hatakeyama also acknowledged that there existed a role for the age-related decrease in hormonal activity in the reduction in testicular mass.[29]

In summary, age-dependent testicular atrophy is the result of interrelated factors including deteriorations in trophic hormone secretion and in vascular integrity.

REFERENCES

1. Langman J: *Medical Embryology*, ed 2. Baltimore, Williams & Wilkins, 1969, pp 148–177.
2. Brocklehurst JC: The bladder, in Brocklehurst JC (ed): *Textbook of Geriatric Medicine and Gerontology*, ed 2. Edinburgh, Churchill Livingstone, 1978, pp 306–325.
3. Anderson WF: Bladder and prostate, in Platt D (ed): *Geriatrics* 2. New York, Springer-Verlag, 1983, pp 222–249.
4. Goldman R: Aging of the excretory system: Kidney and bladder, in Finch CE, Hayflick L (eds): *Handbook of the Biology of Ageing*, New York, Van Nostrand Reinhold Co, 1972, pp 409–431.
5. Pugh RCD: Lower urinary tract, in Anderson WAD, Kissane JM: *Pathology*, ed 7. St. Louis, CV Mosby Co, 1977, pp 977–998.
6. Parvinen M, Sourander LB, Vuorinen P: Cystographic studies in old women. *Gerontol Clin* 1967;7:343–347.
7. Andersen JT, Jacobsen O, Worm-Petersen J, et al: Bladder function in healthy elderly males. *Scand J Urol Nephrol* 1978;12: 123–127.
8. Brocklehurst JC, Dillane JB: Studies of the female bladder in old age. III. Micturating cystograms in incontinent women. *Geront Clin* 1967;9:47–58.
9. Koss LG: *Diagnostic Cytology and Its Histopathologic Basis*, ed 3. Philadelphia, JB Lippincott Co, 1979, pp 711–723.
10. Tweeddale DN: *Urinary Cytology*. Boston, Little, Brown & Co, 1977, pp 23–32.
11. Cortivo R, Pagano F, Passerini G, et al: Elastin and collagen in the normal and obstructed urinary bladder. *Br J Urol* 1981;53:134–137.
12. Susset JG, Servot-Viquiet D, Lamy F, et al: Collagen in 155 human bladders. *Invest Urol* 1978;16:204–206.
13. Steward VM, Brandes D: The accessory male sex glands and their changes with age, in Bourne GH (ed): *Structural Aspects of Ageing*. New York, Hafner, 1961, pp 407–414.
14. Hutch JA, Rambo ON Jr: A study of the anatomy of the prostate, prostatic urethra, and the urinary sphincter system. *J Urol* 1970;104:443–452.
15. Moore RA: The evolution and involution of the prostate gland. *Am J Pathol* 1936;12: 599–624.
16. Talbert GB: Aging of the reproductive system, in Finch CE, Hayflick L (eds): *Handbook of the Biology of Aging*. New York, Van Nostrand Reinhold, 1961, pp 318–356.
17. Leissner KH, Tisell LE: The weight of the human prostate. *Scand J Urol Nephrol* 1979;13:137–142.
18. Hooker CW: Pubertal increase in responsiveness to androgen in male rat. *Endocrinology* 1942;30:77–84.
19. Harbitz TB, Haugen OA: Histology of the prostate in elderly men: a study in an autopsy series. *Acta Pathol Microbiol Scand* [*A*], 1972;80:756–768.
20. Harbitz TB: Testis weight and the histology of the prostate in elderly men. *Acta Path Microbiol Scand* [*A*], 1973;81:148–158.

21. Harbitz TB: Morphometric studies of the seminiferous tubules in elderly men with special reference to the histology of the prostate. *Acta Pathol Microbiol Scand* [*A*], 1973; 81:843–856.
22. Harbitz TB: Morphometric studies of the Leydig cells in elderly men with special reference to the histology of the prostate. *Acta Pathol Microbiol Scand*, [*A*], 1973;81: 301–314.
23. Harbitz TB: Morphometric studies of the Sertoli cells in elderly men with special reference to the histology of the prostate. *Acta Pathol Microbiol Scand* [*A*], 1973;81:5: 703–714.
24. Mostofi FK, Price EB Jr: Tumors of the male genital system. *Armed Forces Insti Pathol*, 1973.
25. Resnick MI, Stubbs AJ: Age-specific electrophoretic patterns of prostatic fluid. *J Surg Res* 1978;24:415–420.
26. Kirk E: The acid phosphatase concentration of the prostatic fluid in young, middle-aged, and old individuals. *J Gerontol* 1948; 3:98–104.
27. Tyukov AI: Age changes in the vessels in the corpora cavernosa of the penis. *Arch Pathol* 1967;29:29–34.
28. Nilsson S: The human seminal vesicle: A morphogenetic and gross anatomic study with special regard to changes due to age and to prostatic adenoma. *Acta Chir Scand [Suppl]*1962;296:1–96.
29. Takizawa T, Hatakeyama S: Age-associated changes in microvasculature of human adult testis. *Acta Pathol Jpn* 1978;28:541–554.
30. Sasano N, Ichijo S: Vascular patterns of the human testis with special reference to its senile changes. *Tohoku J Exp Med* 1969;99: 269–280.
31. Bishop MWH: Aging and reproduction in the male. *J. Reprod Fertil* [*Suppl*]1979;12: 65–87.
32. Hatakeyama S, Sengoku K, Takayama S: On the hernia-like protrusions suggestive of regeneration of the human seminiferous tubule. *Bull Tokyo Med Dent Univ* 1962;9: 471–481.
33. Honore LH: Aging changes of the human testis: A light-microscopic study. *Gerontology* 1978;24:58–65.
34. Suoranta H: Changes in the small blood vessels of the adult human testis in relation to age and to some pathologic conditions. *Virchows Arch Pathol Anat* 1971;352: 165–181.
35. Engle ET: Male reproductive system, in Cowdry EV (ed): *Problems of Aging: Biological and Medical Aspects*. Baltimore, Williams & Wilkins, 1938, pp 434–458.
36. Joffre M, Kormano M: An angiographic study of the fox testis in various stages of sexual activity. *Anat Rec* 1975;183: 599–604.

CHAPTER 18 Voiding Problems in the Elderly: Functional Disorders of the Lower Urinary Tract

Edward T. Zawada, Jr.

Incontinence is well known as a common urologic problem in the elderly. In some series it occurs in 10% to 40% of patients over the age of 65.[1] Incontinence as well as the problem of bladder outlet obstruction can be considered together in a category of problems termed voiding problems. These voiding problems are so common in this population as to represent almost a normal consequence of aging itself rather than a by-product of various disease states. For example, the functional problem of incontinence in males is most often caused by detrusor instability,[2] which consists of uninhibited contractions of the bladder emptying muscle, the detrusor. In women, stress incontinence is the result of anatomic changes in the angle of the posterior bladder wall and the urethra due to either stretching of the pelvic floor due to birth trauma or to loss of support due to atrophy of estrogen-sensitive tissues.[3] In men, bladder outlet obstruction is due to benign prostatic hypertrophy whose incidence steadily increases over the age of 65.[4] Of course many disease states such as diabetes which are common in the elderly can also contribute to voiding problems.[5]

Voiding problems can often be diagnosed accurately by the clinical tool of urodynamic measurements which is a rapidly expanding field within the subspecialty of urology. This is a controversial area in geriatrics as some authors feel that clinical assessment alone will lead to the correct diagnosis and proper selection of a treatment plan in most cases.[6] Nevertheless, urodynamics in general has broadened our understanding of the pathophysiology of these problems and has proved the effectiveness of several treatment plans. Whether the cost/benefit ratio justifies widespread use of urodynamic measurements in individual cases remains to be seen.

The goals of this chapter are to review briefly anatomical changes of the lower urinary tract which occur as a consequence of aging and are responsible for voiding problems. A detailed review of urodynamic procedures and interpretation of urodynamic data will then be undertaken. The urodynamic findings in the common voiding problems will be presented. Finally, the voiding disorders which can occur without an associated secondary or systemic disease will be covered in the greatest detail; the functional problems and urodynamic findings attributable to common diseases of the elderly (diabetes or commonly employed therapeutic agents such as antihypertensive drugs) will also be surveyed.

ANATOMICAL CHANGES OF THE AGING LOWER URINARY TRACT

The anatomical changes that occur with advancing age and contribute to voiding problems in the elderly are depicted in Figures 18-1 and 18-2. In Figure 18-1 it can be seen that birth trauma in women distorts the pelvic floor. As a consequence there is a loss of the normal angle of the posterior wall of the bladder and the proximal urethra. This is believed to be an important factor predisposing to stress incontinence in women.[7] Return of this angle to normal on bimanual examination, by upward pressure from the rectum, will correct the problem. Such findings have led to the development of surgical technics such as the Marshall-Marchetti procedure which restores the angle by suturing paraurethral tissues to the symphysis pubis and the bladder to the posterior rectus sheath.[8] This procedure, shown schematically in Figure 18-3, has a 90% rate of success in eliminating stress incontinence in several series.[9,10] In elderly men, benign prostatic hypertrophy commonly leads to impaired bladder emptying (Figure 18-2) because of obstruction of the bladder outlet. Figure 18-4 shows the relationship of the prostate to the internal sphincter. Transurethral prostatectomy in

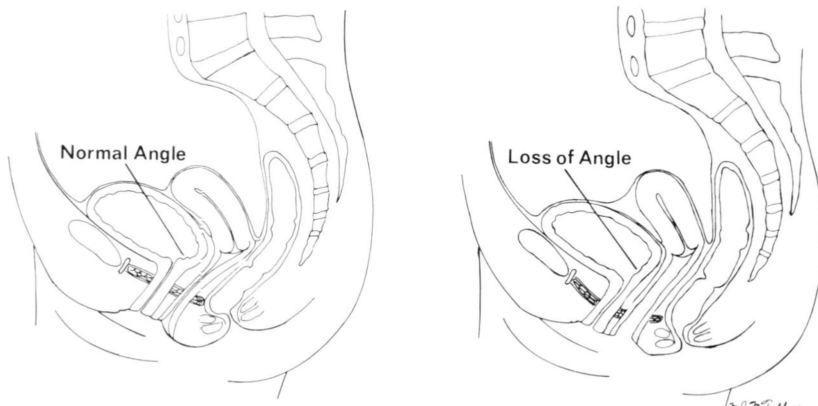

Figure 18-1 Anatomical changes in women due to birth trauma which contribute to stress incontinence.

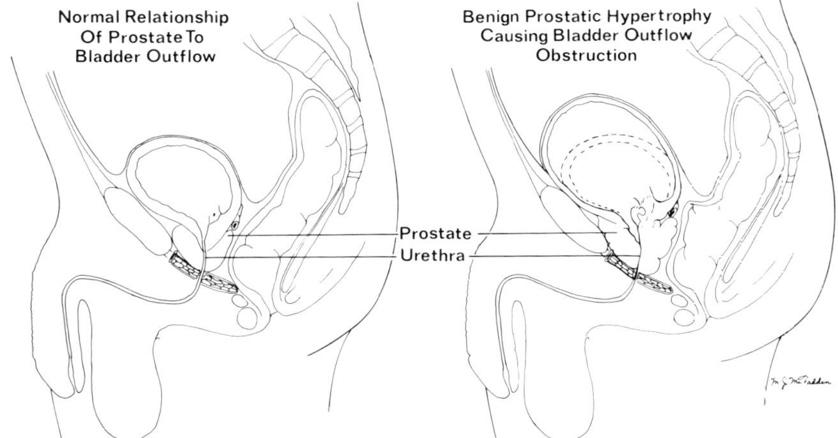

Figure 18-2 Anatomical changes in man causing bladder outflow obstruction.

turn leads to incontinence due to partial surgical curettage of internal sphincter fibers.

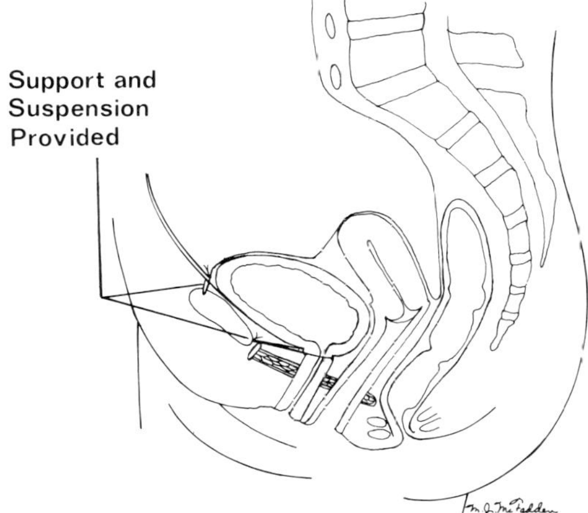

Figure 18-3 Marshall-Marchetti operation to correct stress incontinence.

NORMAL ANATOMY AND PHYSIOLOGY OF THE LOWER URINARY TRACT

Figure 18-4 is a simplified diagram of the important structures of the lower urinary tract which contribute to voiding problems in the elderly. The bladder is a muscular structure whose main force of contraction arises from the thicker outer muscular region known as the detrusor. The detrusor is supplied by the pelvic nerve which arises from the lumbosacral spine. The most important sphincter is the internal sphincter;

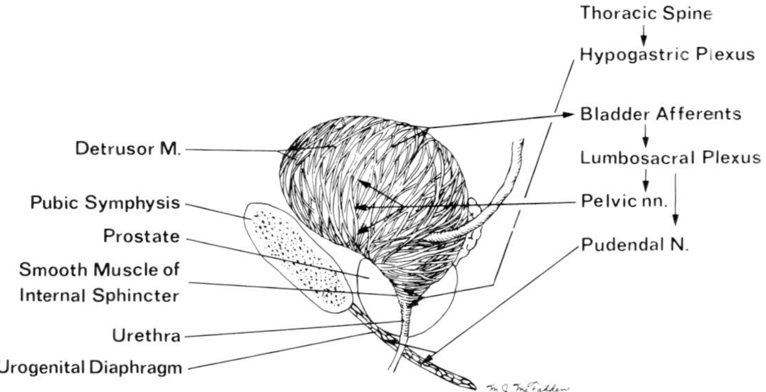

Figure 18-4 Anatomy and neural innervation of the bladder. Relationship of prostate to internal sphincter.

this consists of smooth muscle innervated from sympathetic fibers that originate in the thoracic spine and travel to the sphincter in the hypogastric nerve. Finally, the external sphincter consists of striated voluntary muscle of the pelvic floor which receive its neural supply from the pudendal nerve which arises from the lumbosacral spine. Detrusor contraction originates bladder emptying; at the same time there is cortical inhibition of the external sphincter and no excess activity of the internal sphincter. The net effect is that of a balanced bladder contraction with concomitant sphincteric relaxation.[11]

Neuropharmacology of Voiding Continence

Bladder muscular tone is probably maintained by β-adrenergic fibers (not shown in Figure 18-4) carried through the hypogastric nerve. Detrusor contractions of the bladder are dependent on cholinergic (parasympathetic) neurotransmitters derived from the pelvic nerve. The smooth muscle of the internal sphincter contracts under the influence of α-adrenergic (sympathetic) neurotransmitters from the hypogastric nerve. Finally, the striated muscle of the voluntary external sphincter is innervated by the cholinergic pudendal nerve. The neuropharmacology of this latter innervation is less important to common disorders of voiding and continence. The reason is that the cholinergic detrusor and β-fibers for bladder tone are the main neuropharmacologic mechanism for voiding, whereas the internal sphincter α-adrenergic fibers are the most important neuropharmacologic activity necessary for continence.[12]

Principles of Urodynamics

Cystometry is the oldest means by which quantitative measurements can be obtained to diagnosis disorders of voiding. The technic involves placement of catheters into the bladder and rectum and recording pressures by the necessary physiologic transducers and electronic recording apparatus.[12,13] The rectal catheter measures intra-abdominal pressures. The net pressure obtained by subtracting the bladder catheter pressure and the rectal catheter pressure (this can be done electronically, instantaneously, and recorded simultaneously with the above catheter tracings as a third tracing) is the true voiding pressure generated from intact neuropharmacologic activity. Intact neuropharmacologic events in turn require normal anatomy and physiology of the bladder and urethra. A normal tracing is shown in Figure 18-5. In a typical study the following are recorded: pressure amplitude, activity at rest, activity when the patient is requested to void, and effects of instructions to the patient to voluntarily increase intra-abdominal pressure through coughing. Artifacts due to increased intra-abdominal pressure are discovered by simultaneous increased pressure from the intravesical (IV) measurements as well as the intrarectal (IR) measurements. During a normal voluntary voiding, the voiding pressure obtained results from the integrated activity of bladder-sphincter pharmacology, neuroanatomy and neurophysiology. It should be noted that voiding pressure is independent of intra-abdominal pressure.

Another important urodynamic measurement now incorporated into cystometry is urethral pressures.[14] These measurements are made from a catheter placed in the bladder but with side holes located approximately at the internal urethral sphincter. By similar use of a transducer and recorder, urethral pressures can also be monitored

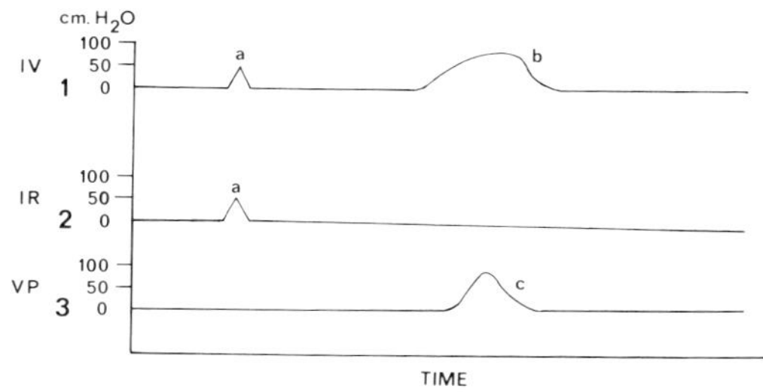

Figure 18-5 Normal cystometric measurements: 1-intravesical pressure tracing; 2-intrarectal pressure tracing; 3-net voiding pressure.

as well as those described during classical cystometry (a fourth tracing). Figure 18-6 illustrates a normal tracing incorporating urethral pressures. This combination tracing facilitates a physiologic understanding of the process of micturition. It can be seen that urethral pressure exceeds voiding pressure at conditions of normal continence. During voiding the urethral pressure decreases and is exceeded by the voiding pressure, resulting in the flow of urine.

Two additional items may be employed in a complete urodynamic study, electromyography (EMG) and contrast radiography (VCUG). The EMG of the internal sphincter is obtained by a typical EMG needle placed in the pelvic floor between the rectum and urethra. Cystoradiography synchronizes contrast radiographs with the previously described measurements. Figure 18-7 displays a normal complete urodynamic study.

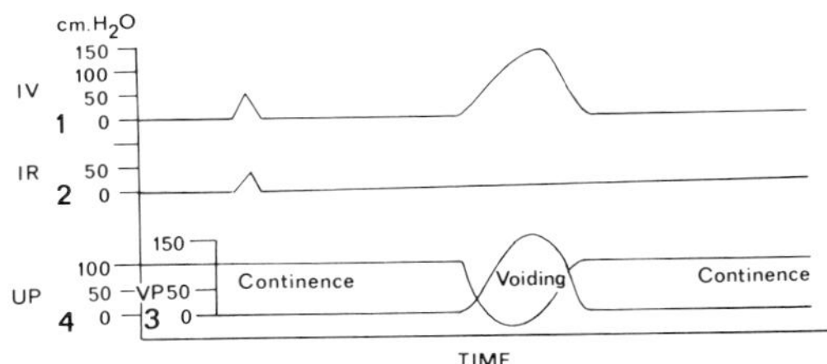

Figure 18-6 Normal cystometric measurements, including urethral pressure tracings (4).

Finally it should be said that the above measurements may need to be repeated several times. In addition, repeat studies after pharmacologic blockade or stimulation may provide additional important information. The study may range from 1 to 3 or 4 hours. The cost of the study may range from $400 to $750, depending upon the extent to which radiography is involved.

VOIDING PROBLEMS IN THE ELDERLY

Primary Voiding Problems

The most common voiding problems in the elderly due to lower genitourinary changes of aging are detrusor instability, increased afferent loop stimuli, stress incontinence, and bladder outlet obstruction. The first three result in incontinence, the last in impaired bladder emptying. Detrusor instability as well as bladder outlet obstruction are more common in men. Stress incontinence occurs almost exclusively in women. Increased afferent loop stimuli are uncommon causes of chronic voiding problems but can occur in both men and women.

Detrusor instability is the uninhibited contraction of the detrusor muscle in the absence of secondary disease or an obvious stimulus. This is the most common cause of incontinence in men and has become

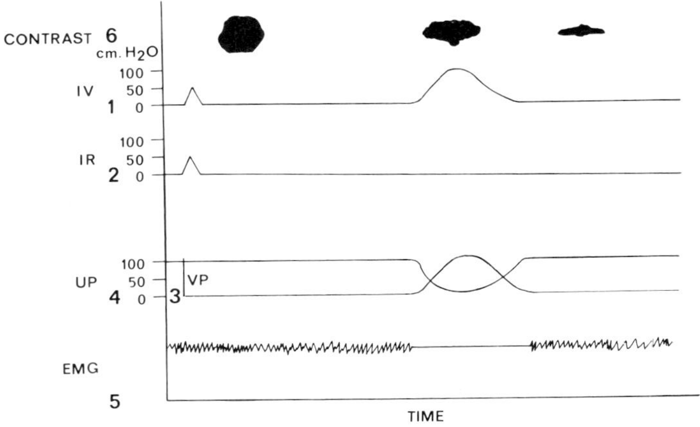

Figure 18-7 Normal optometric measurements including EMG (5) and contrast studies (6). Complete urodynamic study.

better understood because of urodynamic testing.[15] Figure 18-8 reveals a characteristic urodynamic study in a case of detrusor instability. It can be seen that when the patient is instructed to cough there is an increase in intravesical pressure but it is clearly due to increased intra-abdominal pressure (IR tracing) and so the voiding pressure does not change. Urethral pressures are not decreased and continence is maintained with a full bladder being detected by radiography. When instructed to void, the EMG reflects sphincteric inhibition and an increase in intravesical pressure without a change in intra-abdominal pressure. Thus voiding pressure increases. Since it exceeds the urethral pressure, voiding occurs. Radiography reveals an emptying bladder and the flow of contrast material through the urethra. If the patient is instructed to stop voiding, all of the events stop, and continence is restored. Finally, without instruction to void, it can be seen that there is again an increase of vesical pressure due to spontaneous detrusor contraction. This is independent of changes in intra-abdominal pressure and again initiates all the changes leading to bladder emptying and urethral flow. This has obviously been an involuntary detrusor contraction resulting in a bladder-emptying event. A diagnostic maneuver to confirm detrusor instability is the propantheline bromide test. In this test 15 mg of propantheline bromide is administered intramuscularly or intravenously. Ten to fifteen minutes later detrusor contractions disappear due to the anticholinergic activity of the drug. Therapy consists of chronic anticholinergic pharmacotherapy such as propantheline bromide 7.5 mg three times daily.

Increased afferent loop stimulation can result in the voiding problem of incontinence in the elderly.[5] This is depicted in Figure 18-9. In this circumstance some pelvic or bladder process such as urinary tract infection, fecal impaction, neoplasm, uterine prolapse, prostatic hypertrophy, deconditioned voiding reflexes, or surgical manipulation leads to enhanced activity of afferent or sensory nerve traffic. This is transmitted to the motor fibers of the detrusor by a spinal reflex which exceeds any cortical inhibitory flow to the detrusor. The

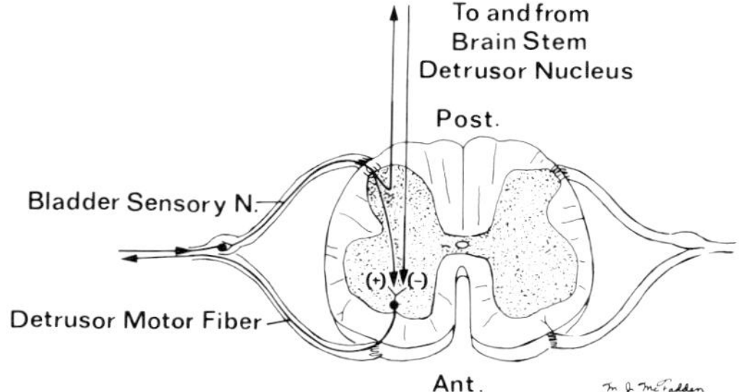

Figure 18-9 Neural pathways mediating increased afferent loop stimulation to the detrusor motor fibers.

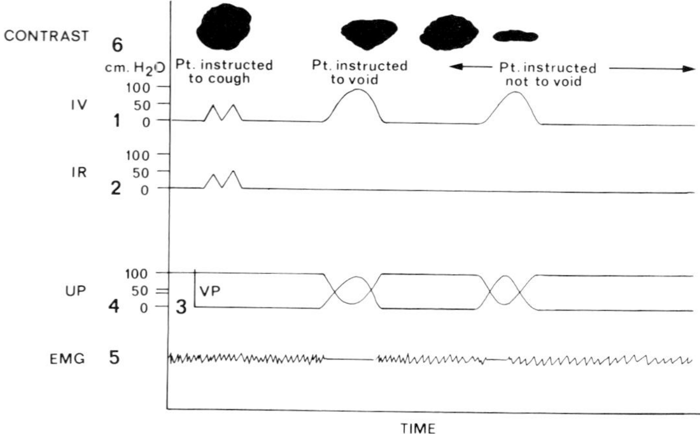

Figure 18-8 Classic urodynamic finding in detrusor instability.

net result is enhanced efferent motor traffic to the detrusor and involuntary bladder contraction and emptying. The importance of this category of voiding problems is that correction of the common problems of the elderly such as infection or constipation will lead to cessation of the incontinence. Urodynamically these appear to be identical to detrusor instability, but are corrected once the pelvic stimuli are eliminated, eg, an enema to relieve fecal impaction. Deconditioned voiding reflexes deserve a special description. Anxiety over any previous episode of a voiding problem may lead to chronic low volume voiding. Such a practice then reduces bladder capacity and increases detrusor tone and bladder wall thickness, all of which aggravate detrusor instability and make future episodes of incontinence more likely.

Stress incontinence demonstrates characteristic urodynamic findings as illustrated in Figure 18-10. It can be seen that increases in intra-abdominal pressure such as coughing, sneezing, Valsalva's maneuver, laughing, all lead to intravesical pressures which exceed urethral pressures and thus cause partial bladder emptying. Therapy with sympathomimetic drugs enhances urethral pressures and can limit the problem. Topical estrogen therapy can enhance the tone of the periurethral tissues in some cases.[16] A final strategy is to employ surgery to improve the valve action of the urethral sphincter. As previously described this restores the angle between the urethra and posterior bladder wall and improves the level of continence.

Figure 18-11 displays the typical urodynamic findings in the voiding problem of bladder outlet obstruction. Fluid is instilled in the bladder until bladder pressure is raised. At a high filling volume there is reflex bladder contraction with urethral pressure falling and the sphincter EMG showing cessation of sphincter activity.

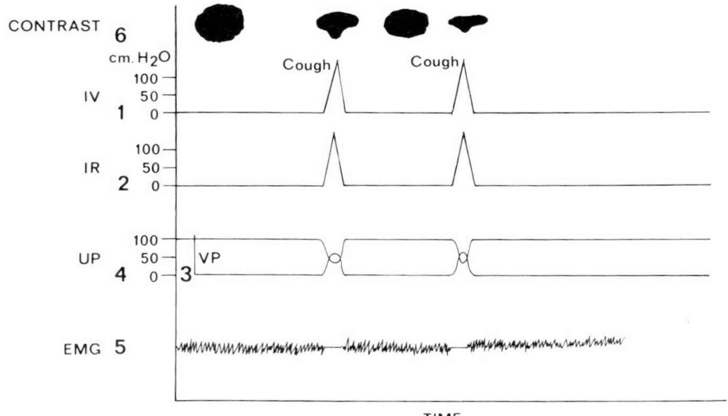

Figure 18-10 Urodynamic findings in stress incontinence.

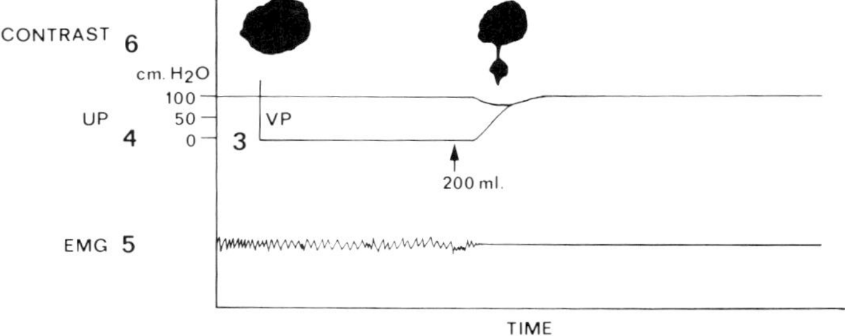

Figure 18-11 Urodynamic findings in bladder outlet obstruction.

Urethral pressure declines but cannot decline sufficiently for adequate voiding. There is radiographic evidence of bladder emptying, but proximal narrowing is evident. Management consists of surgical relief of obstruction when feasible. Otherwise, intermittent catheterization can be employed. Finally, if necessary, bladder contractile force (detrusor contractile strength) can be enhanced with cholinergic agonists such as bethanechol chloride, a representative dose of which might be 10 mg three times daily.

Secondary Voiding Problems

Central nervous system disease in the elderly can cause voiding problems. This set of problems will primarily be developed in another chapter, and only a brief summary will be presented here. Complete cord transection initially causes a flaccid paralysis of the detrusor and compromises inhibitory influences on the external sphincter. The detrusor inadequacy results in bladder distention and inability to void. Overflow incontinence is often the paradoxical clinical presentation of detrusor inadequacy. Most patients will in time develop spontaneous bladder contractions resembling those seen in detrusor instability. Very low (sacral or below T-11) spinal cord lesions may produce lower cord atrophy with permanent detrusor inadequacy. Detrusor inadequacy can also be caused by lower motor neuron diseases; diseases capable of afflicting the motor nerves to the detrusor include diabetes and alcoholism. Additionally, detrusor inadequacy may result from medication use; such medications include the commonly employed muscle relaxants. The urodynamic findings in detrusor inadequacy are shown in Figure 18-12: a gradual rise in bladder pressure is associated with a flat urethral pressure tracing and no change in EMG activity. Leakage of contrast material across a closed sphincter occurs when intravesical pressure exceeds intraurethral pressure. Management consists of discontinuing unnecessary medications, scheduled voiding, and use of agents to stimulate detrusor contractions such as cholinergic agents like bethanechol; if necessary intermittent self-catheterization can be employed.

Lesions of the anteromedial frontal lobe such as intracranial tumors, aneurysms of the anterior cerebral artery, penetrating brain injuries and lobotomy, Parkinson's disease, Alzheimer's disease, multiple sclerosis, thoracic spine transection above T-7, and normal pressure hydrocephalus are all often accompanied by the voiding problem of incontinence. This results from damage to higher cortical centers, which ordinarily transmit inhibitory signals to the detrusor nuclei in the brain stem. The urodynamic findings are consistent with that of detrusor instability. However, unlike idiopathic detrusor instability, the most common cause of incontinence in the elderly, in these diseases the detrusor instability is the direct result of the disease process. The mechanism by which transection of the spinal cord above T-7 causes a syndrome similar to detrusor instability is unknown.[5] Secondary detrusor instability is managed like primary detrusor instability with administration of anti-

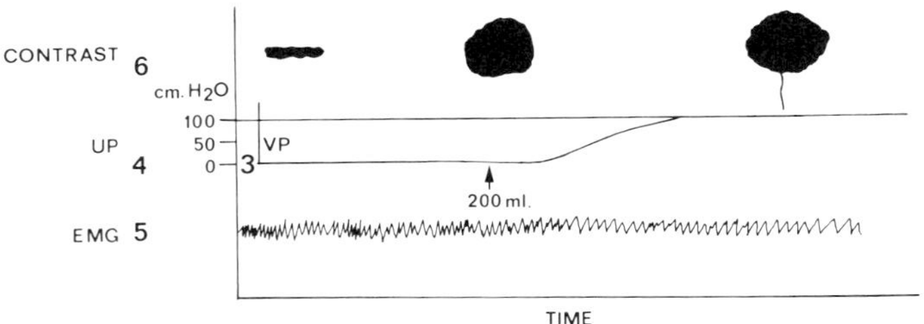

Figure 18-12 Urodynamic findings in detrusor inadequacy.

cholinergic agents such as propantheline bromide.

Finally, impaired sensory input from the bladder due to diabetes mellitus or tabes dorsalis causes a syndrome of overflow incontinence.[5] These persons are frequently not aware of their need to void, but can maintain volitional bladder control. Consequently, as long as they remember or are reminded to void, their overflow incontinence can be controlled. Management consists of training in scheduled voiding routines.

Pharmacologic Agents Causing Voiding Problems

Table 18-1 summarizes the pharmacologic agents which can affect lower urinary tract function. It can be seen that many common drugs used to treat associated conditions like hypertension in the elderly may interfere with function of the lower urinary tract. α-Adrenergic blockade could result in decreased intraurethral pressure which could predispose to incontinence. β-Adrenergic agonists could enhance intravesicular pressures which could contribute to incontinence. Antispasmodics and muscle relaxants by decreasing intraurethral pressure could contribute to incontinence. The exact role concurrent medications play in the voiding problems of the elderly is not known. Based on the known urodynamic consequences of these agents they may at least contribute to voiding problems in a group such as the elderly who are prone to these problems and who are commonly treated with multiple drugs for concomitant medical problems.

Workup for Voiding Problems

The workup for voiding problems in the elderly is summarized in Figures 18-13 and 18-14. It can be seen that the workup will most commonly lead to two management problems for impaired emptying (Figure 18-13): (1A) detrusor inadequacy or insufficiency and (1B) bladder outlet obstruction. Incontinence commonly leads to four management problems (Figure 18-14): (2A) increased afferent loop stimulation, (2B) stress incontinence, (2C) detrusor instability, and (2D) overflow incontinence. Figures 18-13 and 18-14 also demonstrate how drugs may participate in the problems.

Table 18-1
Pharmacologic Agents Affecting Lower Urinary Tract Pressure

	Intra-vesicular Pressure	Intra-urethral Pressure	Clinical Problem
Cholinergic			
Stimulation	Increase	–	Incontinence
Inhibition	Decrease	–	Detrusor insufficiency
α-adrenergic			
Stimulation	–	Increase	Outlet obstruction
Inhibition	–	Decrease	Stress incontinence
β-adrenergic			
Stimulation	Minimal increase	–	Mild stress incontinence possible
Inhibition	Minimal decrease	–	Detrusor insufficiency
Antispasmodics and muscle relaxants	Minimal decrease	Minimal decrease	Detrusor insufficiency

Finally, it can be seen that urodynamic testing appears most useful for diagnosis of detrusor instability and stress incontinence.

Management of Voiding Problems

Eliminating the pharmacologic causes of voiding problems and concentrating on the six problems just described, management will consist of the following: (1) Increased afferent loop stimulation requires correction of the underlying cause. Treatment of urinary tract infection, enemas for fecal impaction, surgical correction of gynecologic fistulas are examples. (2) Detrusor instability is managed with any of the commonly used anticholinergic drugs described in Table 18-2. (3) Overflow incontinence is corrected by surgical correction of outlet obstruction or by voiding schedules. (4) Stress incontinence is treated with sphincter-strengthening exercises (Kegel's exercises), topical estrogens, α-agonists as listed in Table 18-2, or the Marshall-Marchetti operation.

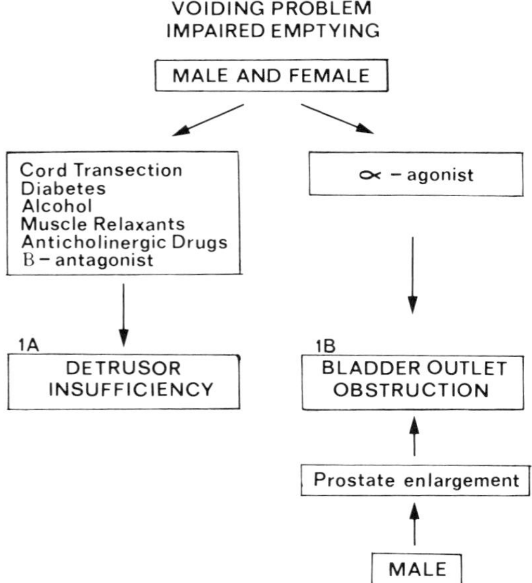

Figure 18-13 Workup for impaired emptying in the elderly.

Impaired emptying is managed by the following: (1) bladder outlet obstruction is managed by surgical correction, by intermittent catheterization, or by manual bladder compression (Credé's maneuver). (2) Detrusor insufficiency is managed by use of the cholinergic drugs described in Table 18-2.

REFERENCES

1. Milne JS: Prevalence of incontinence in elderly age groups, in Willinton WL (ed): *Incontinence in the Elderly*. London, Academic Press, 1976, pp 9–21.
2. Castleden CM, Duffin HM, Ashner MJ:

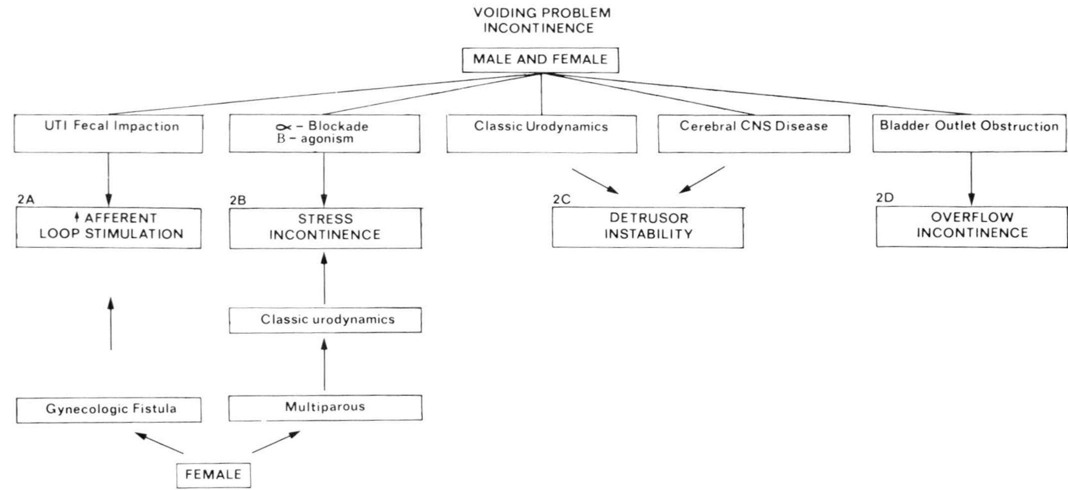

Figure 18-14 Workup for incontinence in the elderly.

Clinical and urodynamic studies in 100 elderly patients. *Br Med J* 1981;282:1103–1105.
3. Salmon UJ, Walter RI, Geist SH: The use of estrogens in the treatment of dysuria and incontinence in postmenopausal women. *Am J Obstet Gynecol* 1941;42:845–851.
4. McDonald DF: Urology, in Schwartz SI (ed): *Principles of Surgery.* New York, McGraw Hill, 1969, pp 1402–1445.
5. Williams ME, Pannill FC III: Urinary incontinence in the elderly. *Ann Intern Med* 1982;97:895–907.
6. Hilton P, Stanton SL: Algorithmic method for assessing urinary incontinence in elderly women. *Br Med J* 1981;282:940– 942.
7. Green TH Jr: Urinary stress incontinence: differential diagnosis, pathophysiology and management. *Am J Obstet Gynecol* 1975; 122:368–400.

Table 18-2
Pharmacologic Agents Used in the Treatment of Incontinence

Agent	Generic Name	Primary Action	Application
Urised	Atropine sulfate, hyoscyamine sulfate methanamine, methylene blue acidifier	Anticholinergic	Detrusor irritability, mild detrusor hyperreflexia
Donnatal	Atropine sulfate hyoscyamine sulfate, scopolamine hydrobromide, methscopolamine bromide, Phenobarbital 16 mg	Anticholinergic, Mild sedative	Same
Pyridium Plus	Phenazopyridine hydrochloride, butabarbital sodium	Anticholinergic, anesthetic-urothelium sedative	Same
Cystospaz	Hyoscyamine	Anticholinergic	Same
Pro-Banthine	Propantheline bromide	Anticholinergic	Moderate to severe detrusor hyperreflexia
Urispas	Flavoxate hydrochloride	Antispasmodic with mild anticholinergic effects	Same
Ditropan	Oxybutynin chloride	Same	Same
Bentyl	Dicyclomine hydrochloride	Same	Same
Ephedrine	Ephedrine sulfate	α-Adrenergic stimulation, increases urethral resistance	Stress incontinence, postprostatectomy incontinence
Ornade	Phenylpropanolamine hydrochloride, chlorpheniramine maleate, isopropamide iodide	Same	Same
Tofranil	Imipramine hydrochloride	α- and β-adrenergic stimulation, increases urethral resistance and bladder capacity; Antidepressant	Stress incontinence, postprostatectomy incontinence, detrusor instability
Urecholine; Duvoid	Bethanecol chloride	Cholinergic-parasympathetic stimulation	Detrusor hyporeflexia, nonobstructive urinary retention

8. Marshall VF, Marchetti AA, Krantz KE: The correction of stress incontinence by simple vesico-urethral suspension. *Surg Gynecol Obstet* 1949;88:509–518.
9. Adult urinary incontinence, in Brown RB (ed): *Clinical Urology Illustrated.* New York, Adis Press, 1982, pp 356–359.
10. Graber EA: Stress incontinence in women. *Obstet Gynecol Surv* 1977;32:565–577.
11. The interpretation of urodynamic findings, in Abrams P, Feneley R, Torens M (eds): *Urodynamics.* Berlin, Springer-Verlag, 1983, pp 97–117.
12. Urodynamic investigations, in Abrams P, Feneley R, Torens M (eds): *Urodynamics.* Berlin, Springer-Verlag, 1983, pp 28–96.
13. Urodynamics, in Brown RB (ed): *Clinical Urology Illustrated.* New York, Adis Press, 1982, pp 120–128.
14. Asmussen M, Ulmsten U: Simultaneous urethro-cystometry with a new technique. *Scand J Urol Nephrol* 1976;10:7–11.
15. Eastwood HDM: Urodynamic studies in the management of urinary incontinence in the elderly. *Age Ageing* 1979;8:41–48.
16. Siegel I, Zelinger BB, Kanter AE: Estrogen therapy for urogenital conditions in the aged. *Am J Obstet Gynecol* 1962;84:505–507.

CHAPTER 19 Central Nervous System Causes of Urinary Incontinence in the Elderly

Anthony J. Furlan

ANATOMY AND PHYSIOLOGY

The central nervous system (CNS) has important facilitory and inhibitory influences on normal bladder function. Numerous and widespread areas of the CNS have been shown to affect bladder control in animals, but the relevance of these findings to man is unclear.[1–3] In cats there is a micturition "center" in the rostral pons which is involved in the normal micturition reflex. Bladder afferent fibers traveling in the pelvic nerves ascend in the lateral spinothalamic tracts, and possibly the dorsal columns, to synapse in the pontomesencephalic reticular formation. Kuru[4] described three descending reticulospinal tracts: (1) the lateral, which facilitates bladder contraction; (2) the ventral, which inhibits bladder contraction; (3) the medial, which causes the external sphincter to contract. Degroat[5] and Bradley et al[3] have proposed other descending pathways which affect normal detrusor function.

The cerebral cortex, hypothalamus, and basal ganglia affect reflex bladder control by influencing the brain-stem reticular activating system. Voluntary control of the external sphincter also relies on intact corticospinal tracts which synapse with the anterior horn cells giving rise to the pudendal nerves in the sacral cord. Areas of the cerebral cortex implicated in bladder control include the superior medial portion of the midfrontal lobe, sensorimotor areas I and II, the genu of the corpus callosum, and the cingulate gyrus (Figure 19-1).[6,7] Inhibition of bladder function has been reported in cats and monkeys with stimulation of the red nucleus, substantia nigra, subthalamic nucleus, medial thalamic nuclei, and the globus pallidus. Although the hypothalamus contains the major CNS autonomic nuclei, its role in bladder control is uncertain.

Loci of facilitation and inhibition have also been reported in various areas of the cerebellum, and Bradley et al[3] suggest the cerebellum is important in the central organization of the micturition reflex.

CLINICAL IMPLICATIONS

Although a form of urinary incontinence in elderly patients which seems to reflect selective dysfunction of central inhibition has been described,[8,9] urinary incontinence is almost never the sole presenting manifestation of brain disease. Peripheral causes must always be sought in patients with brain disease and prominent urinary incontinence. Nonetheless, incontinence can accompany several common neurologic disorders which are generally thought to produce an uninhibited neurogenic bladder.

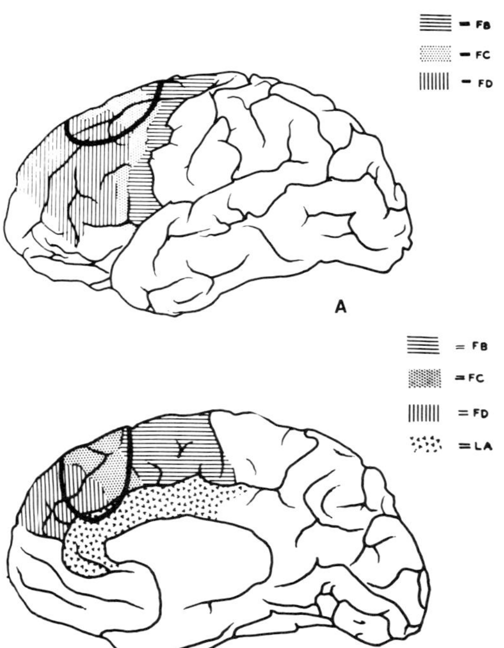

Figure 19-1 Lateral (A) and medial (B) views of cerebral hemisphere with area involved in control of micturition outlined in black. FB and FC = premotor cortex, FD = prefrontal cortex, LA = limbic area/cingulate gyrus. (Reproduced with permission from Andrew and Nathan.[6])

Detailed cystometric studies have rarely been performed in most neurologic conditions so that precise categorization of the urologic disorder is often impossible. Kendall and Karafin[10] have discussed the cystometrogram associated with an uninhibited bladder. There is decreased bladder capacity, an early first desire to void, and uninhibited contractions (Figure 19-2). Voluntary initiation is present but often impaired; inhibition is usually defective. There is no residual urine and vesical sensation is present; in addition, saddle sensation and the bulbocavernous reflex are present. Uninhibited contractions can be eradicated with anticholinergic medications.

There are two unifying concepts of importance in understanding urinary incontinence due to brain disease: (1) The net CNS effect on micturition is inhibition. Thus, CNS lesions tend to produce incontinence rather than retention, although the latter can occur. (2) Brain structures involved in bladder control tend to lie medially or in the deep midline. This explains why incontinence is infrequent with

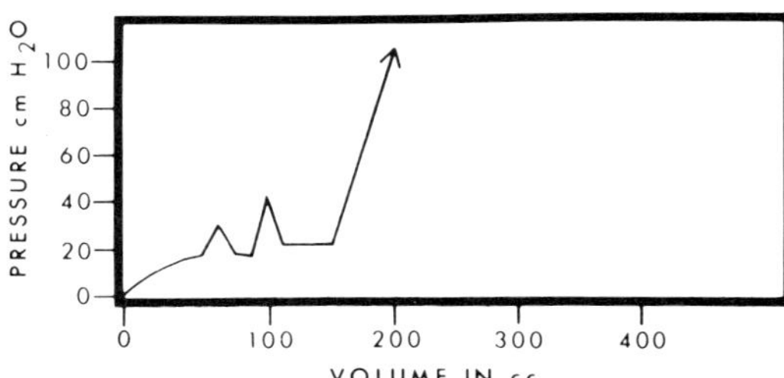

Figure 19-2 Cystometrogram in uninhibited neurogenic bladder. (Reproduced with permission from Kendall and Karaffin.[10])

laterally placed unilateral hemisphere lesions, and why urinary urgency and incontinence are early symptoms of hydrocephalus due to any cause.

Although one can postulate innumerable brain lesions which *might* produce incontinence, in clinical practice significant urinary incontinence due to brain disease is encountered in relatively few situations in the elderly.

Stroke[11]

Urinary incontinence is common in elderly patients with large ischemic or hemorrhagic strokes when there is a depressed level of consciousness. Incontinence is also frequent in patients who are aphasic and unable to communicate the need to void. Multiple or bilateral strokes may cause incontinence, particularly when interruption of the corticobulbar and corticospinal fibers controlling reflex micturition inhibition or voluntary sphincter control has occurred. Urinary incontinence is often seen, for example, as part of the pseudobulbar or lacunar state due to multiple small, deep infarcts in elderly patients with hypertension. Urinary incontinence may also occur in the rare patient with anterior cerebral artery occlusive disease and mesial frontal lobe infarction.

Many patients with brain-stem stroke require catheterization because of depressed level of consciousness or severe neurologic deficits. Because of the proposed pontomesencephalic micturition center, brain-stem stroke might directly affect the central control of micturition, but this possibility has not been systematically studied.

Dementia

Patients with moderately advanced or severe memory dysfunction often develop uninhibited urinary incontinence. The most common cause of dementia is Alzheimer's disease, although there are many other treatable and untreatable forms of dementia. Normal pressure hydrocephalus (NPH) should be suspected in elderly patients with the recent onset of urinary incontinence, dementia, and a gait disorder.[12] The brain computed tomography (CT) scan shows enlarged ventricles with minimal or no cortical atrophy (Figure 19-3), and the cerebrospinal fluid opening pressure is normal. Indium or ytterbium cisternography should demonstrate intraventricular accumulation of isotope at 48 to 72 hours (Figure 19-4). Although patients who fulfill these criteria for NPH are not rare, the response to shunting remains unpredictable and complications of shunting in the elderly occur quite frequently.

Extrapyramidal Disease

Autonomic dysfunction can occur in Parkinson's disease. Two types of bladder dysfunction have been reported in Parkinson's disease.[13,14] One type is a hyperactive bladder characterized by frequency, urgency, and incontinence, and decreased bladder capacity. The other type is a hypoactive bladder with a decreased desire to

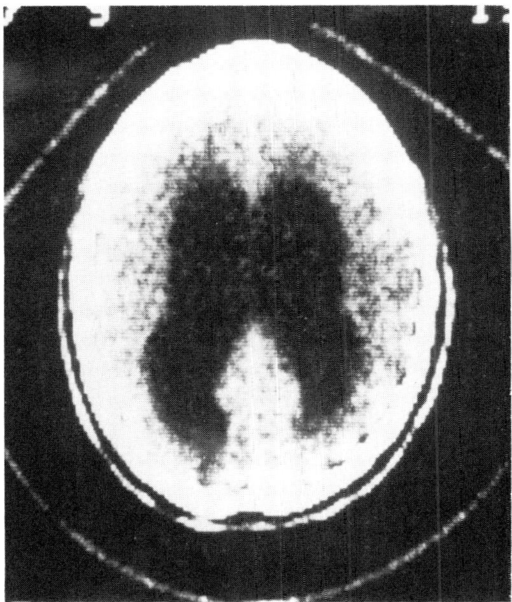

Figure 19-3 Brain CT scan in a patient with normal pressure hydrocephalus. Note the enlarged ventricles without corresponding cortical atrophy.

void which later converts to a pattern of precipitant micturition.

Significant urinary incontinence is rare in Parkinson's disease. Prominent incontinence associated with extrapyramidal signs should raise the possibility of Shy-Drager syndrome, especially when associated with orthostatic hypotension and impotence.[15]

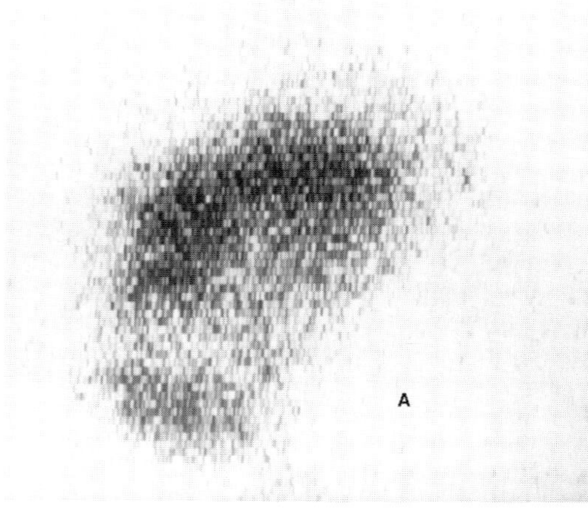

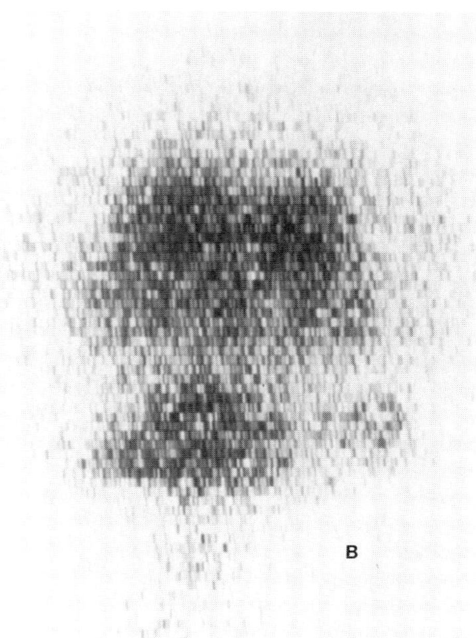

Figure 19-4 Isotope cisternogram in a patient with normal pressure hydrocephalus. The lateral (A) and anteroposterior (B) views show intraventricular accumulation of isotope at 48 hours. The patient improved with shunting.

Extrapyramidal dysfunction and urinary incontinence may be late manifestations of certain types of olivopontocerebellar atrophy, a group of degenerative disorders sometimes causing ataxia in the elderly.[16]

Parasagittal Syndrome

Tumors, often meningiomas, affecting the superior and mesial frontal lobes produce bilateral leg weakness and urinary incontinence. A similar syndrome is seen with bilateral anterior cerebral artery territory infarction, anterior cerebral artery aneurysm,[17] and superior sagittal sinus thrombosis.

Brain Tumor

Watts and Uhle[18] described a number of cystometric patterns in patients with brain tumors. Lesions affecting the corpus callosum and frontotemporal area produce hypertonic bladders and uninhibited urinary incontinence. These findings were later confirmed by Andrew and Nathan[6,7] who found the following associated with superior frontal tumors: (1) Urinary frequency, urgency, and incontinence. (2) loss of desire to void but not necessarily the sensation of imminent micturition; (3) precipitate micturition; (4) reduced bladder capacity. These are, of course, the features of an uninhibited neurogenic bladder and reflect destruction of cortical inhibitory pathways.

REFERENCES

1. Wein AJ, Raezer DM: Physiology and micturition, in Krane RJ, Siroky MB (eds): *Clinical Neuro-Urology.* Boston, Little, Brown & Co, 1979, pp 1–33.
2. Bors E, Comarr AE: *Neurological Urology.* Baltimore, University Park Press, 1971, pp 61–128.
3. Bradley WE, Timm GW, Scott FB: Innervation of the detrusor muscle and urethra. *Urol Clin North Am* 1974;1:3–27.
4. Kuru M: Nervous control of micturition. *Physiol Rev* 1965;45:425–494.

5. DeGroat WC: Nervous control of the urinary bladder of the cat. *Brain Res* 1975; 87:201–211.
6. Andrew J, Nathan PW: Lesions of the anterior frontal lobes and disturbances of micturition and defecation. *Brain* 1964;87: 233–262.
7. Andrew J. Nathan PW: The cerebral control of micturition. *Proc R Soc Med* 1965; 58:553–555.
8. Lapides J, Costello RT Jr: Uninhibited neurogenic bladder: A common cause for recurrent urinary infection in normal women. *J Urol* 1969;101:539–544.
9. Herwig KR: The history and physical examination in neurogenic bladder disease. *Urol Clin North Am* 1974;1:29–35.
10. Kendall AR, Karafin L: Classification of neurogenic bladder disease. *Uro Clin North Am* 1974;1:37–44.
11. Lorenze EJ, Simon HB, Linden JL: Urologic problems in rehabilitation of hemiplegic patients. *JAMA* 1959;169: 1042–1046.
12. Symon L, Hinzpeter T: The enigma of normal pressure hydrocephalus tests to select patients for surgery and to predict shunt function. *Clin Neurosurg* 1977;24:285–315.
13. Murnaghan GF: Neurogenic disorders of the bladder in Parkinsonism. *Br J Urol* 1961;33:403–409.
14. Porter RW: Visceral manifestations of extrapyramidal dysfunction. Read before the 16th Annual Spinal Cord Injury Conference, Long Beach, Calif, Sept 27–29, 1967.
15. Chokroverty S, Barron KD, Katz FH, et al: The syndrome of primary orthostatic hypotension. *Brain* 1969;92:743–768.
16. Critchley M, Greenfield JG: Olivo-ponto-cerebellar atrophy. *Brain* 1948;71:343– 364.
17. Andrew J, Nathan PW, Spanas NC: Disturbances of micturition and defecation due to aneurysms of anterior communicating or anterior cerebral arteries. *J Neurosurg* 1966;24:1–10.
18. Watts JW, Uhle CAW: Bladder dysfunction in cases of brain tumor; cystometric study. *J Urol* 34:10–30, 1935.

CHAPTER 20

Benign Prostatic Hypertrophy

Frank Hinman, Jr.

NATURAL HISTORY

Prostatic enlargement (benign prostatic hyperplasia or hypertrophy; BPH) is a disease of the middle and later years. Pathologically it is very rarely found under the age of 30 years; by age 80 over half of men have frank enlargements, and another third have benign prostatic hyperplasia on microscopic study.[1] All the evidence is that it steadily progresses with age, at a rate different for each individual.

More important is evidence from clinical observations. The number of prostatectomies increase with age.[2] A 50-year-old man has a 1.5% chance for prostatectomy before he is 60, but for a 60-year-old man, the incidence rises to 7% by the time he is 70. These are figures from 1961; with safer surgical procedures, more acquiescent patients, and more urologists, it is estimated that today a 50-year-old man has one chance in four of having such an operation during his lifetime.

The symptoms of prostatic obstruction do not progress uniformly. The chance for acute urinary retention in one United States series was 1 in 10,[3] whereas in Britain it was 4 in 5. In one 3-year study of 26 patients,[3] 15 were worse over the time of observation but eight were improved. If flow rate alone is used, obstructed patients were found to have a decline from 13.9 to 11.9 mL/s, 2 mL/s being a significant change.[4] However, so-called normal men have a decline of 1.5 mL/s over the same period.[5]

Progression is the rule, due to gradual

enlargement of the gland. But variations in the patient's attitude toward his symptoms or from accompanying prostatitis or prostatic infarct, or in the methods of examination, account for the differences and inconstancies in the observed rate of progression.

The occurrence of BPH is not related to sexual activity, and risk factors such as alcohol, drug use, stress, and diet have not been implicated. It is highly improbable that it is related to prostatic cancer.

Its incidence among the black population varies with geography and racial mixtures, but is probably not much different from that among whites. Asians, especially Japanese, show an appreciably lower incidence.

The mortality varies throughout the world. The most developed European countries have the highest rate (23 deaths per 100,000 males). The reason may lie in better reporting, more autopsies, and an older population. Lower rates occur in Japan, where racial characteristics may truly be different, and the United States where differences in surgical diagnosis and methods of recording the first cause of death may be the explanation.

PATHOLOGIC CHARACTERISTICS AND SITE OF DEVELOPMENT

Benign prostatic hypertrophy is not a disease of the prostate proper; rather, it is the involvement of the periurethral tissue in what is best termed benign nodular hyperplasia. As this centrally located growth expands, it compresses the true prostate into a thin fibroglandular structure, the so-called surgical capsule. Between the two is a cleavage plane that permits enucleation of the "gland" (Figure 20-1).

Embryology BPH arises from the transition zone in the preprostatic tissue lying on the floor between the verumontanum and the vesical neck, a zone comprising less than 5% of the entire prostate.[6] Here stromal nodules arise randomly and act as embryo-like inductors for the adjacent ducts. Direct evidence exists for an inductive influence of accessory sex organ stroma on adjacent epithelium.[7] BPH may also involve the expression of the embryo-like inductive properties of prostatic stroma on responsive epithelia.[8] The following steps are involved: diffuse growth in the so-called transition zone, then the development of stromal nodules, followed by glandular proliferation.

Pathology The typical nodule is a fibromyoadenoma in which several distinct histologic patterns can be recognized.

HORMONAL CONTROL OF BPH

Action of endocrine substances Androgens are required to initiate BPH and to allow for its growth. Using the enzyme 5α-reductase, the prostate metabolizes testosterone to dihydrotestosterone. This form of testosterone is bound to a specific cytosolic receptor and transported to the nucleus where an interaction with chromatin occurs producing an androgenic effect on cell differentiation and growth. However, the data do not show clearly that patients with BPH have any lower (or higher) circulating levels of androgen than normal men. The activities of 5α-reductase occur principally in the stroma – an indication of that tissue's importance as the inductive mechanism.

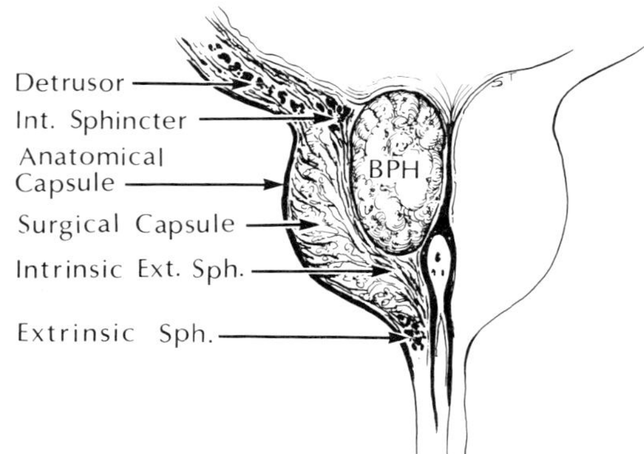

Figure 20-1: Cross section of prostate, showing relation of BPH to the prostate proper.

Hormonal manipulation has been tried. Castration results in rapid involution of the prostate. If done before puberty in man, it prevents the development of BPH, but there is no good evidence that castration significantly affects BPH once it has developed. Some regression in the epithelial component can be seen histologically, but no change occurs in the stroma. A similar differential effect is seen in rats, further suggesting that once stromal growth has occurred, that it is not reversible. Thus a therapeutic approach utilizing hormonal manipulation (by castration or antiandrogens) appears impractical.

Estrogens have a dual effect on the prostate. By suppressing pituitary output of luteinizing hormone (LH) and thus lowering production of testicular androgen, they have an effect similar to castration. Serum estrogen levels are higher in patients with BPH than in age-matched controls.[9] Furthermore, estradiol increases both the uptake and conversion of dihydrotestosterone (DHT) in organ culture.[10] It is possible that the higher levels of active androgen found in BPH are in some way associated with the action of estrogen. Estrogens may play a role in BPH, since their level relative to that of androgens rises with age but perhaps too late to be a factor in the growth. Prolactin may also be involved in the development of BPH. Both the dog and rat prostate involute more completely when castration is supplemented by hypophysectomy,[11] and prolactin receptors have been found in prostatic tissue.[12] It may be that the endocrine hormones are at most facilitative rather than causative for the basic mechanism inherent in stromal-epithelial inductions. Thus it may be concluded that endocrine substances most likely do influence the development of BPH but are not the sole factors in its genesis.

Endocrine effects on established hypertrophy The goals of endocrine treatment are to produce subjective (symptomatic) and objective improvement with acceptable side effects. The standard for comparison is surgical treatment with its usually rapid reversal and long-term relief of obstruction. The effects of medical treatment are difficult to quantitate since the natural history of the disease is so variable in any one patient and among groups of patients. The symptoms may fluctuate, even subsiding completely for long periods. In one series, 60% of the patients showed spontaneous improvement.[13]

This improvement occurs for reasons that have not been fully characterized, including altered adrenergic stimulation, changes in detrusor function, variation in epithelial secretion, or even, although unlikely, temporary reversal of stromal inductive activity. For medical treatment to be acceptable it must not only reduce obstruction but it should be capable of relieving symptoms as well.

Reduction in prostatic size, with resultant decrease in outflow obstruction, must occur to demonstrate that endocrine therapy is effective. However, the size of the prostate relates poorly to both subjective and objective manifestations of obstruction. A hormonal effect on established hypertrophy is not easy to demonstrate. As long ago as 1895, bilateral orchiectomy was reported to have an 87% response rate,[14] but substantiation has not been forthcoming. Stilbestrol therapy has also been tried and has been found to result in a 12% reduction in prostatic size.[15] As would be expected, androgens do not favorably affect BPH. A combination of androgens and estrogens have been tried with the results being quite variable.[16] Antiandrogens, which are progesterone analogues and act by way of pituitary suppression, have had little success. Trials with medrogestone,[17] cyproterone acetate,[18] and flutamide[19] have shown equivocal results at best. Moreover, the side effects of sodium retention, thrombophlebitis, gynecomastia, and impotence make their use impractical, particularly in light of the equivocal results following their use. Even if an effect is obtained, it is frequently lost when treatment is stopped. When compared with surgery, endocrine therapy is neither less expensive nor less morbid. It must be remembered that clinical improvement does not necessarily mean that a reduction in prostatic size has occurred.

Nonhormonal agents that have an effect on the prostate are the cholesterol-lowering substances. The cholesterol level is elevated in BPH tissue and may play a role in its pathogenesis. Cholesterol content can be lowered by polyene macrolides, particularly candicidin, nystatin, and amphotericin B – all antifungal agents.[20-22] However, a double-blind and randomized study of 52 patients utilizing candicidin failed to show any significant clinical improvement although the mean urinary flow rate was seen to increase.[23]

Evidence of regression of prostatic size is necessary if improvement is to be ascribed to any agent. Of the various methods used to measure the size of the prostate, ultrasonography, and computed tomography (CT), which measures the prostate three-dimensionally, are the most accurate (until the magnetic resonance imaging technic is generally available and cost-effective). Even these methods have economic and technical limitations, and have not yet been applied in controlled studies. An additional problem with endocrine therapy is based on its known modulation of smooth muscle function in the urinary tract, thereby sometimes producing improvement unrelated to its effect on prostatic size.

Controlled series are necessary before we can know if any endocrine treatment is truly worthwhile. These entail careful attention to a number of scientific details including (*a*) adequate base-line studies for several weeks prior to treatment to investigate for spontaneous disease variations; (*b*) adrenergic blockade to neutralize adrenergic stimulation; (*c*) carefully performed urodynamic studies before treatment; (*d*) efficient control of medication dosage and monitoring of serum levels; (*e*) continuing drug therapy for at least 3 months; (*f*) evaluation of patient compliance; and (*g*) measurement of the effects of treatment by evaluation of symptoms, by sequential measurements of urodynamic parameters, and by determination of prostatic size by scan. Too many uncontrolled studies have been done; we must wait for results which have been proved by double-blind prospective randomized trials.

NEUROPHYSIOLOGICAL APPROACHES

Storage and emptying The smooth muscle of the bladder and urethra are dually innervated[24] and a functional division exists between the body of the bladder and the vesical neck,[25] the latter acting as the internal sphincter. The striated, so-called external sphincter is somatically innervated, although it may be supplied additionally by autonomic nerves.[26] Important to an understanding of obstruction in BPH is the fact that α-adrenergic excitation of the muscles of the vesical outlet maintains continence throughout the filling phase of the micturition cycle. In turn, the detrusor contraction initiating voiding is accompanied by a massive cholinergic discharge which inhibits the effector sympathetic neurons; α-activity then ceases and the β-adrenergic inhibitory mechanism takes over, which in turn is modulated by both CNS and infraspinal (peripheral) mechanisms. At the end of voiding, α-activity returns and dissipates the parasympathetically induced detrusor contraction.

Drug manipulation Drugs may be useful in the management of BPH in two situations: for relaxation of the unstable bladder, and in particular for relaxation of the vesical neck. Inhibition of bladder contractility may be helpful in patients with bladder instability and symptoms of frequency and precipitant voiding. Since the detrusor is already working against obstruction, it may decompensate if over-inhibited, so drugs must be given with caution. Inhibition can be accomplished by drugs acting on the spinal cord, the ganglia, or directly on the smooth muscle receptors. The detrusor contracts by way of postganglionic cholinergic neurons; anticholinergic activity thus will tend to inhibit this contraction. Also, the prostatic capsule contracts with cholinergic stimulation, and relaxes subsequent to the administration of anticholinergic drugs.[27] Propantheline bromide, an anticholinergic agent, not only acts on the α-receptors but on the ganglia as well. Other drugs effective in the inhibition of contractility are oxybutynin chloride and dicyclomine hydrochloride.

Relaxation of the bladder neck by drugs can be of considerable value in the management of BPH.[27] Studies have shown that the stroma of the adenoma and especially the capsule are rich in α-adrenergic receptors with accompanying short adrenergic neurons.[28,29] The capsule contracts strongly on α-adrenergic stimulation with norepinephrine, an action blocked by the α-blocker phentolamine hydrochloride. From a functional point of view, the contraction resulting from α-sympathetic activity accomplishes emptying of the prostatic acini and expression of the prostatic secretions.[30] In BPH, α-adrenergic activity may induce variations in tone and thus alter the closure pressure, adding a variable dynamic component to any level of pre-existent mechanical obstruction. This accounts for the typical variability in symptoms as observed by the well-known fact that exposure to cold exacerbates the symptoms and that hot baths are beneficial. Allowing the bladder to overfill has the effect of increasing the detrusor-urethra reflexes[31] which then increase tension in the urethra. Mental stress can also increase obstruction. Common to all of these events is an increase in sympathetic activity.

α-Blockers have proved to be of use for the temporary relief of symptoms in those patients with an appreciable increase in the dynamic component of obstruction, since prostatic obstruction is not in itself necessarily progressive. Phenoxybenzamine hydrochloride, a long-acting drug which has been extensively studied, is given in a dose of 10 or 20 mg/d. It often provides relief from hesitancy and weak stream, and it reduces the irritative symptoms of frequency and urgency. Any reduction in obstruction as the result of this drug may then allow the patient to postpone operative intervention until a more convenient time. It must be kept in mind that the effect of this agent does not alter the basic obstructive factors, and that operation may well be inevitable.

In acute urinary retention, which is probably due to overactivation of the adrenergic receptors in the prostate, α-blockers may be helpful. The retention may be actively treated by use of a rapidly acting blocker such as phentolamine hydrochloride; this can be given slowly up to a dose of 10 mg intravenously (IV), while blood pressure and pulse rate are monitored. Its use is limited and may even prove to be dangerous because of both the age and the cardiovascular status of those individuals most likely to suffer acute urinary retention. Moreover, most patients are seen at a time when retention is already well established and thus irreversible by drug therapy alone. When α-blocker therapy is considered the concomitant use of a cholinergic agent such as bethanecol chloride is contraindicated. Studies have shown that although this drug does raise detrusor pressure,[32] it also increases the tension in the prostatic capsule[33] and at least partially counteracts the beneficial effects of α-blockade.

Phenoxybenzamine has been utilized prophylactically in a number of instances. It may prevent acute retention in those patients with otherwise little trouble who may occasionally become completely obstructed. Another prophylactic use is prior to herniorrhapy or hemorrhoidectomy in men with borderline obstruction.[34] It may also prevent return of obstruction after catheter removal.[35] It may help temporarily as many as 60% of patients with obstructive BPH.

A contraindication to the use of phenoxybenzamine is impaired cerebral blood flow as demonstrated in patients who have had a previous cerebral vascular accident or with cerebral arteriosclerosis. Otherwise, cardiovascular disease, even to the extent of myocardial infarction, is not adversely affected. In general, side effects such as orthostatic hypotension, retrograde ejaculation, and weakness are of significance in only about 10% of patients who utilize this agent.

CLINICAL EVALUATION

Vesicourethral response to obstruction If the physician is to conduct a meaningful evaluation of obstructed voiding, he must understand the storage and control mechanisms that are relevant to BPH. Bladder outlet obstruction is currently diagnosed by utilizing both urine flow rate and detrusor pressure; however, these tests are diagnostic in only 65% of patients.[36] Thus it must be said from the outset that the methods at our disposal do not measure obstruction accurately; and furthermore the degree of obstruction is not necessarily proportional to either the size of the prostate or the severity of the symptoms. Pressure and flow are the important clinical factors in BPH because increased pressure may lead to irreversible detrusor damage and, albeit less importantly, because decreased flow greatly delays completion of the voiding act.

A balance exists during voiding between the contractile capability of the detrusor and the conductivity of the urethra. In the normal subject, a low opening pressure in the posterior urethra is associated with a large cross-sectional area, which results in high flow at low pressures. Consequently, the muscular energy expended by the detrusor for each milliliter of urine voided is small. Bladder outlet obstruction, by reducing the cross-sectional area in the urethra and hence the flow rate, reciprocally raises the bladder pressure and places a demand on the detrusor to exert more muscular energy per milliliter of urine voided. Thus detrusor pressure during voiding depends on the flow rate and on the force of the contraction, which in turn is related to the volume of urine in the bladder.

The detrusor can provide a certain limited amount of contractile energy for each voiding, and this energy is related to the volume of urine in the bladder. Because the power of the detrusor depends on the length of the muscle fibers, which is set by the volume in the bladder, lower volumes result in decreased contractile force. As the bladder empties, fiber length shortens and consequently power falls, reaching zero at the end of voiding. The power must be high enough to last all through voiding or the bladder does not empty completely as it might in the normal subject. With obstruction, the detrusor contraction may overcome the increased urethral resistance at the beginning of urination when the bladder is full, but fails to do so as the bladder volume decreases towards the end of voiding, which then results in the retention of urine (residual urine).[37–39] In other words, the detrusor uses more energy per milliliter of urine to void against obstruction, so that the volume of each voiding is lower and hence the volume left behind is higher.

"Compensatory hypertrophy" is the hypertrophy of the muscle fibers that occurs in order to produce an isometrically high force to match the raised outflow resistance. Since the speed of contraction simultaneously decreases, there is little gain in overall power. The muscle is not able to do the prolonged heavy work required throughout one contraction; force is increased but the total work remains virtually the same. With the enlarged prostate compressing the bladder outlet, not only is more power used to open it but also more is needed to "hold it open" throughout urination. As the power of the detrusor fails, voiding tapers off in a dribble and urine is left in the bladder.

The overall force of the detrusor does not change with an operation but residual urine is usually cleared after prostatectomy by the reduction in urethral resistance. With the greater flow rates possible after operation, the same total force can now effectively empty the bladder. The exception to this is following chronic bladder distention; here the resting fiber length is unduly increased, and the vesical wall infiltrated with collagen is unable to contract effectively.

As noted, expenditure of energy by the detrusor is balanced between pressure and flow,[40] but instead of hypertrophying, the bladder may decompensate, resulting in decreased availability of energy. This lowers voiding pressure and further slows the flow. It is not known why opposite patterns such as compensation and decompensation occur; it may be that the deposition of collagen among the muscle bundles acts to restrict the transmission of energy necessary for detrusor contraction.

To summarize, with obstruction from BPH, as the resistance of the bladder outlet increases, flow decreases, with little variation in the total power. Rather, it is the energy spent per unit of time that changes. When, at a certain point of obstruction, the energy need exceeds the supply, the bladder begins to "decompensate," as evidenced by the accumulation of residual urine.

Examination of the BPH patient Patients will seldom be referred merely because of a large prostate but rather seek evaluation because of complaints attributable to obstruction. The following steps allow for an orderly workup:

1. *Flow rate* by observation and timing of voiding, or, better, measured instrumentally. When measured as maximum (peak) flow (Figure 20-2), it is an easy test to perform, requiring only a stopwatch and a graduated receptacle in its simplest form. Electronic uroflowmeters are in common use and although they can give information in addition to maximum flow rate, this parameter is the single most useful one. If maximum flow rate is under 10 mL/s, obstruction is very likely. As such, the test is a useful screening technic if one keeps in mind that psychological inhibition may artificially reduce the flow rate, especially on the initial determinations.[41]

As noted previously, maximum flow rate is regulated by the amount voided, so that each clinical determination should be corrected for volume voided. In the normal male, maximum flow rate increases by 2.5 mL/s for each additional 100 mL voided.[42] A nomogram which gives 1, 2, and 3 SD from the mean may be used to correct the observed rate (Figure 20-3).[43] Since the flow rate decreases with age, a further correction may be made, but if the volume voided is only between 250 and 400 mL,

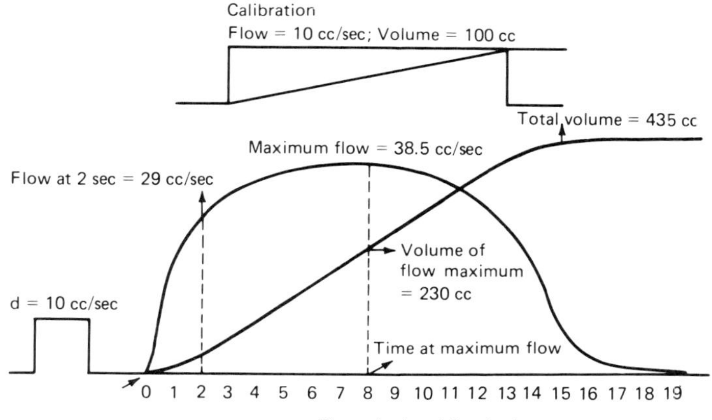

Figure 20-2 Parameters of urinary flow (reproduced with permission from Susset JG, Picker P, Kretz M, et al: Critical evaluation of uroflowmeters and analysis of normal curves. *J Urol* 1973;109:874).

in clinical practice an adjustment is not necessary. At the lesser volumes usually found in prostate patients, correction is usually advisable.[44]

Other parameters may be measured, such as the time to maximal flow rate. This measurement is not particularly useful for BPH patients because much of the increase in total voiding time with obstruction is toward the end of voiding, and not at the beginning. In summary, maximal voiding rate is a useful screening test for prostatic obstruction, and further, is a practical means of following patients for its progression.

2. *Urinalysis* may be used to detect infection or bleeding. This is best performed by the consultant himself since too many laboratories report such equivocal results as 2 to 3 WBC or 1 to 2 RBC. In case of doubt, a midstream specimen may be sent for culture.

3. *Palpation of the abdomen* for bladder fullness. If the bladder is firm or tender on suprapubic palpation, retention is likely.

4. *Rectal examination* with attention to both size, and the presence of discrete densities (malignancy). This procedure is most important, not merely to identify prostatic enlargement but in addition to detect abnormal areas suggestive of carcinoma which might then require needle biopsy. Rectal examination also allows the surgeon to decide on the use of either an open or a transurethral operation, the latter not being employed when very large glands are present.

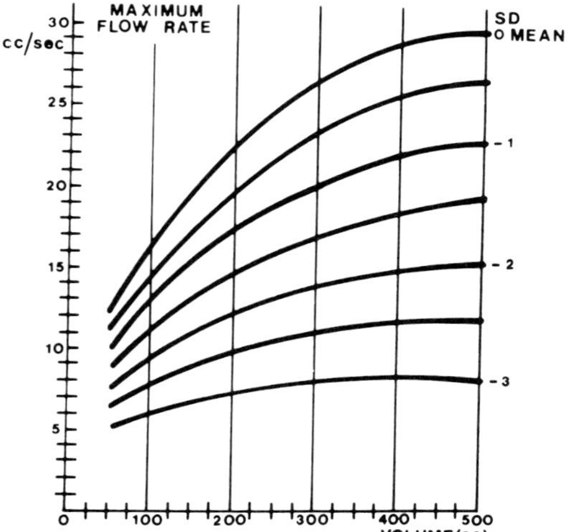

Figure 20-3 Flow rate nomogram, use of which allows correction of the patient's maximal flow rate for any volume (reproduced with permission from Siroky, et al[43]).

It must be appreciated that prostatic size does not demonstrate a direct relationship to the degree of obstruction; small glands may be highly obstructive and large ones hardly obstructive at all, since obstruction is as much due to a response of the capsule and vesical neck to the adenoma as it is to the encroachment of the growing lobes themselves on the urethral lumen. Ultrasonography may also be used to demonstrate prostatic size and configuration but is not in general clinical use.

5. *Residual urine determination* by means of sonography, phenolsulfonphthalein (PSP) test, or catheterization, is important in the evaluation of potential prostatic obstruction since it reflects the result of the imbalance between detrusor capability and outflow resistance. Its use for the diagnosis of BPH has been criticized because residual urine occurs not only in the presence of appreciable obstruction but also from abnormalities of the detrusor itself. This difference should not be ignored in clinical practice, since the results from reducing outlet resistance by transurethral resection (TUR) in the presence of a poorly contractile detrusor are not as good as when the resection occurs when a strong detrusor is present working against a high degree of obstruction. In most cases the detrusor becomes weakened by obstruction, which is usually slowly progressive in nature, and the removal of the obstruction only tends to improve the situation but not to totally correct it. Even if detrusor weakness with consequent urinary retention are due to another primary cause (eg, diabetic neuropathy) in older men outlet obstruction is often superimposed, in which case resection of the prostate or incision of the outlet is indicated.

Serial determinations of residual urine over the years can prove useful with values extrapolable into the future. If, in the absence of neuropathy, the residual volume gradually increases, a decision can be made for prostatectomy before irreversible changes result. For practical purposes 50 or 60 mL is a significant amount since this is enough to be easily measured by clinical methods, and to serve as evidence for early decompensation.

The late consequence of incomplete emptying during active detrusor contraction is obstruction and distortion of the ureterovesical junction (UVJ) and consequent ureterectasis with or without accompanying reflux, hydronephrosis, and renal impairment. These effects are due to detrusor hypertrophy with repeated instances of high intravesical pressure. It is important in these patients to periodically measure serum creatinine in their follow-up with a rise in its level serving as an even stronger indication for operation then increasing residual urine volumes.

Several methods are used to determine residual urine volume. For the phenolsulfonphthalein (PSP) test, a known amount of dye is given IV and the amount recovered after 30 and 60 minutes is related to the volume of urine voided. This test is noninterventional and in some hands very useful,[45] but it is inconvenient and imprecise, and has consequently fallen out of favor. Estimation from the postvoiding film after intravenous excretion pyelography (IVP) is not reliable except when large residual volumes are found since there may exist uncertainty on the time between voiding and film exposure. Residual urine determination itself is not enough to justify performing an IVP, which as mentioned below is otherwise not a cost-effective procedure. If catheterization is resorted to, it probably should not be done so as a routine procedure because of the discomfort it entails, and the possibility of initiating infection; other methods, such as sonography, are probably too costly for general use.

6. *Excretory urography* (IVP) is done only if the result of the urinalysis is abnormal or if the patient has some localizing sign. It is a test uniformly performed by some and seldom utilized by others. It should be done if a history of symptoms of upper tract disease can be elicited or if the urinalysis is abnormal. Information may be obtained from this procedure on a number of anatomical findings including: the presence and severity of vesical trabeculation or diverticula, the incidence of upward displacement of the ureters (J-ureters), the presence of ureteral dilatation from reflux (in 14% of cases), or the demonstration of ureterovesical junction (UVJ) obstruction, which may be manifest by poor renal concentrating ability.

An IVP will detect abnormalities in other parts of the urinary tract in 15% of patients, but these findings are not such as

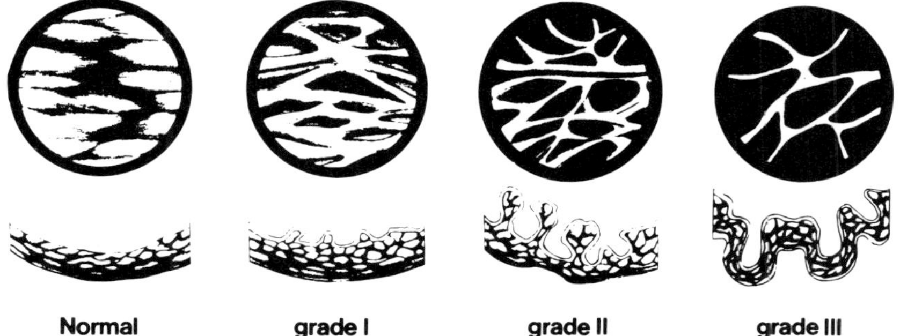

Figure 20-4 Vesical trabeculation, depicted in four grades (reproduced with permission from Andersen JT, Nordling J: Relation of prostatic lobes to degree and rate of obstruction, in Hinman F Jr (ed): *Benign Prostatic Hypertrophy.* New York, Springer-Verlag, 1983, pp 678–681).

to affect the management of the patient in a noteworthy manner.[46] In the general population a good statistical correlation exists between the IVP and a number of clinicopathologic findings; these include urodynamic findings, trabeculation or bladder diverticula, detrusor instability, basal prostatic filling defects, and bladder area (residual urine) with obstruction. Unfortunately, any such correlations in the individual patient have proved to be quite poor. If a very delayed film of the bladder is obtained when it is full, followed by a postvoiding film,[47] some additional information may be obtained. However, it must be stated that the IVP is probably not a cost-effective part of the routine workup for prostate-related obstruction.[48]

7. *Panendoscopy* (urethrocystoscopy) is usually not done prior to the time of operation, since the information obtained by direct inspection of the bladder and urethra usually is not needed either to decide when to operate or to determine the type of operation, and the structures will be examined eventually as part of the operative procedure.

Panendoscopy when performed does allow for an assessment of the degree of trabeculation (Figure 20-4), and the form taken by the lobar intrusion. BPH takes five characteristic forms, ranging from simple bilateral lobar hypertrophy to various combinations at and under the vesical neck (Figure 20-5).[49] These configurations under the vesical neck are due more to adaptation to the surrounding structures than to their actual sites of origin, since all forms of BPH arise from the periurethral glands and stroma. Panendoscopic identification of the BPH form in any given patient may suggest the prognosis. For example, bilateral lobar hypertrophy is usually associated with frequent attacks of acute retention, but with minimal residual urine; whereas with a lobe at the vesical neck, residual urine proves to be the rule. These characteristics are seldom useful in determining the necessity for operation.

8. True *urodynamic studies* will be reserved for those complicated cases where the findings from the procedures just described do not correlate among themselves or do not agree with the patient's symptoms. They are more suitable as research tools than for clinical evaluation. One such urodynamic study, the urethral pressure profile, attempts to measure the local occlusive force of the prostate by means of a pressure-measuring device passed through the posterior urethra; this is in contrast to the previously described methods which use the global information of bladder pressure and flow to deduce the actual extent of local obstruction. The profile is obtained by withdrawing a catheter through the urethra which contains a pressure pickup device though there is considerable variability in how this technic might be employed by its users. A static or total pressure profile can also be obtained dur-

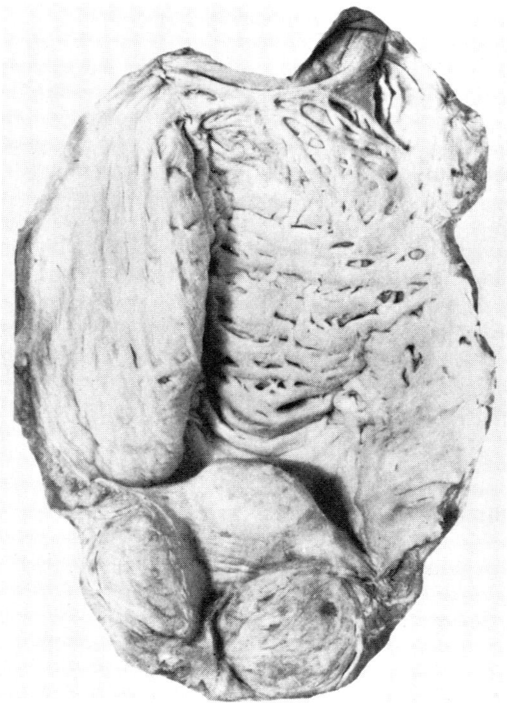

Figure 20-5 Trilobar prostatic hypertrophy, gross specimen (reproduced with permission from Randall A, Hinman F Jr: Surgical anatomy of the prostatic lobes, in Hinman F Jr (ed): *Benign Prostatic Hypertrophy.* New York, Springer-Verlag, 1983, pp 672–677).

ing micturition. These technics have little present-day application in clinical practice, but must be regarded as tools for study of special problems.

The exit velocity may be determined with a special device placed in the urinary stream. Velocity is related to bladder pressure, urethral geometry, and energy losses within the stream. Energy loss is related to the degree of obstruction, and the stream velocity and flow rate fall despite compensatory increases in bladder pressure. Normally 50% to 70% of the bladder energy is lost during voiding; with prostatic obstruction, more than 95% is dissipated. After prostatectomy, velocities tend to increase, along with flow rate and volume voided. However, velocity as a lone determinant is not as good a measure of obstruction as the flow rate alone.[50]

Several urodynamic studies can be combined by simultaneously recording pressure and flow along with viewing the configuration of the bladder and urethra by cinefluorography.[51] An even more sophisticated device, the urinary drop spectrometer, which measures and analyses the size and frequency of the drops of urine in the voided stream, may be 95% accurate in identifying patients with prostatic obstruction. Again, none of these technics are of direct use to the clinician.

Relation of urodynamic findings to symptoms Since prostatic size alone is not a useful indicator of obstruction and since symptoms are subject to misinterpretation, some urodynamic findings must be used in order to determine if obstruction is actually present. This is especially important as over 60% of patients seen for "prostatism" have an overactive or hypersensitive detrusor,[52] in addition to the usual effects of obstruction.

To begin with, it is convenient to distinguish irritative (reflexive) from obstructive symptoms. Nocturia, frequency, small voided volumes, and urgency and urgency incontinence are irritative symptoms. Hesitancy, weak stream, prolonged voiding time, and perhaps the feeling of incomplete emptying (even to acute retention) are symptoms of obstruction.

Irritative symptoms come from detrusor hypersensitivity with combined poor control by the local and central (inhibitory) nerve reflexes. The term "unstable detrusor" has come into use to describe the activity of the detrusor that is not being completely inhibited. Detrusor instability has been defined urodynamically as an elevation of bladder response on filling cystometry of 15 cm H_2O or more at a filling rate of 100 mL/min. Although the natural tendency of the sacrovesical nerve mechanism is to cause bladder contraction, this is normally inhibited centrally. In perhaps a fifth of all men and women, inhibition is poorly accomplished and both frequency and urgency result. With BPH, for some yet undetermined reason, as the detrusor reacts to obstruction it transmits through the sacral centers signals making central inhibition more difficult. This results in the symptoms of frequency and urgency. It often leads to a conditioned response to certain voiding stimuli, such as running water or arrival home (the "garage door syndrome"). There is little correlation between these symptoms and the presence or severity of obstruction since they are principally the result of detrusor hyperirritability and inadequate central inhibition of these contractions.[53]

Nearly half the patients with symptoms of prostatism have a so-called unstable detrusor in spite of having normal resistance to voiding, ie, no objective evidence of outflow obstruction. Of patients with demonstrated obstruction, two thirds will show detrusor instability.[54]

Frequency and nocturia occur in almost all patients with prostatism.[52] Effective bladder capacity is often decreased (in 41% of patients) but not sufficiently to explain the symptoms. Urgency is an indicator of detrusor overactivity[55,56] and is also a fairly good indicator of outflow obstruction.[52]

Obstructive symptoms are hesitancy, weak stream, and dribbling. Hesitancy is associated with a higher residual urine volume than that found in patients without this symptom, and these patients also have a lower urine flow rate. On a plot, the real stream initiation time and the opening time are prolonged (Figure 20-6). How much hesitancy is psychological (paruresis) and how much myoneural and obstruction may be hard to determine in an individual case.

Weak stream, as a complaint, cannot be directly correlated with the measured maximal flow rate, but does correlate statistically with outflow obstruction.[54] Terminal dribbling is an exclusive characteristic of BPH. It is the consequence of the decreasing power of the detrusor toward the end of the stream as energy dissipates and thus is barely able to maintain the bladder outlet open. As passage through the constricting zone occurs, urine accelerates and local pressure drops, which allows the proximal urethra to prematurely collapse.

These symptoms are in contrast to those resulting from stricture. A stricture merely limits the cross-sectional area of the urethra. Detrusor power can readily open the urethra and can keep it open until the end of voiding. The flow rate is low but remains constant throughout and no residual urine is left. The sensation of incomplete emptying, on the other hand, is too subjective to be of value in diagnosis, although in one group studied, half the patients with this complaint had residual urine volumes above 50 mL.[52]

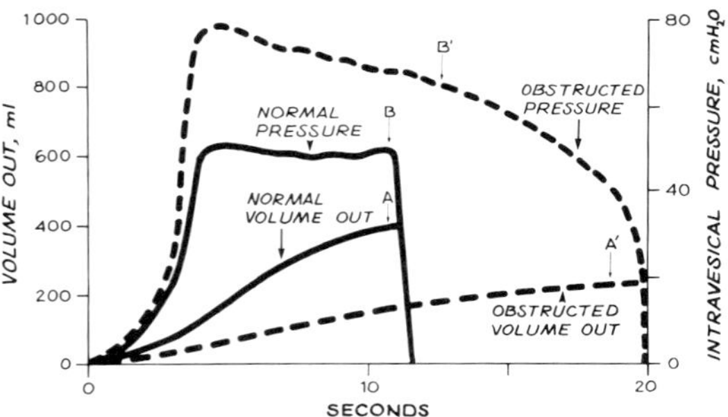

Figure 20-6 Depiction of volume and pressure during normal and obstructed flow. Normal (solid line) and obstructed (dashed line) voiding. Curves A: volume over time. At A, the bladder is empty; at A,′ half the volume remains (residual urine). Curves B: intravesical pressure. at B, voiding ends and pressure falls to resting level; at B,′ the detrusor contracts less effectively against the obstruction so urination slows.

In summary, the symptoms are the cornerstone in diagnosis of BPH, aided by determination of flow rate and/or residual urine. Operations will rarely be done unless the symptoms and findings are in agreement.

The course of BPH The patient more than 50 years old may not notice the insidious increase in his symptoms of frequency and the small volume voidings and will often present with both residual urine and diminished renal function. Alternatively, he may present with acute retention if the vesical neck mechanism is stimulated by overfilling or exposure to cold. In the majority of patients, difficulty in contractile inhibition (detrusor instability) induces frequency and nocturia with or without significant obstruction. In these patients, urgency, perhaps accompanied by incontinence, is a prominent symptom.

Typically, as the disease progresses, the detrusor is unable to cope with the increasing resistance, resulting in incomplete bladder emptying. Tidal volume, defined as the difference between capacity and residual volume, will fall with consequent increase in frequency and nocturia. The symptom of nocturia is of special importance because its rate is fairly constant, the patient can count the number of episodes accurately, and if it seriously interferes with sleep can become an indication for operative intervention. The detrusor reacts to continuing obstruction by hypertrophy of the smooth muscle bundles in its wall, producing trabeculation more or less in proportion to the degree of obstruction. With trabeculation some of the muscle bundles may be microscopically normal, but as it increases they become markedly infiltrated with collagen and elastic fibers. It is obvious that these changes adversely affect detrusor contractility, and will give rise to the "decompensated detrusor."

Finally, when the detrusor can no longer open the vesical neck, retention occurs. In contrast to the acute form of retention where failure of the neck to open is as important as failure of the detrusor to develop an effective contraction, with chronic retention the detrusor slowly stretches the neck open, rendering it incompetent. Wetting at night (overflow incontinence) is the first symptom of chronic retention since the patient may be able to hold his urine when awake.

That prostatic obstruction progresses is a common observation, with subjective symptoms seeming to progress more slowly than objective ones. Half of patients become worse within 3 years,[57] although both symptoms and signs fluctuate and there is great variation from patient to patient. In one study[58] of 208 patients, using 23 symptoms and findings, no statistical difference could be found among these parameters between those patients who subsequently required surgery and those who did not. Acute urinary retention cannot be predicted, since as mentioned earlier it is brought on by myoneural forces acting at the bladder neck rather than by progressive obstruction itself.

OTHER DISEASES AND BPH

Prostatitis Inflammation of the prostate may be diagnostically confused with BPH because frequency is a symptom common to both. In fact, BPH and chronic bacterial prostatitis seldom coexist, and it is even possible that chronic prostatitis may inhibit the development of BPH.[59] Bacterial prostatitis may result from the conservative treatment of BPH, especially if a catheter has been left indwelling.

Bladder infection The obstruction of BPH may promote infection in four ways. Obstruction may (1) foster residual urine and thereby decrease bacterial exchange and washout; (2) increase intravesical pressure, which reduces capillary flow to the vesical mucosa; (3) decrease the rate of flow and hence the effectiveness of urethral washout; and, (4) by creating a need for instrumentation, invite trauma and contamination. Bacteria introduced into the normal bladder are quickly eliminated by its mechanical and intrinsic defense mechanisms;[60] only when these defenses are breached can infection become established. Infection is particularly dangerous in the presence of severe renal failure with obstruction, for here the functional renal reserve may be very small[61] and overt uremia can be precipitated.

Impaired renal function Renal function is found to be decreased in 15% to 25% of patients with BPH, and BPH is the cause of at least 10% of all cases of renal failure.[62,63] Aging is an additional factor, since renal mass is 20% to 50% less at age 70 than at age 40 years.[64] Catheter drainage reverses the process in 80% of cases, although the physician must be alert to the risks of postobstructive diuresis in cases where total obstruction exists. With severe uremia, operation is probably inadvisable.

Other diseases In the older male, in general, unrelated diseases may complicate the management of BPH. Particularly worthy of mention are obesity and musculoskeletal disorders of the lower extremities which make surgical procedures riskier and more awkward: abnormalities of the blood, particularly those relating to impaired coagulation; venous thrombosis; cardiovascular disease, especially associated with electrolyte abnormalities; and chronic obstructive pulmonary disease.

DIFFERENTIAL DIAGNOSIS

When an otherwise healthy older man has a poor urinary flow rate, outlet obstruction is the obvious diagnosis. Its site must be determined. Fortunately the possibilities are few and most can be eliminated by a careful history which inquires into the previously described symptoms. The obstruction may be at the level of the bladder neck, in the prostatic region, or in the more distal urethra.

Vesical neck obstruction Obstruction at the vesical neck may be caused by the prostate obstructing. It may occasionally be seen after transurethral prostatic resection as "vesical neck contracture." In addition, important to the accurate diagnosis of BPH, is the recognition that obstruction may be due to dyssynergia between the detrusor and the musculature at the vesical neck,[65] since normally the vesical neck relaxes as the detrusor contracts as the result of a reflex response initiated by the sympathetic nervous system.[66]

Some patients can recall having a slower than normal stream for much of their lives. As they reach an age at which prostatic hypertrophy is common their normal voiding pattern may be confused with symptoms attributable to BPH itself: these symptoms include poor stream, frequency, urgency, nocturia, and an increased difficulty in voiding when the bladder is overly distended, particularly after incidental operations. In general, the symptoms of vesical neck obstruction are quite similar to those of BPH though the former may present at an earlier age and with symptoms more characteristically irritative in nature. Since these symptoms occur in younger men, they are often ascribed to prostatitis, neurogenic bladder, or a psychodynamic disorder.[67]

It is difficult by objective tests to separate these patients from those with obstructive BPH. Despite flow being near normal as the bladder develops higher pressures, this entity of vesical neck obstruction may be detected by the simultaneous measurement of intravesical pressure and flow. That the obstruction is actually at the bladder neck can be shown by voiding cystourethrography.

Some patients benefit from a urodynamic workup. This may disclose poor flow despite adequate detrusor contraction and good external sphincter relaxation; the additional finding of holdup at the vesical neck on voiding cystography (or on urethral profilometry) may add additional diagnostic information.

In practice endoscopic examination is helpful: if little or no BPH is present in the absence of overt neuropathy one may deduce that the obstruction is from dyssynergia. Confirmation may be obtained by administering an α-blocking agent such as phenoxybenzamine; this same agent can be utilized for short-term treatment.

If the symptoms are severe, or if either infection or retention recurs, surgical treatment is indicated even if BPH is not a factor. Transection of the full thickness of the bladder neck ring at the 7- or 8-o'clock position releases the obstruction and is considered to be minimal surgery. Occasionally retrograde ejaculation may follow, but in almost all cases the bladder neck will close efficiently but no longer acts as an obstructing area.

If prostatic enlargement occurs in these patients, it results in the so-called "trapped prostate,"[68] when the growth is held below the tight vesical neck. Characteristically, the BPH is small, and this finding on rectal palpation in patients with other findings of obstruction leads to the consideration of the diagnosis of double obstruction.[69] After such a gland is resected, it is important to incise the neck deeply or secondary contracture will occur. Sometimes several deep incisions alone are sufficient to avoid actual prostatic resection.[70]

Carcinoma of the prostate Prostatic cancer when large enough obstructs in the same way as BPH might. In fact, since it arises in the capsule around the adenoma, obstruction usually occurs by the lobes merely being compressed inward. Since carcinoma grows more rapidly than BPH, its presence is suspected when the symptoms of obstruction significantly increase over a few months' time. Rectal examination usually will detect the very firm neoplasm, surrounded by the more rubbery capsule containing the BPH, and perineal needle biopsy will establish the diagnosis. If the obstruction is high-grade, immediate resection may be warranted; if less, treatment may be directed at the carcinoma itself. Seldom is total prostatectomy sufficient if the tumor is the cause of the obstruction, since by then it may be too far advanced.

Urethral obstruction Stricture formation is rare without a prior history of instrumentation, and can be identified by retrograde urography or panendoscopy.

Impaired detrusor contractility A damaged detrusor may be a later consequence of severe obstruction. Although not common, once it is detected other causes of obstruction must be considered. Neurologic lesions which interrupt the pathways at the second, third, and fourth sacral segments may produce sacral areflexia. These include the effects of trauma, multiple sclerosis, herniated discs, and diabetic neuropathy. Since these produce additional neurologic defects, they can be detected on physical examination. This might include testing for perineal sensation, anal tone and contractility, and the bulbocavernosus reflex (elicited by vigorously squeezing the glans penis while digitally monitoring anal contraction).

Psychogenic voiding disturbances Anxiety may produce voiding symptoms which mimic those of BPH.[71,72] The patient may have a poorly sustained detrusor contraction on urodynamic study and often has paruresis or difficulty voiding in public places. Conversely, lesser degrees of bladder neck obstruction may be accompanied by psychologic problems. Cause and effect is usually not clear, but thorough study is needed in these cases to detect the physical and psychological elements so that treatment may be properly directed.[73]

Inflammatory conditions Symptoms like those of BPH can be caused by bacterial, interstitial, radiation, and tuberculous cystitis, as well as by the nonbacterial prostatitis syndromes.

Neurological disturbances A hyperreflexic detrusor secondary to a cord lesion may produce symptoms similar to those accompanying BPH. These neurologic patients must be selectively excluded if a poor operative result is to be avoided. The addition of a cystometrogram to the usual tests will detect the hyperreflexic detrusor secondary to a neurologic defect such as a cord lesion (eg, from a herniated disc), Parkinson's disease (about a third of cases show hyperactive detrusors)[74] or multiple sclerosis.

CONSERVATIVE MANAGEMENT

The decision for operation, in spite of careful analysis of symptoms and the performance of tests, remains a subjective one. In general if the patient does not perceive his life to be disturbed and the obstruction is not damaging his bladder or kidneys, he should merely be followed. Nonoperative management consists of re-examination every 6 months to detect incipient renal failure and infection, to assess adverse effects of symptoms (eg, is the patient's health affected by nocturia?), to estimate the rate of progression of the obstruction (is operation inevitable?), and, finally, to detect early prostatic neoplasia.

The role of α-blocking agents in therapy is not well established. Medications such as phenoxybenzamine hydrochloride (10 mg/d) may be used to assist a patient through a difficult period[75] but are probably not as safe as surgery for long-term control. Advice to avoid exposure to cold and overfilling may be helpful, but if the obstruction is found to be progressive, operation will ultimately be necessary.

Self-catheterization Clean intermittent catheterization (CIC) is an alternative to prostatectomy. If the bladder pressure is kept down by sufficiently frequent emptying, the introduction of bacteria is harmless and invasive infection does not occur.[76] Nonsterile "clean" technics can be used by the patient himself. Those elderly men who are either too ill for or too averse to operation are candidates. As is the man who, for personal reasons, must defer the time for prostatectomy. In a small group of patients who demonstrate insufficient detrusor contractility even despite adequate reduction of urethral resistance by TUR, CIC may serve an important role. It is not feasible if the bladder capacity is limited, if the patient is incontinent, or if he is unable to manipulate the catheter. Complications are rare though bladder calculi can form about a pubic hair inadvertently introduced on the catheter tip. Bacteriuria is present in 12% to 15% of patients, and in cases of infection some 27% can be controlled with antibacterial agents; despite this bacteriuria persists in 58%.[77] Although this is harmless if the bladder is not allowed to overfill, an attempt should be made to sterilize the urine by administration of such "urinary tract" drugs as nitrofurantoin and trimethoprim-sulfamethoxazole (TMP-SMX) for 2 or 3 weeks.

OPERATIVE MANAGEMENT

Selecting candidates for operation Patient selection may be done by a point system in which each symptom or finding is weighted.[78] This point system attaches particular importance to the severity of symptoms, large volumes of residual urine, urinary retention, and hydronephrosis. Operation is advised if the score exceeds a certain number. Alternatively, the degree of impairment in the flow rate or the amount of residual urine may serve as a determining factor in the assessment for operative need. In practice, the thoughtful clinician will meld the patient's general condition and his symptoms and desires with the objective findings in order to reach a practical solution to the patient's particular set of circumstances. Indications for surgery may be classified as either mandatory, positive, or optional.

Mandatory indications include complete obstruction or overflow incontinence. Total outflow obstruction is a strong indication for surgery since it is only in the unusually ill or aged that chronic catheter drainage would be tolerated better than operation; this same population for that matter might also be the one to select CIC. A rule of thumb might be: if life expectancy is greater than 1 year, operation is warranted. A second good indication is chronic overflow incontinence. Here the symptom of leakage demands some treatment since the overflow signifies that severe back pressure on the kidneys exists. The patient will generally have a poor appetite, a low hemoglobin level, an elevated creatinine level, and a very large residual urine volume. The effort to void forces feces from the rectum, and certainly exploits any predisposition to the development of hernias. Catheter drainage (either urethrally or by suprapubic punch) is maintained until renal function and the patient's general condition have stabilized. Renal function may not immediately return to normal, since the thickened bladder wall that occludes the ureteral orifices requires sufficient time to respond to continuous drainage. The renal parenchyma itself in certain instances may be so aged and damaged that full recovery is near impossible.

Positive indications for operation include infection, the presence of vesical calculi, and severe bleeding. Persistent infection warrants operation. Vesical decompensation with consequent residual urine fosters the perpetuation of infection once it has been introduced (usually by catheterization or other urethral instrumentation). Bacteria double every 20 or 30 minutes, their number increasing in a geometric fashion. Bladder evacuation normally removes almost all of the accumulated bacteria[79] with the remainder being eliminated by the intrinsic defense mechanisms of the bladder.[80] As some infected urine remains behind after each voiding in the severely obstructed patient, the effectiveness of both the bladder washout and surface defense mechanisms are nullified and any bacteriuria present becomes difficult to eliminate. Even though bladder pressure may be higher than normal with each void, it is unusual for the bacteria to actually invade the vesical wall.[81] The greater risk is that of pyelonephritis if and when the ureterovesical valvular mechanism has been damaged by the obstruction, and reflux up the ureter can occur.

Prostatectomy is also indicated for the infection associated with chronic bacterial prostatitis. Purulent infection of the prostatic acini, often around calculi, occurs at a younger age than BPH but may produce similarly severe symptoms as the prostate periodically swells and the bacteria ascend into the bladder. Complete resection prevents the acute symptomatic episodes but rarely eliminates the bacteria from the remaining prostatic tissue.

Vesical calculi serve as evidence that the vesical neck obstruction was great enough to block passage of small stones of renal origin which normally would be passed with voiding. They may be crushed and passed at the time of prostatic resection (litholapaxy) if sufficiently small or they may be removed directly if an open operation is performed. The large mucosal veins on the protruding lobes may occasionally bleed severely enough (causing clot retention) to require prostatectomy.

Optional indications are not as easy to define. Such factors as the quality of life demanded by the patient as well as the quality of the surgical care he could receive affect the decision. What would be proper in a metropolitan area in an advanced country would be the wrong approach in a rural village in some parts of the third world. The best starting point is the patient's complaint. Does he consult you because he had been told he has a large prostate or because he has an underlying fear of occult malignancy? Neither of these complaints bears a relationship to the need for operation. Or does he complain of severely interrupted sleep (especially if he has heart disease) or such frequency of urination that he cannot carry on his everyday business? Is he fearful of experiencing acute retention while travelling or a repetition of episodes of acute cystitis? For these patients, operation may be indicated. Alternatively, in spite of symptoms, is he fearful of operation in general and one in the area of the genitalia in particular; or is he concerned about the possibility of incontinence or impotency? Operation is least likely to be advocated for these patients; they can usually endure until mandatory indications develop.

Next, the consultant must be certain that the symptoms are in fact caused by prostatic obstruction. In the discussion of the urodynamic aspects of BPH, the key tests were presented, flow rate and residual urine being the most valuable of these. A normal flow rate rules out the diagnosis of obstruction from BPH. The absence of residual urine does not mean there is no obstruction but its presence if accompanied by an appropriate history serves as an indication for operation. Patients whose symptoms are solely "irritative," ie, frequency, urgency, and urge incontinence, due to detrusor instability or even to some degenerative neurologic disorder, may require more complex urodynamic studies. When these symptoms are accompanied by the "obstructive" symptoms of hesitancy, slow stream and postvoid dribbling, they need no special evaluation since operation is then indicated for the obstruction. Because the obstruction is responsible for the detrusor instability in half of the cases, prostatectomy is in this way indicated for relief of the complex of irritative symptoms.

Prostatic obstruction may add to the voiding imbalance in patients with neurogenic bladder disorders. If conservative, principally anticholinergic treatment, proves unsuccessful and residual urine volume is appreciable, prostatic resection (or in extreme cases of neurogenic bladder, external sphincterotomy) is required to improve bladder balance. As would be expected, the results of prostatic resection in these patients is not as good as those for simple BPH. The mortality rate is higher and the persistence of irritative symptoms greater.

Counseling the patient A thorough discussion is necessary because of the patient's fears and the possibility of complications. He may fear loss of sexual potency. Impotency does not follow any but the perineal prostatectomy, although it may be a problem psychologically because of either abstinence or lack of a partner. It has been shown that preoperative counselling will reduce its incidence.[81] Retrograde ejaculation occurs in a majority of cases after operation, and even though the sensation at climax remains intact, a patient may worry about the absence of ejaculate. He should be instructed as to this possibility preoperatively.

Fear of cancer can be assuaged by describing the operation to him as one removing a benign growth from the center of the prostate. Incontinence is a rare complication but its possibility must be mentioned to the patient. The urologist should not guarantee either a perfect result or that he will be able to relieve all symptoms, for then he could be liable for any residual complaints.

It is important that the patient give his informed consent to operation. Thus he must receive enough information to make his own decision. He must have knowledge of the alternatives, prognosis, complications, sequelae, discomforts, risks, and costs.

Operative treatment Since the purpose of operation is to relieve the obstruction which is the result of an interaction between the BPH itself and the capsule-vesical neck structures surrounding the BPH, two options are open. The conventional one, which goes back to the turn of the century, is to remove the BPH. This was formerly done by open finger enucleation, but currently is performed most frequently by transurethral resection; thus either extracting it or trimming it from its bed in the true prostate, the surgical capsule.

Less well accepted but apparently applicable for smaller glands, is the additional option: to incise the surrounding structures (vesical neck and posterior capsule) and "release" the prostate.[70] This procedure is especially useful when chronic incoordination of the smooth sphincter mechanism (detrusor-sphincter dyssynergia) results in occlusive hypertrophy of the vesical neck, often "trapping" a small BPH within it.

Transurethral prostatectomy is the method preferred by most urologists for most glands. Many actively practicing urologists may perform one open operation for BPH a year, while doing from 100 to 200 resections. The operation is made possible by combining a light source (now glass fiber–conducted), a forward-looking endoscope, and an electrically activated wire loop that can be moved in the field of vision. Small pieces are cut with a sine-wave current as the actuated loop is drawn through the tissue; pieces are then washed from the bladder at the end of the procedure. As vessels are transected, they are fulgurated under vision with a damped current. Visibility is maintained by a continuous flow of water (or other irrigant) past the lens. At the end, a catheter is inserted and usually remains in place for two days.

Spinal anesthesia is preferred, since most patients are elderly and the operation seldom lasts much more than an hour. Hazards include poorly controlled blood loss, and the intravascular entry of irrigating fluid if the surgical capsule is penetrated and the loose periprostatic tissue is exposed. Such extravation results in increased intravascular volume and in the dilution of serum sodium. The distilled water used as an irrigant may result in hemolysis which is not necessarily harmful, so that any benefit gained by the use of a nonhemolytic nonelectrolytic solution is probably from its early diuretic effect. Since such nonhemolytic solutions cost more and reduce visibility, they are not universally used instead of distilled water.[82] Uncontrolled water intoxication causes mental confusion, a temporarily elevated blood pressure with bradycardia, followed by hypotension, oliguria, and cyanosis. Any treatment utilized is based on administering diuretics to increase free water loss[82] as well as to infuse a concentrated saline solution (5%) to return the serum sodium level toward normal.[83] Monitoring the serum sodium level is a useful if somewhat delayed method of gauging the effectiveness of therapy.

Before operation, bacteriuria must be eradicated by specific antibiotic therapy.[84] Patients with chronic prostatitis are at special risk, and therapy should be continued for at least 24 hours postoperatively. Whether antibacterials are needed for the routine, uninfected case has yet to be proved, but prudent urologists may give a medication such as TMP-SMX just prior to operation and continue it until the catheter is removed. Maintenance of a "closed" drainage system is important and all irrigation is performed in an aseptic manner.

Alternately, gentamicin sulfate or tobramycin sulfate may be given intramuscularly (IM) the evening before and the morning of operation, and for two additional doses eight hours apart after the operation. Then TMP-SMX is given at the time of and for 5 to 10 days after catheter removal unless cultures have shown need for an alternative agent. Transurethral prostatectomy has a very low mortality rate (0.4% in the hands of experienced urologists)[85] which is considerably less than that observed for open procedures.

Suprapubic prostatectomy is an alternative to transurethral resection for prostates felt to be too large for safe resection. The operating time of this procedure is usually limited to one hour. It is the oldest practical method and is still the routine operation utilized by surgeons not yet trained in transurethral resection. In most centers, an open operation is done in less than 10% of cases, but sometimes other problems such as large bladder stones, severe urethral strictures, or fixed hips preventing proper positioning make the suprapubic approach preferable. Vasectomy is advocated by some prior to open prostatectomy to prevent epididymitis from ascending bacteria, especially if the urine is infected. The chance for such infection after transurethral resection in uninfected patients is so small (2.3%) that routine vasectomy is not warranted.[86]

Suprapubic prostatectomy is performed with the patient lying supine. A low abdominal incision exposes the bladder just above the bladder neck where an incision into the partially filled bladder is made to expose the outlet. The mucosa may then be incised around the protruding prostatic lobes or the commissure torn by the finger being inserted down the roof of the urethra. In either case, the finger enters the cleavage plane between adenoma and true prostate, so that the enlargement may be shelled out. The freed lobes are grasped and removed with large forceps after blunt division of the urethra at the apex. The fossa is packed with gauze to control bleeding during insertion of hemostatic sutures about the prostatic arteries near the bladder neck. A large balloon catheter is inserted through the urethra to a location above the bladder neck and inflated to the estimated size of the adenoma. If bleeding appears to be a problem, a tube may also be left to exit suprapubically. The urethral catheter is removed on the second postoperative day and the suprapubic tube on the fifth day, so that the patient may be discharged on the seventh or eighth day. This is usually three or four days later than after transurethral resection.

Perineal prostatectomy is now used principally for total removal of an early prostate cancer, but a "simple" perineal prostatectomy can be employed to remove only an adenoma. This approach is preferred by some for use in the elderly poor-risk patient, because hemostasis is more exact, dependent drainage can be obtained, and it is the safest operation for large prostates.

The operation is done through an inverted U-shaped incision anterior to the rectum which exposes the posterior surface of the prostate. A second inverted U-incision is made through the prostate to expose the adenoma, which is then digitally removed very much as in the suprapubic operation. Hemostasis is secured by insertion of mattress sutures at the vesical neck or by suturing the vesical neck to the surgical capsule. Complications include rectal injury, inefficient catheter drainage and, rarely, ureteral injury. Impotency is more common with the perineal operation than with the others, so this operation is usually reserved for elderly men who might already be impotent.

Retropubic prostatectomy is more modern than the other open technics, and offers more control of the blood vessels and the sphincters than the suprapubic operation; thus the risk of hemorrhage and incontinence is reduced. Since the bladder is not opened, postoperative discomfort is less, and leakage through the wound is not as likely. The vesical neck and the anterior surface of the prostate is approached through a lower midline incision. The prostate is incised transversely between stay sutures, exposing the anterior surface of the adenoma. Finger enucleation is done to the level of the external sphincter, which is then carefully divided under visual inspection. Hemostasis is secured by suturing the vesical neck on either side down into the fossa. A catheter is introduced and the surgical capsule closed. A herniorrhaphy, if needed, can then be done through the same incision. Complications are similar to those with other open operations, but impotence is rare.

Problems after prostatectomy Incontinence can be a problem. After the catheter is removed, usually on the second day after transurethral resection, the patient may experience some urgency and dysuria but this soon clears. A few may have uncontrollable urgency with incontinence but this also is a temporary phenomenon. The incidence of stress incontinence is low, less than 1%,[87] but if incontinence persists for more than 2 or 3 weeks, especially if unaccompanied by urgency, weakness of the external passive sphincter mechanism, overflow, or detrusor instability should be suspected.

Since the internal sphincter at the bladder neck is removed at the time of prostatectomy, continence is maintained solely by the distal sphincter, which consists of both an intrinsic mechanism controlled by smooth muscle, elastic, and vascular tissue which provides "passive" continence, and an external striated mechanism which gives "active" continence. It is usually the passive mechanism that is damaged, the patient being able to hold his urine voluntarily for a short time, but becoming wet with a constant drip when ambulatory. Overflow incontinence is uncommon, but can occur with low compliance bladders which demonstrate a slow progressive rise in pressure during filling and reach a point where this pressure rise overcomes outlet resistance. Detrusor instability, so common preoperatively, is less often seen following operation and unless accompanied by some weakness of the sphincters, probably only produces urgency and frequency, not incontinence.

Diagnosis of sphincter damage can be made by panendoscopy, which allows direct visualization of the sphincteric area. Another study that may be needed is measurement of urethral pressure through the continence zone by urethral pressure profilometry, a procedure preferably done while in the upright position. With sphincteric incontinence, profilometry will show a very short smooth muscle component which produces little or no closure pressure, even though a command to hold the urine will produce a vigorous rise in pressure. In a patient with incontinence from detrusor hyperreflexia profilometry will show a normal profile but hyperactive detrusor contractions. Overflow will be identified by the finding of a very large residual urine volume after voiding.

Treatment begins with active exercise by utilizing "stop-and-go" voiding. If incontinence persists and is found to be due to sphincter damage, several types of incontinence procedures are currently available. One is reconstruction of the bladder neck by forming a tube from the bladder and anastomosing it to the top of the prostate.[87] Alternatively, an artificial sphincter can be implanted around the urethra, activated by a pump inserted in the scrotum.[88-90] Operations which elevate or continuously compress the urethra have proved less successful.

Impotence occurs in 16% to 30% of patients postoperatively.[91] It may be organic from surgical interference with the erector nerves, drug-induced as seen with antihypertensive medications, or as the result of psychological factors. Workup of such a patient would include assessment of spontaneous nocturnal erections by nocturnal tumescence plethysmography (NPT). This test helps to differentiate between organic and psychogenic causes, since in the latter, erections will continue to occur.

Treatment may entail reassurance, alteration in medications employed, and in an established case, insertion of a prosthesis may become necessary. After counselling both patient and partner, a choice is made between a flexible rod or an inflatable prosthesis. The rod is cheaper, safer, and less prone to problems; the inflatable prosthesis is more "normal" in function and appearance. Perhaps the latter should be reserved for younger men.

Difficulties with micturition may continue. Some patients complain postoperatively of hesitancy, poor stream, and terminal dribbling and may still be obstructed. Others may have decompensated bladders with low detrusor pressure which is augmented by straining. Residual adenoma may cause continued symptoms and can require a second resection. Bladder neck contracture, a result of delayed healing in an area where re-epithelialization occurs late, may be prevented by an adequate ventral incision through the neck fibers at the termination of the resection. Contracture is evidenced by a poor stream 1 month or more postoperatively, and requires dilatation if not incision.

Urethral strictures occur in 6% of patients after TUR.[92] Preoperative urethral calibration, and urethrotomy if the urethra is tight, will help prevent them, as will the use of small instruments, short operations, and small catheters. Operating through a perineal urethrostomy will prevent strictures altogether. The most common site for stricture formation is in the fossa navicularis (the smallest section of the urethra) and may occur in the curvature of the bulb where the instrument is held up by the suspensory ligament of the penis. They are treated by simple dilatation, or if that fails, by visual internal urethrotomy.

Low detrusor pressure/low flow voiding can occur if the patient had long-standing retention preoperatively. Voiding by straining may help empty the bladder but intermittent catheterization may be necessary. Motor urgency may be a problem following a good operation, although detrusor instability is relieved in two thirds of patients by prostatectomy. Sensory urgency is suspected when symptoms persist but the detrusor is shown to be stable by cystometry. The causes may range from persistent infection to infiltrating carcinoma of the bladder.

CONCLUSIONS

Benign prostatic hypertrophy is a common disease that not only produces morbidity and often requires operation, but also is costly in time because of the extra seconds spent at micturition. One can calculate that if there are 20,022,000 men over age 55 in this country who void 4 times a day and are delayed ten seconds by hesitancy, slow voiding, and care for the postvoid dribbling, some 22,225 hours are lost per day. This adds up into wasted dollars: at a median hourly wage of $8.47, $394 million are lost yearly.

Research into the etiology of BPH has yet to provide a medical treatment but the future is promising. In the meantime, the instrumentation and technics for operative removal are being constantly improved, with consequent decreases in morbidity and mortality. Even now, prostatic resection is neither a painful nor dangerous procedure. The outlook is for even better selection of patients actually needing operation and consequently for a reduction in adverse effects of obstruction and its release.

REFERENCES

1. Franks LM: Benign nodular hyperplasia of prostate: a review. *Ann R Coll Surg Engl* 1954;14:92–106.
2. Lytton B, Emery JM, Harvard BM: The incidence of benign prostatic hypertrophy. *J Urol* 1969;99:639–645.
3. Birkhoff JD, Weiderhorn AR, Hamilton ML, et al: Natural history of benign prostatic hypertrophy and acute urinary retention. *Urology* 1976;7:48–52.
4. Ball AJ, Feneley RCL, Abrams PH: The natural history of untreated "prostatism." *Br J Urol* 1981;53:613–616.
5. Drach GW, Layton JN, Binard WJ: Male peak urinary flow rate: relationship to voided volume and age. *J Urol* 1979;122: 210–214.
6. McNeal JE: Relationship of the origin of benign prostatic hypertrophy to prostatic structure of man and other mammals, in Hinman, F Jr (ed): *Benign Prostatic Hypertrophy*. New York, Springer-Verlag, 1983, pp 152–166.
7. Cunha GR: Epithelio-mesenchymal interactions in the developing accessory sexual glands of embryonic mice. *Anat Rec* 1970; 166:295.
8. Neubauer BL: Endocrine and cellular inductive factors in the development of human benign prostatic hypertrophy, in Hinman F Jr (ed): *Benign Prostatic Hypertrophy*. New York, Springer-Verlag, 1983, pp 179–192.
9. Skoldefors H, Blomstedt B, Carlstrom K: Serum hormone levels in benign prostatic hyperplasia. *Scand J Urol Nephrol* 1978;12: 111–114.
10. Bard DR, Laznitzki I: The influence of oestradiol on the metabolism of androgens by human prostatic tissue. *J Endocrinol* 1977;74:1–9.
11. Grayhack JT, Bunce PL, Kearns JW, et al: Influence of the pituitary on prostatic response to androgen in the rat. *Bull Johns Hopkins Hosp* 1955;96:154–163.
12. Witorsch RJ: Immunohistochemical studies of prolactin binding in sex accessory organs of the male rat. *J Histochem Cytochem* 1978;26:565–580.
13. Clark R: The prostate and the endocrines: A control series. *Br J Urol* 1937;9:254–271.
14. White JW: The results of double castration in hypertrophy of the prostate. *Am Surg* 1895;22:1.
15. Peirson EL: A study of the effect of stilbestrol therapy on the size of the benignly hypertrophied prostate gland. *J Urol* 1946;49:73–78.
16. Kaufman JJ, Goodwin WE: Hormonal management of the benign obstructing prostate; use of combined androgen-estrogen therapy. *J Urol* 1959;81:165–171.
17. Rangno RE, McLeod PJ, Ruedy J, et al: Treatment of benign prostatic hypertrophy with medrogestone. *Clin Pharmacol Ther* 1971;12:658–665.
18. Scott WW, Wade JC: Medical treatment of benign nodular prostatic hyperplasia with cyproterone acetate. *J Urol* 1969;101:81–85.
19. Caine M, Perlberg S, Gordon R: The treatment of BPH with flutamide (SCH 13521): a placebo controlled study. *J Urol* 1975; 114:464–568.
20. Keshin JG: Effect of candicidin on the human hypertrophied prostate gland. *Int Surg* 1973;58:116–122.
21. Orkin LA: Efficacy of candicidin in benign prostate hypertrophy. *Urology* 1974;4: 80–84.
22. Sporer A, Cohen S, Kamat MH, et al: Candicidin: physiological effect on prostate. *Urology* 1975;6:298–305.
23. Abrams PH: A double-blind trial of the effects of candicidin on patients with benign prostatic hypertrophy. *Br J Urol* 1977;49: 67–71.
24. Mobley TL, Elbadawi A, McDonald DF, et al: Innervation of the human urinary bladder. *Surg Forum* 1966;27:505.
25. Elbadawi A: Histochemical studies of the construction of the peripheral autonomic innervation apparatus. *Fed Proc* 1967; 26:234.
26. Elbadawi A: Neuromorphologic basis of vesicourethral functions. *Neurourol Urodyn* 1982;1:3.
27. Caine M, Raz S, Zeigler M: Adrenergic and cholinergic receptors in the human prostate, prostatic capsule and bladder neck. *Br J Urol* 1975;47:293–302.
28. Owman C, Sjostrand NO: Short adrenergic neurons and catecholamine-containing cells in vas deferens and accessory male genital glands of different mammals. *Z Zellforsch Mikrosk Anat* 1965;66:300–320.

29. Gosling JA, Thompson SA: A neurohistochemical and histological study of peripheral autonomic neurons of the human bladder neck and prostate. *Urol Int* 1977;32:269–276.
30. Bruschini H, Schmidt RA, Tanagho EA: Neurological control of prostatic secretion in the dog. *Invest Urol* 1978;15:288–290.
31. Jonas U, Tanagho EA: Study of vesicourethral reflexes. I. Urethral sphincteric responses to detrusor stretch. *Invest Urol* 1975;12:357–373.
32. Osius TG, Hinman F Jr: Dynamics of acute urinary retention: A manometric, radiographic and clinical study. *J Urol* 1963; 90:702–712.
33. Cardus D, Quesada EM, Scott FB: Use of an electromagnetic flowmeter for urine flow measurements. *J Appl Physiol* 1963;18: 845–847.
34. Leventhal A, Pfau A: Pharmacologic management of postoperative over-distention of the bladder. *Surg Gynecol Obstet* 1978; 146:347–348.
35. Caine M, Perlberg S, Shapiro A: Phenoxybenzamine for benign prostatic obstruction: review of 200 cases. *Urology* 1982;17: 542–546.
36. Abrams PH, Griffiths DJ: The assessment of prostatic obstruction from urodynamic measurements and from residual urine. *Br J Urol* 1979;51:129–134.
37. Von Garrelts B: Intravesical pressure and urinary flow during micturition in normal subjects. *Acta Chir Scand* 1957;114:41–66.
38. Coolsaet BLRA: Detrusor energy factors, in Hinman F Jr (ed): *Benign Prostatic Hypertrophy.* New York, Springer-Verlag, 1983, pp 443–449.
39. Schäfer W: The contribution of the bladder outlet to the relation between pressure and flow rate during micturition, in Hinman F Jr (ed): *Benign Prostatic Hypertrophy.* New York, Springer-Verlag, 1983, pp 470–496.
40. Schäfer W: Detrusor as the energy source of micturition, in Hinman F Jr: *Benign Prostatic Hypertrophy.* New York, Springer-Verlag, 1983, pp 450–469.
41. Susset JG: Development of nomograms for application of uroflowmetry, in Hinman F Jr (ed): *Benign Prostatic Hypertrophy.* New York, Springer-Verlag, 1983, pp 528–538.
42. Drach GW, Layton TN, Binard WJ: Male peak urinary flow rate: relationships to volume voided and age. *J Urol* 1979; 122:210–214.
43. Siroky MB, Olsson CA, Krane RJ: The flow rate nomogram. I. Development. *J Urol* 1979;122:210–214.
44. Layton TN, Drach GW: Urinary flow rates: measurement and adjustment, in Hinman F Jr (ed): *Benign Prostatic Hypertrophy.* New York, Springer-Verlag, 1983, pp 523–527.
45. Hinman F Jr: Residual urine: Measurement and influence on management of obstruction, in Hinman F Jr (ed): *Benign Prostatic Hypertrophy.* New York, Springer-Verlag, 1983, pp 589–596.
46. Marshall V, Singh M, Blandy JP: Is urography necessary for patients with acute retention of urine before prostatectomy? *Br J Urol* 1974;47:73–76.
47. Turner Warwick R, Whiteside CG, Milroy EJG, et al: The intravenous urodynamogram. *Br J Urol* 1979;51:15–18.
48. Pinck BD, Corrigan MJ, Jasper P: Preprostatectomy excretory urography: does it merit the expense? *J Urol* 1980;123: 390–391.
49. Randall A: *Surgical Pathology of Prostatic Obstructions.* Baltimore, Williams & Wilkins, 1931.
50. Gleason DM, Bottaccini MR, Drach GW, et al: Urinary velocity in prostatism, in Hinman F Jr (ed): *Benign Prostatic Hypertrophy.* New York, Springer-Verlag, 1983, pp 539–544.
51. Miller ER: Combined monitoring for the study of continence and voiding, in Hinman F Jr (ed): *Hydrodynamics of Micturition.* Springfield, Ill, Charles C Thomas, 1971, pp 5–17.
52. Melchior H, Jaschke W: Urodynamic interpretation of symptoms, in Hinman F Jr (ed): *Benign Prostatic Hypertrophy.* New York, Springer-Verlag, 1983, pp 627–641.
53. Arnold EP: A urodynamic analysis of detrusor dysfunction, thesis, London, 1973.
54. Abrams PH, Feneley RCL: The significance of the symptoms associated with bladder outflow obstruction. *Urol Int* 1978;33: 171–174.
55. Fischer J: Cystometrische: Erhebungen bei Prostatikern. *Z Urol* 1955;48:743–751.
56. Schoenberg HW, Gutrich JM, Cote R: Urodynamic studies in benign prostatic hypertrophy. *Urology* 1979;14:634–637.
57. Birkhoff JD, Wiederhorn AR, Hamilton

MC, et al: Natural history of benign prostatic hypertrophy and acute urinary retention. *Urology* 1976;7:48–52.
58. Barnes RW, Marsh C: Progression of obstruction and symptoms, in Hinman F Jr (ed): *Benign Prostatic Hypertrophy.* New York, Springer-Verlag, 1983, pp 711–713.
59. Sharer WC, Fair WR: Bacterial prostatitis and benign prostatic hypertrophy, in Hinman F Jr (ed): *Benign Prostatic Hypertrophy.* New York, Springer-Verlag, 1983, pp 721–726.
60. Cox CE, Hinman F Jr: Experiments with induced bacteriuria, vesical emptying and bacterial growth on the mechanism of bladder defense to infection. *J Urol* 1961;86: 739–748.
61. Janson KL, Roberts JA: Experimental pyelonephritis. V. Functional characteristics of pyelonephritis. *Invest Urol* 1978;15: 397–400.
62. Beck AD: Benign prostatic hypertrophy and uraemia. *Br J Surg* 1970;57:561–565.
63. Chisholm GD: Obstructive uropathy–a review of 146 patients with postrenal uraemia. *S Afr Med J* 1967;41:962–964.
64. Byrd L, Sherman RL: Radiocontrast-induced acute renal failure: a clinical and pathophysiologic review. *Medicine* 1979; 58:270–279.
65. Turner Warwick R, Whiteside CG, Worth PHL, et al: A urodynamic view of the clinical problems associated with bladder neck dysfunction and its treatment by endoscopic incision and transtrigonal posterior prostatectomy. *Br J Urol* 1973; 45:44–59.
66. Raz S, Zeigler M, Caine M: Pharmacological receptors in the prostate. *Br J Urol* 1973; 45:663–667.
67. Webster GD, Lockhart JL, Older RA: The evaluation of bladder neck dysfunction. *J Urol* 1980;123:196.
68. Turner Warwick R: The spincter mechanisms: their relation to prostatic enlargement and its treatment, in Hinman F Jr (ed): *Benign Prostatic Hypertrophy.* New York, Springer-Verlag, 1983, pp 809–828.
69. Turner Warwick R, Whiteside CG: Urodynamic studies and their effect upon management, in Williams DI, Chisholm G (eds): *Scientific Foundations in Urology.* London, William Heinemann, Ltd, 1982, pp 442–457.
70. Turner Warwick R, Whiteside CG, Worth PHL, et al: A urodynamic view of clinical problems associated with bladder neck dysfunction and its treatment by endoscopic incision-trans-trigonal posterior prostatectomy. *Br J Urol* 1973;45:44–59.
71. George N, Slade N: Hesitancy and poor stream in men without flow obstruction–the anxious bladder. *Br J Urol* 1979;51: 506.
72. Siroky MB, Goldstein I, Krane RJ: Functional voiding disturbances in men. *J Urol* 1979;126:665–668.
73. Blaivas JG: Differential diagnosis, in Hinman F Jr (ed): *Benign Prostatic Hypertrophy.* New York, Springer-Verlag, 1983, pp 747–762.
74. Porter R, Bors E: Neurogenic bladder in parkinsonism: effect of thalamotomy. *J Neurosurg* 1972;34:27–32.
75. Caine M, Perlberg S, Meretyk S: A placebo-controlled double-blind study of the effect of phenoxybenzamine in benign prostatic obstruction. *Br J Urol* 1978;50:551–554.
76. Lapides J: Mechanisms of urinary tract infection. *Urology* 1979;14:217–225.
77. Lapides J, Diokno AC, Gould FR, et al: Further observations on self-catheterization. *J Urol* 1976;116:169–179.
78. Madsen PO, Iversen P: A point system for selecting operative candidates, in Hinman F Jr (ed): *Benign Prostatic Hypertrophy.* New York, Springer-Verlag, 1983, pp 763–765.
79. Cox CE, Hinman F Jr: Incidence of bacteriuria with indwelling catheter in normal bladders. *JAMA* 1961;178:919–921.
80. Orikasa S, Hinman F Jr: Reaction of the vesical wall to bacterial penetration: resistance to attachment, desquamation, and leukocytic activity. *Invest Urol* 1977; 15:185–193.
81. Zohar J, Meiraz D, Maoz B, et al: Factors influencing sexual activity after prostatectomy: A prospective study. *J Urol* 1976; 116:332–334.
82. Pitts HH, Hinman F Jr: The safety of water irrigation in transurethral prostatectomy. *J Urol* 1954;72:925–927.
83. Wakim KG: The pathophysiologic basis for the clinical manifestations and complications of transurethral prostatic reaction. *J Urol* 1971;106:719–728.
84. McLin PH, Fisher R, Hinman F Jr: Rapid sensitivity testing in the prevention of sep-

sis from genitourinary instrumentation. *J Urol* 1968;100:787–791.

85. Bergman RT, Turner R, Barnes RW, et al: Comparative analysis of 1000 consecutive cases of transurethral prostatic resection. *J Urol* 1955;74:533–545.
86. Mebust WK, Valk WL: Transurethral prostatectomy, in Hinman F Jr (ed): *Benign Prostatic Hypertrophy.* New York, Springer-Verlag, 1983, pp 829–846.
87. Tanagho EA: Bladder neck reconstruction for total urinary incontinence: 10 years of experience. *J Urol* 1981;125:321–326.
88. Scott FB, Bradley WE, Timm GW: Treatment of urinary incontinence by an implantable prosthetic sphincter. *Urology* 1973; 1:252–259.
89. Scott FB, Light JK, Fishman IJ, et al: Implantation of an artificial sphincter for urinary incontinence. *Contemp Surg* 1980; 18:11–34.
90. Kaufman JJ: Treatment of post-prostatectomy urinary incontinence using a silicone gel prosthesis. *Br J Urol* 1973;45:646.
91. Gold FM, Hotchkiss RS: Sexual potency following simple prostatectomy. *NY State J Med* 1969;69:2987–2989.
92. Lentz HC Jr, Mebust WK, Foret JD, et al: Urethral strictures following transurethral prostatectomy: review of 2,223 resections. *J Urol* 1977;117:194–196.

CHAPTER 21 Urinary Tract Infections in the Elderly

Charles J. Schleupner

Urinary tract infections comprise a spectrum of clinical entities whose common denominator is the presence of bacteriuria. They are second only to respiratory infections as causes of febrile illness among the elderly.[1] Furthermore, the urinary tract is the most common source of community-acquired bacteremia in elderly patients.[2] Urinary infections occur throughout life, primarily in females, but reach their peak prevalence in the older age groups.[1,3] This change in prevalence is a reflection of complex and multiple interactions occurring during the aging process. This chapter will include a review of the epidemiology, pathogenesis, and etiology of cystitis (acute and recurrent) and pyelonephritis in the elderly, along with a discussion of their diagnosis and management. The topics of prostatitis and catheter-associated infection will also be discussed.

EPIDEMIOLOGY

The prevalence of bacteriuria among adult females rises from 1% to 4% before age 50 years to 7% to 20% of postmenopausal women after the sixth decade of life. Among adult males, the low incidence of bacteriuria before age 50 (less than 1%) has been shown in some surveys to rise in the 60- to 70-year age group to levels comparable to the female population. After age 60 the incidence of symptomatic infection among males may actually exceed that of females.[1] Despite these data, Williamson et al have shown that family physicians are unaware of the presence of chronic urinary tract infections in many of their patients.[4] This is probably related to the lack of symptoms in such an elderly population.[5,6]

Along with the aging process itself, debility plays a significant role in the acquisition of urinary infections among the elderly.[7] As shown in Table 21-1, while the incidence of urinary tract infections among the elderly who reside at home is higher than that of comparable younger adults, this incidence increases at an even greater rate for similarly aged men and women who are nursing home residents or patients in acute care or long-term care hospital settings. Recent studies have accented the frequency of both asymptomatic and symptomatic bacteriuria and their association with catheterization in nursing home residents.[8,9] Similar to the findings of Sherman et al,[8] others have also reported that the urinary tract was the most common site of infection in long- term care facilities for the elderly.[10,11] However, Sourander and Kasanen have shown that, while the prevalence of bacteriuria is constant over time in an elderly population, the individuals affected vary.[12] Five years after their initial evaluation of 405 elderly persons, these authors found similar prevalences of bacteriuria among men and women; however, they noted that most of those with bacteriuria during their initial study were no long bacteriuric. Therefore, initial bacteriuria was not a predictor of the individual's subsequent status. Dontas et al have reported a statistically significant shortened survival of elderly asymptomatic bacteriuric patients during a 10-year follow-up of 342 ambulatory nursing home residents; this altered survival was more marked among women.[13] Overall, patients without bacteriuria survived 20 to 41 months longer than bacteriuric patients. The causes of death did not differ between bacteriuric and nonbacteriuric patients, except for an increased incidence of stroke and "senile cachexia" in the former group. While a cause-and-effect relationship was not established, these authors did demonstrate an association of bacteriuria with diminished survival. Sourander and Kasanen have noted similar findings.[12] Aside from these data, there is little information on the long-term consequences of bacteriuria in the elderly. Several authors have recently documented urosepsis to be the most common cause of community-acquired bacteremia seen at their hospitals.[14,15]

PATHOGENESIS AND PATHOPHYSIOLOGY

The elderly exhibit an increased susceptibility to a variety of diseases, including those affecting the vascular system, the heart and the lungs, as well as immunologic disorders and infections. There is currently no generally accepted and comprehensive theory of aging which can explain each of these developments.[16,17] The predisposition of the elderly to urinary infections is due to an interaction of a variety of factors, including (*a*) altered physiology, (*b*) mechanical wear-out or degenerative changes, (*c*) an altered immu-

Table 21-1
Prevalence of Urinary Infection in the Elderly in Relation to Residence

Residence	Incidence (%)	
	Men	*Women*
Living at home	6–13	17–33
Nursing home residents	17–26	23–27
Acute care hospital admissions	30–33	32–34
Long-term care patients	34	34–50

Adapted from Williamson et al,[4] Brocklehurst et al,[5] Lye,[7] Sourander and Kasanen,[12] Gladstone and Recco,[18] Akhtar et al,[37] and Klarskov.[45]

nologic status, and (*d*) the concomitant occurrence of other disease processes.[16]

While prolonged immobilization associated with debility may result in bone demineralization, hypercalciuria, and stone formation, these sequelae account for only a small number of urinary infections related to debility.[18] Other more significant factors predisposing the elderly to urinary tract infections are outlined in Table 21-2.

The elderly have a diminished response to stress and have a higher incidence of poor nutrition (eg, deficiencies of vitamins or zinc), which may be related causally to the damped or delayed cell-mediated immune responses in vitro and in vivo observed among the elderly.[19,20] Skin test responses to common microbial antigens have been generally found to be depressed in the elderly,[16,17] as have in vitro lymphocyte responses to mitogens.[20–22] These abnormalities may relate only to urinary infections in the aged due to pathogens which rely partially or totally upon intact cell-mediated immune responses for host defense (eg, tuberculosis, fungi, cytomegalovirus, other viruses). Polymorphonuclear leukocyte functions, which may more directly relate to urinary tract defenses, have been found to be intermittently abnormal in the aged with underlying diseases, such as diabetes mellitus,[17,20,22] and more consistently abnormal in those with myeloproliferative and lymphoproliferative disorders.[18] A decline of circulating IgM levels has been found in the aged.[18,20,23] Furthermore, the elderly generally form lower levels of antibody than younger controls in response to

Table 21-2
Factors Possibly Predisposing the Elderly to Urinary Tract Infections

1. Diminished response to stress
2. Poor nutritional status
3. Decreased cell-mediated immunity and neutrophil dysfunction
4. Decline of IgG and IgM levels
5. Chronic diseases
   a. Neurologic diseases and associated debility[26,27]
   b. Diabetes mellitus[28]
   c. Chronic renal disease[26]
   d. Malignancies[26]
   e. Diseases for which cytotoxic agents, steroids, and radiation therapy are used[26]
6. Chronic prostatitis[3,7,26,34,35]
7. Diminished outflow from urinary bladder due to:
   a. Urethral stenosis, cystocele, urethrocele[3,5,7,26,37,38]
   b. Prostatic hypertrophy[39]
   c. Prostatic carcinoma[39]
   d. Bladder diverticula or tumors[3,26,38]
   e. Neurogenic bladder[38]
8. Urinary calculi[26]
9. Vesicoureteral reflux[3,26,41,42]
10. Colovesical fistula
11. Indwelling urinary catheters; catheter manipulation[2,3,5,26,14,15,43]
12. Other GU instrumentation[26]

various vaccines. [24,25] A role for these alterations of immunoglobulin levels in urinary infections has not been evaluated.

A number of chronic disease states, more common in the elderly and in part due to accompanying debility, have been associated with an increased incidence of urinary tract infections.[26] Various neurologic diseases, including stroke and senile dementia, predispose the elderly to fecal incontinence with associated poor personal hygiene. In elderly women, perineal soiling in this fashion has been associated with an increased incidence of bacteriuria.[27] Female patients with diabetes mellitus appear to have a higher incidence of lower urinary tract infections with secondary pyelonephritis, while the overall rate of urinary tract infections in male diabetics does not differ appreciably from a control population.[27] Factors possibly related to the increased incidence of pyelonephritis among diabetic women are abnormalities of polymorphonuclear leukocyte function associated with hyperglycemia, recurrent vaginitis, bladder dysfunction, and possibly the frequency of urinary catheterization in this group of patients.[28] The increased incidence of renal infection in patients with chronic renal disease cannot be explained by their increased frequency of instrumentation and is probably related to deficient local defense mechanisms within the kidney itself.[26] Associations of increased frequency of urinary tract infections with malignancies and the use of chemotherapeutic agents are probably indirectly due to related complications and their management.

While Stamey and Sexton have causally related introital colonization with pathogens in women to the development of recurrent urinary infections,[29] others have suggested only a permissive relationship of such colonization with infections.[30,31] In addition to the possible role of cervicovaginal antibody in periurethral and introital colonization in women[32] (see above), Schaeffer et al have demonstrated increased adherence of *Escherichia coli* to vaginal epithelial cells of women with recurrent bacteriuria when compared to controls; this enhanced adherence of bacteria to vaginal epithelial cells was reversed when women with recurrent urinary infections were given antibiotic prophylaxis.[33] Various factors interplaying further with these host-pathogen interactions undoubtedly remain to be defined.

In males, recurring urinary tract infections (usually relapses) are commonly related to chronic bacterial prostatitis. Chronic prostatitis presents a difficult therapeutic problem because antimicrobials penetrate the prostate poorly, thereby allowing survival of bacteria which subsequently reinfect the urine.[3,26,34] The presence of prostatic calculi, which are radiographically visible in 14% of aging men, further precludes successful therapy.[34] The loss of the antibacterial activity of prostatic secretions with aging has been invoked to explain the increased incidence of urinary infections and prostatitis in elderly males.[7,34] Furthermore, increasing alkalinity with age, worsened by infection, as well as alterations of cation levels (Zn^{+}, Mg^{++}, Ca^{++}) in prostatic fluid, may also play a role in the development of these infections with aging.[34,35] Although acute bacterial prostatitis may precede chronic bacterial prostatitis, most men are unaware of a previous acute episode.[34]

In these cases, invasion of the prostate by rectal bacteria via direct extension of lymphatic routes and hematogenous spread of microorganisms to the prostate are unlikely to be common routes of infections. Rather, ascending urethral infection or reflux of infected urine into the prostate through the prostatic ducts can be more easily supported through investigative data as mechanisms of infection.[34] The bacterial causative agents of chronic prostatitis are the same as those of urinary infections and epididymitis in this age group, including *E coli*, *Proteus* organisms, members of the family Enterobacteriaceae, and *Pseudomonas* species.[34,36] The enterococcus is the only gram-positive organism believed to have a significant etiologic role in prostatitis.[34] However, unlike epididymitis in the elderly,[36] most cases of chronic prostatitis in younger men are nonbacterial in etiology; *Chlamydia trachomatis* and *Ureaplasma urealyticum* are candidates but unproven agents in this setting.[34]

Anatomical factors and abnormal bladder physiology often relate to the occurence of "complicated" urinary infections. Throughout life, females are predisposed to the acquisition of urinary infections due to their shorter urethral length and the lack of prostatic secretions which have antibacterial activity.[3,7,26] Parity has been inconstantly related to the development of bacteriuria.[5,37] Additionally, obstruction to urinary outflow and incomplete emptying of the bladder are frequent and important causes of urinary tract infections in the elderly, the latter being especially important in women. These abnormalities may be related to urethral stenosis (due to prior instrumentation or surgery), the presence of cystocele, urethrocele, or uterine prolapse secondary to relaxation of pelvic musculature, prostatic hypertrophy or carcinoma, urinary bladder diverticula or tumors, or CNS disease, primarily cerebrovascular disease, with secondary bladder dysfunction.[3,26,38] Prostatic hypertrophy has been reported to lead to obstruction in up to 75% of males by the age of 65.[39] Abnormal cystometrograms have been documented in elderly women both with and without CNS disorders.[38] Incomplete emptying of the urinary bladder may result from any of these abnormalities and thereby impair mechanical washout, which is the bladder's most effective defense mechanism against infection. Secondary urinary stasis allows for replication of microorganisms and local infection. Additionally, some authors believe that bladder distention results in bladder wall ischemia and a secondary reduction of local resistance to infection with consequent tissue invasion.[7,40] Urinary or prostatic calculi, frequently composed of magnesium ammonium phosphate (struvite) or calcium phosphate (apatite), harbor bacteria that are difficult to eradicate. Their presence causes therapeutic problems because of the high frequency of recurrent infection. Furthermore, the presence of urinary calculi may result in obstruction and lead to sepsis and destruction of renal parenchyma.[26] While vesicoureteral reflux is common in children as a result of urinary infections, its occurrence in the adult often signifies the presence of a congenital abnormality or severe bladder distention.[3,26] Whatever the cause, reflux allows for bacteria from the lower urinary tract to enter the upper tract with resultant renal infection. The renal medulla is especially prone to infection; this may be related to the fact that the hypertonicity of the medulla inactivates the fourth component of complement, retards the inflammatory response, and inhibits granulocyte chemotaxis and phagocytosis.[41,42] The development of a colovesical fistula due to a perforated diverticulum or carcinoma of the colon may uncommonly be the cause of urinary infection.

Urinary catheterization is frequent in the elderly, especially in skilled nursing homes, where 5% to 12% of patients are catheterized.[9,10] Catheterization and other genitourinary (GU) instrumentation and surgery, which are often necessary procedures in the elderly, allow for ready entry of microorganisms and account for many community- and hospital-acquired urinary infections.[2,3,5,14,15,26] Even a single brief urethral catheterization for diagnostic purposes in hospitalized or bedridden patients carries a greater risk of subsequent bacteriuria (5% to 10%) than the same procedure in healthy outpatients, which is associated with only a 1% to 3% risk.[1,26] With meticulous attention to maintenance of a closed urinary drainage system during continuous urinary catheterization, the risk of bacteriuria is 50% at ten days, but eventually all patients will develop bacteriuria with continued catheterization.[43]

ETIOLOGIC AGENTS

With this background about the factors predisposing the elderly to urinary tract infections, a comparison of the etiologic agents of urinary tract infections in the young and aged population is presented in Table 21-3. An individual's own enteric flora are believed to colonize the perineal and periurethral areas and result in urinary infections. The presence of fecal incontinence among the elderly due to dementia and other forms of CNS dysfunction may further predispose this group to urinary infections, especially in women.[27] The role of introital colonization by fecal flora in the pathogenesis of recurrent urinary infections in females has been demonstrated by Stamey et al.[32] These findings are corroborated by the fact that *E coli* causes 75% to 80% of urinary infections in young adults and ambulatory elderly patients.[3,7,26,37] However, other gram-negative organisms, including *Proteus* organisms, *Ps aeruginosa*, and members of the Enterobacteriaceae, assume importance among the elderly who are in nursing homes or hospitalized.[8,9,11] These organisms are often catheter-associated.[8,9] The reason for the predilection of *Proteus* organisms, especially for elderly males, is unclear. Several authors have also reported that *Proteus* organisms were the most common individual bacterial isolate when polymicrobial bacteriuria was found in a population of elderly women.[15,44] This organism is also associated with an alkaline urine and urinary calculus formation due to its urea-splitting property. Many of the gram-negative bacilli isolated from elderly patients in nursing homes or hospitals display increased antibiotic resistance.[8,9,37,44,45] Undoubtedly, involvement of resistant gram-negative isolates in hospital-acquired and recurrent urinary infections is a reflection of antimicrobial-induced selection. Cell wall–deficient bacteria are not believed to play a role in recurrent urinary infections among the elderly.[46] While enterococci also play a role in urinary infections among the elderly, *Candida* species, *Trichomonas vaginalis, C trachomatis, U urealyticum*, and viruses (adenovirus, mumps virus, cytomegalovirus, and measles virus) are not usual pathogens in this age group. Gram-negative bacilli inhibit the replication of yeasts, such as *Candida* species. When gram-negative organisms are suppressed by antibiotics, yeasts may colonize the urinary tract, occasionally in association with gram-positive bacteria.[40]

CLINICAL MANIFESTATIONS

Symptoms occasionally associated with acute cystitis in the elderly are given in Table 21-4. Fever is usually absent with cystitis. While dysuria, urgency, frequency, lower abdominal pain, and incontinence have classically been linked with

Table 21-3
Frequency of Organisms Isolated from Different Population Groups with Urinary Tract Infections

	Frequency (%) in Each Population				
				Elderly in Hospital	
Organism	*Young Men*	*Elderly in Community*	*Elderly in Nursing Home*	Men	Women
E coli	75	78	17–21	29	38–52
Proteus sp	8	7	32–50	50	18–22
Klebsiella sp	4	2	11	0	1–28
Pseudomonas sp	1	2	11	4	2–8
Staphylococcus sp	6	3	0	5	0–2
Others	6	8	7–33	12	10

Adapted from Lye,[7] Sherman et al,[8] Garibaldi et al,[9] Akhtar et al,[37] McMillin,[45] and Klarskov.[45]

Table 21-4
Frequency of Symptoms of Acute Cystitis in the Elderly

	Frequency (%)	Reference
Painful (burning) micturition	8–10	5,37
Frequency	11–67	5,37
Urgency	12–41	5,37
Lower abdominal pain		7
Incontinence	14–26	5,37
Confusion	Occasional	7

lower urinary tract infections and are usually more common in an ambulatory elderly population with urinary infection,[6] Brocklehurst et al found no symptoms which correlated with the presence of urinary infection among 172 elderly males in a geriatric practice.[5] Furthermore, only precipitancy and difficulty in urination were linked with lower urinary infection among 334 elderly females in their study; noteworthy was a lack of correlation of frequency, incontinence, or nocturia with urinary infection for either sex due to the prevalence of these symptoms in the uninfected elderly population. Asymptomatic bacteriuria is especially common in the hospitalized elderly with underlying diseases (especially diabetes mellitus and cerebrovascular disease), with physiologic or anatomic GU tract abnormalities, or with an indwelling urinary catheter.[6] Interestingly, confusion in an elderly individual may occasionally be a manifestation of lower urinary infection.[7] The absence of specific symptoms in this age group undoubtedly accounts for the lack of physician awareness of urinary infections among the elderly.[4] An appropriate caveat in geriatric medicine is "to consider urinary infection whenever an unexplained change in clinical status occurs."

Symptoms and signs of pyelonephritis are given in Table 21-5. While acute pyelonephritis appears to be uncommon in the elderly,[7] the same cautions about anticipating a typical complex of signs and symptoms for cystitis in the elderly applies as well for acute pyelonephritis. Upper tract infection (or tissue invasion) is most common (*a*) in men with "complicated" urinary infections, (*b*) in women who present six or more days after the onset of symptoms (ie, with a more protracted clinical course), (*c*) in patients with signs of upper tract infections, and (*d*) in patients whose bacteriuria reappears within a few days of single-dose therapy.[47] Dysuria and frequency are unreliable indicators of any urinary infection in the aged; however, even rigors, fever, systemic toxicity, and flank pain, while often present, may be mild or absent in elderly individuals with acute pyelonephritis due to their poor response to stress. The physician's attention may first be gained by the patient's manifestations of dehydration.[7,26] Elderly patients may be bacteremic and lapse into septic shock with minimal signs or symptoms. Furthermore, the symptoms and signs of acute pyelonephritis may abate after several days despite continued infection. The latter observation is believed to be a manifestation of patient tolerance to endotoxin, believed to be the mediator of many of the classical signs and symptoms

Table 21-5
Symptoms and Signs of Pyelonephritis in the Elderly

1. Acute pyelonephritis
   a. Dysuria, frequency (not specific)
   b. Rigors, fever, and toxicity (may be absent)
   c. Flank pain (may be absent)
   d. Bacteremia and shock
2. Chronic pyelonephritis
   a. Low-grade fever, malaise, weight loss, or
   b. Same symptoms complex as with acute pyelonephritis, or
   c. Without classic symptoms (may be asymptomatic)

of this syndrome.[26] Therefore, both appropriate diagnosis and documentation of adequacy of therapy require bacteriologic support.

Gleckman et al have recently noted the insidious presentation of community-acquired urosepsis in the elderly.[14,15] These authors reported a group of patients with urinary obstruction and catheterization who were generally more disabled and living in nursing homes; this group was prone to develop polymicrobic bacteriuria of which *P mirabilis* was present in 90% of cases.[15] The development of bacteremia in these cases was frequently associated with urinary tract manipulation or trauma. A second group of 23 patients without catheters was also presented who had bacteremic pyelonephritis confirmed radiologically or by ultrasonic imaging in 17 of 18 evaluated cases.[14] Both of these groups of patients were typified in their clinical presentation (*a*) by neurologic disease, altered mental status or associated dominant gastrointestinal (GI) or respiratory signs and symptoms obscuring the diagnosis, and (*b*) by the absence of leukocytosis in 21% of cases. The authors noted that the presentation of these patients so obscured their diagnosis that house officers often omitted the elicitation of costovertebral tenderness from their examinations. Urinalysis was especially valuable in directing physician attention to the affected organ system.

Chronic pyelonephritis in the elderly is often insidious, though it may present with the same symptom complex typical of acute pyelonephritis. More often, patients either complain of malaise, weight loss, low-grade fever, recurrent urinary tract infections, or have symptoms of urinary obstruction. Moreover, they may be entirely asymptomatic and the disease discovered due to an abnormal urinalysis or an elevated BUN. Chronic pyelonephritis should be suspected in any patient who has chronic bacteriuria associated with obstruction to urine flow, an indwelling urinary catheter, or a neurogenic bladder.

While some patients with chronic prostatitis are asymptomatic, most complain of varying amounts of dysuria, urgency, frequency, nocturia, discomfort at various sites (low back, perineal, suprapubic, scrotal, penile, inner thighs), myalgias and/or arthalgias.[34] Postejaculatory pain and hematospermia have also been noted. Occasional accompanying low-grade fever is more frequent with acute exacerbations of chronic prostatitis. Rectal examination of the prostate is often not helpful. In addition to recurrent cystitis, upper urinary infections and epididymitis are also complications and historically suggestive of chronic bacterial prostatitis.

DIAGNOSIS

The approach to the diagnosis of urinary tract infections in the elderly does not differ from that used in younger adults and depends upon the demonstration of significant bacteriuria by quantitative culture of an appropriately collected specimen. After discarding the first 10 mL of voided urine, a midstream specimen should be collected in a sterile container. Patients require instruction about careful cleansing of the periurethral area before voiding. More detailed discussions of these procedures can be found elsewhere.[1,48] However, despite careful instruction, the elderly may be less able to comply than younger adults due to declining mental and physical abilities. Moore-Smith has noted that 57% of midstream urine specimens obtained from elderly women are falsely positive, presumably related to contamination during collection.[49] Furthermore, Stamey et al have shown (Table 21-6) that, of 54 females (age unstated) with sterile urine obtained via suprapubic bladder aspiration, only one (1.9%) could void a sterile midstream urine specimen after careful instruction.[48] Perhaps more significantly, four (7.4%) of these women with sterile suprapubic aspirates voided urine specimens containing greater than 10^5 organisms/mL. In contrast, when 151 females with sterile suprapubic bladder aspirations were aided by a nurse in obtaining midstream urine specimens for culture, 54 (36%) were able to void a sterile urine specimen and none voided a urine contaminated with $\geq 10^5$ organisms/mL. It is clear that the care with which a voided urine specimen is obtained from any population of patients, especially the elderly, will have a direct influence upon the accuracy of the culture results obtained and upon the appropriateness of care rendered. All of these comments presume prompt handling of these specimens, which is another necessity for appropriate interpretation of culture results. Urine specimens should remain at room temperature for no longer than 15 to 30 minutes before being cultured or may be refrigerated overnight for processing.

As shown in Table 21-7, criteria for diagnosis of significant bacteriuria vary depending upon the sex of the patient, presence or absence of symptoms, and method of collection. For the asymptomatic female, one midstream urine culture containing $\geq 10^5$ organisms/mL of one species is diagnostically accurate in eight of ten occasions. Second and third specimens containing similar numbers of the same species of organism increase specificity, as shown in Table 21-7. At least two specimens are necessary for the diagnosis of asymptomatic bacteriuria in the female.[3] If a female is symptomatic, a single midstream urine culture containing $\geq 10^5$ organisms/mL of one species has been the diagnostic norm.[1] Stamm et al have suggested that $\geq 10^2$ organisms/mL of midstream urine from a symptomatic woman should be adopted as the criterion for infection because of the enhanced sensitivity of this number (0.95) with little loss of specificity.[50] This suggested alteration of the diagnostic criterion for symptomatic women would undoubtedly result in the inclusion of those women with the "acute urethral syndrome" who have bladder bacteriuria but fewer than the diagnostic standard of 10^5 organisms/mL of urine.[51] Whether such a criterion will have applicability to elderly women due to their difficulty in voiding a clean midstream urine is unclear (see above).

For the asymptomatic and symptomatic male most authorities will accept $\geq 10^4$ organisms/mL as a quantitative criterion for midstream urine culture.[3,52] If a brief urethral catheterization is necessary to obtain urine for culture, the presence of $\geq 10^4$ organisms/mL of one species is

Table 21-6
Midstream Urine Bacterial Counts in 54 Females with Sterile Suprapubic Urinary Bladder Aspirates

Bacteria/mL	Total Patients (%)
Sterile	1.9
1–100	16.7
100–1000	38.9
1000–10,000	24.1
10,000–100,000	11.1
>100,000	7.4

Adapted from Stamey et al.[48]

Table 21-7
Methods for Diagnosis of Significant Bacteriuria

1. Clean-catch midstream urine culture with $\geq 10^5$ organisms/mL of one species in the female
   a. One specimen: 80% specificity if asymptomatic, diagnostic if symptomatic
   b. Two specimens: 92% specificity if asymptomatic
   c. Three specimens: 98% specificity if asymptomatic
2. Midstream urine culture with $\geq 10^4$ organisms/mL of one species in the male
   a. One specimen: diagnostic if symptomatic
   b. Two specimens: diagnostic if asymptomatic
3. Urine culture obtained by urethral catheterization containing $\geq 10^4$ organisms/mL of one species
4. Urine culture obtained by suprapubic aspiration should be sterile

diagnostic of a urinary infection.[52] As mentioned, the risk of secondary bacteriuria developing related to this procedure must be considered when it is elected. In this regard, suprapubic bladder aspiration, an underutilized procedure in adult and geriatric medicine, can obviate the risks associated with a brief urethral catheterization and provide the most reliable urine specimen for diagnostic culture. Any growth in such a specimen is significant, but in the presence of a urinary infection, organism numbers usually exceed 5000/mL urine.[1,3,48,52] This procedure, described elsewhere, is often less traumatic to the patient than urethral catheterization.[48] The presence of polymicrobic bacteriuria in any urine specimen should suggest inappropriate collection or handling of the specimen. Should adequately collected specimens consistently reveal multiple identical pathogens in significant numbers in the absence of a chronic urinary catheter or ileal bladder, serious urinary tract pathology should be suspected.[3,7,26] Additionally, the quantitative criteria outlined in Table 21-7 apply to common gram-negative bacilli only. Quantitative criteria have not been established for gram-positive and other more fastidious bacteria or the fungi[3]; these organisms commonly do not replicate to high titers, and when cultured, their significance must be established with repeated specimen collection.

In addition to quantitative urine culure, there are numerous bacteriologic and chemical screening tests for bacteriuria, as reviewed by Kunin,[53] suitable for use in office practice or for performing surveys. These tests have varying degrees of sensitivity and specificity. The dip slide and pad culture with the Greiss nitrite dipstick are probably the most useful of these tests for the office or clinic setting due to their acceptable levels of sensitivity and specificity, and ease of handling. Other indirect methods for diagnosing urinary infections utilize urine microscopy. The presence of greater than five leukocytes per high-power microscopy field in the sediment of a centrifuged urine specimen has a variable correlation with the presence of urinary infection and is especially unreliable in the elderly.[37,45] The detection of one or more bacteria in the gram-stained smear of a drop of uncentrifuged, freshly voided urine has been shown to have an 80% to 90% correlation with the presence of $\geq 10^5$ organisms/mL of urine.[54,55] Similarly, the presence of one or more bacteria per oil immersion microscopy field in each of five fields examined using uncentrifuged, unstained urine or $>10^4$ leukocytes/mL of uncentrifuged urine have been shown to correlate well with urinary infection.[56–58] However, these technics are tedious and impractical for routine office use.

While the presence of a urinary tract infection can be documented with appropriately obtained urine cultures, the differentiation of renal from bladder infection is often difficult on the basis of symptoms and signs alone, especially in the elderly; however, the distinction is therapeutically important. The presence of a positive blood culture containing a pathogen identical to that in the urine culture in the absence of recent lower urinary tract instrumentation defines with high probability a renal source for the infection. Gleckman et al have recommended that at least three sets of blood cultures be obtained, in addition to urinalysis and culture, when urosepsis is suspected in an elderly patient (*a*) because of the low levels of gram-negative rod bacteremia, and (*b*) because bacteriuria and pyuria are such common findings in the elderly that their presence alone does not define the urinary tract as the source of fever and sepsis in an individual patient.[14,15]

In addition, there are a number of indirect and direct techniques for making the distinction between upper and lower tract infection which have been described and reviewed elsewhere.[1,26,40,48] These include renal biopsy, selective ureteral catheterization, the bladder washout technic and the detection of antibody-coated bacteria (ACB) in the urine. Each of these invasive technics is associated with significant inaccuracies or risks; perhaps the most practical and rewarding is the bladder washout technic.[1] The most promising recent development is an indirect test which determines the presence or absence of ABC.[59,60] The presence of immunoglobulin-coated bacteria in the urine correlated well with the presence of renal infection, while its absence defined lower urinary tract infection. However, subsequent studies have shown lesser degrees of sensitivity and specificity.[61–63] Most significant for the elderly male is the false positivity of the ACB determination caused by prostatitis.[64] Merritt and Keys have also documented high rates of false positivity and negativity for this test in patients with neurogenic bladders.[65] The clinical usefulness of the ACB test may reside in its limited ability to predict the presence of lower urinary tract infection in women and the likelihood of their response to single-dose antibiotic therapy[66–69] (see below). The failure of such single-dose therapy invariably predicts the presence of upper tract infection or prostatitis.[66–70]

The diagnosis of prostatitis is best established by the simultaneous quantitative bacteriologic culture of urethral (first voided 10 mL, VB1) and bladder (midstream, VB2) urine, expressed prostatic secretions (EPS), and the first voided 10 mL of urine (VB3) after obtaining expressed prostatic secretions.[34] The colony counts of EPS and VB3 should be at least tenfold above those of VB1 and VB2. Quantitative culture of an ejaculate may be substituted for EPS. The measurement of quantitative leukocyte counts in these specimens can be misleading in the diagnosis of prostatitis and the histologic evaluation of prostatic biopsy is subject to sampling errors.[34]

THERAPY

Preliminary comments about the therapy of urinary infections in the elderly are appropriate. The rate of adverse drug reactions, including ototoxicity, nephrotoxicity, neurotoxicity, volume overload, and hypersensitivity, is two- to sevenfold higher in elderly adults than in their younger counterparts.[71,72] This results primarily from increased blood levels of antibiotics related to decreased renal excretory capacity due to both intrinsic renal disease and obstructive uropathy.[3,18] Additionally, a decreased lean body weight, often present in the elderly, may result in overdosage with potentially toxic, lipid-insoluble aminoglycoside antimicrobials, which are often required to treat the more resistant gram-negative isolates encountered in these patients. While elimination of urinary infection in the elderly is no more difficult than in comparable young adults, the frequency of recurrence is higher, up to 43% in one study.[27] If these infections are symptomatic, and thereby necessitate repeated therapy, this implies the possibility of numerous exposures to potentially toxic antimicrobials with each recurrence. Therefore, it is important to choose not only an antimicrobial to which the pathogen is sensitive, but also one which is least toxic and has the most narrow spectrum of activity to avoid selection of more resistant organisms.[3,26] Generally, bacteriocidal agents are preferred theoretically over bacteriostatic drugs to reduce the need for retreatment. The duration of therapy should be minimized while being efficacious.

Acute Infections

In addition to the above considerations, the decision must be made whether to treat an individual patient. Every episode of symptomatic bacteriuria in the elderly should be treated.[3,7,26] With regard to the first episode of acute cystitis, oral therapy with a sulfonamide (eg, sulfisoxazole), ampicillin, amoxicillin, nitrofurantoin, or, in the case of penicillin allergy, a cephalosporin would be reasonable due to the likelihood of a sensitive *E coli* in this setting.[3,18,26] These choices are also dictated by the relatively low frequency to toxicity of these agents and, except for the oral cephalosporins, their low cost. In an elderly woman with an initial episode of bacteriuria, treatment without a urologic workup and even without a urine culture is reasonable.[6,73] In an elderly male with a first episode of symptomatic bacteriuria, a urine culture, as well as a urologic evaluation, is appropriate.[6] Culture results may necessitate a revision of therapy. Therapy should be continued for no more than seven to ten days;[3] a number of studies suggest the efficacy of a single dose or up to a three-day course of therapy with uncomplicated acute cystitis.[3,26,47,66–70] Souney and Polk have reviewed the results of a number of controlled trials of single-dose *v* conventional, more prolonged therapy.[70] They have concluded that amoxicillin, sulfisoxazole, and trimethoprim-sulfamethoxazole are effective single-dose regimens for uncomplicated lower urinary tract infections in women. This may also be true for men. Lacy et al have compared a single dose (200 mg) to five days of therapy with trimethoprim alone (200 mg twice a day) for acute urinary infections in elderly men.[74] While the cure rate was only 67% for the single-dose therapy, compared to 94% with five days of therapy, single-dose therapy was associated with less suppression of fecal Enterobacteriaceae. The merits of single-dose trimethoprim requires further evaluation in the elderly. The absence of ACB in the urine does have usefulness, although limited, for identifying candidates for single-dose therapy.[66–70] An often forgotten adjunct to antimicrobial therapy in the elderly is the use of urinary analgesics for symptomatic relief. While urine cultures should be sterile at 48 to 72 hours after initiating therapy,[3] if symptoms persist three to four days into therapy, the urine should be recultured; if this culture reveals a resistant organism, therapy should be changed. If, however, the organism persists and is sensitive to the antibiotic which the patient is taking, a urologic workup should be initiated.[6] In any event, follow-up urine cultures should be obtained 2 weeks after discontinuing therapy and at 6 weeks and 6 months after therapy is completed when infection has been related to renal damage by past experiences (as with obstructive uropathy).[3,18]

Recurrent Infections

Bacterial *persistence* throughout therapy usually reflects (*a*) therapy with an antimicrobial to which the organism is not sensitive, (*b*) an inadequate course of therapy (ie, too brief a duration or poor patient compliance) or, (*c*) use of an agent which is not excreted in the urine (possibly due to renal failure). *Relapse* of infection, which usually occurs within 2 to 4 weeks after cessation of therapy, may be due to the presence of renal calculi, prostatitis, pyelonephritis, urinary structural abnormalities, or obstruction.[3,26,75] Relapse is also typical of catheter-related bacteriuria, unless the catheter is removed.[14,15] The development of cell wall–deficient organisms during therapy accounting for recurrent infections is largely a theoretical concern and has only been demonstrated for enterococci.[76] *Persistence or relapse* of infection justifies therapy, whether it is symptomatic or asymptomatic, unless it is catheter-related and asymptomatic.[3,26] In addition to alteration of previously inappropriate or inadequate therapy and performance of appropriate urologic, radiographic, and surgical evaluation, some authors believe that patients with persistence or relapse of a urinary infection after a brief course of therapy should be treated for 3 to 6 weeks with an antimicrobial to which their infecting organism is sensitive.[3,26,47] The goal of such prolonged therapy is the eradication of renal parenchymal infection. In the case of prostatitis, the most frequent cause of relapsing infection or apparent reinfection in older men, up to 3 months of therapy with trimethoprim-sulfamethoxazole may be indicated and is curative in 32% to 71% of cases caused by susceptible pathogens.[34,77]

Reinfection after initial therapy of a urinary infection is seen more often in females, and occurs within 6 months of prior infection in two thirds of cases; such reinfection has been related to colonization of the introital area with endogenous fecal flora.[3,26,32] The possible relationships of such colonization to cervicovaginal antibody and bacterial adherence to introital epithelial cells have been discussed (see above). Screening women for recurrent urinary infections is not necessary or cost-effective since 94% of recurrences are symptomatic.[78] Infrequent, symptomatic reinfections in women (no more frequently than two per year) should be treated as acute episodes with a seven-day course of an appropriate antimicrobial.[3] For women with more frequent symptomatic reinfections, long-term, low-dose trimethoprim-sulfamethoxazole prophylaxis (half tablet daily, every other day or thrice weekly for 6 months), begun after the second infection has been treated with organism-specific therapy, has been shown to decrease these recurrences significantly and to be less costly than treating each individual recurrence.[78-84] Efficacy in this setting is apparently related to the ability of trimethoprim to enter vaginal secretions and reduce introital colonization with potential pathogens.[85] While the appearance of drug-resistant organisms has not been a problem, such women should be followed monthly for a recurrence of symptoms or with urine culture to monitor for the emergence of resistant organisms.[3] Other potential prophylactic regimens in this setting include: (*a*) nitrofurantoin 100 mg/d,[78] (*b*) trimethoprim 100 mg/d,[83] and (*c*) cinoxacin 500 mg/d.[86] While recurrences of urinary infection are low during such 6-month prophylaxis regimens (zero to one infection per patient year), recurrences (usually reinfections) occur in 50% to 60% of women after prophylaxis is stopped.[79,84] When recurrences do occur during or after prophylaxis with trimethoprim-containing regimens, the enterococcus is more commonly involved.[81,82,84] Harding et al have reported the long-term (2-year) prophylaxis with trimethoprim-sulfamethoxazole of women subject to recurrent infections after prophylaxis for 6 months with this agent.[87] No complications were noted in this study with 40 mg trimethoprim and 200 mg sulfamethoxazole given thrice weekly for 2 years, while recurrent infections were reduced to 0.14 per patient year. However, eight of 13 women experienced recurrences during the first year after prophylaxis was discontinued. Clearly, further studies are needed to evaluate therapeutic regimens to prevent infections in this recurrence-prone subset of women.

While advice concerning reinfection bacteriuria in the female seems to have a rational basis, our understanding of this problem in the male is less clear and the recommendations more complex. The most complete recent study of chronic bacteriuria in males (both symptomatic and asymptomatic) and its therapy was performed by a Public Health Service–sponsored program that evaluated 249 men (85% >50 years of age) with reinfection or "late relapse" of bacteriuria.[76] After initial organism-specific therapy, these men were randomized to receive continuous therapy with either a placebo, sulfamethizole, nitrofurantoin, or methenamine mandelate for up to 10 years of follow-up. This study revealed that: (*a*) long-term prophylactic therapy for chronic bacteriuria delays, but does not prevent, the recurrence of bacteriuria after an initial course of organism-specific therapy; (*b*) urologic sepsis was prevented in the group receiving prophylaxis while they were on therapy; and (*c*) in the absence of severe urologic abnormalities or noninfectious renal disease, chronic bacteriuria was unrelated to the progression of renal failure. After data analysis these authors recognized a number of good and poor prognostic signs that can be used as a guide to the management and therapy of elderly males with bacteriuria (Table 21-8).

They concluded that men with infrequent recurrences of symptomatic bacteriuria should be treated briefly with organism-specific therapy for each recurrence, if these patients have all of the good prognostic factors listed in Table 21-8 and none of the poor prognostic factors. The authors additionally recommend that, regardless of symptoms, any elderly male with infrequent recurrences of bacteriuria and "possible" poor prognostic signs should be managed with short-term, specific therapy and careful follow-up urine cultures without continued prophylaxis. They also concluded that men with frequent recurrences of symptomatic bacteriuria and males with two or more of the "possible" poor prognostic factors or with a "definite" poor prognostic factor (Table 21-8) should be considered for continued prophylaxis after a brief, specific course of therapy. The decision for prophylaxis must be made after consideration of the potential benefits and toxicities from such therapy, especially if there is pre-existing renal compromise.

Smith et al have reported the results of therapy of 38 men (mean age 69 years) with recurrent urinary infections who were positive for ACB[88]; 13 of these men had "complicated" infections and 22 had prostatic infection documented by quantitative bacteriologic localization technics. After initial organism-specific therapy followed by relapse, these men were randomized to receive either 10 days or 12 weeks of daily trimethoprim-sulfamethoxazole. Prolonged therapy was better statistically than ten days of treatment (60% *v* 20% cure, respectively); 50% of those without prostatic infection were cured, compared to 29% with prostatitis. These authors concluded that a ten-day course of therapy for recurrent infections in men with ACB is inadequate. Alternative agents to trimethoprim-sulfamethoxazole evaluated for prophylaxis of recurrent, symptomatic infections in elderly men include nitrofurantoin (50 to 100 mg daily), sulfisoxazole, or sulfamethoxazole (500 mg daily), and methenamine mandelate (2 g daily, with ascorbic acid, 2 g daily).[76]

Prostatitis

Any consideration of the therapy of recurrent urinary tract infection in elderly males must deal with the therapy of chronic bacterial prostatitis, which is associated causally with these recurrences. Meares has shown that two tablets twice daily of trimethoprim-sulfamethoxazole given for 12 weeks permanently cured one third of a group of 16 patients with chronic bacterial prostatitis documented by segmented localization cultures of lower urinary tract specimens.[34] While this regimen is the most effective current therapy, Fair et al have recently challenged the theoretical basis for its success and have proposed a reappraisal of other antimicrobials for use in this setting.[35] Because of enhanced diffusion into alkaline prostatic secretions, minocycline and erythromycin have received recent interest in the therapy of chronic prostatitis.[34,89] An added advantage to erythromycin is its increased activity in an alkaline environment.[90] A report on the efficacy of carbenicillin orally for prostatitis is inestimable because of the brief (< 1 month) follow-up of patients.[91] If bacterial pathogens are not isolated from quantitatively cultured urine and EPS and *Chlamydia* or *Mycoplasma* species are suspected, a single trial of therapy with minocycline or erythromycin in maximal doses for 14 days is appropriate.[34] A favorable response might dictate further use of these drugs. Sitz baths are also useful for symptomatic relief of chronic prostatitis.[34] However, therapeutic prostatic massage and radical transurethral prostatectomy for prostatitis are not generally practiced.[34]

An occasional patient with symptoms consistent with prostatitis will have a negative culture of EPS and no history of prior urinary tract infection. If inflamma-

Table 21-8
Patient Characteristics of Value in Predicting Response to Therapy in Bacteriuric Men

I. Good prognosis
- *a.* Symptoms present 12 months or less
- *b.* No previous therapy for urinary tract infections (UTI)
- *c.* Normal prostate clinically and radiologically
- *d.* Normal IVP
- *e.* Pure *E coli* infection

II. Poor prognosis
- *a.* Definite
  1. Calculus disease of the upper urinary tract
  2. Prostatic calculi
  3. Focal renal atrophy with subadjacent calyceal deformity
  4. Mixed infection
  5. Enterococcal infection
- *b.* Possible
  1. Symptoms for 20 years or more
  2. Four or more previous courses of therapy for UTI
  3. Prostatic enlargement clinically and radiologically
  4. Recurrent bacteriuria with the same organism (relapse)
  5. Serum creatinine, 2 mg/dL or more

Adapted from Freeman et al.[76]

tory cells are repeatedly absent from EPS, the patient may be said to have prostadynia.[34] Additionally, the patient with negative EPS cultures who fails to respond to minocycline or erythromycin may also be considered to have this syndrome. Some of these men have been found to have detrusor-sphincter dyssynergia, which may respond to phenoxybenzamine hydrochloride, an α-blocker. Other men with this syndrome have been thought to have muscular disorders in the pelvis, or emotional disturbances. Regardless, this group of men does not need antibiotic therapy.

Asymptomatic Bacteriuria

Despite considerable past debate, many authorities today agree that asymptomatic bacteriuria should not be treated in elderly patients without vesicoureteral reflux, a neurogenic bladder, or urinary obstruction, or in elderly patients who lack those poor prognostic signs outlined in Table 21-8.[3,7,18,45,76,92] In addition to the fact that it is not practical to treat all elderly patients with asymptomatic bacteriuria, other reasons for not treating include (*a*) the lack of definitive evidence for deterioration of renal function or the development of hypertension in this subset of the elderly despite untreated bacteriuria and (*b*) the frequency of isolation of drug-resistant organisms that require the use of potentially toxic antimicrobials.[3,7,37,76,92] However, several authors have associated chronic bacteriuria with decreasing creatinine clearance in the elderly.[8,13] Should the urinary bacterial isolate in the asymptomatic elderly patient be sensitive to nontoxic agents, some authorities have favored therapy for ten to 14 days.[18] Furthermore, there is agreement that in any patient with chronic bacteriuria in whom urinary tract instrumentation is planned, organism-specific antimicrobial therapy should be initiated prior to the procedure to attempt sterilization of the urine in order to minimize the likelihood of a secondary bacteremia.

Pyelonephritis

While acute pyelonephritis is uncommon among the elderly,[7] its therapy is no different from that in other age groups.[26]

Depending upon the severity of illness, an individual without a prior history of urinary infection, urologic abnormalities, or instrumentation may be treated in the outpatient or inpatient setting.[26] Therapy for an initial episode of pyelonephritis without signs of systemic toxicity can be treated on an outpatient basis with oral sulfonamides, tetracycline, ampicillin, nitrofurantoin, or a cephalosporin given for ten to 14 days.[26] A prior history of urinary problems dictates the need for hospitalization because of the possibility of the presence of an antimicrobial-resistant organism, which necessitates that initial therapy be parenteral with broad-spectrum agents (usually ampicillin or a cephalosporin plus an aminoglycoside). Patients who relapse after an initial oral or parenteral therapy should be retreated for 6 weeks with an antimicrobial to which the organism remains sensitive, while appropriate urologic and radiologic evaluations are completed.[26]

The management of chronic pyelonephritis necessitates complete urologic and radiologic evaluation of the urinary tract.[26] Organism-specific therapy frequently requires a parenteral antimicrobial because selection of resistant organisms by prior treatment has occurred. If the urine culture is sterilized within 72 hours of initiation of therapy, specific antimicrobials should be continued for 10 days, when the patient should be placed on an oral agent for a minimum of 3 months (eg, trimethoprim-sulfamethoxazole, nitrofurantoin, or methenamine mandelate with ascorbic acid). Periodic urine cultures should be obtained during continuous therapy. Results of therapy for chronic pyelonephritis may be gratifying because of the improvement of deteriorating renal function seen with successful treatment.

All of these comments about the work up and therapy of urinary infection in the elderly should be tempered by the clinical status of the patient. If the patient and/or the patient's family or guardian believe that an extensive evaluation is inappropriate due to the patient's age or deteriorating mental or physiologic status, the physician will need to decide the extent of such a workup, after careful consultation with those involved.

Catheter-Associated Infections

Comments about the management of catheter-associated bacteriuria are especially relevant in the discussion of urinary infections in the elderly due to their frequent debility requiring prolonged catheterization. Guidelines for catheter placement and maintenance as a closed system are thoroughly discussed elsewhere.[1,93,94] The rate of acquisition of bacteriuria during indwelling urethral catheterization with a closed drainage system has been defined at 50% by ten days after catheterization.[44] Despite adherence to guidelines, acquisition of bacteriuria is inevitable with increased duration of catheterization.[43] Antibiotic irrigation of the catheter and bladder does not reduce the rate of acquisition of infection.[95] The instillation of hydrogen peroxide into the drainage bag is, likewise, of no value in preventing the acquisition of bacteriuria.[96] Antibiotic prophylaxis during short-term catheterization has not been shown to be of definite value; the prolonged administration of antibiotics to chronically catheterized patients has not been adequately studied and may lead to colonization or infection with resistant organisms.[43,97,98] Only acute symptomatic infections should be treated with organism-specific antimicrobials because relapse of infection despite therapy is inevitable with continued catheterization.[26,97] Therapy of asymptomatic, monomicrobic bacteriuria with bacterial suppressants (nitrofurantoin or a sulfonamide) may be elected,[93] but specific therapy may be readily justified for catheter-associated polymicrobic bacteriuria because of its documented association with spontaneous bacteremia.[43,99] Additionally, any manipulation of a urinary catheter in the presence of bacteriuria should be preceded by organism-specific therapy.[18] Noteworthy is the fact that methenamine compounds are ineffective in catheterized patients because 60 to 90 minutes in an acid urine are needed for the hydrolysis of methenamine to formaldehyde; continuous catheter drainage precludes this.[97] Other potential sequelae of chronic urethral catheterization include urethral irritation and stricture, vesicoureteral reflux, urinary tract stones, bladder cancer, prostatitis, epididymitis, orchitis, and pyelonephritis with or without associated gram-negative rod bacteremia and sepsis.[97,100] Mechanical complications include balloon rupture with latex fragments remaining in the bladder, failure of the balloon to deflate, and encrustation of the catheter. The elderly are less able to handle such stresses.

The use of intermittent catheterization has avoided many of these complications in spinal cord injury patients, but the use of this technic does not have broad applicability in the elderly.[97] The condom catheter collection system has been utilized in incontinent elderly male patients to avoid the need for catheterization and the associated risks of bacteriuria; however, in uncooperative patients, as encountered in a geriatric population, even this collection system has been associated with urinary infections.[101] As with an indwelling Foley catheter, the condom catheter drainage tube should always be secured to the patient's thigh to prevent traumatic manipulation and obstruction to drainage by twisting of the balloon portion of the condom. Another alternative urinary drainage system in the elderly is the suprapubic catheter; however, its benefit in terms of reducing infections is unproven.[94]

Prostatectomy

A common clinical problem in the elderly male is the use of antibiotics at the time of prostatectomy. Williams and Hole have reported data on 248 elderly men undergoing transurethral or open prostatectomy.[102] The presence of pre- and postoperative bacteriuria correlated in their patients with the use and duration of preoperative catheterization. The enterococcus was the most common cause of postprostatectomy bacteriuria. These authors, and others, have supported the use of a single preoperative dose of antibiotics for prostatectomy. The use of ampicillin with an aminoglycoside is a reasonable choice of agents.

CONCLUSION

From the foregoing information, the complexities related to the pathophysiology and management of urinary tract infections in the elderly offer an example of the challenge and potential gratification to the internist practicing geriatric medicine.

REFERENCES

1. Kunin CM: *Detection, Prevention and Management of Urinary Tract Infections*, ed 2, Philadelphia, Lea & Febiger, 1974.
2. Esposito AL, Gleckman RA, Cram S, et al: Community-acquired bacteremia in the elderly: An analysis of one hundred consecutive episodes. *J Am Geriatr Soc* 1980;20:315–319.
3. Santoro J, Kay D: Recurrent urinary tract infections: Pathogenesis and management. *Med Clin North Am* 1978;62: 1005–1020.
4. Williamson J, Stokoe IH, Gray S, et al: Old people at home: Their unreported needs. *Lancet* 1964;1:1117–1120.
5. Brocklehurst JC, Dillane JB, Griffiths L, et al: The prevalence and symptomatology of urinary infection in an aged population. *Gerontol Clin* 1968;10:242–253.
6. Yoshikawa TT, Guze LB: UTI: Special problems in the elderly. *Geriatrics* 1982; 37:109–118.
7. Lye M: Defining and treating urinary infections. *Geriatrics* 1978;33:71–77.
8. Sherman FT, Tucci V, Libow LS, et al: Nosocomial urinary-tract infections in a skilled nursing facility. *J Am Geriatr Soc* 1980;28:456–461.

9. Garibaldi RA, Brodine S, Matsumiya S: Infections among patients in nursing homes. *N Engl J Med* 1981;305:731- 735.
10. Cohen ED, Hierholzer WJ, Schilling CR, et al: Nosocomial infections in skilled nursing facilities: A preliminary survey. *Public Health Rep* 1979;94:162–165.
11. Magnussen MH, Robb SS: Nosocomial infections in a long-term care facility. *Am J Infect Control* 1980;8:12–17.
12. Sourander LB, Kasanen A: A 5-year follow-up of bacteriuria in the aged. *Gerontol Clin* 1972;14:274–281.
13. Dontas AS, Kasviki-Charvati P, Panayiotis CL, et al: Bacteriuria and survival in old age. *N Engl J Med* 1981;304:939–943.
14. Gleckman R, Blagg N, Hibert D, et al: Community-acquired bacteremic urosepsis in the elderly patients: A prospective study of 34 consecutive episodes. *J Urol* 1982;128:79–81.
15. Gleckman R, Blagg N, Hibert D, et al: Catheter-related urosepsis in the elderly: A prospective study of community-derived infections. *J Am Geriatr Soc* 1982;30: 255–257.
16. Gardner ID: The effect of aging on susceptibility to infection. *Rev Infect Dis* 1980; 2:801–810.
17. Doggett DL, Chang MP, Makinodan T, et al: Cellular and molecular aspects of immune system aging. *Mol Cell Biochem* 1981;37:137–156.
18. Gladstone JL, Recco R: Host factors and infectious diseases in the elderly. *Med Clin North Am* 1976;60:1225–1240.
19. Palmer DL, Reed WP: Delayed hypersensitivity skin testing. II: Clinical correlates and allergy. *J Infect Dis* 1974; 130:138–143.
20. Phair JP, Kauffman CA, Bjornson A, et al: Host defenses in the aged: Evaluation of components of the inflammatory and immune responses. *J Infect Dis* 1978; 138:67–73.
21. Goodwin JS, Searles RP, Tung KSK: Immunological responses of a healthy elderly population. *Clin Exp Immunol* 1982;48: 403–410.
22. MacDonald SM, Goldstone AH, Morris JE, et al: Immunological parameters in the aged and in Alzheimer's disease. *Clin Exp Immunol* 1982;49:123–128.
23. Buckley CS III, Buckley EG, Dorsey FC: Longitudinal changes in serum immunoglobulin levels in older humans. *Fed Proc* 1974;33:2036–2039.
24. Howells CHL, Vesselinova-Jenkins CK, Evans AD, et al: Influenza vaccination and mortality from bronchopneumonia in the elderly. *Lancet* 1975;1:381–383.
25. Phair J, Kauffman CA, Bjornson A, et al: Failure to respond to influenza vaccine in the aged: Correlation with B-cell number and function. *J Lab Clin Med* 1978;92: 822–828.
26. Riff LJM: Evaluation and treatment of urinary infections. *Med Clin North Am* 1978;62:1183–1199.
27. Brocklehurst JC, Bee P, Jones D, et al: Bacteriuria in geriatric hospital patients, its correlates and management. *Age Ageing* 1977;6:240–245.
28. Forland M, Thomas V, Shelokov A: Urinary tract infections in patients with diabetes mellitus. *JAMA* 1977;238: 1924–1926.
29. Stamey TA, Sexton CC: The role of vaginal colonization with enterobacteriaceae in recurrent urinary infections. *J Urol* 1975;11:214–217.
30. Kunin CM, Polyak F, Postel E: Periurethral bacterial flora in women. Prolonged intermittent colonization with *Escherichia coli. JAMA* 1982;43:134–139.
31. Cooper J, Brumfitt W, Hamilton-Miller JMT, et al: The role of periurethral colonization in the aetiology of recurrent urinary infections in women. *Br J Obstet Gynaecol* 1980;87:1145–1151.
32. Stamey TA, Wehner N, Mihara G, et al: The immunologic basis of recurrent bacteriuria: Role of cervicovaginal antibody in enterobacterial colonization of introital mucosa. *Medicine* 1978;57:47–56.
33. Schaeffer AJ, Jones JM, Dunn JK: Association of *in vitro Escherichia coli* adherence to vaginal and buccal epithelial cells with susceptibility of women to recurrent urinary-tract infections. *N Engl J Med* 1981;304:1062–1066.
34. Meares EM Jr: Prostatitis syndromes: New perspectives about old woes. *J Urol* 1980;123:141–147.
35. Fair WR, Crane DB, Schiller N, et al: A re-appraisal of treatment in chronic bacterial prostatitis. *J Urol* 1979;121:437–441.

36. Berger RE, Alexander ER, Harnisch JP, et al: Etiology, manifestations and therapy of acute epididymitis: Prospective study of 50 cases. *J Urol* 1979;121:750–754.
37. Akhtar AJ, Andrews GR, Caird FI, et al: Urinary tract infection in the elderly: A population study. *Age Ageing* 1972; 1:48–54.
38. Brocklehurst JD, Dillane JB: Studies of the female bladder in old age. II. Cystometrograms in 100 incontinent women. *Gerontol Clin* 1966;8:306–319.
39. Jaffe JW: Common lower urinary tract problems in older persons, in *Clinical Aspects of Aging.* Baltimore, Williams & Wilkins Co, 1978, p 228.
40. Merritt JL: Urinary tract infection, causes and management, with particular reference to the patient with spinal cord injury: A review. *Arch Phys Med Rehabil* 1976; 57:365–373.
41. Andriole VT: Water, acidosis and experimental pyelonephritis. *J Clin Invest* 1970;49:21–30.
42. Andriole VT: Acceleration of inflammatory response of renal medulla by water diuresis. *J Clin Invest* 1966;45:847–854.
43. Garibaldi RA, Burke JP, Dickman ML, et al: Factors predisposing to bacteriuria during indwelling urethral catheterization. *N Engl J Med* 1974;291:215–219.
44. McMillin SA: Bacteriuria of elderly women in hospital: Occurrence and drug resistance. *Lancet* 1972;1:452–455.
45. Klarskov P: Bacteriuria in elderly women. *Dan Med Bull* 1973;23:200–204.
46. Gleckman RA, Crowley MM, Natsios GA, et al: Recurrent urinary tract infections in men: A role for aberrant bacterial forms? *J Clin Microbiol* 1980;11: 650–653.
47. Kunin CM: Duration of treatment of urinary tract infections. *Am J Med* 1981; 71:849–854.
48. Stamey TA, Govan DE, Palmer JM: The localization and treatment of urinary tract infections: The role of bactericidal urine levels as opposed to serum levels. *Medicine* 1965;44:1–36.
49. Moore-Smith B: Bacteriuria in elderly women. *Lancet* 1972;1:827.
50. Stamm WE, Counts GW, Running KR, et al: Diagnosis of coliform infection in acutely dysuric women. *N Engl J Med* 1982;307:463–468.
51. Stamm WE, Wagner KF, Amsel R, et al: Causes of the acute urethral syndrome in women. *N Engl J Med* 1980; 303:409–415.
52. Meares EM Jr: Asymptomatic bacteriuria: Current concepts in management. *Postgrad Med* 1977;62:106–111.
53. Kunin CM: New methods in detecting urinary tract infections. *Urol Clin North Am* 1975;2:423–432.
54. Bulger RJ, Kirby WM: Simple tests for significant bacteriuria. *Arch Intern Med* 1963;112:742–746.
55. Kass EH: Asymptomatic infections of the urinary tract. *Trans Assoc Am Physicians* 1956;69:56–63.
56. Barbin GK, Thorley JD, Reinarz JA: Simplified microscopy for rapid detection of significant bacteriuria in random urine specimens. *J Clin Microbiol* 1978;7: 286–291.
57. Kunin CM: The quantitative significance of bacteria visualized in the unstained urinary sediment. *N Engl J Med* 1961; 265:589–590.
58. Musher DM, Thorsteinsson SB, et al: Quantitative urinalysis: Diagnosing urinary tract infection in men. *JAMA* 1976;236:2069–2072.
59. Thomas V, Shelokov A, Forland M: Antibody-coated bacteria in the urine and the site of urinary tract infection. *N Engl J Med* 1974;290:588–590.
60. Jones SR, Smith JW, Sanford JP: Localization of urinary tract infections by detection of antibody-coated bacteria in urine sediment. *N Engl J Med* 1974;290: 591–593.
61. Rumans LW, Vosti KL: The relationship of antibody-coated bacteria to clinical syndromes as found in unselected populations with bacteriuria. *Arch Intern Med* 1978; 138:1077–1081.
62. Harding GKM, Marrie TJ, Ronald AR, et al: Urinary tract infection localization in women. *JAMA* 1978;240:1147–1150.
63. Hawthorne JJ, Kurtz SB, Anhalt JP, et al: Accuracy of antibody-coated-bacteria test in recurrent urinary tract infections. *Mayo Clin Proc* 1978;53:651–654.
64. Jones SR: Prostatitis as cause of antibody-coated bacteria in urine. *N Engl J Med* 1974;291:365.
65. Merritt JL, Keys TF: Limitations of the antibody-coated bacteria test in patients

with neurogenic bladders. *JAMA* 1982; 247:1723–1725.
66. Fang LST, Tolkoff-Rubin NE, Rubin RH: Efficacy of single-dose and conventional amoxicillin therapy in urinary tract infection localized by the antibody-coated bacteria technic. *N Engl J Med* 1978; 298:413–416.
67. Rubin RH, Fang LST, Jones SR, et al: Single-dose amoxicillin therapy for urinary tract infection. *JAMA* 1980;244: 561–564.
68. Savard-Fenton M, Fenton BW, Reller LB, et al: Single-dose amoxicillin therapy with follow-up urine culture. *Am J Med* 1982;73:808–813.
69. Buckwold FJ, Ludwig P, Harding GKM, et al: Therapy for acute cystitis in adult women. *JAMA* 1982;247:1839–1842.
70. Souney P, Polk BF: Single-dose antimicrobial therapy for urinary tract infections in women. *Rev Infect Dis* 1982; 4:29–34.
71. Smith IM: Cephalexin: Clinical effectiveness in geriatric patients. *Geriatrics* 1977;32:91–99.
72. Berk SL, Smith JK: Infectious diseases in the elderly. *Med Clin North Am* 1983; 67:273–293.
73. Fowler JE Jr, Pulaski ET: Excretory urography, cystography, and cystoscopy in the evaluation of women with urinary-tract infection. *N Engl J Med* 1981; 304:462–465.
74. Lacey RW, Simpson MHC, Lord VL, et al: Comparison of single-dose trimethoprim with a five-day course for the treatment of urinary tract infections in the elderly. *Age Ageing* 1981;10:179–185.
75. Turck M, Ronald AR, Petersdorf RG: Relapse and reinfection in chronic bacteriuria. II. The correlation between site of infection and pattern of recurrence in chronic bacteriuria. *N Engl J Med* 1968; 278:422–427.
76. Freeman RB, Smith WM, Richardson JA, et al: Long-term therapy for chronic bacteriuria in men: U.S. Public Health Service Cooperative Study. *Ann Intern Med* 1975;83:133–147.
77. Meares EM: Long-term therapy of chronic bacterial prostatitis with trimethoprim-sulfamethoxazole. *Can Med Assoc J* 1975;112:22S–25S.
78. Kraft JK, Stamey TA: The natural history of symptomatic recurrent bacteriuria in women. *Medicine* 1977;56:55–60.
79. Stamey TA, Condy M, Mihara G: Prophylactic efficacy of nitrofurantoin macrocrystals and trimethoprim-sulfamethoxazole in urinary infections: Biologic effects on the vaginal and rectal flora. *N Engl J Med* 1977;296:780–783.
80. Stamm WE, McKevitt M, Counts GW, et al: Is antimicrobial prophylaxis of urinary tract infections cost effective? *Ann Intern Med* 1981;94:251–255.
81. Harding GKM, Ronald AR: A controlled study of antimicrobial prophylaxis of recurrent urinary infection in women. *N Engl J Med* 1974;291:597–601.
82. Harding GKM, Buckwold FJ, Marrie TJ, et al: Prophylaxis of recurrent urinary tract infection in female patients. Efficacy of low-dose, thrice-weekly therapy with trimethoprim-sulfamethoxazole. *JAMA* 1979;242:1975–1977.
83. Light RB, Ronald AR, Harding GKM, et al: Trimethoprim alone in the treatment and prophylaxis of urinary tract infection. *Arch Intern Med* 1981;141: 1807–1810.
84. Stamm WE, Counts GW, Wagner KF, et al: Antimicrobial prophylaxis of recurrent urinary infections. *Ann Intern Med* 1980;92:770–775.
85. Stamey TA, Condy M: The diffusion and concentration of trimethoprim in human vaginal fluid. *J Infect Dis* 1975;131: 261–266.
86. Scheckler WE, Burt RAP, Paulson DF: Comparison of low-dose cinoxacin therapy and placebo in the prevention of recurrent urinary tract infections. *J Fam Pract* 1982;15:901–904.
87. Harding GKM, Ronald AR, Nicolle LE, et al: Long-term antimicrobial prophylaxis for recurrent urinary tract infections in women. *Rev Infect Dis* 1982;4:438–443.
88. Smith JW, Jones SR, Reed WP, et al: Recurrent urinary tract infections in men. *Ann Intern Med* 1979;91:544–548.
89. Paulson DF, White RD: Trimethoprim-sulfamethoxazole and minocycline-hydrochloride in the treatment of culture-proved bacterial prostatitis. *J Urol* 1978;120:184–185.
90. Zinner SH, Sabath LD, Casey JI, et al: Erythromycin and alkalinisation of the

urine in the treatment of urinary-tract infections due to gram-negative bacilli. *Lancet* 1971;1:1267–1268.

91. Oliveri RA, Sachs RM, Caste PG: Clinical experience with geocillin in the treatment of bacterial prostatitis. *Curr Ther Res* 1979;25:415–421.
92. Gleckman R: The controversy of treatment of asymptomatic bacteriuria in non-pregnant women—resolved. *J Urol* 1976;116:776–777.
93. Stamm WE: Guidelines for prevention of catheter-associated urinary tract infections. *Ann Intern Med* 1975;82:386–390.
94. Wong ES, Hooton TM: Guidelines for prevention of catheter-associated urinary tract infections. *Infect Control* 1981;2: 125–130.
95. Warren JW, Platt R, Thomas RJ, et al: Antibiotic irrigation and catheter-associated urinary trace infections. *N Engl J Med* 1978;299:570–573.
96. Thompson RL, Haley CE, Gröschel DM, et al: Effect of periodic instillation of hydrogen peroxide into urinary drainage systems in the prevention of catheter-associated bacteriuria. Read before the 22nd Interscience Conference on Antimicrobial Agents and Chemotherapy, Oct 4–6, Miami Beach, 1982, abstract No. 769.
97. Warren JW, Munci HL Jr, Bergquist EJ, et al: Sequelae and management of urinary infection in the patient requiring chronic catheterization. *J Urol* 1981; 125:1–7.
98. Britt MR, Garibaldi RA, Miller WA, et al: Antimicrobial prophylaxis for catheter-associated bacteriuria. *Antimicrob Agents Chemother* 1977;11:240–243.
99. Gross PA, Flower M, Barden G: Polymicrobic bacteriuria: Significant association with bacteremia. *J Clin Microbiol* 1976;3:246–250.
100. Schabel SI, Rittenberg GM: Complications of the Foley catheter. *CRC Crit Rev Diagn Imaging* 1981;16:219–237.
101. Hirsh DD, Fainstein V, Musher DM: Do condom catheter collecting systems cause urinary tract infection? *JAMA* 1979; 242:340–341.
102. Williams M, Hole DJ: Bacteriuria in patients undergoing prostatectomy. *J Clin Pathol* 1982;35:1185–1189.

CHAPTER 22 Urinary Calculus Diseases in the Elderly

Edward T. Zawada, Jr.
Domenic A. Sica

While the world's literature is replete with extensive reviews of urinary stone disease, to date there have been no specific reviews germane to this problem in the elderly patient. It is only after careful scrutiny of the broad literature of urolithiasis that an understanding can be gained of the significant impact of this problem on those over 60 years of age. This chapter synthesizes much prior work in an attempt to focus on the specific aspects of stone disease applicable to the elderly.

Surprisingly, stone disease and obstructive events from crystal deposits within the urinary system are not rare occurrences in the elderly. The consequences of such urinary calculi are more significant in this group of patients than for individuals in younger age groups. This reflects the loss of renal reserve that occurs naturally as a consequence of the aging process. Because these patients often have other systemic illnesses, frequently of a vascular nature, standard management principles may sometimes not apply. The use of state of the art technologies, such as noninvasive dissolution of stones, may be indicated to avoid surgical intervention. This chapter is not intended as an extensive review of stone disease; its purpose rather is to characterize the types of stones particular to the aged and their management in the elderly. The chapter begins with a review of the incidence and prevalence of stones in the aged, followed by a discussion on the etiology, consequences, and management of such calculi.

INCIDENCE

A number of reports suggest that urinary tract stone formation is a problem principally limited to patients during their middle decades of life.[1–3] These reports indicate that about 80% of all patients with stones have had their initial stone prior to the age of 60 years (Figure 22-1). Despite this, statistics indicate that hospital admissions for stone disease do not decline until beyond the age of 70. In a study from Sweden by Ljunghall et al[4] there was demonstrated higher hospital admission rates per stone episode in the 65- to 69-year-olds than in any other age group. This fact is not surprising since urinary calculi often lead to greater morbidity in the elderly than in other age groups.[5] In addition, when recurrence of stones is considered, some reports demonstrate a *prevalence* rate that is still rising in patients at age 60.[4] Thus, although urinary calculus disease is most frequent in the middle years, it remains a problem meriting attention in persons more than 60 years of age.

ETIOLOGY

Calcium Stones

The most common type of stone found in the elderly is a calcium-containing stone[6,7] of the upper urinary tract (Figure 22-2). In a recent report by Otnes[8] analyzing the type and site of presentation of stones over a 5-year-period, 125 calcium-containing stones were passed by those 60 years and older (total number of stones in study = 500). These stones were localized to the upper urinary tract. Of the 100 bladder stones studied, about 85 were obtained from patients more than 60 years of age and were about equally distributed in their composition between calcium oxalate and triple phosphate (struvite).[8]

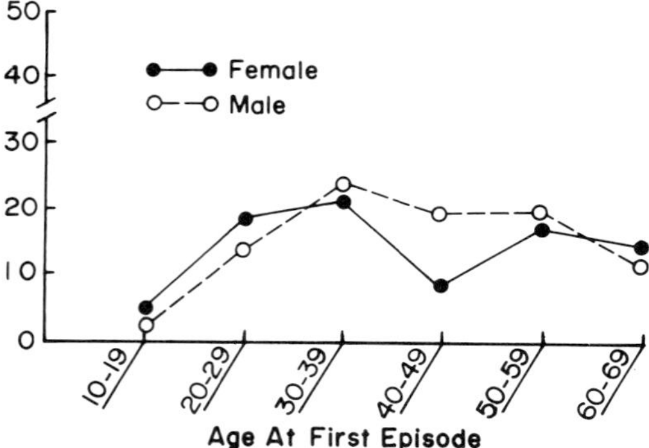

Figure 22-1 Age at first stone episode according to sex (adapted from Johnson et al[3]).

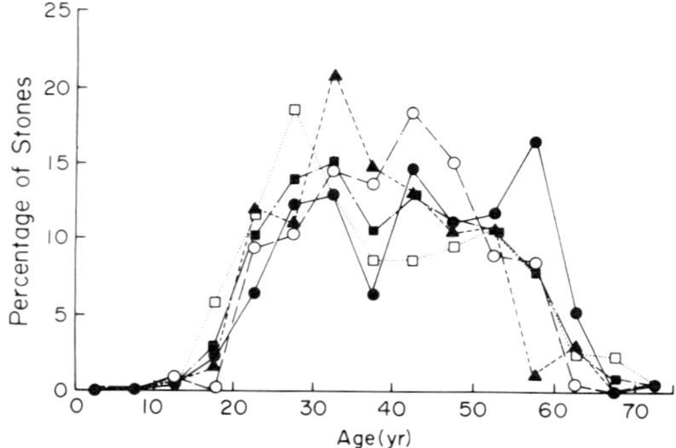

Figure 22-2 Distribution of stone types by age: triangle indicates idiopathic hypercalciuria; open circle=hyperuricosuria; closed circle=marginal hyperuricosuria; closed square=hypercalciuric and hyperuricosuria; open square=no metabolic disorder (Reproduced with permission from Coe et al[6]).

Calcium stones may be secondary to a number of disorders (Table 22-1). A common denominator in most cases of calcium-containing stones is that there exists either a raised serum calcium and thereby an increased filtered load or a normal serum calcium with concurrent increased tubular rejection of that calcium filtered. The end result is then a raised tubular calcium concentration where alterations in urine volume, pH, or inhibitors of crystallization may then effect a change in the solubility of calcium and result in supersaturation of the urine.

Idiopathic hypercalciuria is the most common metabolic disorder leading to recurrent calcium stones in individuals under the age of 60 years.[9,10] The pathogenesis of idiopathic hypercalciuria is unresolved though it involves in varying degrees either excessive intestinal calcium

Table 22-1
Clinical Disorders Associated with Calcium Stones

Idiopathic hypercalciuria (>4 mg/kg on unrestricted diet)
Hyperuricosuria (≥800 mg in males, ≥750 mg in females)
Hypercalciuria and hyperuricosuria
Primary hyperparathyroidism
Renal tubular acidosis
Inflammatory bowel disease
Medullary sponge kidney
Sarcoidosis
Malignancy
Vitamin A or D excess
Paget's disease with immobilization

Adapted and modified from Coe.[9]

absorption (absorptive hypercalciuria types I and II) or depressed renal tubular calcium reabsorption (renal hypercalciuria).

Both stone incidence and the number of calcium-containing stones decrease with age.[6] This decrease in calcium-containing stones may reflect the alterations in calcium homeostasis that occur with aging. Intestinal calcium absorption falls with age,[11,12] conceivably representing diminished levels of 25-hydroxyvitamin D [25(OH)D][13] or 1,25-dihydroxyvitamin D [1,25$(OH)_2$D] in the elderly.[14] In addition, with age there occurs a decline in renal function; this in turn leads to hypocalciuria[15] which is in part related to the decrease in 1,25$(OH)_2$D[14] levels that occurs with renal impairment.

A significant calcium stone-forming disease in the elderly is primary hyperparathyroidism.[16–18] This disease results in upper tract stones composed of hydroxyapatite or calcium oxalate. Though hyperparathyroidism remains an important etiology of stones, the incidence of stone disease in primary hyperparathyroidism has declined. This is the result of an apparent increase in the prevalence of primary hyperparathyroidism based on the more frequent diagnosis of asymptomatic hyperparathyroidism by use of biochemical screens. These biochemical screens have been particularly noteworthy in the diagnosis of primary hyperparathyroidism in the elderly.[18]

Primary hyperparathyroidism is primarily found in females, a finding that is no different in the elderly. The incidence of stones in elderly patients with hyperparathyroidism has been reported as 16%.[16] From clinical material consisting of 400 patients treated surgically for primary hyperparathyroidism during a 10-year-period, Tibblin et al studied 158 (38%) patients who were older than age 64.[16] The surgical response in this group was excellent with the large majority (80%) of patients having a solitary adenoma.

There is little available information regarding the frequency with which sarcoidosis, vitamin A or D intoxication, or renal tubular acidosis causes nephrolithiasis in the elderly. Paget's disease (osteitis deformans) is usually observed between the ages of 40 and 60 and may present with stone disease in up to 5% of cases.[19,20] Stone disease is more likely to occur when an elderly patient with Paget's disease is immobilized and has a simultaneous high rate of bone resorption. Malignancy may frequently present with hypercalciuria and/or hypercalcemia. Despite this, the incidence of stones is low in patients with the hypercalcemia of malignancy reflecting the limited life expectancy of most patients once hypercalcemia has developed.

The diagnosis of the majority of hypercalciuric conditions relies on both the magnitude of urinary calcium excretion as well as the presence or relative absence of parathyroid hormone. Caution should be exercised in the interpretation of parathyroid hormone levels in the elderly since normal values appear to run in a higher range in this patient population.[21-23] Some authors have felt that this represents parathyroid hormone fragment retention as the result of age-related renal insufficiency.[21] Other authors have found that a significant residual correlation of age with immunoreactive parathyroid hormone exists despite controlling for creatinine clearance.[23] The exact cause of the rise in parathyroid hormone with age awaits further characterization.

Bladder Calculi

After calcium stones of the upper urinary tract, bladder and prostate calculi represent the next most common variety of urinary calculus disease in the elderly. In some series vesical calculi have represented 6% of all stones analyzed.[24] Vesical calculus disease is rare prior to the age of 50 (except for endemic calculi); it reaches a peak incidence in the 60- to 80-year-old age range.[8]

There are few causes of vesical calculi and they fall into three etiologic categories: endemic calculi, stasis calculi, and foreign body nidus calculi:

Endemic calculi are usually found in children and occur with no prerequisite for obstruction, infection, or other calculogenic factors. Whereas in eighteenth century Europe and North America these stones were common in children this is no longer so. Now, these stones, which are usually composed of ammonium hydrogen urate, are commonly seen in the lower socioeconomic classes of Middle and Far Eastern countries.[25] Their development probably relates to peculiarities in the type of diet ingested in these areas.[26]

Stasis calculi are primarily seen in adults and occur in conditions which impede the normal bladder outflow of urine. A number of these conditions exist among elderly patients (Table 22-2). Prostatic obstruction is a very common event in the elderly male and when combined with infection by a urea-splitting organism may lead to the development of bladder stones.[24] A bladder diverticulum may be the site of calculus formation, related in part to the urine stasis it promotes and to the urine infection that may be present.[27] Though cystoceles caused by uterine prolapse were previously common causes of bladder stones,[28] this is no longer the case.[24] Stasis calculi may be composed of any of a number of substances including calcium oxalate, magnesium ammonium phosphate, calcium phosphate, or uric acid.[8] In a series of 100 bladder stones analyzed by Otnes 10% were predominantly composed of uric acid.[8] This proportion of bladder stones caused by uric acid is much greater than that observed in other locations in the urinary tract in the elderly.

Foreign body nidus calculi result from phosphatic encrustation on a foreign body within the bladder or bladder wall. Commonly encountered nidi include nonresorbed suture material from prior prostate surgery, retained fragments from Foley catheter balloons, prostatic chips, or bone fragments from pelvic fractures

Table 22-2
Predisposing Causes of Urinary Stasis in the Elderly*

Prostatic obstruction
Bladder diverticula
Neurogenic bladder
Cystocele due to uterine prolapse
Urethral stricture

*Stone development is more common when infection co- exists with a stasis condition.

which had penetrated the bladder wall.[29]

In the elderly, in the absence of infection, bladder stones are often asymptomatic. The presenting symptoms are those related to the predisposing condition as illustrated by difficulty in initiating a urinary stream with prostatic hypertrophy. The development of fever and urinary tract infections may serve as the impetus to seek an anatomical cause for infections. Careful roentgenographic evaluation may then discover an underlying vesical calculus.

Prostate Calculi

Prostatic calculi are common findings in middle age and in older men. In a review of 3510 pelvic x-ray films, Fox found evidence of prostatic calculi in 484 resulting in an overall incidence of 13.8%.[30] The incidence of stones is probably much higher than this since small stones frequently escape detection. In a series of autopsy specimens examined by Hassler[31] 71 of 100 cases had calcification within the prostatic gland. The location of these calculi is depicted in Figure 22-3.

Calcification in the prostate results from calcification of corpora amylacea. The calcification does not occur in prostatic nodules and is primarily localized to prostatic acini and ducts, particularly in the posterolateral aspects of the gland. These stones are generally multiple, 1 to 2 mm across, moderately opaque on pelvic films (Figure 22-4) and composed of either calcium phosphate[31] or calcium hydroxyapatite.[24]

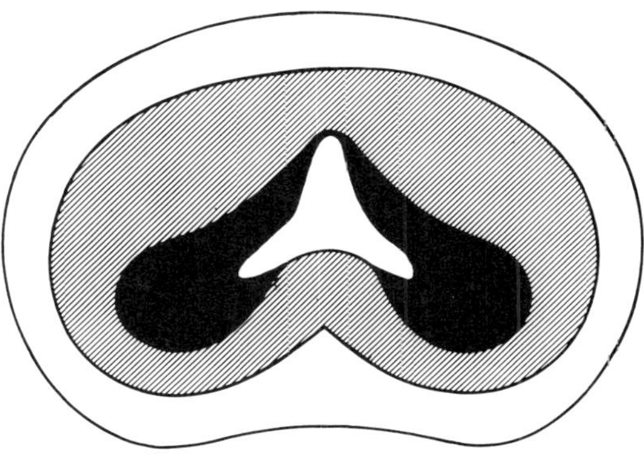

Figure 22-3 Distribution of calcifications within the prostate gland. The diagram represents a cross section forming a right angle with the urethra. Black area represents location of calcifications in 20 or more of the 100 cases. Hatched area is the location of calcifications in 10 to 19 of the 100 cases. White area is site of calcifications in nine or less of the 100 cases. (Reproduced with permission from Hassler.[31])

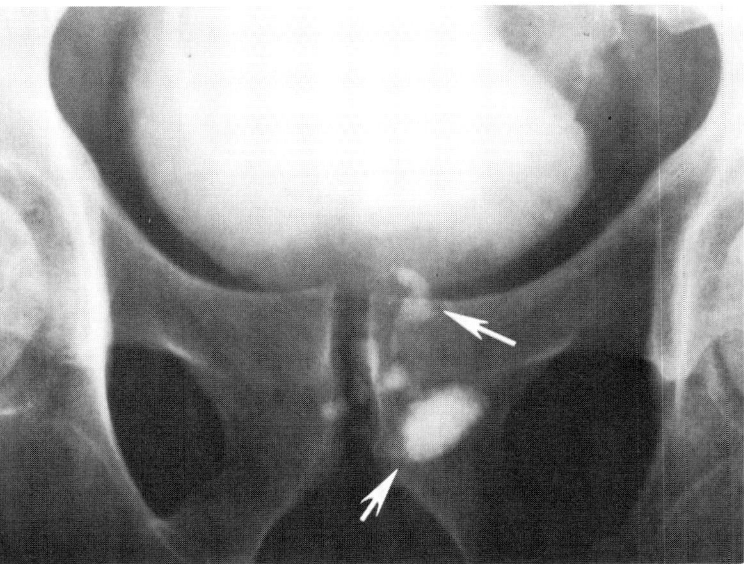

Figure 22-4 Plain film of the pelvis. Arrows indicate calcifications within the prostate.

Prostatic stones increase in frequency with age. They are usually sterile and seldom evoke any symptoms, but once infected they prove extremely difficult to sterilize without surgical intervention.[32] The major significance of prostatic stones involves differential diagnosis with prostatic carcinoma since these entities are easily confused on rectal examination.

Two other types of prostatic calculi may be observed in the elderly. In one type, calcification is dystrophic developing after the early use of radiation therapy after transurethral resection for carcinoma of the prostate.[33] In the other type, calculi develop postoperatively within a prostatic fossa devoid of tissue. These stones are not truly in the prostate since they usually rest between the bladder neck and the lower portion of the excavated prostatic urethra.

Infection Stones

Struvite ($MgNH_4PO_4 \cdot 6H_2O$) stones form in the renal pelvis, calyces, or bladder only when the urine is infected by a urea-splitting organism, usually a *Proteus* species.[34] These stones grow rapidly, frequently filling the collecting systems and assuming a "staghorn" shape. They can be quite refractory to therapy and frequently regrow since surgical removal is commonly incomplete.

Struvite stones are predominantly found in women; some series report 80% of the patients with infection stones being female.[35] This reflects the higher incidence of urinary tract infections in women. In fact, any patient group susceptible to urinary tract infections may develop struvite stones. Elderly patients requiring either an indwelling catheter or intermittent catheterization are considered at risk for the development of struvite stones. Bacterial urease hydrolyzes urea by the following reaction[36]:

$$H_2N-\overset{\overset{\displaystyle O}{\|}}{C}-NH_2 \xrightarrow[H_2O]{Urease} CO_2+NH_3$$

The NH_3 hydrolyzes to NH_4OH whereas the $CO_2+H_2O \rightleftharpoons H_2CO_3 \rightleftharpoons HCO_3^-+H^+$. The urine pH rises with the hydrolysis of NH_3 and at the higher pH HCO_3^- loses a proton to become $CO_3^=$. At this point conditions are optimal for struvite formation. That is, there exists at the same time increased concentrations of $CO_3^=$, NH_4^+, and an elevated urine pH. The presence of a urease-

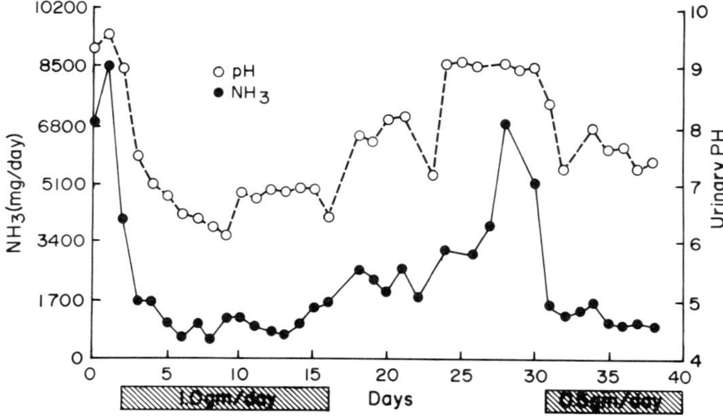

Figure 22-5 Urinary pH and ammonia in a 21-year-old paraplegic with an ileal conduit and chronic *Proteus* urinary infections and staghorn renal calculi treated with two doses of acetohydroxamic acid (cross-hatched bars). Though urinary pH and ammonia were reduced they were not normalized (normal pH < 6.5 and ammonia < 800 mg/d). (Reproduced with permission from Griffith et al.[37])

producing organism is a central component of stone development by this mechanism. From 92% to 99% of clinical isolates of *Proteus* and *Providentia* species possess urease,[37] while *Klebsiella* and *Serratia marcescens* isolates are urease-positive 60% and 29% of the time respectively.

Infection-induced stones may grow on a pre-existent stone. In some series up to 50% of the infection stones have as an underlying basis a coexistent metabolic stone or biochemical abnormality.[38] Infection stones may form with few, if any, symptoms. The patient may initially present with pyelonephritis with a urease-producing bacterial species cultured from the urine.

Treatment of staghorn calculi is neither simple nor uniformly effective. Surgical removal suffers from a high recurrence rate and persistence of urinary tract infections. Medical management frequently includes prolonged antibiotic use in an attempt to eradicate infection and the simultaneous treatment of any underlying metabolic disturbance. In either instance the choice between surgical and conservative care is both difficult and frequently unsatisfactory. A promising agent recently marketed is acetohydroxamic acid, a compound capable of inhibiting bacterial urease. This agent decreases both urinary pH and daily urinary ammonia excretion (Figure 22-5) thereby stabilizing stone growth. Acetohydroxyamic acid seems best suited for palliative treatment of patients with good renal function and urine flow whose infection is particularly recalcitrant.

Uric Acid Stones

Uric acid calculi occur in the elderly though they are not common. They account for 5% to 10% of all renal stones in the United States. Herring found that 9.4% (940/10,000) of stones contained uric acid; in 740 of these the stone was pure uric acid and in the remainder it was an admixture of uric acid and other substances.[39]

Uric acid stones are more common in patients with gout. While there is a prevalence of 0.01% of uric acid stones in the general adult population, Yü and Gutman found that 22% of 1258 gouty patients passed stones.[40] In large population surveys the risk of gout and uric acid lithiasis appears to be directly correlated with the level of serum urate. In one series of patients whose mean age was 58 years, 12.7% of the men with serum urate values between 7 and 8 mg/100 mL developed renal stones, while in those individuals whose serum urate exceeded 9 mg/100 mL, 40% developed stones.[41] Gouty patients may develop stones prior to the onset of articular symptoms though this occurs less frequently after the age of 60.[40] Finally, the quantity of uric acid in the urine is directly correlated with the frequency of stones. In 888 patients reported by Yü, urine excretion rates of 300 to 699 mg, 700 to 1100 mg, and greater than 1100 mg/24 h were associated with stone formation rates of 21%, 35%, and 50% respectively.[40]

Uric acid stones are radiolucent and have a tendency to form staghorn calculi. Uric acid crystalluria may manifest as stones, crystal formation, or obstruction. The particular variant of uric acid crystalluria that causes obstruction commonly does so by bilateral intratubular obstruction. Sufficient uric acid to result in this syndrome only occurs when cell turnover has accelerated rapidly as in the tumor lysis syndrome. Treatment of a tumor with chemotherapeutic agents liberates large quantities of intracellular nucleoprotein, much of which is converted to uric acid.[42,43] If the appropriate urine conditions prevail (acid and concentrated urine) then precipitates of the relatively insoluble uric acid occur within tubular lumina.

Crystal formation in the urine is largely determined by the urine pH. Uric acid is a weak base with two dissociable protons, with pK values of 5.57 and 10, only the former being dissociable. The quantity of uric acid in the urine does not have the same impact on stone formation as does the urinary pH. The average daily uric acid excretion could be tripled (500→1500 mg/24 h) and not obtain the same effect on stone formation as when the urinary pH is lowered from 6 to 5. In this latter instance, lowering the urinary pH by 1 pH unit will alter the concentration of the more poorly soluble uric acid moiety sixfold. Therefore, the major determinants of uric acid lithiasis are urine pH, followed by the quantity of uric acid excreted, and finally the urine volume.

A number of causes of uric acid lithiasis exist. They relate either to hyperuricemia, hyperuricosuria, or to urinary conditions which prove favorable to crystallization. Of these causes few are seen with any degree of frequency in the elderly. Either primary or secondary gout may lead to uric acid lithiasis in the elderly. Myeloproliferative disturbances are common in the elderly and often require chemotherapy. This in turn increases cell turnover which can be manifested as hyperuricosuria. Finally, the elderly patient is prone to dehydration which raises the urine concentration of uric acid.

The mainstays of therapy for uric acid lithiasis are fluids, alkali, diet, and the xanthine oxidase inhibitor allopurinol. The purpose of all of these treatment modalities is to lower urine uric acid concentration below the saturation point. The optimal condition sought should be that of a urine volume of 2 L/d and a urine pH of 6.0 to 6.5. Allopurinol is widely used though its major role should be in limiting uric acid production when uric acid excretion is excessive (>700 mg/d).

Medullary Sponge Kidney

Medullary sponge kidney (MSK) is by far the most common renal structural abnormality associated with calcium nephrolithiasis. MSK is a congenital anomaly of the renal medullary pyramids characterized by ectatic collecting ducts with associated cystic changes. The radiographic appearance of this entity is that of radial and linear striations in the dye-filled ectatic tubules in one or more of the renal pyramids (Figure 22-6).

In several series the age at presentation for MSK was usually below 40.[44–47] Though the typical appearance of MSK may be noted on an incidental abdominal x-ray film it is more often discovered during evaluation for a recent stone episode. The stones that occur with MSK are predominantly composed of either calcium oxalate or calcium phosphate.[44]

Patients with MSK may have metabolic abnormalities predisposing to stone formation. These defects are similar in nature to those found in the overall population of stone formers.[46] The assertion that a relationship exists between MSK and primary hyperparathyroidism can be found frequently in the literature, but this awaits further documentation.[47] Other renal functional abnormalities may exist with MSK including defects in urinary acidification and concentration.[44]

Treatment for MSK is directed toward

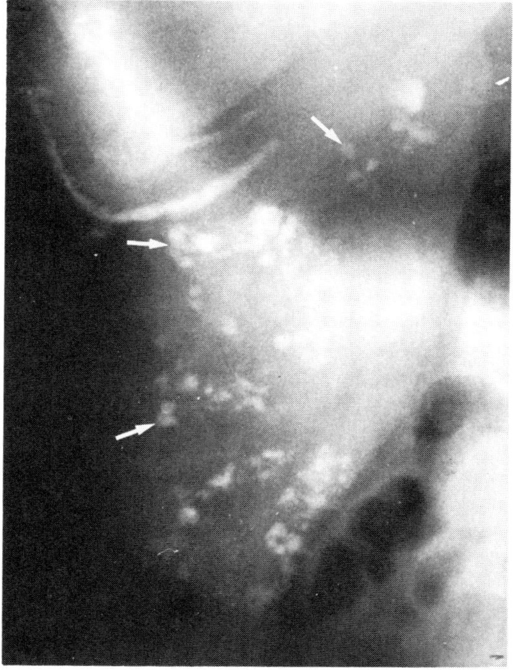

Figure 22-6 Flat plate of the abdomen with numerous radial calcifications. Radiopaque areas (arrows) represent calcifications within the renal pyramids in medullary sponge kidney.

management of any underlying metabolic abnormality. If either urinary tract obstruction or urinary tract infection occurs, standard treatment regimens should be employed.

TREATMENT

An absolute prerequisite to the management of the elderly patient with recurrent nephrolithiasis is a thorough medical assessment. It is only by this approach that the proper therapeutic agent can be selected for the associated medical condition. In addition, documentation of all medications is necessary to ascertain if concurrent medications are contributing to the occurrence of stones. Two such examples exist that are germane to the elderly. Glaucoma treatment commonly entails use of the carbonic anyhdrase inhibitor acetazolamide which is capable of causing stones.[48] Also, the elderly are often administered aluminum containing antacids for the treatment of peptic ulcer disease. These antacids precipitate sizable quantities of aluminum phosphate in the gut if taken in sufficient quantities, thereby leading to phosphate depletion. Phosphate depletion in turn leads to hypercalciuria and decreased urinary pyrophosphate,[49] both of which increase stone risk.

An important question as regards stone management in the elderly is whether or not conservative measures such as increasing urinary volume and correcting dietary excesses are sufficient therapy. As previously noted, stones do not commonly occur as primary events in the elderly. The passage of one stone need not presage the passage of another. The natural history of stone disease in the elderly is unknown so that the benefit of any therapeutic strategy devised must clearly exceed its risk.

A high fluid intake has been repeatedly advocated as helpful in stone prevention. Though the rationale of this approach is sound its efficacy as a sole form of therapy has not been clearly demonstrated. Use of fluid intake as monotherapy presents some potential problems. Hypodipsia in geriatric patients is not uncommon[50] so compliance to this regimen may be limited. If an increase in fluid intake is utilized then it should be of a sufficient magnitude to increase the urine volume to about 2 L/d. This will then decrease the chance of dilutional hyponatremia or bladder distention in the male with benign prostatic hypertrophy.

Urinary alkalinization is most important in the management of uric acid stones. Uric acid is poorly soluble in urine when the pH is below 5.6. Its solubility rises steeply above a pH of 6.5. If alkali therapy is employed it should be used in a way that limits urinary pH to the range of 6 to 7. Most alkali usage entails a significant sodium intake. In the elderly, this can precipitate congestive heart failure or worsen pre-existent hypertension. This form of therapy may also exacerbate pre-existing infection or calcium phosphate stones.

Dietary manipulation is difficult in elderly patients. Socioeconomic constraints frequently dictate very rigid diets. Elimination of calcium and oxalate from the diet is frequently not practical and may in fact be harmful. The use of calcium supplementation with or without vitamin D is a common treatment for osteoporosis. It is possible that calcium restriction, if sufficiently prolonged, may worsen metabolic bone disease.

Thiazide diuretics are commonly employed in the management of recurrent calcium urolithiasis. They primarily act by decreasing urinary calcium excretion. They accomplish this by a direct distal tubular effect to increase calcium reabsorption[51] and by inducing volume depletion and thereby increasing proximal tubular reabsorption.[52] These agents also increase the urinary loss of magnesium[53] and zinc[54] which may also contribute to stone prevention. The standard dose of thiazides employed is 50 mg twice daily. This is associated with complications in 30% to 35% of young patients[53] and this figure is probably appreciably higher in the elderly.[55,56] The elderly may be more likely to develop hypotension with diuretic use. In addition, diuretic use can lead to urinary incontinence or acute urinary retention.

A variety of electrolyte disturbances may occur with thiazide use. Hypokalemia and/or hypomagnesemia occur and if not corrected can manifest as cardiac arrhythmias, particularly if digoxin is being administered at the same time. Potassium supplements are frequently prescribed for the elderly, but the unpalatable nature of these supplements makes noncompliance the rule in most populations studied including the elderly. An alternative solution may be the simultaneous administration of a potassium-sparing diuretic with the thiazide. A particularly effective combination is that of Moduretic which contains 5 mg amiloride hydrochloride and 50 mg hydrochlorothiazide.[57] It has even been suggested that the amiloride-hydrochlorothiazide combination is more effective than hydrochlorothiazide alone in the prevention of calcium stones.[58] The use of potassium-sparing diuretics, however, may be limited to those patients with normal renal function. Hyperuricemia may develop with thiazide use but fortunately this rarely evolves into secondary gout. Finally, diuretics may precipitate overt diabetes mellitus,[59] especially when causing potassium deficiency. Fortunately, this syndrome of aggravating diabetes with thiazide use is one that often is responsive to correction of the potassium deficit. If thiazide use is to be considered in the elderly, proper supervision of the patient is essential.

The administration of inorganic phosphate has proved efficacious in the management of calcium-containing stones. The mechanism of action of phosphate administration is unclear. Phosphate administration lowers urinary calcium excretion and increases urinary pyrophosphate, but the magnitude of both of these events appears insufficient to explain its efficacy.[60] Phosphate therapy is contraindicated in the presence of struvite stones which may become appreciably larger during treatment. An effective dose of phosphate is about 1.5 g/d administered in three to four divided doses. The elderly may not tolerate the common phosphate-related side effect of diarrhea. Also, some phosphate mixtures contain sodium which may limit the extent of their use if sodium restriction is necessary. Finally, many elderly have impaired renal function. Since the excretion of phosphate is dependent on the extent of its glomerular filtration, its use, unless serum values are carefully monitored, can result in dangerously elevated levels of phosphate.

Cellulose phosphate is administered two or three times daily in a dose of 5 g. It acts to decrease gastrointestinal (GI) calcium absorption and thereby limit urine calcium excretion. It can cause diarrhea and has a high sodium content (14.5 mEq/5 g) both of which may be undesirable in the elderly. Since this agent has not had extensive testing, it has not been determined if its long-term administration has deleterious skeletal effects. This is of particular concern in the elderly population who often have osteoporosis.

When drug therapy is indicated for recurrent calcium stone disease, the agent of first choice will be either inorganic phosphate or a thiazide. Whichever agent is selected has side effects which may be more prominent in the elderly patient. Therefore, follow-up at regular intervals is critical in order to assess both the efficacy of the regimen and to treat side effects.

Finally, the elderly often suffer from concomitant diseases such as diabetes, heart failure, or malignancy and are consequently at greater risk for operative intervention as is sometimes necessary for removal of calculi and/or correction of predisposing anatomical conditions. Thus, this group will benefit from the use of noninvasive measures to remove calculi. In addition to direct nephrotomy, urethrotomy, or retrograde removal by a ureteral basket, there has been the recent development of strategies that disrupt calculi and have the resultant gravel exit harmlessly with normal passage of urine. These procedures employ a minimum of anesthesia and little surgical instrumentation.

This subject has received increasing attention[61–67] with two technics especially becoming more commonly employed. In one, an ultrasonic probe is placed in direct approximation to a stone either via a retrograde or by direct nephrotomy. This is followed by the transmission of ultrasonic waves from the probe to the stone (Figure 22-7). The other technic is completely external and involves focusing of ultrasonic waves stereotactically. The crossing of waves from two probes aimed at the stone will then result in its dissolution (Figure 22-8).

These strategies are thought to be beneficial to the elderly for the management of upper tract calculi for a number of reasons. They do not require general anesthesia, and they can be done in a same-day surgery suite without the need for hospital admission. Finally, there has been very low morbidity reported with these strategies.

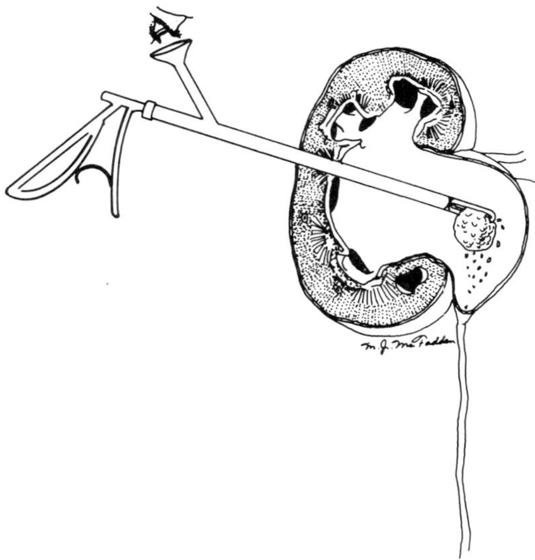

Figure 22-7 Dissolution of renal pelvis stone by an ultrasonic probe directly approximated to the stone by nephrotomy.

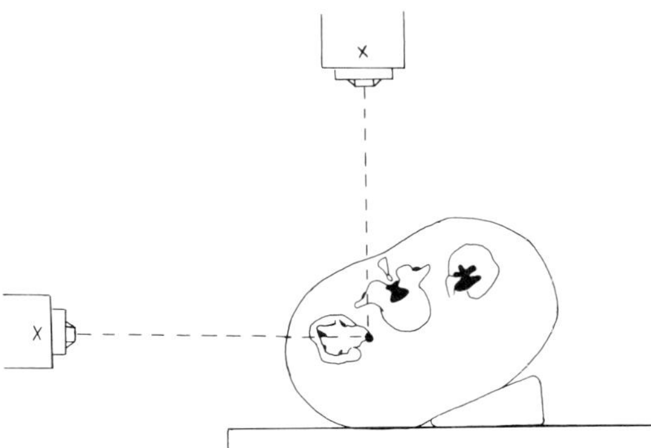

Figure 22-8 Stereotactic ultrasonic stone dissolution.

CONCLUSION

Though stone disease in the elderly occurs, it is not common. Its presence may result from either an underlying metabolic or anatomical abnormality. Younger individuals frequently tolerate nephrolithiasis quite well. The elderly on the other hand are lacking in renal reserve and thus can be quite devastated by the events surrounding the passage of a stone. With respect to therapy, the physician should be mindful of the fact that the elderly tolerate surgical procedures poorly. Alternatively, the use of medical treatment for stone disease is not without risk. Drug therapy should be carefully weighed as to its risk/benefit ratio since the elderly are less tolerant of the expected side effects of such medications.

REFERENCES

1. Rao DS, Kleerekoper M, Littleton R, et al: Kidney stones 1983: A preventable cause of morbidity. *Henry Ford Hosp Med J* 1983;31:182–183.
2. Sierakowski R, Finlayson B, Landes RR, et al: The frequency of urolithiasis in hospital discharge diagnoses in the United States. *Invest Urol* 1978;15:438– 441.
3. Johnson CM, Wilson DM, O'Fallon WM, et al: Renal stone epidemiology: A 25-year study in Rochester, Minnesota. *Kidney Int* 1979;16:624–631.
4. Ljunghall S, Backman V, Danielson BG, et

al: Epidemiology of renal stones in Sweden, in Brockis JG, Finlayson B (eds): *Urinary Calculus.* Littleton, Mass, PSG Publishing Co, pp 13–24.

5. Rosen H: Renal disease in the elderly. *Med Clin North Am* 1976;60:1105–1119.
6. Coe FL, Keck J, Norton ER: The natural history of calcium urolithiasis. *JAMA* 1977;238:1519–1523.
7. Elliot JS: Calcium oxalate urinary calculi: Clinical and chemical aspects. *Medicine* 1983;62:36–43.
8. Otnes B: Crystalline composition of urinary stones in Norwegian patients. *Scand J Urol Nephrol* 1983;17:85–92.
9. Coe FL: Hyperuricosuric calcium oxalate nephrolithiasis. *Kidney Int* 1978;13:418–426.
10. Pak CY, Britton F, Peterson R, et al: Ambulatory evaluation of nephrolithiasis: Classification, clinical presentation and diagnostic criteria. *Am J Med* 1980;69: 19–30.
11. Bullamore JR, Wilkinson R, Gallagher JC, et al: Effect of age on calcium absorption. *Lancet* 1970;2:535–537.
12. Nordin BE, Wilkinson R, Marshall DH, et al: Calcium absorption in the elderly. *Calcif Tissue Res* 1976;21:442–451.
13. Baker MR, Peacock M, Nordin BE: The decline in vitamin D status with age. *Age Ageing* 1980;9:249–252.
14. Francis RM, Peacock M, Barkworth SA: Renal impairment and its effects on calcium metabolism in elderly women. *Age Ageing* 1984;13:14–20.
15. Bulusu L, Hodgkinson A, Nordin BE, et al: Urinary excretion of calcium and creatinine in relation to age and body weight in normal subjects and patients with renal calculus. *Clin Sci* 1970;38:601–612.
16. Tibblin S, Palsson N, Rydberg J: Hyperparathryoidism in the elderly. *Ann Surg* 1983;197:135–138.
17. Mundy GR, Cove DH, Fisken R: Primary hyperparathyroidism: Changes in the pattern of clinical presentation. *Lancet* 1980;1:1317–1319.
18. Pearson MW: Asymptomatic primary hyperparathyroidism in the elderly–a review. *Age Ageing* 1984;13:1–5.
19. Ridlon HC: Urinary calculi associated with Paget's disease of bone. *J Urol* 1962; 87:499–503.
20. Deuxchaisnes de CN, Krone SM: Paget's disease of bone; clinical and metabolic observations. *Medicine* 1964;43:233–266.
21. Marcus R, Maduig P, Young G: Age-related changes in parathyroid hormone and parathyroid hormone action in normal humans. *J Clin Endocrinol* 1984;58: 223–230.
22. Wiske PS, Epstein S, Bell NH, et al: Increases in immunoreactive parathyroid hormone with age. *N Engl J Med* 1979; 300:1419–1421.
23. Gallagher JC, Riggs BL, Jerpbak CM, et al: The effect of age on serum immunoreactive parathyroid hormone in normal and osteoporotic women. *J Lab Clin Med* 1980; 95:373–385.
24. Taylor TA, Bowyer RC: Bladder and prostatic calculi–clinical presentation and composition, in Brockis JG, Finlayson B (eds): *Urinary Calculus.* Littleton, Mass, PSG Publishing Co, pp 57–63.
25. Valyasevi A, Dhanamitta S: Epidemiology and pathogenesis of bladder stone disease in Thailand, in Brockis JG, Finlayson B (eds): *Urinary Calculus.* Littleton, Mass, PSG Publishing Co, pp 185–194.
26. Brockis JG, Bowyer RC, McCulloch RK, et al: Physiopathology of endemic bladder stones, in Brockis JG, Finlayson B (eds): *Urinary Calculus.* Littleton, Mass, PSG Publishing Co, pp 225–236.
27. Crenshaw JL, Crompton CBR: Calculus and diverticulum of the bladder. *J Urol* 1922;8:185–195.
28. Varnier H: Des cystocèle vaginales avec du sans chute de l'utérus compliquées de calculus. *Ann Gynaecol Obstet* 1885;24: 201–219.
29. Banner MP, Pollack HM: Radiologic evaluation of urinary calculi, in Roth RA, Finlayson B (eds): *Stones: Clinical Management of Urolithiasis.* Baltimore, Williams & Wilkins, pp 53–167.
30. Fox M: The natural history and significance of stone formation in the prostate gland. *J Urol* 1963;89:716–727.
31. Hassler O: Calcifications in the prostate gland and adjacent tissues. *Pathol Microbiol* 1968;31:97–107.
32. Meares E: Infection stones of prostate gland: Laboratory diagnosis and clinical management. *Urology* 1974;4:560–566.
33. Jones WA, Miller EV, Sullivan LD, et al:

Severe prostatic calcification after radiation therapy for cancer. *J Urol* 1979;121: 828–830.
34. Chute R, Suby HI: Prevalence and importance of urea-splitting bacterial infections of the urinary tract in the formation of calculi. *J Urol* 1943;44:590–595.
35. Sleight MW, Wickham JE: A long term followup of 100 cases of renal calculi. *Br J Urol* 1977;49:601–604.
36. Griffith DP: Infection-induced renal calculi. *Kidney Int* 1982;21:422–430.
37. Griffith DP, Gibson JR, Clinton CW, et al: Acetohydroxamic acid: Clinical studies of a urease inhibitor in patients with staghorn renal calculi. *J Urol* 1978;119:9–115.
38. Smith LW: Medical evaluation of urolithiasis. *Urol Clin North Am* 1974;1:241–260.
39. Herring LC: Observations in the analysis of ten thousand urinary calculi. *J Urol* 1962;88:545–562.
40. Yü TF, Gutman A: Uric acid nephrolithiasis in gout: Predisposing factors. *Ann Intern Med* 1967;67:1133–1148.
41. Hall AP, Berry PE, Dawber TR, et al: Epidemiology of gout and hyperuricemia: A long-term population study. *Am J Med* 1967;42:27–37.
42. Klinenberg JR, Kippen I, Bluestone R: Hyperuricemic nephropathy: Pathologic features and factors influencing urate deposition. *Nephron* 1975;14:88–98.
43. Kjellstrand CM, Campbell DC, von Hartitzsch B, et al: Hyperuricemic acute renal failure. *Arch Intern Med* 1974;133:349–359.
44. Harrison AR, Rose GA: Medullary sponge kidney. *Urol Res* 1979;7:197–207.
45. Parks JH, Coe FL, Strauss AL: Calcium nephrolithiasis and medullary sponge kidney in women. *N Engl J Med* 1982;306: 1088–1091.
46. O'Neill M, Breslau NA, Pak CY: Metabolic evaluation of nephrolithiasis in patients with medullary sponge kidney. *JAMA* 1981;245:1233–1236.
47. Maschio G, Tessitore N, D'Angelo A, et al: Medullary sponge kidney and hyperparathyroidism – a puzzling association. *Am J Nephrol* 1982;2:77–84.
48. Gordon EE, Shepps SG: Effect of acetazolamide on citrate excretion and formation of renal calculi. *N Enlg J Med* 1957; 256:1215–1219.
49. Cooke N, Teitelbaum S, Avioli L: Antacid-induced osteomalacia and nephrolithiasis. *Arch Intern Med* 1978;138:1007–1009.
50. Miller PD, Krebs RA, Neal BJ, et al: Hypodipsia in geriatric patients. *Am J Med* 1982;73:354–356.
51. Costanzo LS, Windhager E: Calcium and sodium transport by the distal convoluted tubule of the rat. *Am J Physiol* 1978;235: F492–506.
52. Brickman AS, Massry SG, Coburn JW: Changes in serum and urinary calcium during treatment with hydrochlorthiazide: studies on mechanisms. *J Clin Invest* 1972;51:945–954.
53. Yendt ER, Guay FG, Garcia DA: The use of thiazides in the prevention of renal calculi. *Can Med Assoc J* 1970;102:614–620.
54. Cohanim M, Yendt ER: The effects of thiazides on serum and urinary zinc in patients with renal calculi. *Johns Hopkins Med J* 1975;136:137–141.
55. Diuretics in the elderly, editorial. *Br Med J [Clin Res]* 1978;1:1092–1093.
56. Ashraf N, Locksley R, Arieff AI: Thiazide-induced hyponatremia associated with death or neurologic damage in outpatients. *Am J Med* 1981;70:1163–1168.
57. Maronde RF, Milgram M, Vlachkis ND, et al: Response of thiazide-induced hypokalemia to amiloride. *JAMA* 1983;249: 237–241.
58. Maschio G, D'Angelo A, Fabris A, et al: Prevention of calcium nephrolithiasis with low-dose thiazide, amiloride and allopurinol. *Am J Med* 1981;71:623–626.
59. Grunfeld C, Chappell DA: Hypokalemia and diabetes mellitus. *Am J Med* 1983;75: 553–554.
60. Thomas WC Jr: Use of phosphates in patients with calcareous renal calculi. *Kidney Int* 1978;13:390–396.
61. Segura JW, Patterson DE, LeRoy AJ, et al: Percutaneous removal of kidney stones: Preliminary report. *Mayo Clin Proc* 1982; 517:615–619.
62. Alkin P, Hutschenreiter G, Günther R, et al: Percutaneous stone manipulation. *J Urol* 1981;125:463–466.
63. Chaussy C, Brendel W, Schmiedt E: Extracorporeally induced destruction of kidney stones by shock waves. *Lancet* 1980;2: 1265–1268.
64. Fernström I, Johansson B: Percutaneous

pyelolithotomy: A new extraction technique. *Scand J Urol Nephrol* 1976;10: 257–259.
65. Alken P: Percutaneous ultrasonic destruction of renal calculi. *Urol Clin North Am* 1982;9:145–151.
66. Smith AD: Endourology. *Urol Clin North Am* 1982;9:3–201.
67. Vallancien G, Capdeville R, Charton M, et al: Ablation percutaneé des calculs rénaux. *Presse Med* 1983;12:2997–3000.

CHAPTER **23**

Surgical Considerations in the Elderly

Barry Stults

As the population ages, increasing numbers of elderly individuals will require some type of surgery, including urologic procedures. Many of these elderly patients will have significant medical and psychosocial problems which will require careful assessment and management in the perioperative period. A successful outcome may necessitate the joint skills and cooperation of the surgeon, anesthesiologist, and internist. This chapter reviews preoperative medical assessment and postoperation medical management pertinent to the elderly patient undergoing urologic surgery.

DEMOGRAPHIC CONSIDERATIONS

Although persons over age 65 comprise only 11% of the United States population, one third of elective and one half of emergency surgical procedures are performed on them.[1,2] This results from the increased prevalence of disease and disability in the elderly population, especially in the "old, old" elderly over age 75.[3] Over the next 50 years, the total population of the United States is expected to increase by 40%. However, the population over ages 65, 75, and 85 years will increase by 150%, 200%, and 300%, respectively.[3] There will thus be a dramatically increased need for surgical care of the elderly.

Urologic surgeons will be particularly affected by this shift in population demographics, since the peak incidence of symptomatic presentation of benign prostatic hypertrophy and prostatic and bladder carcinoma is in the seventh and eighth decades of life.[4] Already, for men over 65 years old, benign prostatic hypertrophy is the fourth most common cause of hospitalization and accounts for 5% of all hospital days of care.[5] With improvements in anesthesia, surgical technic, postoperative intensive care, and immunosuppressive therapy, there may also be increasing consideration of elderly patients for the more high-risk surgical procedures of renovascular reconstruction and renal transplantation.

SURGICAL RISK IN THE ELDERLY

General Considerations

Operative mortality in most studies refers to deaths occurring within 30 days of the induction of anesthesia or to deaths occurring during the initial surgical hospitalization.[6,7] Deaths due to errors in anesthetic or surgical technic are relatively uncommon and account for only 5% to 10% of total operative mortality.[8,9] Most operative mortality is due to one of two factors. Irreversibility of the underlying surgical illness (eg, patients with diffuse malignancy, mesenteric infarction, ruptured aortic aneurysm) accounts for a significant proportion of deaths, particularly in the first 48 hours after anesthesia induction.[8,9] Postoperative complications such as myocardial infarction, infection (pneumonia, peritonitis, septicemia), venous thromboembolism, and respiratory failure cause a majority of deaths after the first 48 postoperative hours.[9,10]

Both the severity of the surgical illness and pre-existing chronic medical illness predispose patients to postoperative mortality and morbidity. This is demonstrated by the close correlation of operative mortality with the patient's preoperative physical status as described by the American Society of Anesthesiologists' (ASA) Physical Status Scale (Table 23-1). Patients are classified according to the presence or absence of mild to moderate, severe, or life-threatening medical and surgical illnesses. Operative mortality increases progressively as the classification rises from 1 to 5.[8,10] For example, in a large study of general surgery patients, operative mortality at 6 weeks was 0.18%, 1.4%, 5.4%, 12.4%, and 27.3% in classes 1 to 5, respectively.[10] Emergency surgery doubles the expected mortality for classes 1 to 3.[9,11] Although vague, classification using this scale is reproducible and is the best available predictor of noncardiac deaths and a fair predictor of cardiac deaths in surgical patients.[10,11]

Age and Surgical Risk

General surgery Available studies demonstrate a progressive eight- to tenfold increase in operative mortality between the third and ninth decades when all surgical procedures are considered together.[12–14] Although only one third of elective surgical procedures are performed in patients over age 65,[1,2] 60% to 90% of the total postoperative deaths occur in this age group.[1,15,16] The increased operative mortality is especially marked for patients over age 75[7,13,15] which may relate to the increased prevalence of chronic disease and disability in this segment of the population.[3] Emergency surgical procedures in the elderly carry a three- to fivefold greater operative mortality than the same procedures done electively.[6] This compares to an only twofold increase with emergency surgery when patients of all ages are considered.[8] In both unselected and elderly general surgery patients, the causes of operative mortality are equally divided among cardiac complications (myocardial infarction, congestive heart failure, and sudden death), infection (especially peritonitis and pneumonia) and miscellaneous causes (venous thromboembolism, respiratory failure, stroke, gastrointestinal (GI) hemorrhage).[7,9,17]

Urologic surgery Operative mortality also increases with age for most urologic procedures (Table 23-2).[4,13,18–24] With re-

Table 23-1
American Society of Anesthesiologists' (ASA) Physical Status Scale

Class 1.	No organic, physiologic, biochemical or psychiatric disturbance. The pathologic process for which operation is to be performed is localized and does not entail a systemic disturbance.
Class 2.	Mild-to-moderate systemic disturbance caused either by the condition to be treated surgically or by other pathophysiologic processes. Neonates and octogenarians may be included even though no discernible systemic disease is present.
Class 3.	Severe systemic disturbance or disease from whatever cause, even though it may not be possible to define the degree of disability with finality.
Class 4.	Severe systemic disorders that are already life-threatening and not always correctable by operation.
Class 5.	The patient is moribund with little chance of survival.
Emergency operation (E).	Any patient in one of the classes listed above who is operated upon as an emergency is considered to be in poorer physical condition than normal. The letter E is placed beside the numerical classification.

Adapted from Dripps et al.[45]

spect to prostate surgery, operative mortality for transurethral resections is 2% or more in patients over 80 years of age compared to less than 1% in younger patients.[13,18,19] Open prostatectomy procedures, which require an abdominal or perineal incision, carry a much higher operative mortality which may reach 4% to 12% in patients over age 80.[4,13] Total cystectomy with urinary diversion for treatment of bladder carcinoma has also been reported to carry a higher mortality in elderly patients[20] although some series have failed to find this correlation.[21] Two recent series noted only a 2% to 5% operative mortality for total cystectomy for patients in the eighth and ninth decades.[22,23] For salvage cystectomies for patients with recurrent bladder cancer following radical radiotherapy, postoperative mortality at 3 months in patients over 70 years of age may reach 70%, compared to 15% in patients under 70.[24] It is suggested that this procedure be avoided in patients over 70 years old unless simpler measures have failed.[24] With respect to renal surgery, the operative mortality for nephrectomy appears to be threefold greater for patients over 80 years old as compared with younger patients.[13] Unfortunately, there is very little published data concerning operative mortality and morbidity in patients over age 65 who undergo renovascular surgery. Operative mortality was 9.3% in a major series of patients aged 50 to 65 years undergoing renal artery reconstruction for atherosclerotic disease; however, the operative mortality in this series approach 22% when the patients also had clinically manifest coronary artery

Table 23-2
Operative Mortality for Urologic Procedures

Operation	Age (yr)	Mortality (%)
Transurethral prostatectomy	<80	0.5–0.8
	≥80	1.7–2.0
Open prostatectomy	<80	0.6–3.3
	≥80	4.3–12.5
Radical prostatectomy	<70	0–1.9
	≥70	5.8–16.6
Nephrectomy	<80	1.6–6.8
	≥80	9.0–16.6
Total cystectomy	<65	2.4–3.4
	≥65	2.0–12.0
Salvage cystectomy	<70	15.6 (at 3 months)
	≥70	71.0 (at 3 months)

Adapted from Shaldon,[4] Ziffren,[13] Wheatley,[19] Thomas and Riddle,[20] Johnson and Lamy,[21] Drago and Rohner,[22] Zincke,[23] and Osborn et al.[24]

disease.[25] Fortunately, it appears that surgical correction of coronary artery disease prior to renovascular surgery may reduce operative mortality to 2%, at least in patients with a mean age of less than 60 years old.[26] For those elderly patients with clinically significant renal artery disease but in whom surgery is contraindicated due to severe vascular disease elsewhere or poor general medical condition, percutaneous transluminal renal angioplasty may be a viable alternative mode of therapy.[27,28] Although few patients over 70 years of age have been studied, 54% to 84% of those in the age range of 55 to 70 have either improvement or cure of their hypertension during the initial 1- to 4-year follow-up period.[27,28] There appears to be little or no mortality associated with the procedure, but there is an approximately 10% complication rate (renal artery dissection, puncture site trauma requiring surgery, microcholesterol emboli resulting in acute renal failure), primarily in the more elderly patients with extensive atheromatous disease.[27-29]

Very few centers currently consider renal transplantation for patients over age 60.[30] The little data available suggest that in patients aged 50 years or more, there is little effect on either patient or graft survival when the donor is a histocompatibly well matched living relative.[31] However, in these patients there is a prohibitive decrease in survival using cadaveric transplants due to sepsis, myocardial infarction, and cerebrovascular accidents.[31] It has been suggested that transplantation might be more feasible in elderly patients if the degree of immunosuppression could be reduced.[30]

Among patients undergoing urologic surgery, cardiac complications are responsible for 20% to 50% of the operative mortality, and infections (especially septicemia from urinary tract sources) account for another 12% to 30%.[32-35] The relative frequency of pulmonary embolism as a cause of operative mortality appears to be greater in urologic surgery than in general surgery.[36] The exact incidence of lethal pulmonary embolism in urologic surgery is difficult to determine due to variable and often inadequate or unspecified diagnostic criteria. Reported incidences have varied from 5% to 60% of all operative deaths.[32,36-38]

Causes of increased operative risk in the elderly Increased operative risk in the elderly appears to be due in large part to a greater prevalence of chronic systemic illness in this segment of the population, especially cardiopulmonary diseases.[17,39,40] In those elderly patients who have lost considerable cardiopulmonary reserve, further decrements in function induced by anesthesia and surgery may result in organ failure and/or death.

It is not clear whether advanced chronologic age alone is an independent risk factor for operative mortality. Several studies suggest that those elderly patients without clinically manifest, coexisting systemic disease may be at no greater operative risk than their younger counterparts.[12,14,17] In these studies, operative mortality rates within a given ASA physical status class did not differ significantly according to age. Other investigations have come to opposite conclusions. In one large study of patients undergoing general surgery, age over 70 years was an independent risk factor for postoperative cardiac death even after multivariate discriminant analysis was applied to the data.[41,42] Additionally, there appears to be an age-related physiologic decline in cardiopulmonary function[43,44] which may predispose the elderly to postoperative complications in these two organ systems. For this reason, the ASA Physical Status Scale places all patients over age 80 in class II–mild to moderate systemic disturbance–even in the absence of recognizable disease.[9,45]

It may be that both disease and age-related, physiologic decline in critical organ function contribute to the increase in operative mortality with age. Those elderly patients who have lost considerable cardiopulmonary reserve, for whatever reason, will be at increased risk for postoperative complications. In contrast, those elderly patients with well-preserved organ function may tolerate surgery as well as younger patients. Elderly patients clearly must be assessed individually according to their biological age rather than their chronologic age alone. An effective assessment of operative risk in the elderly requires a knowledge of those physiologic effects of aging which are pertinent to the functional insults induced by surgery.

PHYSIOLOGIC CHANGES WITH AGE RELEVANT TO SURGICAL STRESS

From the fourth through the eighth and ninth decades, many organ systems demonstrate a progressive decline in function in the absence of recognizable disease.[43,44] For some organs (eg, kidney, lung) resting organ function is lost. For other organs (eg, heart), only maximal organ function under conditions of stress (eg, exercise) declines significantly. The rate and extent of this decline vary considerably among different organ systems and, importantly, among different individuals with respect to a given organ system.[43] Some individuals have minimal loss of function and maintain relatively high and stable performance. Others lose function more rapidly with normal aging. These latter individuals with less functional reserve may be more likely to experience organ failure as a result of a given functional insult from disease or surgery. Cardiovascular, pulmonary, renal, and thermoregulatory systems all lose functional capacity with age,[46-51] and each of these organ systems is further compromised by anesthesia and surgery.[52,53]

Cardiovascular Function

Cardiovascular performance under conditions of stress such as maximal exercise may decrease with age.[46,47] This may result from an age-related decrease in cardiovascular responsiveness to endogenous catecholamines, from cardiovascular deconditioning from relative inactivity, and/or from clinically occult cardiovascular disease.[46,47] Maximal cardiac output, oxygen delivery, and total body oxygen consumption in response to exercise may decline by 40% between the ages of 20 and 70.[46,47] Maximal pulmonary capillary wedge pressure during exercise increases from 15 mmHg in the third decade to 22 mmHg in the eighth decade.[54]

Major surgery, even when uncomplicated, is a significant stress on the cardiovascular system, imposing increased demands for oxygen transport.[52] Intraoperatively and during the first postoperative week there is a marked increase in total body oxygen consumption which must be matched by an increase in oxygen delivery. The latter is accomplished primarily by an increase in cardiac output which in turn increases myocardial oxygen consumption. The magnitude of increased oxygen consumption depends on the type and extent of surgery, being greatest for thoracic and upper abdominal procedures and least for nonthoracoabdominal procedures. Postoperative oxygen demands and consumption may be further increased by pain, fever, and infection. Unfortunately, the ability to transport oxygen in the postoperative period may be compromised by complications such as arterial hypoxemia, anemia, and decreased cardiac output resulting from intravascular volume depletion due to blood loss or third space losses into damaged tissues. Because of the age-related reduction in cardiovascular reserve described above, elderly surgical patients may be less able than their younger counterparts to compensate for increased oxygen demands by increasing oxygen transport. As a result, they may be relatively predisposed to develop tissue and organ hypoxia. Those elderly patients with underlying cardiac disease will be at even greater risk to develop end-organ ischemia.

Pulmonary Function

The pulmonary system also loses functional reserve with age.[48,49] The elastic recoil of the lung decreases with age, ie, the lung becomes more compliant. This reduces the stability of small airways in gravity-dependent portions of the lung and may cause their closure with subsequent ventilation/perfusion mismatch and inefficient arterial oxygenation.[49] As a result, arterial pO_2 decreases with age. In the third decade of life, arterial pO_2 is 90 to 95 torr at sea level and 70 to 80 torr at an altitude of 1600 m. By the ninth decade, arterial pO_2 has diminished to the 70- to 75-torr range at sea level and to the 55 to 60 torr range at 1600-m altitude.[55,56] With advancing age there is also a decrease in chest wall compliance (ie, stiffening), a decrease in the motor strength of the diaphragm and accessory muscles of breathing, and a major reduction in the ventilatory response to hypoxemia and hypercarbia.[48,49] These changes increase the work of breathing and reduce the ability of the elderly patient to maintain high levels of ventilation when there is an increased demand for oxygen transport and/or carbon dioxide removal. Mucociliary clearance and the cough reflex also lose efficacy with age, resulting in decreased clearance of secretions and inhaled particles.[48]

Anesthesia, the surgical incision, postoperative analgesia, and postoperative immobilization together cause profound alterations in the pulmonary system in patients of all ages.[53,57,58] These factors alter postoperative ventilatory pattern by decreasing tidal volume, increasing respiratory rate, and importantly, by eliminating the eight to ten large volume or sigh breaths normally taken each hour. These sigh breaths are critical to the prevention of microatelectasis in the gravity-dependent portions of the lung. Cough and mucociliary clearance, which together clear secretions from the large and small airways, are also diminished. As a result, diffuse microatelectasis or alveolar collapse develops within the lung postoperatively. Microatelectasis causes a reduction in lung volumes, air flow rates, and gas exchange, and thereby predisposes the patient to the postoperative pulmonary complications of hypoxemia, atelectasis, bronchitis, and pneumonia. The magnitude and frequency of postoperative pulmonary function decrements and pulmonary complications depend significantly on the proximity of the incision to the diaphragm–the nearer the incision to the diaphragm, the greater the compromise.[53] In descending order, pulmonary compromise is greatest for upper abdominal, thoracic, lower abdominal, and nonthoracoabdominal incisions, respectively. In the first one to two days after surgery, vital capacity decreases by 50% to 75% after upper abdominal surgery, by 40% to 50% after lower abdominal surgery, and negligibly after nonthoracoabdominal surgery.[57-59] For the same surgical procedures, arterial pO_2 on the first postoperative day shows mean decrements from preoperative values of 19, 10, and 6 torr, respectively.[60] Arterial pO_2 generally normalizes within 24 hours or less of nonthoracoabdominal surgery, since the predominant causes of the hypoxemia are the effects of general anesthesia and narcotic analgesic therapy.[61] For thoracoabdominal procedures, however, incisional pain, narcotic analgesics, and immobilization also contribute to arterial hypoxemia. With these procedures arterial pO_2 may not reach its lowest value until 48 hours postoperatively.[61] Therefore, with respect to urologic surgery, those procedures not requiring abdominal or flank incisions–primarily transurethral resections of prostate and bladder pathology–should alter pulmonary function minimally in the postoperative period.

Because of the base-line preoperative reductions in pulmonary function and gas exchange described above, elderly patients would be expected to have more compromised pulmonary function postoperatively than younger patients. Available studies suggest that postoperative arterial pO_2 is indeed lower in elderly patients than in younger patients.[49,61,62] Following general surgical procedures, arterial pO_2 in the first few postoperative hours is inversely related to age and independent of the site of surgery.[62] In one study room air arterial pO_2 two hours following surgery was predicted by the equation $pO_2 = 103 - 0.54 \times \text{age}$.[62] Elderly patients might also be expected to have lower arterial pO_2 values than younger patients for the first several days following surgical procedures, especially those involving thoracic or abdominal incisions. However, there are no available studies concerning this point.

Renal Function

The decline in renal function with normal aging may also have important consequences for elderly surgical patients. Major reductions in glomerular filtration rate (GFR) and in the ability to both conserve and excrete sodium make elderly patients more liable to both hypovolemia and hypervolemia in the postoperative period.[50] The reduction in GFR with age must also be considered whenever renally eliminated medications are given to elderly patients. Finally, the ability to clear free water decreases with age.[50] Elderly patients are therefore more susceptible to dilutional hyponatremia than younger patients.

Thermoregulatory Function

Thermoregulatory function diminishes with age.[51] Decreased numbers of cutaneous capillaries, diminished vasoconstrictor responsiveness of dermal arterioles, and thinning of the epidermis, dermis, and subcutaneous fat layers all predispose elderly patients to hypothermia.[51,63] As a result, during anesthesia and in the recovery room, elderly patients develop more severe and prolonged hypothermia than do younger patients.[64,65] With postoperative rewarming, elderly patients will therefore require a greater endogenous heat production to return the body to normothermia. This increased heat production is accompanied by major increases in both total body and myocardial oxygen consumption.[65,66] It has been postulated that this increase in myocardial oxygen consumption may be an important contributing factor to perioperative myocardial infarction,[67] which is four times more common in patients over age 70 than in younger patients.[42]

PERIOPERATIVE MEDICAL MANAGEMENT

Effective perioperative medical management of the elderly patient requires accurate and thorough preoperative assessment, appropriate postoperative monitoring, and treatment of postoperative complications which may arise. Anesthesia management is appropriately left to the anesthesiologist. His decisions will be facilitated by access to a complete medical and surgical data base. Geriatric anesthesia has recently been reviewed elsewhere and is not discussed further in this chapter.[63,68]

Preoperative Assessment of the Elderly Patient

Preoperative assessment of the elderly patient may reveal more problems and present more difficulties to the physician than are usually encountered with younger patients. Therefore, for elective surgery, a thorough preoperative assessment will ideally be accomplished in the outpatient setting. This will help avoid costly delays in scheduling the surgical procedure which may otherwise occur if a complicated elderly patient is first evaluated after admission to the hospital.

The cornerstones of an effective preoperative assessment are a complete history and physical examination. Unfortunately, the ability to obtain an adequate history may be limited in many elderly individuals. Some are reticent historians who under-report their illnesses, believing their problems to be due to "old age" rather than to potentially remediable disease processes.[69] Nearly 30% of elderly individuals have significant hearing deficits which may make effective communication between patients and physician either difficult or impossible.[5] Another 10% of elderly patients may have significant cognitive deficits from organic brain syndromes of various etiologies and as a result provide unreliable histories.[70] In these patients, critical historical data may have to be obtained from a spouse, close relative, or friend. Physical examination may also be more difficult and time-consuming with many elderly patients. Limited patient mobility and, in some, difficulty following instructions, may prove frustrating to both patient and physician.

Preoperative assessment of the elderly patient should routinely include a complete blood count, measurements of renal function, serum electrolytes and glucose, liver function tests, urinalysis, chest radiograph, and ECG. In younger surgical patients with a normal history and physical examination, there is both concern and evidence that many of these tests yield few significant abnormalities and are wasteful of limited health resources.[71,72] Whether all of these tests have a desirable cost/benefit ratio in elderly patients with a normal history and physical examination is not currently known. However, the yield of abnormalities on preoperative laboratory screening is much higher in elderly patients than in younger patients, and it appears that some of this information is clinically useful. For example, the frequency of significant abnormalities (eg, arrhythmias, ST segment and T wave abnormalities, left ventricular hypertrophy, evidence of myocardial infarction, conduction abnormalities, etc) on routine ECGs in hospitalized medical and surgical patients is only 5% in those under age 65, but is 50% or more in patients aged 65 years and over.[73,74] An abnormal routine preoperative ECG only occasionally results in a delay or cancellation of surgery, generally in those patients found to have had a silent myocardial infarction (1% of all patients over age 65 in a recent surgical series).[74] However, the preoperative ECG does serve as a very useful base line which can be compared with postoperative ECGs obtained when complications occur. Additionally, arrhythmias[41,42] and perhaps ST segment abnormalities on preoperative ECGs[75] may help to further stratify elderly surgical patients into a higher postoperative cardiac risk category and thereby guide the intensity of postoperative monitoring of these patients.[74,76]

Many elderly patients will require a preoperative chest film to help evaluate known cardiac or pulmonary disease. However, even in those elderly preoperative patients lacking apparent medical indication for a chest film, nearly 40% may prove to have significant, unsuspected abnormalities.[77] Although it is not known how much discovery of these abnormalities influences perioperative management, it is probably worthwhile at this time to obtain routine preoperative chest films on all patients over age 70.

Routine urinalysis is an important screening procedure for elderly patients who are to undergo urologic surgery. The prevalence of urinary tract infections, many of which are asymptomatic, is 20% in the ambulatory elderly and 30% to 50% in the institutionalized elderly.[78] Urinary tract infections are a major source of bacteremia in urologic and other surgical patients and may also contribute to postoperative wound infections.[79,80] Those discovered preoperatively should be vigorously treated.

Some clinicians have recommended more extensive medical preoperative assessment for all elderly patients, including either routine preoperative invasive monitoring with pulmonary artery catheters[81] or extensive radiologic evaluations with upper and lower GI series, intravenous pyelograms (IVP), and gallbladder visualization, even in the absence of suspicious symptoms.[81] There is clearly insufficient evidence to recommend either of these approaches on a routine basis.

Preoperative assessment of elderly patients should uncover not only medical illnesses but also psychological disturbances and social problems which may influence surgical and postoperative management. Some form of significant psychological disturbance is found in 25% of the ambulatory elderly over age 65, including 10% with clinically manifest depression and 5% with senile dementia.[3,82] These illnesses could have an important bearing on postoperative recovery. Social problems may also be of major importance in many elderly patients. Among the noninstitutionalized elderly, 20% of those aged 75 to 84 years and 31% of those over age 85 are essentially housebound and unable to carry on major activities such as housework.[5] Up to 18% of the elderly over age 85 are unable to adequately perform activities of daily living.[5] The effects of surgery and hospitalization may further compromise the ability of these patients to function independently when they return home. Such high-risk patients must be recognized preoperatively and appropriate arrangements made to assure they will have adequate social as well as medical support on discharge from the hospital.

The physician preparing an elderly patient for urologic or general surgery must pay special attention to several problem areas. The sections that follow review each problem area with respect to preoperative assessment, necessary postoperative monitoring, and potential postoperative complications and their management.

Cardiovascular Disorders

Cardiovascular complications (myocardial infarction, congestive heart failure, and sudden death) account for about one third of the operative mortality in elderly patients undergoing either general or urologic surgery.[7,9,17,32–35] Twelve percent of patients over 65 years of age and more than 20% of patients over 75 may experience serious postoperative cardiac complications following general surgery.[83] This frequency is primarily related to the high prevalence of organic heart disease in the elderly population in combination with the functional insults to the cardiovascular system induced by anesthesia and surgery. In autopsy series, 70% of individuals over age 70 show evidence of significant cardiac pathology, primarily coronary artery disease (20% to 40%), hypertensive heart disease (20%), and significant valvular heart disease (10% to 12%); one third of these subjects have more than one type of cardiac pathology.[84,85] The clinically manifest prevalence of heart disease is slightly lower and estimated to be 40% in the population over age 65.[86,87] It is not clear whether age, in the absence of clinically manifest heart disease, is an independent risk factor for postoperative cardiac complications. Some studies have noted a correlation,[41,42] while others have found none.[88]

The ASA Physical Status Scale (Table 23-1) correlates well with overall operative mortality and morbidity but is only a fair predictor of cardiovascular complications.[41] A multifactorial cardiac risk index developed by Goldman and coworkers may provide a better assessment of perioperative cardiac risk in patients of all ages.[41,42,89] From a prospective study of 1001 surgical patients, one third of whom were over 70 years old, they identified nine independent risk factors for perioperative cardiac mortality and morbidity using multivariate discriminant analysis.[41,42] These are listed in Table 23-3 according to their predictive value. Surgery in the face of gross preoperative congestive heart failure (S_3 gallop, elevated jugular venous pressure) or a recent myocardial infarction in the previous 6 months carried the greatest risk. The arrhythmias listed in Table 23-3 do not appear to be intrinsically dangerous, but instead derive their risk correlations from their association with underlying organic heart disease. Age was an independent risk factor in this study, with a frequency of perioperative cardiac death ten times greater in patients over 70 years old than under age 70. Nonthoracoabdominal surgery carried a three- to fourfold lower risk than procedures which invaded the thoracic or peritoneal cavities, perhaps due in part to lesser increases in postoperative total body

Table 23-3
Cardiac Risk Factors for Noncardiac Surgery

Factors	Relative Risk Points
Preoperative S_3 gallop or jugular venous distention	11
Myocardial infarction in previous 6 months	10
Five or more premature ventricular beats/min at any time before surgery	7
Rhythm other than sinus or presence of premature atrial beats on preoperative ECG	7
Age >70 years	5
Emergency surgery	4
Intrathoracic, intraperitoneal, or aortic surgery	3
Significant aortic stenosis	3
Poor general medical condition *a.* pO_2 <60, P_{CO_2} >50 *b.* Potassium <3.0 mEq/L, HCO_3 <20 mEq/L BUN >50 mg/dL, creatinine >3.0 mg/dL *c.* Elevated liver function tests or chronic liver disease *d.* Chronic bedridden status	3

Adapted from Goldman et al.[41]

and myocardial oxygen consumption. Perioperative cardiac death was four times more common after emergency surgery than after elective operations. With respect to valvular heart disease, only significant aortic stenosis was correlated with perioperative cardiac death; other valvular heart disease did, however, increase the risk of postoperative congestive heart failure. Poor general medical condition, defined in this study as electrolyte abnormalities, azotemia, liver dysfunction, hypoxemia or hypercarbia, or a chronically bedridden status, was also a risk factor. Chronic stable angina pectoris was not a significant independent risk factor in this study or in several other investigations.[88,90] Though little data are available, most clinicians consider the patient with unstable angina to be at high risk, similar to the risk of a patient with a recent myocardial infarction.[89] From these nine independent risk factors, the investigators devised a quantitative "risk index" to estimate perioperative cardiac morbidity and mortality (Table 23-4).[41] Points are assigned to each risk factor according to its predictive value on multivariate discriminant analysis. Patients are stratified according to their point totals into one of four classes, I to IV, of progressively increasing cardiac risk. Preliminary reports of recent prospective studies suggest that this risk index is clinically useful.[89] Because of their tremendous risk of death, class IV patients should probably undergo an operative procedure only when the surgical illness is life-threatening. Many class III and all class IV patients should have intraoperative and postoperative hemodynamic monitoring.[89]

Several excellent monographs are available which further review the management of patients with cardiac disease who undergo noncardiac surgery.[52,67,89,91]

Ischemic heart disease in the postoperative period As previously discussed, during the postoperative period total body and myocardial oxygen consumption may increase significantly while oxygen transport decreases. As a result, those patients with already compromised myocardial blood flow from coronary artery disease may be further predisposed after surgery to the development of myocardial ischemia. The overall incidence of postoperative myocardial infarction following general surgery in patients over age 65 to 70 years is in the range of 2% to 4%.[41,42,83] This incidence is more than four times higher than that found in younger patients[42] and reflects the high prevalence of coronary artery disease in the elderly population. Most elderly persons with coronary artery disease are asymptomatic. While only 10% of unselected elderly subjects in the community give a history consistent with symptomatic angina pectoris,[92] nearly 50% of persons over age 70 have evidence of ischemic heart disease when subjected to exercise stress testing.[93] This large reservoir of asymptomatic coronary artery disease in the elderly may explain why age appears to independently increase the risk of postoperative myocardial infarction and cardiac death.

The incidence of postoperative myocardial infarction in elderly persons following urologic surgery is not well defined. While cardiac complications account for 20% to 50% of the operative mortality of urologic procedures,[32-35] most studies do not state what percentage of the cardiac mortality is due specifically to myocardial infarction or what criteria were used to make the diagnosis. The incidence likely varies considerably with the type of surgery performed. Urologic procedures involving an abdominal or flank incision increase total body and myocardial oxygen consumption to a greater extent than transurethral procedures and will more likely be complicated by postoperative myocardial ischemia.

It is important for the physician to be aware of the clinical characteristics of

Table 23-4
Multifactorial Cardiac Risk Index in Noncardiac Surgery

Class	Total Points	No or Minor Cardiac Complications	Life-threatening Cardiac Complications	Cardiac Death
I	0–5	99%	0.7%	0.2%
II	6–12	93%	5%	2%
III	13–25	86%	11%	2%
IV	≥26	22%	22%	56%

Adapted from Goldman et al.[41]

postoperative myocardial infarctions.[89] Fifty percent occur without chest pain, perhaps due in part to the pain-suppressing effects of analgesic medications given for incisional pain. Postoperative myocardial infarction may instead present as new or increased congestive heart failure, hypotension, arrhythmias (especially sinus tachycardia and atrial or ventricular arrhythmias), altered mental status, or stroke. It is not known whether these atypical presentations are more commonly seen in elderly patients. The peak time risk for myocardial infarction is between the third and fifth days following surgery when total body and myocardial oxygen consumption are usually maximal; 90% of the infarctions occur during the first week.[89] Elderly patients considered to be at high risk for myocardial ischemia should therefore be followed carefully for at least the first week after surgery.[89]

The multifactorial risk index developed by Goldman et al is the best available predictor of postoperative myocardial infarction risk (Table 23-4).[89] Of these factors, myocardial infarction within 6 months of surgery is the most important single risk. In several studies, the risk of reinfarction and cardiac death following surgery performed within 3 months of infarction is about 30%.[42,88,90] This decreases to 15% at 3 to 6 months and stabilizes at 5% to 10% beyond 6 months.[89] These figures compare to a 0.2% to 0.6% risk of postoperative myocardial infarction in the entire surgical population.[94] The mortality of postoperative reinfarction is a staggering 50% to 70%.[89] Recent studies suggest that intensive intraoperative and postoperative management using hemodynamic monitoring may decrease the mortality rate to under 10% for surgery performed within 6 months of infarction.[89] With respect to urologic surgery, it is notable that transurethral procedures carried only a 4% operative mortality when performed within 6 months of infarction, probably reflecting the reduced need for an increase in myocardial oxygen consumption in nonthoracoabdominal procedures.[88,95] Still, this is a fourfold greater risk than these procedures usually carry, and they should not be performed within 6 months of an infarction unless the benefit clearly exceeds the risk.

A number of preventive measures should be taken to decrease the risk of postoperative myocardial infarction. These measures are summarized in Table 23-5. Preoperatively, elderly patients at risk for cardiac morbidity and mortality should be identified by history, physical examination, and ECG, according to the criteria of Goldman et al (Table 23-4).[41] If possible, those risk factors which are correctable or partially correctable should be adequately treated prior to surgery. Spinal anesthesia is no safer than general anesthesia.[89] For patients with class IV risk, and for those with class III risk with congestive heart failure, significant aortic stenosis, or myocardial infarction within 6 months, hemodynamic monitoring with an arterial line and Swan-Ganz catheter should be in-

Table 23-5
Prevention of Postoperative Myocardial Infarction After Noncardiac Surgery

Identification of patients at risk

Prophylactic hemodynamic monitoring and postoperative intensive care management if high risk

Serial postoperative ECGs

Maintenance of oxygen transport
- Hct > 30 vol %
- pO_2 > 60 torr
- Adequate intravascular volume replacement
- Inotropic therapy when necessary

Minimization of postoperative myocardial oxygen consumption
- Avoidance of hypothermia in recovery room
- Control of severe hypertension
- Adequate analgesia
- Prompt treatment of fever, infection

Continuance of preoperative antianginal medications postoperatively

Prior coronary arteriography and bypass surgery only if otherwise indicated

itiated prior to surgery and continued for at least 48 hours postoperatively.[89] Elderly patients with prolonged intraoperative hypotension (defined as a drop in systolic blood pressure from base line of ≥30% and a persistence for ≥10 minutes) are at considerable risk of postoperative infarction and should be monitored in an intensive care setting for several days. All class IV patients and the above listed class III patients with any significant postoperative complications should be observed in an intensive care unit for the first three to five days postoperatively.[52,88,89] Class III and IV patients should have routine ECGs on several, if not all, of the first three to five postoperative days.[52,89] Careful attention should be paid to maintenance of adequate oxygen transport whether or not hemodynamic monitoring is used. The hematocrit should be monitored frequently and maintained above 30% with transfusions. Such transfusions are frequently required for prostatic surgical procedures.[96] Arterial pO_2 should be measured and kept above 60 torr. Oxygen demand and myocardial oxygen consumption should be minimized postoperatively in high-risk patients. This may be accomplished by: (1) Avoidance of hypothermia in the operating and recovery rooms. As previously noted, hypothermia is more common in elderly patients.[64] (2) Monitoring blood pressure postoperatively and treating hypertension. (3) Maintaining adequate postoperative analgesia, but not at the expense of excessive sedation.[67] This will require careful titration of analgesics. (4) Prompt diagnosis and therapy of both fever and infection. Any antianginal medications prescribed preoperatively should be continued postoperatively. If the GI tract is functional, these may be administered orally or by nasogastric tube. If not, topical nitrates with appropriate monitoring may be administered, or even intravenous (IV) propranolol may be given, if necessary.[89]

Coronary arteriography and bypass surgery are generally recommended prior to noncardiac surgery only if they are already indicated independently of the noncardiac procedure.[89] Any contemplated corrective surgery, should be accomplished prior to the noncardiac surgery. However, for atherosclerotic renovascular surgery, some investigators have suggested prior surgical correction of any anatomically significant coronary and cerebrovascular lesion.[26]

Congestive heart failure in the postoperative period For patients over 65 years old undergoing general surgery, there is a 10% incidence of postoperative congestive heart failure.[83] The incidence may increase to 15% to 20% in patients over age 75.[83] Age over 60 years appears to be an important predictor of both postoperative congestive heart failure and/or pulmonary edema even in those patients with no prior history of heart failure.[42] Other important risk factors include the presence of congestive heart failure in the preoperative period, valvular heart disease of any type (20% incidence of new or worsening congestive heart failure), and surgery which requires either a thoracic or abdominal incision.[42,89] The severity of preoperative heart failure is a particularly important predictor of the occurrence of both postoperative cardiogenic pulmonary edema and cardiac mortality.[42,89] Even patients with a past history of congestive heart failure which might not be evident on preoperative evaluation still have a 6% incidence of pulmonary edema postoperatively.[42] However, patients with mild-to-moderate left ventricular failure before surgery may have a 16% incidence of postoperative pulmonary edema, and those with gross congestive heart failure (S_3 gallop and jugular venous distention) may have up to a 30% incidence of pulmonary edema and a mortality rate of 20%.[41,42,89]

Less data are available concerning the incidence of congestive heart failure following urologic surgery, and as expected the incidence may vary among the different urologic procedures. Congestive heart failure has occurred in from 4% to 8% of elderly patients having undergone total cystectomy for bladder carcinoma.[97,98] Even though it does not involve an abdominal incision, transurethral prostatic resection may also contribute to the development of postoperative congestive heart failure in those elderly patients with pre-existing heart disease. During this procedure, patients may rapidly absorb several liters of irrigant fluid or more with immediate postoperative weight gains of 2.5 kg or more.[32,99]

Postoperative congestive heart failure most frequently occurs either in the recovery room or 24 to 48 hours after surgery when sufficient time has elapsed for mobilization of third space fluid losses.[89] The most common precipitant proves to be excessive intravascular volume replacement,[89] often exacerbated by anemia due to blood loss. Despite these obvious perioperative events, the physician must be fully alert to the possibility of a silent myocardial infarction. If the new onset of heart failure is not readily explained by excessive fluid administration, serious consideration should be given to monitoring patients in an intensive care unit for 24 to 48 hours to rule out a myocardial infarction. Therapy to correct congestive heart failure would best be undertaken in the intensive care unit as well. Blood urea nitrogen and postural blood pressure measurements should be monitored to avoid excessive diuresis.[89] There remains considerable controversy about the use of digitalis preparations for congestive heart failure in the surgical setting.[52,89,100] Some recommend digitalization not only for patients with preoperative evidence of heart failure, but also for all those with a history of heart failure, valvular heart disease, or known pump dysfunction, even in the setting of a normal heart size.[52] Others suggest stopping digoxin preoperatively in patients with compensated heart failure and restarting it just prior to hospital discharge.[100] Patients with significant preoperative heart failure who must undergo major urologic procedures requiring an abdominal or flank incision should have intraoperative and postoperative hemodynamic monitoring.

Heart murmurs and management of valvular heart disease in the perioperative period The physician evaluating an elderly patient for surgery is frequently confronted by the presence of a heart murmur. Sixty percent of patients over 70 years and 80% of patients over 80 years have a systolic murmur heard at the base, apex, and/or left sternal border of the heart.[101,102] The physician must determine whether the murmur reflects hemodynamically significant valvular pathology which might require either intraoperative and postoperative hemodynamic monitoring or even cardiac catheterization and surgical correction prior to proceeding with the noncardiac surgical procedure. Additionally, the physician must decide whether to provide antibiotic prophylaxis against endocarditis prior to surgery.

Over 90% of the systolic murmurs heard in elderly patients do not reflect hemodynamically significant pathology.[102] Instead, they are generated by minor degenerative calcific or fibrotic changes in the aortic and/or mitral valves.[102] Several other entities which are clinically significant can also produce systolic murmurs in the elderly patient. These include mitral valve prolapse, mitral annular calcification, papillary muscle dysfunction, and hypertrophic obstructive cardiomyopathy.[103–105] Any of these lesions may be associated with hemodynamically significant mitral regurgitation. Patients with significant valvular heart disease have an overall 20% risk of developing new or increased congestive heart failure after general surgery.[89] As previously discussed, the risk and degree of monitoring required for an individual patient will depend on the presence and severity of preoperative heart failure and the type and extent of the surgical procedure.[89]

Aortic stenosis, however, is the most frequent form of serious valvular heart disease in the elderly with a prevalence of

4% in individuals over age 65.[87] In the series of Goldman et al, this lesion was an independent risk factor for postoperative cardiac death and carried an operative mortality of 13%.[42] Most patients with important aortic stenosis are symptomatic with angina pectoris, syncope, or congestive heart failure.[106] However, elderly patients may also have the same symptoms due to other kinds of organic heart disease,[106] and the classic signs of significant aortic stenosis (low systolic blood pressure, narrow pulse pressure, slow carotid upstroke, and long duration of murmur) are frequently absent in patients over age 65.[107] Echocardiography may be helpful in determining whether significant aortic stenosis is present. Goldman suggests the following approach to suspicious systolic ejection murmurs[89]:

1. If clinical and echocardiographic evaluation suggests insignificant aortic stenosis, the patient requires only antibiotic prophylaxis for endocarditis.
2. If the patient is asymptomatic but has potentially severe aortic stenosis, the type and extent of the surgery will dictate whether catheterization and possibly aortic valve replacement should precede noncardiac surgery. For most noncardiac surgery, these patients will not require catheterization. However, they should have hemodynamic monitoring during and after surgery. Some clinicians also suggest that these patients be digitalized preoperatively to prevent postoperative supraventricular tachyarrhythmias.
3. Patients who are symptomatic with potentially severe aortic stenosis should undergo catheterization and, if appropriate, should have valve replacement prior to noncardiac surgery.

Elderly patients with either valvular heart disease (including mitral valve prolapse when a systolic murmur is present), hypertrophic cardiomyopathy, or mitral annulus calcification require antibiotic prophylaxis against endocarditis prior to general surgery, particularly if there is drainage of an infected site or entry into the biliary or GI tract. The risks of endocarditis after urologic surgery are probably greater than for general surgery because of the increased frequency of transient bacteremia following a variety of urologic procedures (Table 23-6).[108] Prostatectomies and urinary catheterizations and dilatations are considered high-risk procedures for endocarditis, especially in the presence of infected urine. As previously noted, the elderly have a very high incidence of urinary tract infection even in the absence of urologic disease or manipulation.[78] The incidence of bacterial endocarditis following transurethral prostatic resection in the 1940s–prior to the use of antibiotic prophylaxis–was estimated at 0.1% in patients without valvular heart disease as opposed to nearly 10% in patients with valvular lesions.[108] For these reasons, elderly patients with valvular heart disease should routinely have a urine culture prior to urologic manipulation and appropriate antibiotic prophylaxis for endocarditis. Since the most common bacterial etiology of endocarditis following urologic surgery is the enterococcus,[108,109] the antibiotic regimen should consist of ampicillin (or vancomycin hydrochloride if

Table 23-6
Incidence of Bacteremia with Common Urologic Procedures

Procedure	Incidence (%)
Urethral catheterization	8
Catheter removal	2–30
Urethral dilation	10–33
Transurethral prostatic resection	32–46
Sterile urine	11
Infected urine	58
Retropubic prostatectomy	68
Sterile urine	13
Infected urine	82
Cystoscopy	0–22
Transrectal prostate biopsy	76

Adapted from Brown.[111]

the patient is penicillin-allergic) and gentamicin sulfate according to the recommendations of the American Heart Association.[109]

A more difficult question concerns whether elderly patients with systolic murmurs due to degenerative, fibrocalcific aortic and mitral valves should receive antibiotic prophylaxis against endocarditis. The incidence of infection of these valves, which are responsible for more than 90% of systolic murmurs in the elderly,[102] is not known. However, recent reviews of endocarditis in the elderly note that one quarter of the cases are nosocomially acquired with the most frequent predisposing factors being genitourinary (GU) surgery and contaminated IV lines.[110] The majority of these elderly patients did not have pre-existing, recognizable valvular heart disease. Some clinicians, therefore, have suggested antibiotic prophylaxis for all elderly individuals with murmurs due to "degenerative valvular disease."[111] Other authorities note that no firm guidelines are available.[112] The physician must individualize his decision empirically as to which patients with systolic murmurs require antibiotic prophylaxis or further evaluation to determine whether prophylaxis is needed.[112]

Blood pressure abnormalities in the perioperative period Perioperative problems with blood pressure regulation are more likely to be encountered in elderly patients than in younger patients. This is due to the increased prevalence of both hypertension and orthostatic hypotension with advancing age.[113]

Thirty percent of individuals over age 65 have diastolic hypertension and another 10% to 12% have pure systolic hypertension.[113] In more than one quarter of these elderly patients, the hypertension is either untreated or in poor control.[114] It is controversial whether mild to moderate hypertension at the time of surgery is a risk factor for postoperative cardiac complications.[42,75,88] Several recent studies suggest that preoperative hypertension is a significant risk factor.[75,88] In contrast, Goldman and coworkers found that hypertension alone, at least with preoperative diastolic blood pressure up to 110 mmHg, did not increase perioperative cardiac risk after controlling for other factors with multivariate analysis.[42,115] However, patients with treated or untreated hypertension do have increased lability of blood pressure both during the intraoperative and postoperative periods.[115,116] Nearly 25% of these patients will develop intraoperative hypotension requiring therapy, while another 25% will develop postoperative hypertension, usually in the recovery room or 24 to 48 hours after surgery.[89] Intraoperative hypotension especially appears to be an important risk factor for postoperative cardiac complications.[41,42,117] Elderly patients with hypertension must therefore be carefully monitored for both hypotension and hypertension during and for the first 72 hours after surgery, especially in the setting of known coronary or cerebrovascular disease.[52,89]

Ideally, patients should be made normotensive prior to surgery, but surgery need not be delayed as long as the diastolic pressure is less than 110 mmHg.[89] Antihypertensive medication should be continued up to the time of surgery and reinstituted postoperatively by mouth or by nasogastric tube when possible. Some patients may require parenteral antihypertensive therapy.[89] Because of alterations in intravascular volume status, the dose of antihypertensive medication may need to be readjusted postoperatively. Blood pressure control may also be improved by maintaining adequate analgesia and sedation.

Elderly patients should also be monitored preoperatively and postoperatively for postural hypotension. Thirty percent of ambulatory individuals over age 75 have a ≥20 mmHg drop in systolic blood pressure from the supine to the standing position.[113,118] Postural blood pressure decrements of this magnitude cause no symptoms under normal circumstances.

However, the blood pressure decrement may be greatly exacerbated postoperatively by prolonged bed rest and/or intravascular volume depletion, potentially resulting in orthostatic syncope or dizziness and a serious fall. The nursing staff should monitor supine, sitting, and standing blood pressures prior to ambulating elderly surgical patients.

Cardiac arrhythmias in the perioperative period It has been suggested that the presence of certain preoperative cardiac arrhythmias, including any baseline rhythm other than sinus mechanism, atrial ectopic beats, or documentation at any time of more than five ventricular ectopic beats per minute, may be associated with an increased risk of postoperative cardiac complications and death.[42] As the deaths in this series were due to myocardial infarction and/or congestive heart failure, it is presumed that these arrhythmias were markers of severe underlying organic heart disease, generally ischemic, rather than being intrinsically dangerous themselves.[89] Only one third of the patients in this series were over 65 to 70 years old. Moreover, the prevalence of all types of arrhythmias is greatly increased in the elderly population,[119-121] even in those elderly who appear to be free of significant organic heart disease.[119] It is therefore not known whether the correlation of preoperative arrhythmias and postoperative cardiac complications remains significant in the elderly population. Fleg and Kennedy found an 11% incidence of premature atrial contractions on the resting ECGs of healthy elderly subjects with no evidence of underlying ischemic heart disease as based on their normal maximal treadmill exercise tests and thallium scintigraphy.[119] Twenty percent of these subjects were also found to have more than 30 to 60 ventricular ectopic beats per hour during at least some hours of the day.[119] Other studies have also noted a lack of correlation between major ventricular arrhythmias and long-term cardiovascular prognosis in apparently healthy elderly subjects.[120,121] On the basis of this limited, indirect evidence, it would appear that elderly patients with these arrhythmias but no clinical evidence of heart disease may not be at greatly increased surgical risk.

Many elderly patients presenting for surgery have a prior history of arrhythmias for which they are taking antiarrhythmic medications. In general, these medications should be continued up to the time of surgery and restarted as soon as the patient is able to resume oral intake.[89] Use of prophylactic parenteral antiarrhythmic medications should be limited to those patients with a prior history of serious, symptomatic ventricular arrhythmias.[89] Some investigators also suggest that elderly patients with any prior history of paroxysmal supraventricular arrhythmias be treated prophylactically with digoxin before and after surgery even if they have not been maintained on this drug chronically.[89]

Age over 70 years may be a risk factor for the development of postoperative supraventricular arrhythmias. Goldman and coworkers found a 10% incidence of these arrhythmias following general surgery in patients over 70 years old as compared with a 4% incidence in their entire patient population.[42] These arrhythmias occurred most often after major thoracic or abdominal surgery and generally in the setting of other cardiopulmonary, infectious, or fluid-electrolyte complications.[89] Such complications should be searched out in patients experiencing postoperative supraventricular arrhythmias and corrected, if possible; this therapy may revert the arrhythmia back to sinus rhythm and eliminate the need for cardioversion with drugs or electricity.[89]

Venous Thromboembolism Following Urologic Surgery

The incidence of postoperative venous thromboembolism increases with age.[122]

This may result from several factors, including increased peripheral venous dilatation, decreased fibrinolytic activity, and greater venous stasis from more prolonged and severe immobility in elderly postoperative patients.[122]

Venous thromboembolism in urologic surgery patients has recently been reviewed.[36] The incidence of lethal pulmonary embolism is estimated at 1.1% to 2.2% and the incidence of nonlethal pulmonary embolism at 10% to 20% among patients undergoing urologic surgery.[36] As previously noted, pulmonary embolism has been reported to cause anywhere from 5% to 60% of the total operative mortality in urologic surgery.[32,37,38] Risk factors for venous thromboembolism following urologic surgery include age over 60 years, duration of anesthesia greater than one hour, obesity, presence of malignant disease, estrogen use, and the magnitude and duration of postoperative immobility.[36] The type of surgery is also an important determinant of venous thromboembolic risk. Open prostatectomy carries the greatest risk, with an incidence of deep venous thrombosis diagnosed by contrast venography of 16% to 21%.[36] Using radiofibrinogen leg scanning as the diagnostic technic, the incidence of deep venous thrombosis is 30% to 50% following open prostatectomy and 10% to 20% after transurethral resections.[36] Urologic surgery procedures involving the abdomen may also carry a greater thromboembolic risk than other general surgery procedures.[36,123]

It is not clear what form of prophylaxis for venous thromboembolism is most effective and least toxic in high-risk patients undergoing urologic surgery. Low-dose heparin sodium prophylaxis (5000 units subcutaneously two hours before surgery and every eight to 12 hours after surgery for several days) has been effective and well tolerated in some studies but ineffective and associated with increased hemorrhage in other studies.[36] Similar variability in results has been observed with the use of warfarin preoperatively and/or postoperatively.[36] Several investigators believe the most effective and least toxic prophylactic method for high-risk urologic surgery patients to be continuous external mechanical compression of the calves using a pneumatic compression sleeve initiated during surgery and maintained thereafter until the patient is fully ambulatory.[36,123] Unfortunately, this device is not always available. For those patients considered to be at high risk according to the previously listed risk factors, external mechanical compression should probably be utilized if available; otherwise, the physician must choose between low-dose heparin or warfarin and utilize simpler methods such as early ambulation and graded elastic antiembolism stockings.[124]

Venous thromboembolism should be diagnosed objectively. Contrast venography or the combination of impedance plethysmography and radiofibrinogen scanning may be used to diagnose deep venous thrombosis.[122] Pulmonary angiography may be required in addition to ventilation-perfusion scanning to confirm pulmonary embolism. Initial therapy for venous thromboembolism will generally be with heparin since thrombolytic agents are relatively contraindicated within ten days of surgery.[125] The risk of both major and minor hemorrhagic complications with heparin therapy is two to threefold greater in patients over age 60 than in younger patients.[126,127] The risk of hemorrhage is particularly increased in elderly females and in patients with serious underlying illness.[126,127] Specific orders should be written that heparinized patients receive no antiplatelet compounds and no intramuscular (IM) injections. Elderly postoperative patients on heparin should be monitored for blood loss with daily postural blood pressure measurements, hematocrits, platelet counts, and urine and stool specimens for heme. As discussed later in this review, special precautions should be taken with anticoagulated elderly patients to prevent potentially disastrous falls.

Infectious Complications

Infections are a major source of operative mortality and morbidity in both general and urologic surgery patients.[1,80] They are responsible for nearly one third of the mortality in elderly general surgery patients[7,9] and 12% to 30% of the mortality in series of urologic surgery patients.[32,35] Some of these infections may antedate the surgical procedure, but a majority are acquired nosocomially. There is a 13% incidence of nosocomially acquired infections in urologic surgery patients: 8% with urinary tract infections, 3.5% with wound infections, 1% with pneumonia, and 0.5% with bacteremia.[128] Age is strongly associated with the acquisition of nosocomial infections. Between the ages of 18 and 85 there is a fivefold increase in the incidence of urinary tract infections, a threefold increase in pneumonias, and a twofold increase in wound infections and bacteremia.[128] However, when subjected to multivariate analysis, age is much less a risk for nosocomial infections than other factors such as the nature and severity of the underlying illness, duration of preoperative hospitalization, duration of the surgical procedure, location of the operative incision, duration of urinary catheterization, and the presence of pre-existing infection.[129]

Urinary tract infections are the most common nosocomial infection and the primary source of bacteremia in urologic surgery patients.[79,128] This is likely related to the high prevalence of preoperative urinary tract infections in these patients, especially in those who are elderly,[78] the site of surgery, and the frequent need for prolonged postoperative urinary catheterization. Elderly urologic patients should routinely have preoperative urine cultures and appropriate antibiotic therapy for infection prior to instrumentation and surgery of the urinary tract. In those patients without a concurrent urinary tract infection, there is increasing evidence that prophylactic antibiotics given preoperatively may decrease the incidence of postoperative urinary tract infection and perhaps septic complications as well.[130,131] Catheters must be inserted aseptically and removed as soon as possible; daily meatal care by a variety of methods may be more harmful than helpful.[132] Gram-negative aerobic bacteria and enterococci are the most frequent pathogens.

The most important risk factor for postoperative pneumonia appears to be the site of the operative incision, with pneumonia incidence of 40%, 17%, and less than 5% after thoracic, upper abdominal, and lower abdominal or nonthoracoabdominal incisions, respectively.[133] Other risk factors include smoking, chronic pulmonary disease, serum albumin less than 2 g/dL, prolonged preoperative hospitalization, and duration of surgery greater than two hours; age may not be an independent risk factor.[133] Since a large proportion of urologic surgery procedures do not involve either an abdominal incision, or at least an upper abdominal incision, it is not surprising that the incidence of postoperative pneumonia is less than 5% after urologic surgery.[128] However, when it does occur, postoperative pneumonia carries a significant fatality rate of 15% to 50%.[9,133,134] Therefore, when suspected, the diagnosis should be promptly and vigorously pursued. Gram-negative aerobic bacteria, *Staphylococcus aureus*, and *Diplococcus pneumoniae* account for about 50%, 10%, and 5% of these pneumonias, respectively.[134]

The incidence of bacteremia after urologic surgery is about 0.5%.[128] The primary source of this bacteremia is the urinary tract. The clinical presentation of bacteremia in the elderly may be quite subtle.[135] The major presenting signs may be limited to unexplained confusion, lethargy, or only nonspecific, generalized deterioration. In one study, nearly 13% of elderly patients with bacteremia were afebrile; 40% of these patients were already on antibiotic therapy and 30% did not have an associated leukocytosis.[135] The physician must therefore suspect bacteremia in all elderly surgical patients with unexplained deterioration, even in the absence of fever and leukocytosis. These patients should be carefully evaluated by history, physical examination, and appropriate laboratory studies, including blood cultures. In many cases, consideration should be given to empiric antibiotic therapy pending culture results.[135,136]

Pulmonary Complications

Postoperative pulmonary complications (PPCs) include hypoxemia, acute bronchitis, atelectasis, pneumonia, and respiratory failure. The incidence of PPCs reported in studies in the literature varies widely, depending upon several factors including: (1) preoperative status of the patients, especially with respect to their pulmonary function; (2) type and distribution of surgical procedures performed, particularly the location of the incision relative to the diaphragm; (3) possibly the intensity of preoperative and/or postoperative pulmonary care; and (4) exactly how the PPCs are defined.[137,138] For example, with respect to the definition of PPCs, abnormalities noted on auscultation of the chest are twice as common as radiographic abnormalities on chest film, and four times as common as the occurrence of fever associated with a productive cough.[138]

Risk factors Chronic respiratory disease, particularly chronic obstructive pulmonary disease, is the most important risk factor and is associated with an overall three- to fourfold increase in risk of PPCs.[57,139] Among these patients, those with chronic hypercapnia ($P_{CO_2} > 45$ torr) appear to experience the most frequent and severe PPCs; some clinicians consider chronic hypercapnia a contraindication to all but lifesaving surgery if a thoracic or abdominal incision is required.[139] While spirometrically documented airway obstruction clearly predisposes to PPCs, there is no correlation between the magnitude of the obstruction detected and the frequency of PPCs, as long as preoperative hypercapnia is not present.[140,141] The location of the surgical incision is also an important determinant of the incidence of PPCs. For example, the incidence of atelectasis is 20% to 40% after upper abdominal surgery, 10% after lower abdominal surgery, and 1% after nonthoracoabdominal surgery.[53] Cigarette smoking alone, without associated obstructive lung disease, may double the frequency of PPCs.[142] Some investigators do not believe that age and obesity are risk factors independent of the other listed factors.[40,49,142] Age is associated with an increased prevalence of chronic obstructive pulmonary disease[143] and probably with greater postoperative immobility, and this may explain the association of age with PPCs. While regional anesthesia carries a lesser risk of PPCs, it is not clear that a difference exists between general and spinal anesthesia.[57]

Following general surgery in patients over age 65, the incidence of PPCs – specifically defined as two or more of the following: productive cough, fever of 38° C or over, and/or physical signs on examination of the chest not present preoperatively – has been reported as 40% in a recent prospective study.[83] In this study,PPCs were no more common in patients over age 75 than in the 65- to 74-year-old age group.[83] Unfortunately, the incidence of PPCs following urologic surgery has not been well defined by careful prospective investigation.[144] The risk will likely vary according to the factors described above. With respect to the type of procedure, the risk of PPCs should be greater with upper abdominal incisions than with flank or lower abdominal incisions, which in turn carry greater risks than transurethral procedures. The incidence of PPCs – often not defined – has been reported at 4% to 12% following cystectomy procedures involving a lower abdominal incision.[20,97,98,142] In contrast, the incidence of PPCs (defined as fever, purulent sputum, and altered chest physical findings) has been reported as less than 1% following transurethral procedures.[142]

Maneuvers to reduce PPCs Preoperatively, elderly patients should be screened carefully for pulmonary disease using the history, physical examination, and chest radiograph. Those with abnormal findings by any of these parameters and who will undergo flank or abdominal incisions should have preoperative spirometry and arterial blood gas measurements. Recent proposals that all patients over age 70 have preoperative screening spirometry,[139] regardless of the clinical findings and type of surgery to be performed, seem excessive.[141] Elderly patients who smoke should be strongly encouraged to stop for a few weeks or at least a few days prior to elective surgery. Elective surgery should be delayed for several weeks following any acute respiratory tract infection.[139] Elderly patients with significant chronic obstructive pulmonary disease should be treated with inhaled bronchodilators and perhaps theophylline preparations (with monitoring of serum theophylline concentrations) for at least 48 hours prior to elective surgery; however, it should be noted that there are conflicting results as to whether this therapy decreases the incidence of PPCs.[140,141,145] Prior to surgery, the elderly patient at high risk for PPCs because of underlying pulmonary disease and/or type of surgery planned and his family should be carefully educated about the importance of early ambulation, frequent position changes, coughing, deep breathing, chest physiotherapy, and the use of incentive spirometry.[57,139]

Postoperatively, elderly patients are at greater risk of hypoxemia because of their age-related increase in closing volume and reduction in arterial pO_2.[61] After nonthoracoabdominal surgery, arterial pO_2 will return to base line within 24 hours. In contrast, after abdominal surgery, arterial pO_2 may not reach its lowest value until 48 hours after surgery and may not return to base-line values for three to seven days.[61] Elderly patients, especially those with other risk factors for PPCs, should be maintained on oxygen therapy until arterial blood gas measurement confirms it is safe to discontinue the oxygen.[61]

It is important that analgesics be carefully titrated in the postoperative period. Elderly patients must have sufficient relief of incisional pain to facilitate coughing and deep breathing maneuvers. However, excessive sedation may further suppress cough and sigh mechanisms as well as inhibit or prevent early ambulation and cooperation with chest physiotherapy. Elderly patients appear to achieve more prolonged analgesia with a given dose of narcotic analgesic such as morphine or meperidine hydrochloride than do younger patients.[146] It is not clear if the magnitude of analgesia is greater in elderly patients.[147] It has been suggested that age be used as a guide to the dosing interval for narcotic analgesics rather than as a determinant of the dosage size.[146]

The efficacy of chest physiotherapy in the prophylaxis and treatment of atelectasis in surgical patients has not been confirmed; however, the trends in most studies suggest some benefit.[137] It is currently recommended that chest physiotherapy be initiated prophylactically in patients who produce copious amounts of sputum (>30 mL/d).[137,148,149] Chest physiotherapy is also likely to be beneficial in patients with established atelectasis.[148,149] Its routine use in other patients may not be indicated.[148,149] Because hypoxemia may follow the treatment, patients with obstructive lung disease should receive supplemental oxygen during and after chest physiotherapy for at least several hours.[48]

There are conflicting results about the efficacy of incentive spirometry in the prophylaxis and therapy of postoperative atelectasis.[144] However, it is inexpensive, easy to perform, and may be beneficial if performed properly.[150] Effective use requires that the patient mimic the normal sigh mechanism which is often inactive in the postoperative period. The patient should take at least ten breaths with the incentive spirometer each hour, with volumes documented to be at least 50% of the predicted normal vital capacity (ie, each breath should be at least 2.0 to 2.5 L).[150] Physicians, nurses, respiratory therapists, and family members will often have to encourage the patient to fulfill these minimal requirements.

Central Nervous System Complications

Postoperative delirium and depression Psychiatric symptoms and signs following surgery are a serious problem for several reasons.[151] Delirium and confusion may constitute the first indication of a complicating physical illness such as a postoperative infection or electrolyte abnormality. Second, the postoperative psychiatric illness may itself require treatment. Finally, postoperative psychiatric problems, either delirium or depression, may diminish the patient's ability to comply with postoperative therapy such as ambulation, chest physiotherapy, IV lines, and urinary catheters. In one large study of elderly general surgery patients where overall operative mortality was 10%, operative mortality in the setting of preoperative dementia was nearly 45%.[16] The high mortality in these patients may have been due in part to decreased compliance with postoperative rehabilitation measures.

The reported incidence of postoperative delirium in elderly patients following general surgery varies from 5% to 30%,[16,40,152–157] with several recent studies noting incidences in the range of 10% to 15%.[16,83,151] The frequency of postoperative depression in the elderly has been less well studied; a recent study noted an incidence of about 7%.[151] Few studies are available specifically concerning psychiatric morbidity in elderly patients following urologic surgery. Rollason et al reported a 7.4% incidence of postoperative confusion in patients undergoing prostatectomy, but the mean age of the patients in this study was just above 60 years.[153]

The natural history of postoperative delirium will, of course, vary with its etiology. When it occurs, delirium most often has its onset between one and four days following surgery, lasts two to five days, and resolves within 1 week.[40,151,154] On occasion, postoperative delirium may persist for several weeks.[151,155] Nearly two thirds of these patients may remain "quietly confused," while the other one third are more agitated and cause serious management difficulties.[151]

The pathogenesis of postoperative delirium has not been fully delineated and is likely multifactorial with respect to both causative and potentiating factors. Advancing age appears to be an important predisposing factor.[83,151,152] It is not clear whether this association is due to coexisting preoperative cognitive dysfunction since some studies have not found a relationship between preoperative intellectual status and postoperative psychiatric morbidity.[151] Significant dementia is a predisposing factor to postoperative delirium in most studies.[16,152] Elderly patients with even mild dementia may develop severe confusion in response to usually well-tolerated stimuli such as postoperative fever, mild-to-moderate anemia or hypoxemia, or simple change in environmental surroundings. Cerebral hypoxia may also be a contributing factor to postoperative delirium.[16,154] In elderly general surgery patients Palmberg and Hirsjärvi[16] found that postoperative confusion correlated strongly with intraoperative blood loss and somewhat less strongly with the occurrence of intraoperative hypotension. The incidence was 10.7% for intraoperative blood loss less than 400 mL but increased to 50% for 800 to 1200 mL blood loss.[16] The high frequency of sensory impairment in the elderly—nearly two thirds have significant impairment of vision or hearing—may predispose elderly patients to postoperative sensory deprivation and subsequent delirium.[69,70] The type and duration of anesthesia may not correlate with the incidence of postoperative delirium.[16,83]

It is important to thoroughly evaluate all patients with postoperative delirium for a variety of causative and potentiating factors (Table 23-7). In nearly one half of elderly patients with postoperative delirium, the syndrome is the initial presenting manifestation of complicating physical illness.[151] Fever and infections are common etiologies. As previously discussed, bacteremia may present with postoperative confusion or lethargy even in the absence of fever and leukocytosis.[135] Silent myocardial infarction may present with confusion in the elderly.[158] In susceptible elderly patients, cerebral hypoxia and confusion may result from various combinations of hypoxemia, anemia, and congestive heart failure. Because of altered pharmacokinetics and increased intrinsic sensitivity, elderly patients (especially those with base-line cognitive impairments) may develop confusional syndromes from narcotic analgesics, benzodiazepines, and barbiturates.[70] Alcoholism is relatively prevalent among the elderly and the possibility of alcohol withdrawal must also be considered in confused postoperative elderly patients.[159]

In elderly patients undergoing transurethral resection of the prostate, hyponatremia is a common cause of postoperative delirium.[160] The hyponatremia is dilutional resulting from the excessive absorption of prostate irrigant fluid. Some patients may absorb between 1 and 8 L of irrigant fluid abruptly dropping serum sodium to values as low as 88 to 124 mEq/L.[160] Risk factors for this complication include advancing age, increasing prostate size, and prolonged resection time.[160] Two to ten hours following surgery, patients may develop nausea, vomiting, confusion, and agitation, or may even progress to seizures and coma from the cerebral edema. Prompt diagnosis and treatment with hypertonic saline will generally reverse these manifestations.[160]

Table 23-7
Factors Which May Contribute to Postoperative Delirium

Preoperative cognitive impairment
Major sensory impairments in hearing, vision
Cerebral hypoxia
Intraoperative blood loss and/or hypotension
Anemia
Arterial hypoxemia
Silent myocardial infarction with heart failure
Fever
Infection
Drug toxicity from analgesics or sedative-hypnotics
Electrolyte disorders
Stroke
Alcohol withdrawal

Maneuvers to reduce postoperative delirium Preoperatively, elderly patients should be carefully assessed for cognitive impairment as a risk factor for postoperative delirium. This evaluation constitutes an important but often neglected base line for later reference. Ten percent of individuals over age 65 and 30% over age 85 will be found to have some form of cognitive impairment.[70,82] Families should be advised prior to surgery of the possible occurrence of postoperative confusion. Prophylactic measures of potential, but not proven, benefit in the postoperative period include frequent orientation of the patient to his surroundings, minimizing sensory impairments by early restoration of hearing aids and spectacles, asking family members to stay close at hand to increase the patient's sense of security, and placement of high-risk elderly patients in rooms close to the nurses' station.[161] To the degree possible, the exacerbating factors listed in Table 23-7 should be avoided or corrected, should they occur. Should serious confusion appear, evaluation should be prompt and thorough. Only severely agitated patients should receive major tranquilizers (for example, haloperidol or thioridazine) and then in low doses and for limited periods of time; benzodiazepines are probably best avoided, although there are no solid data to support the use of major as opposed to minor tranquilizers.[161] Restraints are rarely necessary, but if used, must be continuously monitored by a staff member who reassesses their need each shift.[161]

Cerebrovascular complications There are no specific data concerning the incidence of perioperative stroke in patients undergoing urologic surgery, but it is probably similar to the 0.3% incidence reported in general surgery patients.[162] Risk factors for perioperative stroke in general surgery patients have not been well delineated. Most recent studies suggest that the presence of an asymptomatic carotid bruit does not predict perioperative stroke risk, which is equal in patients with and without bruits.[162–164] Similarly, noninvasive evaluation of the carotid arteries of patients with asymptomatic bruits does not reveal subgroups of patients at higher risk for perioperative stroke. This is important information, since the prevalence of carotid bruits is about 12% in patients with a mean age of 70 years about to undergo a general surgical procedure.[164]

It is not known if patients with recent or frequent transient ischemic attacks are at increased risk of perioperative stroke. These patients may require neurologic consultation and more extensive cerebrovascular evaluation and therapy prior to undergoing major general or urologic surgical procedures.[164]

Drug Therapy

As reviewed in a previous chapter, elderly patients are at increased risk for adverse drug reactions. On general surgical wards, there is a progressive increase with age in the number of drug exposures.[165] The incidence of adverse drug reactions on surgical wards has been reported at 2.5% when patients of all ages are considered[165] and 6.0% in elderly patients over age 65.[157] While nausea, vomiting, constipation, and diarrhea are the most common adverse drug effects, there is also a nearly 10% incidence of drowsiness and disorientation.[165] The drugs most commonly responsible for adverse drug reactions on surgical wards include hydrochlorothiazide, warfarin, codeine, and a variety of antibiotics.[165] Most fatal drug reactions in surgical patients are due to heparin therapy, usually in elderly females.[166,167]

With all drugs given to elderly surgical patients, the specific geriatric pharmacology and possible adverse effects of the drug must be carefully considered prior to initiating therapy. For some drugs, like gentamicin, monitoring of serum levels, if available, may be invaluable.[168]

Iatrogenic Complications

Thirty to forty percent of elderly patients will experience iatrogenic complications during hospitalization.[157,169,170] These complications and their reported incidences are listed in Table 23-8. The incidence clearly increases with age in medical patients,[157,169] although no definite relation to age has yet been documented in surgical patients.[157] Some iatrogenic complications in elderly patients may not be entirely avoidable. However, the incidence of falls in particular may be minimized by identifying patients at high risk who have confusion, difficulties with balance and vision, or postural blood pressure decrements.[171] These patients and their families should be cautioned about the danger of falls should they arise

Table 23-8
Iatrogenic Complications in Hospitalized Elderly Patients

Complications	Incidence (%)
Adverse reaction to diagnostic or therapeutic procedure	18
Hospital-acquired infection	16
Falls	13
Adverse drug reactions	6
Decubitus ulcers	4.5

Adapted from Jahnigen et al,[157] Reichel,[170] and Rueler and Cooney.[172]

during the early postoperative period without assistance. They should be closely monitored in rooms near the nursing station, and bed rails should be maintained in the upright position. Postural blood pressure should be measured daily. Sedation and analgesia should be cautiously titrated to avoid confusion. Elderly patients should routinely have assistance with postoperative ambulation. The incidence of decubitus ulcers may be reduced by daily inspection of sacrum, hips, ankles, and heels for evidence of cutaneous irritation, frequent turning, elimination of excessive moisture (using temporary urinary catheters and rectal tubes, if necessary), and use of sheepskin pads and/or water mattresses.[172] The potential adverse reactions to all diagnostic and therapeutic procedures must always be considered prior to initiating them, especially in elderly patients.

Discharge Planning

Postsurgical convalescence and rehabilitation in the elderly may be seriously hampered by the interaction of adverse social and medical circumstances. Even without surgery, among the noninstitutionalized elderly, 20% of those aged 75 to 84 years and 30% of those over 80 years are essentially housebound and unable to carry on major activities such as housework or driving a car.[3] Nearly 20% of elderly individuals over age 85 and living at home have serious difficulties with basic activities of daily living including dressing, ambulating, preparing and eating food, and regulating excretory functions.[3] Following surgery, it may require elderly patients 4 to 6 months to fully recover medically, psychologically, and socially.[2,65] As a result, some elderly patients previously able to function on an independent basis at home may no longer be able to do so after surgery, either on a temporary or permanent basis.

Physicians caring for elderly surgical patients must determine the optimal disposition for each patient on discharge from the hospital. This requires careful assessment of the patient's functional as well as disease status before and following surgery. The physician must have precise knowledge of what activities the patient can and cannot accomplish including correct administration of medications, care of wound dressings, and performance of activities of daily living. It is also important for the physician to determine the home circumstances to which the patient will return. Specifically, the following questions need to be answered[2]:

1. How much care will the patient require?
2. Who at home will be able to provide this care? Is the spouse living, able, and willing to accomplish the necessary tasks? Are there children who may help, and if so, to what degree?
3. Are there environmental hazards in the home (eg, stairs) which may present a danger to the patient?
4. How reliable will the patient and his family be in administering needed medications and wound dressings?

These questions should be addressed as soon as possible after admission to the hospital. It appears that a considerable number of days in acute care hospitals are needlessly wasted by delays in disposition planning for elderly patients.[3] The physician's functional assessment and discharge planning may frequently benefit from consultation with an expert social worker, occupational therapist, and clinical pharmacist.

Many elderly patients will be able to return home without outside assistance, while others will require mobilization of family and/or community resources such as home nursing, homemakers, and/or meals on wheels. A few elderly patients may benefit from nursing home placement for a period of time. However, discharge to a nursing home should be utilized only after a thorough assessment suggests the patient cannot get adequate care at home even with outside assistance.

THE DECISION TO OPERATE

The eventual decision on whether to perform surgery on an elderly patient requires careful analysis of a number of factors.[2] There are several critical considerations to be answered by the physicians caring for an elderly patient[2]:

1. What is the elderly patient's life expectancy if surgery is not done? This will depend on the patient's chronologic age and on the nature and severity of his surgical and medical illnesses.
2. Will successful surgery significantly improve the patient's quality of life? If surgery is not done, will the patient's quality of life further deteriorate?
3. What are the risks of surgery in terms of mortality and morbidity? This will depend not just on the mortality figures for a procedure published in the literature, but also on the surgical experience and expertise at a given institution and on the health status of the individual patient at the time of surgery.
4. Should the operation be elective and soon, or should it wait until an acute problem or complication develops?

In many cases, the answers to these questions are not known with certainty for individual patients. Here, the clinical judgment of the surgeon, anesthesiologist, and internist must be effectively communicated to the elderly patient and his family, so that an informed decision can be made.

REFERENCES

1. Greenburg AG, Saik RP, Farris JM, et al: Operative mortality in general surgery. *Am J Surg* 1982;144:22–28.
2. Vowles KDJ: Surgery for the aged, in Vowles KDJ (ed): *Surgical Problems in the Aged.* Bristol, John Wright, 1979, pp 1–11.
3. Ouslander JG, Beck JC: Defining the health problems of the elderly. *Annu Rev Public Health* 1982;3:55–83.
4. Shaldon C: Urological problems, in Vowles KDJ (ed): *Surgical Problems in the Aged.* Bristol, John Wright, 1979, pp 127–137.
5. Lowenstein SR, Schrier RW: Social and political aspects of aging, in Schrier, RW (ed): *Clinical Internal Medicine in the Aged.* Philadelphia, WB Saunders, 1982, pp 1–23.
6. Linn BS, Linn MW, Wallen N: Evaluation of results of surgical procedures in the elderly. *Ann Surg* 1982;195:90–96.
7. Seymour DG, Pringle R: A new method of auditing surgical mortality rates: application to a group of elderly general surgical patients. *Br Med J [Clin Res]* 1982;1:1539–1542.
8. Hirsh RA: An approach to assessing perioperative risk, in Goldmann DR, Brown FH, Levy WK, et al (eds): *Medical Care of the Surgical Patient.* Philadelphia, JB Lippincott, 1982, pp 31–39.
9. Djokovic JL, Hedley-Whyte J: Prediction of outcome of surgery and anesthesia in patients over 80. *JAMA* 1979;242:2301–2306.
10. Feigal DW, Blaisdell FW: The estimation of surgical risk. *Med Clin North Am* 1979;63:1131–1143.
11. Goldman L: Letter. *N Engl J Med* 1978; 298:340.
12. Marx GF, Mateo CV, Orkin LR: Computer analysis of postanesthetic deaths. *Anesthesiology* 1973; 39:54–58.
13. Ziffren SE: Comparison of mortality rates for various surgical operations according to age groups, 1951–1977. *J Am Geriatr Soc* 1979;27:433–438.
14. Mohr DN: Estimation of surgical risk in the elderly: a correlative review. *J Am Geriatr Soc* 1983;31:99–102.
15. Palmberg S, Hirsjärvi E: Mortality in geriatric surgery with special reference to the type of surgery, anesthesia, complicating diseases and prophylaxis of thrombosis. *Gerontology* 1979;25:103–112.
16. Palmberg S, Hirsjärvi E: Surgical management of the very old, in Andrews J, von Hahn HP (eds): *Geriatrics for Everyday Practice.* Basel, S Karger, 1981, pp 168–184.

17. Lewin I, Lerner AG, Green SH, et al: Physical class and physiologic status in prediction of operative mortality in the aged sick. *Ann Surg* 1971;174:217–231.
18. Mason JH, Gau FC, Byrne MP: General surgery, in Steinberg, FU (ed): *Cowdry's the Care of the Geriatric Patient*, ed 6. St Louis, CV Mosby, 1983, pp 299–326.
19. Wheatley JK: Urology, in Lubin MF, Walker HK, Smith RB (eds): *Medical Management of the Surgical Patient.* Boston, Butterworths, 1982, pp 811–830.
20. Thomas DM, Riddle PR: Morbidity and mortality in 100 consecutive radical cystectomies. *Br J Urol* 1982;54:716–719.
21. Johnson DE, Lamy SM: Complications of a single stage radical cystectomy and ileal conduit diversion: Review of 214 cases. *J Urol* 1977;117:171–173.
22. Drago JR, Rohner TJ: Cystectomy and urinary diversion: a safe procedure for elderly patients. *Urology* 1983;21:17–19.
23. Zincke H: Cystectomy and urinary diversion in patients eighty years or older. *Urology* 1982;19:139–142.
24. Osborn DE, Honan RP, Palmer MK, et al: Factors influencing salvage cystectomy results. *Br J Urol* 1982;54:122–125.
25. Franklin SS, Young JD, Maxwell MH, et al: Operative morbidity and mortality in renovascular disease. *JAMA* 1975;231:1148–1153.
26. Novick AC, Straffon RA, Stewart BH, et al: Diminished operative morbidity and mortality in renal revascularization. *JAMA* 1981;246:749–753.
27. Geyskes GG, Paylaert CBA, Oei HY, et al: Follow up study of 70 patients with renal artery stenosis treated by percutaneous transluminal dilatation. *Br Med J [Clin Res]* 1983;287:333–336.
28. Sos TA, Pickering TG, Sniderman K, et al: Percutaneous transluminal angioplasty in renovascular hypertension due to atheroma or fibromuscular dysplasia. *N Engl J Med* 1983;309:274–279.
29. Grim CE, Luft FC, Yune HY, et al: Percutaneous transluminal dilatation in the treatment of renal vascular hypertension. *Ann Intern Med* 1981;95:439–442.
30. Steinmuller DR: Evaluation and selection of candidates for renal transplantation. *Urol Clin North Am* 1983;10:217–229.
31. Sommer BG, Sutherland DER, Simmons RL, et al: Prognosis after renal transplantation: Cumulative influence of combined risk factors. *Transplantation* 1979;27:4–7.
32. Wittels E, Wright KE: Cardiovascular complications of urologic surgery. *Urol Clin North Am* 1976;3:225–237.
33. Natoli C: Causes of death in urologic patients. *J Urol* 1960;84:420–423.
34. Lurie A, Fischelovitch J, Lazebnik J: Overall mortality in urologic patients. *J Urol* 1971;106:409–411.
35. Sakati I, Marshall V: Postoperative fatalities in urology. *J Urol* 1966;95:412–420.
36. Moser KM: Thromboembolic disease in the patient undergoing urologic surgery. *Urol Clin North Am* 1983;10:101–108.
37. Antila LE, Markkula H, Iisalo E: Ten years' experience of geriatric aspects in surgery of patients with benign prostatic hyperplasia. *Acta Chir Scand* 1966;357 (suppl):95–97.
38. Erlik D, Valero A, Birkham J, et al: Prostatic surgery and the cardiovascular patient. *Br J Urol* 1968;40:53–61.
39. Blake R, Lynn J: Emergency abdominal surgery in the aged. *Br J Surg* 1976;63:956–960.
40. Johnson JC: Surgery in the elderly, in Goldman DR, Brown FH, Levy WK, et al (eds): *Medical Care of the Surgical Patient.* Philadelphia, JB Lippincott, 1982, pp 578–590.
41. Goldman L, Caldera DL, Nussbaum SR, et al: Multifactorial index of cardiac risk in noncardiac surgical procedures. *New Engl J Med* 1977;297:845–850.
42. Goldman L, Caldera DL, Nussbaum SR, et al: Cardiac risk factors in noncardiac surgery. *Medicine* 1978;57:357–370.
43. Shock NW: Aging of physiological systems. *J Chronic Dis* 1983;36:137–142.
44. Gilchrest BA, Rowe JW: The biology of aging, in Rowe JW, Besdine RW (eds): *Health and Disease in Old Age.* Boston, Little Brown & Co, 1982, pp 15–24.
45. Dripps RD, Eckenhoff JE, Vandam LD: Physical status and risk, in Dripps RD, Eckenhoff JE, Vandam LT (eds): *Introduction to Anesthesia,* ed 5. Philadelphia, WB Saunders 6, 1977, pp 13–15.
46. Lakatta EG: Determinants of cardiovascular performance: modification due

to aging. *J Chronic Dis* 1983;36:15–30.

47. Lakatta EG, Gerstenblith G: Cardiovascular system, in Rowe JW, Besdine RW (eds): *Health and Disease in Old Age.* Boston, Little Brown & Co, 1982, pp 369–380.
48. Weiss ST: Pulmonary system, in Rowe JW, Besdine RW (eds): *Health and Disease in Old Age.* Boston, Little Brown & Co, 1982, pp 369–380.
49. Wahba WM: Influence of aging on lung function–clinical significance of changes from age twenty. *Anesth Analg (Cleve)* 1983;62:764–776.
50. Rowe JW: Renal system, in Rowe JW, Besdine RW (eds): *Health and Disease in Old Age.* Boston, Little Brown & Co, 1982, pp 165–184.
51. Gilchrest BA: Skin, in Rowe JW, Besdine RW (eds): *Health and Disease in Old Age.* Boston, Little Brown & Co, 1982, pp 381–392.
52. Logue RB, Kaplan JA: The cardiac patient and noncardiac surgery. *Curr Probl Cardiol* 1982;7:1–49.
53. Peters RW: Routine respiratory care and support and acute respiratory insufficiency, in Hardy JD (ed): *Rhoad's Textbook of Surgery,* ed 5, Philadelphia, JB Lippincott, 1977, pp 133–148.
54. Gerstenblith G, Lakatta EG, Weisfeldt ML: Age changes in myocardial function and exercise response. *Prog Cardiovasc Dis* 1976;19:1–22.
55. Murray JF: *The Normal Lung.* Philadelphia, WB Saunders, 1976.
56. Pierson DJ: Respiratory care of the elderly, in TL Petty (ed): *Intensive and Rehabilatative Respiratory Care,* ed 3. Philadelphia, Lea & Febiger, 1982.
57. Tisi GM: Preoperative evaluation of pulmonary function. *Am Rev Respir Dis* 1979;119:293–310.
58. Craig DB: Postoperative recovery of pulmonary function. *Anesth Analg (Cleve)* 1981;60:46–52.
59. Hensley MJ, Fencl V: Lungs and respiration, in Vandam L (ed): *To Make the Patient Ready for Surgery.* Menlo Park, Calif, Addison-Wesley, 1980, pp 18–43.
60. Diament ML, Palmer KNV: Postoperative changes in gas tensions of arterial blood and in ventilatory function. *Lancet* 1966; 2:180–182.
61. Fairley HB: Oxygen therapy for surgical patients. *Am Rev Respir Dis* 1980;122 (pt 2):37–44.
62. Kitamura H, Sawa T, Ikezono E: Postoperative hypoxemia: the contribution of age to the maldistribution of ventilation. *Anesthesiology* 1972;36:244–252.
63. Zamost B, Benumof JL: Anesthesia in the geriatric patient, in Katz J, Benumof J, Kadis LB, (eds): *Anesthesia and Uncommon Diseases,* ed 2. Philadelphia, WB Saunders Co, 1981, pp 98–118.
64. Vaughn MS, Vaughn RW, Cork RC: Postoperative hypothermia in adults: relationship of age, anesthesia, and shivering to rewarming. *Anesth Analg (Cleve)* 1981;60:746–751.
65. Renck H: The elderly patient after anesthesia and surgery. *Acta Anaesth Scand* 1969;34(suppl):1–136.
66. Bay J, Nunn JF, Prys-Roberts C: Factors influencing arterial PO_2 during recovery from anesthesia. *Br J Anaesth* 1968;40: 398–406.
67. Tinker JH, Noback CR, Vlietstra RE, et al: Management of patients with heart disease for noncardiac surgery. *JAMA* 1981;246:1348–1350.
68. Dodd RB: Anesthesia, in Steinberg FU (ed): *Cowdry's The Care of the Geriatric Patient,* ed 6. St Louis, CV Mosby Co, 1983, pp 327–338.
69. Besdine RW: The data base of geriatric medicine, in Rowe JW, Besdine RW, (eds): *Health and Disease in Old Age.* Boston, Little Brown & Co, 1982, pp 1–14.
70. Besdine RW: Dementia, in Rowe JW, Besdine RW (eds): *Health and Disease in Old Age.* Boston, Little Brown & Co, 1982, pp 97–114.
71. Carson JL, Eisenberg JM: The preoperative screening examination, in Goldman DR, Brown FH, Levy WK, et al (eds): *Medical Care of the Surgical Patient.* Philadelphia, JB Lippincott Co, 1982, pp 16–30.
72. Robbins JA, Mushlin AI: Preoperative evaluation of the healthy patient. *Med Clin North Am* 1979;63:1145–1156.
73. Fisch C: The electrocardiogram in the aged, in Noble RJ, Rothbaum DA (eds): *Geriatric Cardiology.* Philadelphia, FA Davis, 1981, pp 65–74.
74. Seymour DG, Pringle R, Maclennan WJ:

The role of the routine preoperative electrocardiogram in the elderly surgical patient. *Age Ageing* 1983;12:97–104.

75. VonKnorring J: Postoperative myocardial infarction: a prospective study in a risk group of surgical patients. *Surgery* 1981; 90:55–60.
76. Rabkin SW, Horne JM: Preoperative electrocardiography: Effect of new abnormalities on clinical decisions. *Can Med Assoc J* 1983;128:146–147.
77. Tornebrandt K, Fletcher R: Preoperative chest x-rays in elderly patients. *Anesthesia,* 1982;37:901–902.
78. Schneider EL: Infectious diseases in the elderly. *Ann Intern Med* 1983;98:395–400.
79. Sullivan N, Sutter VL, Mims MM, et al: Clinical aspects of bacteremia after manipulation of the genitourinary tract. *J Infect Dis* 1973;127:49–55.
80. Allo M, Simmons RL: Surgical infectious disease and the urologist, *Urol Clin North Am* 1983;10:131–137.
81. Del Guercio LRM, Cohn JD: Monitoring operative risk in the elderly. *JAMA* 1980;243:1350–1355.
82. Gurland BJ, Cross PC: Epidemiology of psychopathology in old age. *Psychiatr Clin North Am* 1982;5:11–26.
83. Seymour DG, Pringle R: Post-operative complications in the elderly surgical patient. *Gerontology* 1983;29:262–270.
84. Pomerance A: Cardiac pathology in the elderly, in Noble RJ, Rothbaum DA (eds): *Geriatric Cardiology.* Philadelphia, FA Davis, 1981, pp 9–54.
85. Noble RJ, Rothbaum DA: History and physical examination, in Noble RJ, Rothbaum DA (eds): *Geriatric Cardiology.* Philadelphia, FA Davis, 1981, pp 55–64.
86. Caird FI, Kennedy RD: Epidemiology of heart disease in old age, in Caird FI, Dall JLC, Kennedy RD (eds): *Cardiology in Old Age.* New York, Plenum Press, 1976, pp 1–10.
87. Kannel WB, Gordon T: Evaluation of cardiovascular risk in the elderly: The Framingham Study. *Bull NY Acad Med* 1978;54:573–591.
88. Steen PA, Tinker JH, Tarhan S: Myocardial reinfarction after anesthesia and surgery. *JAMA* 1978;239:2566–2570.
89. Goldman L: Cardiac risks and complications of noncardiac surgery. *Ann Intern Med* 1983;98:504–513.
90. Tarhan S, Moffitt EA, Taylor WF, et al: Myocardial infarction after general anesthesia. *JAMA* 1972;220:1451–1454.
91. Silverstein DK, Karliner JS: Perioperative cardiac care. *Urol Clin North Am* 1983;10:51–63.
92. Kitchin AH, Louther CP, Milne JS: Prevalence of clinical and electrocardiographic evidence of ischemic heart disease in the older population. *Br Heart J* 1973; 35:946–953.
93. Gerstenblith G, Fleg JL, Vantosh A, et al: Stress testing redefines the prevalence of coronary artery disease in epidemiologic studies, abstracted. *Circulation* 1980;62 (3):308.
94. Portal RW: Elective surgery after myocardial infarction. *Br Med J [Clin Res]* 1982; 284:843–844.
95. Thompson GJ, Kelatis PP, Connolly DC: Transurethral prostatic resection after myocardial infarction. *JAMA* 1962;182: 908–911.
96. Kattlove HE: Hematologic complications associated with urologic surgery, in Smith RB, Skinner DG (eds): *Complications of Urologic Surgery.* Philadelphia, WB Saunders, 1976, pp 39–53.
97. Kursh ED, Rabin R, Persky L: Is cystectomy a safe procedure in elderly patients? *J Urol* 1977;118:40–42.
98. Kutscher HA, Leadbetter GW, Vinson RK: Survival after radical cystectomy for invasive transitional cell carcinoma of the bladder. *Urology* 1981;17:231–234.
99. Garcias VA, Mallough C, Park T, et al: Depressed myocardial function after transurethral resection of the prostate. *Urology* 1981;17:420–427.
100. Pritchett ELC, Orgain ES: Evaluation and management of patients with heart disease who undergo noncardiac surgery, in Hurst JW (ed): *The Heart.* New York, McGraw Hill, 1982, pp 1630–1636.
101. Burch GE, Depasquale NP: Geriatric cardiology. *Am Heart J* 1969;78:700–708.
102. Wong M, Tei C, Shah P: Degenerative calcific valvular disease and systolic murmurs in the elderly. *J Am Geriatr Soc* 1983;31:156–163.
103. Selzer A, Paternak RC: Congenital and valvular heart disease, in Noble RJ, Roth-

baum DA (eds): *Geriatric Cardiology.* Philadelphia, FA Davis, 1981, pp 169–184.

104. Mintz GS, Kottler MN: Are you overlooking IHSS in your elderly patients? *Geriatrics* 1981;36:95–102.
105. Lindenfeld J, Groves BM: Cardiovascular function and disease in the aged, in Schrier RW (ed): *Clinical Internal Medicine in the Aged.* Philadelphia, WB Saunders, 1982, pp 87–123.
106. Noble RJ, Rothbaum DA: Heart disease in the elderly, in Hurst JW (ed): *Update I. The Heart.* New York, McGraw Hill, 1979, pp 211–234.
107. Roberts WC, Perloff JK, Constantino T: Severe valvular aortic stenosis in patients over 65 years of age. *Am J Cardiol* 1971; 27:497–506.
108. Merrit W: Bacterial endocarditis as a complication of transurethral prostatic resection. *J Urol* 1951;65:100–107.
109. Committee for Prevention of Rheumatic Fever and Bacterial Endocarditis of the American Heart Association: Prevention of bacterial endocarditis. *Circulation* 1977; 56:139A–143A.
110. Robbins N, Demaria A, Miller MH: Infective endocarditis in the elderly. *South Med J* 1981;73:1335–1338.
111. Brown FH: Antibiotic prophylaxis in infective endocarditis, in Goldmann DR, Brown FH, Levy WK, et al: *Medical Care of the Surgical Patient.* Philadelphia, JB Lippincott Co, 1982, pp 40–58.
112. Bisno AL: Antimicrobial prophylaxis of infective endocarditis, in Bisno AL: *Treatment of Infective Endocarditis.* New York, Grune & Stratton, 1981, pp 281–306.
113. Franklin SS: Geriatric hypertension. *Med Clin North Am* 1983;67:395–417.
114. Hale WE, Marks RG, Stewart RB: Screening for hypertension in an elderly population: report from the Dunedin program. *J Am Geriatr Soc* 1981;29:123–125.
115. Goldman L, Caldera DL: Risks of general anesthesia and elective operation in the hypertensive patient. *Anesthesiology* 1979;50:285–292.
116. Prys-Roberts C: Hypertension and anesthesia–50 years on. *Anesthesiology* 1979; 50:281–284.
117. Schoeppel SL, Wilkinson C, Waters J, et al: Effect of myocardial infarction on perioperative cardiac complications. *Anesth Analg (Cleve)* 1983;62:493–498.
118. Caird FI, Andrews GR, Kennedy RD: Effect of posture on blood pressure in the elderly. *Br Heart J* 1973;35:527–530.
119. Fleg JL, Kennedy HL: Cardiac arrhythmias in a healthy elderly population. *Chest* 1982;81:302–307.
120. Taylor IC, Stout RW: The significance of cardiac arrhythmias in the aged. *Age Ageing* 1983;12:21–28.
121. Camon AJ, Evans KE, Ward DE, et al: The rhythm of the heart in active elderly subjects. *Am Heart J* 1980;99:598–603.
122. Hirsch J, Genton E, Hull R: *Venous Thromboembolism.* New York, Grune & Stratton, 1981.
123. Coe NP, Collins REC, Klein LA, et al: Prevention of deep venous thrombosis in urological patients: a controlled, randomized trial of low-dose heparin and external pneumatic compression boots. *Surgery* 1978;83:230–234.
124. VanArsdalen KN, Barnes RW, Clarke G, et al: Deep venous thrombosis and prostatectomy. *Urology* 1983;21:461–463.
125. Sasahara AA, Sharma GRVK, Tow DE, et al: Clinical use of thrombolytic agents in venous thromboembolism. *Arch Intern Med* 1982;142:684–688.
126. Nelson PH, Moser KM, Stoner C, et al: Risk of complications during intravenous heparin therapy. *West J Med* 1982; 136;189–197.
127. Deykin D: The risks and benefits of heparin therapy. *West J Med* 1982;136: 241–242.
128. Haley RW, Hooton TM, Culver DH, et al: Nosocomial infections in United States hospitals 1975–76: estimated frequency by selected characteristics of patients. *Am J Med* 1981;70:947–959.
129. Hooton TH, Haley RW, Culver DH, et al: The joint associations of multiple risk factors with the occurrence of nosocomial infection. *Am J Med* 1981;70:960–970.
130. Childs SJ, Wells WG, Mirelman S: Antibiotic prophylaxis for genitourinary surgery in community hospitals. *J Urol* 1983; 130:305–308.
131. Shah PJR, Williams G, Chaudhary M: Short-term antibiotic prophylaxis and prostatectomy. *Br J Urol* 1981;53:339–343.
132. Burke JP, Garibaldi RA, Britt MR, et al:

Prevention of catheter-associated urinary tract infections. *Am J Med* 1981;70: 655–658.
133. Garibaldi RA, Britt MR, Coleman ML, et al: Risk factors for postoperative pneumonia. *Am J Med* 1981;70:677–680.
134. LaForce FM: Hospital-acquired gram negative rod pneumonias: an overview. *Am J Med* 1981;70:664–669.
135. Gleckman R, Hibert D: Afebrile bacteremia: a phenomenon in elderly patients. *JAMA* 1982;248:1478–1481.
136. Smith IM: Afebrile septicemia. *JAMA* 1982;248:1502.
137. Peters RM, Turnier E: Physical therapy: indications for and effects in surgical patients. *Am Rev Respir Dis* 1980;122(5, pt 2):147–154.
138. Hansen G, Drablos PA, Steinert R: Pulmonary complications, ventilation, and blood gases after upper abdominal surgery. *Acta Anaesthesiol Scand* 1977;21: 211–215.
139. Arabian AA, Spagnolo SV, Rohatgi PK: Evaluation and therapy of pulmonary problems in surgical patients. *Clin Notes Respir Dis* 1982;27:3–14.
140. Gracey DR, Divertie MB, Didier EP: Preoperative pulmonary preparation of patients with COPD: a prospective study. *Chest* 1979;76:123–129.
141. Cain HD, Stevens PM, Adaniya R: Preoperative pulmonary function and complications after cardiovascular surgery. *Chest* 1979;76:130–135.
142. Wightman JAK: A prospective study of the incidence of postoperative pulmonary complications. *Br J Surg* 1968;55:85–91.
143. Thurlbeck WM: *Chronic Airflow Obstruction in Lung Disease.* Philadelphia, WB Saunders Co, 1976.
144. Pontoppidan H: Mechanical aids to lung expansion in nonintubated surgical patients. *Am Rev Respir Dis* 1980;122(5, pt 2):109–119.
145. Stein M, Cassara EL: Preoperative pulmonary evaluation and therapy for surgery patients. *JAMA* 1970;211:787–790.
146. Kaiko RF: Age and morphine analgesia in cancer patients with postoperative pain. *Clin Pharmacol Ther* 1980;28:823–826.
147. Bellville JW, Forrest WH, Miller E: Influence of age on pain relief from analgesics. A study of postoperative patients. *JAMA* 1971;217:1835–1841.
148. Rochester DF, Goldberg SK: Techniques of respiratory physical therapy. *Am Rev Respir Dis* 1980;122(5, p 2):133–146.
149. Sutton PP, Pavia D, Bateman JRM, et al: Chest physiotherapy: a review. *Eur J Respir Dis* 1982;63:188–201.
150. Bartlett RH: Postoperative pulmonary prophylaxis; breathe deeply and read carefully. *Chest* 1982;81:1–3.
151. Millar HR: Psychiatric morbidity in elderly surgery patients. *Brit J Psychiatry* 1981;138:17–20.
152. Mesulam M, Gerschwind N: Disordered mental status in the postoperative period. *Urol Clin North Am* 1976;3:199–216.
153. Rollason WN, Robertson GS, Cordimer CM, et al: A comparison of mental function in relation to hypotensive and normotensive anesthesia. *Br J Anaesth* 1971; 43:561–565.
154. Riis J, Lomholt B, Haxholdt O, et al: Immediate and long-term mental recovery from general versus epidural anesthesia in elderly patients. *Acta Anaesthesiol Scand* 1983;27:44–49.
155. Hole A, Terjesen T, Breivik H: Epidural versus general anesthesia for total hip arthroplasty in elderly patients. *Acta Anaesthesiol Scand* 1980;24:279–287.
156. Titchener JL, Zwerling I, Gottschaltk L, et al: Psychosis in surgical patients. *Surg Gynecol Obstet* 1956;102:59–65.
157. Jahnigen D, Hamnon C, Laxson L, et al: Iatrogenic disease in hospitalized elderly veterans. *J Am Geriatr Soc* 1982;30: 87–390.
158. Pathy M: Clinical presentation of myocardial infarction in the elderly. *Br Heart J* 1967;29:190–199.
159. Liptzin B: Psychiatric aspects of aging, in Rowe JW, Besdine RW, (eds): *Health and Disease in Old Age.* Boston, Little Brown & Co, 1982, pp 85–96.
160. Henderson DJ, Middleton RG: Coma from hyponatremia following transurethral resection of prostate. *Urology* 1980;15: 67–271.
161. Liston EH: Delirium in the aged. *Psychiatr Clin North Am* 1982;5:49–66.
162. Hart RG, Easton JD: Management of cervical bruits and carotid stenosis in preperative patients. *Stroke* 1983;14:290–297.

163. Yatsu FM, Hart RG: Asymptomatic carotid bruit and stenosis: a reappraisal. *Stroke* 1983;14:301–304.
164. Ropper AH, Wechsler LR, Wilson LS: Carotid bruit and the risk of stroke in elective surgery. *N Engl J Med* 1982;307: 1388–1390.
165. Danielson DA, Porter JB, Dinan BJ, et al: Drug monitoring of surgical patients. *JAMA* 1982:248;1482–1485.
166. Armstrong B, Dinan B, Jick H: Fatal drug reactions in patients admitted to surgical services. *Am J Surg* 1976;132:643–645.
167. Jick H, Sloane D, Burden IT, et al: Efficacy and toxicity of heparin in relation to age and sex. *N Engl J Med* 1968;279: 284–286.
168. Zaske DE, Irvine P, Strand LM, et al: Wide interpatient variations in gentamicin dose requirements for geriatric patients. *JAMA* 1982;248:3122–3126.
169. Steel K, Gertman PM, Crescenzi C, et al: Iatrogenic illness on a general medical service at a university hospital. *N Engl J Med* 1981;304:638–642.
170. Reichel W: Complications in the care of 500 elderly hospitalized patients. *J Am Geriatr Soc* 1965;13:973–981.
171. Rubenstein LZ: Falls in the elderly: a clinical approach. *West J Med* 1983;136: 189–197.
172. Rueler JB, Cooney TG: The pressure sore: pathophysiology and principles of management. *Ann Intern Med* 1981;94:661–666.

CHAPTER 24 Cancer of the Prostate

Frederick A. Klein

Prostatic carcinoma is the third most common malignant disease in males and is surpassed only by carcinoma of the lung and colon-rectum. It is estimated that from birth males have approximately a 5% risk of developing prostatic cancer and an approximately 2% risk of dying from it.[1] The American Cancer Society estimates that in 1984 there will be 76,000 new cases diagnosed in the United States with 25,000 deaths.[2] Prostatic cancer is responsible for 18% of all malignancies occurring in men and 10% of all cancer fatalities in men. When comparing incidence and death rates over the past three decades, there have been fluctuations all through the period; but overall there has been a moderate increase.[2] It cannot be overemphasized, as stated by Johnson, that because of the increase in the frequency with which physicians encounter the disease and the wide variety of its manifestations, it is mandatory to know more about its clinical presentations, diagnosis, and treatment.[1] This is emphasized by the fact that today less than 25% of potentially curable patients are receiving treatment with the intention of cure.[3]

EPIDEMIOLOGY

From examination of prostate glands during autopsy studies the presence of carcinoma seems to be the same worldwide. The clinical incidence, however, is high in the United States and Western Europe and low in the Orient. Likewise the incidence is low in Filipinos, Mexicans, Hawaiians, American Indians, and members of the Mongoloid race.[4]

The role of diet and/or environmental carcinogens in the causation and expression of prostate cancer may be reflected by the fact that there exists a low incidence of this disease among European-born Jewish males residing in the United States; when the Jewish male is a native-born American the incidence rates rise becoming similar to those of other native-born[1] whites. Similarly, higher death rates from prostate cancer have been demonstrated for first generation sons of immigrants from Japan and Eastern Europe.[1] A more interesting epidemiologic feature may be the difference in incidence and mortality rates between American whites and blacks. The age adjusted death rate for prostate cancer in the United States for whites is 23/100,000/yr compared to 41/100,000/yr for blacks, and the incidence rate for the black population is about 50% greater than that for the total population.[1] The reasons for these differences are unknown.

There is no question that the risk of developing prostate cancer increases with age. Stamey compared the incidence of prostate cancer found incidentally at transurethral resection (TURP) and at autopsy.[5] The overall incidence at TURP was about one-half that seen at autopsy and at least in the series by Franks by the age of 90 years, 100% of men had demonstrable cancer.[6] The clinical diagnosis of prostatic malignancy, however, ranges from 0.02% in patients aged 50 to approximately 0.8% of patients 80 years old.[7] This discrepancy between the incidence of clinical and latent disease raises several points in the natural history of this disease. First, there is a latency period of several decades between the malignant transformation phase and the appearance of clinical symptoms. This observation has led to the conclusion that prostate cancer in the elderly should have a more favorable prognosis. Second, the number of men who die each year from prostate cancer represents only a small proportion of those who are living with the disease.

Although there has been at least one study that suggested that men who develop prostatic cancer have been more sexually active than other men with regard to number of partners, frequency of coitus, greater frequency of venereal disease, and less satisfaction with the amount of coitus that has occurred,[8] epidemiologic studies have consistently failed to demonstrate differences between groups with cancer and control groups with regard to socioeconomic status, education, alcohol, cigarettes, and body habitus.[1] Likewise, inconsistent data have been reported concerning the association between prostatic cancer and urbanization, religion, fertility, blood type, and occurrence of second primary cancer.[8–11]

ETIOLOGY

The etiology of adenocarcinoma of the prostate remains uncertain. Because of the straight-line relationship between incidence and patient age, it is logical to conclude that the prostate is constantly being insulted by carcinogens. Thus, given enough time most and probably all prostates will develop histologic evidence of malignancy.[6,12] A genetic influence is suggested by the higher incidence in American blacks, a lower incidence among Asians, and a more frequent history of prostate cancer in families of men who develop it than in controls.[10]

The role of sex hormones in prostatic cancer has been considered for several reasons: (1) the experimental and clinical demonstration of regression following castration or estrogen therapy,[13] (2) the findings that patients with prostatic cancer excrete less androsterone, have a lower estrogen-etiocholanolone ratio, and excrete a higher proportion of total estrogen as estrone and estradiol than normal controls,[8] (3) the absence of prostate cancer in eunuchs,[14] and (4) the relative infrequency in patients with cirrhosis of the liver, a disease in which estrogen levels are high.[10]

Chemical exposure has been implicated as a cause of prostate cancer as the result of reports of an increased incidence in workers exposed to cadmium salt dusts, and an above-average mortality in workers in the rubber industry.[15-17] Similarly, diets rich in animal fat have been suggested as a possible initiating agent[1]; whereas diets rich in green and yellow vegetables have been reported to significantly lower the age-standardized death rate from prostate cancer in Japanese men aged 40 years and more.[18] Supporting evidence for this theory is available in reports by Phillips who showed a lower risk of prostate cancer in vegetarians living in the United States.[19]

The relationship between benign prostatic hypertrophy (BPH) and the development of prostate cancer remains somewhat controversial with some investigators considering BPH to be a possible precursor of carcinoma. When comparing age-matched normal controls and patients with BPH, those with BPH not only have a higher incidence of prostate cancer but also have a higher death rate from prostate cancer.[20,21] On the other hand, Greenwald et al,[22] Moore,[23] and Mostofi and Price[24] have not found any such relationship.

Although no definite causal relationship for oncogenic viruses[4] has been demonstrated in prostatic carcinogenesis, viruslike structures have been seen in human prostatic cancers[25] and in the malignant change seen in in vitro hamster prostatic tissue following the introduction of oncogenic viruses.[26] Similarly, Heshmat et al[27] suggested an association between gonorrhea and death from prostatic cancer. They postulated that the bacteria act as vectors allowing viruses to enter prostate cells and to subsequently develop cancer. Since the latency period in this study ranged between 42 and 45 years an increased incidence of prostate cancer might be expected in this decade as a result of the high rate of gonorrhea after World War II.[1]

HISTOPATHOLOGY

Adenocarcinoma accounts for 95% of prostatic malignancy with transitional cell carcinoma, squamous cell carcinoma, and sarcomas accounting for the remainder. Adenocarcinoma arises from the acini or ducts in the periphery of the gland from where it spreads centrally toward the urethra eventually penetrating the capsule. Benign prostatic hyperplasia, in comparison, arises not in the periphery but rather in the periurethral portion of the gland. Byar and Mostofi,[28] step-sectioned 208 radical prostatectomy specimens and found only one to have arisen in the central tissue alone, confirming the above view of tumor origin and spread. They also found that 85% of tumors were multifocal or extensive, while only 9% existed as single nodules. These data are quite compatible with the low incidence of the prostatic nodule (B_1, T_{2a}) of between 5% and 10%.

The histologic criteria for making the diagnosis of prostate cancer include the presence of microacini in a back-to-back or cribiform pattern, an absent basal layer with single cells lining the acini, prominent nucleoli, cellular anaplasia, stromal invasion, perineural infiltration, and a positive reaction on staining for prostate-specific acid phosphatase. Since the original classification or grading (I–IV) of prostate cancer by Broders in 1925,[29] the degree of differentiation has been used as a base for prognosis. Traditionally, this classification has been limited to well, moderately, or poorly differentiated variants. More recently, other major grading systems have been devised based upon different nuclear and/or glandular features of the tumor cells. These include the system devised by Gleason, Mellinger, and the Veterans Administration Co-operative Urological Research Group (VACURG) in 1974,[30] the system described by Mostofi and employed at the Armed Forces Institute of Pathology,[31] the system described by Gaeta et al[32] and used by the National Prostate Cancer Project, and the Mayo Clinic system reported by Utz and Farrow.[33] A good correlation exists with a tumor grade or score and the presence of lymph node metastases as well as the ultimate survival in some reports.[34-36] Despite this, the assignment to a specific grade or score remains subjective, qualitative, not entirely reproducible, heavily reliant on the expertise and interest of an individual pathologist, and not uniformly accurate in predicting tumor behavior or prognosis in an individual patient.

On the other hand, there are two newer automated technics, computerized image analysis and flow cytometry, that allow quantitative, relatively objective, and reproducible determinations of specific nuclear or cellular features of tumor cells which may have more prognostic significance for a specific tumor in a given individual. Diamond et al[37] in 1982 reported results on 27 patients using a relative nuclear roundness factor. In this study a distinct difference was demonstrated in this factor when comparing those patients with and without metastatic disease. There have been several reports of flow cytometric quantification of the DNA content of prostatic adenocarcinoma.[38-45] The potential advantage of this technic is that as the percentage of aneuploid tumor cells increases, differentiation decreases and the presence or absence of aneuploid tumor, diploid or tetraploid tumor will correspond to eventual endocrine response. These technics, therefore, become an important adjunct in prognosis and in determining for an individual patient who should have earlier more aggressive treatment.

Squamous Cell and Transitional Cell Carcinoma

Squamous cell and transitional cell carcinoma comprise approximately 3% of prostatic epithelial neoplasms.[46,47] While adenocarcinomas usually arise from the tubuloalveolar glands, transitional cell carcinomas arise from the distal prostatic ducts. Squamous carcinoma is rare and occurs most commonly as secondary involvement from a primary urethral or bladder neoplasm. Squamous carcinoma, however, can arise from either adenocarcinoma, metaplasia, or as a primary tumor.[48]

The average age of onset for transitional cell carcinoma is about 10 years less than for adenocarcinoma.[47] The most common symptoms at presentation are severe prostatitis, hematuria, and obstructive symptoms. Acid phosphatase levels are usually normal and bone metastases, if they occur, are usually osteolytic. The diagnosis is best made by transurethral resection. The best chance for cure is anterior pelvic exenteration as the tumor is generally unresponsive to endocrine or radiation therapy. The prognosis is poor.[47]

Sarcoma

Primary sarcomas of the prostate are very rare and account for less than 1% of prostatic neoplasms. The majority of these are myosarcomas with embryonal rhabdomyosarcomas more common in children and young adults and leiomyosarcomas more common in the middle-aged or older male.[48] These tumors usually present with symptoms of urinary obstruction. They are best diagnosed by transurethral resection and best treated by anterior exenteration.

STAGING

Once the diagnosis of prostatic carcinoma has been confirmed histologically it becomes necessary to assess the extent of disease as accurately as possible. The orderly planning of therapy, prognosis, and ultimately the comparison of results of various therapies from multiple institutions depends on this staging assignment. Although there have been several staging systems proposed in the past[49-53] usage is generally limited to the Union Internationale Contre le Cancer (UICC) system and a modification of the Jewett system[53] (Table 24-1).

Stage A (T_1) refers to clinically unrecognized carcinoma found incidentally in a prostatectomy specimen done for benign disease. If three or fewer microscopic foci of disease are found the stage is considered A_1 or T_{1a}. If more than three foci are

Table 24-1
Staging Classifications for Prostate Cancer

Staging System				
Jewett[53]	*MSKCC*	*UICC*		Definition
A_1	A_1	T_{1a}	(clinically unrecognized)	Focal (<3 foci, well differentiated)
A_2	A_2	T_{1b}		Diffuse (≥3 foci)
B_1	B_1	T_{2b}		Intraprostatic nodule <1.5 cm
B_2	B_2	T_{2b}		All other intracapsular disease
C	C_1	T_{3a}		Periprostatic extension ± one seminal vesicle.
	C_2	T_{3b}		Periprostatic extension ± one or both seminal vesicles and >6 cm in diameter
	C_3	T_4		Tumor fixed or involving neighboring structures
D_1	D_1	N-1,-2,-3		Regional lymph node involvement
D_2	D_2	M specific site		Distant nodal, bony, or visceral metastases

MSKCC = Memorial Sloan Kettering Cancer Center.
UICC = Union Internationale Contre le Cancer.

found or if there is dedifferentiation the stage is A_2 or T_{1b}.

Stage B_1 (T_{2a}) refers to an asymptomatic palpable nodule 1.5 cm in size or less and confined to one lobe. There must be normal prostatic tissue completely surrounding the nodule.

Stage B_2 (T_{2b}) refers to any other prostatic carcinoma clinically confined within the prostatic capsule. Memorial Sloan-Kettering Cancer Center (New York) more carefully classifies a B_2 lesion as unilobar involvement, but a lesion larger than 1.5 cm and a B_3 lesion as all other intracapsular disease.[50]

Stage C (T_3–T_4) lesions refer to those patients who have localized disease with extension through the prostatic capsule to involve any combination of seminal vesicles, bladder neck, or extension to the lateral side wall of the pelvis or other pelvic organs. This classification may be further subdivided according to Memorial Hospital criteria into C_1, C_2, or C_3, representing involvement of the lateral sulcus alone (C_1), the base of the seminal vesicle with or without sulci involvement (C_2), and a tumor which involves more than just the base of the seminal vesicle with or without involvement of other adjacent structures (C_3). The UICC defines a T_{3a} lesion as a tumor extending through the capsule or involving one seminal vesicle, a T_{3b} lesion as a tumor extending into the periprostatic tissues, involving one or both seminal vesicles and more that 6 cm in diameter, and a T_4 lesion as a tumor fixed or involving neighboring structures.[49]

Stage D cancer is metastatic disease. D_1 refers to pelvic lymph node involvement below the bifurcation of the aorta. D_2 refers to lymph node involvement above the aortic bifurcation, bony metastases, or metastases to other visceral organs. For the UICC classification lymph node involvement is referred to as N-0 (no involvement of regional lymph nodes), N-1 (involvement of a single homolateral regional lymph node), N-2 (involvement of contralateral, bilateral, or multiple regional nodes) and N-3 (a fixed mass present on the pelvic wall with a free space between the wall and the tumor). Distant metastases are referred to as M with mention of the specific metastatic site (M bone).[49]

DIAGNOSIS

Symptoms

The early diagnosis of prostate cancer is made infrequently as approximately 80% of patients will be initially diagnosed with either locally advanced or metastatic disease. Initial symptoms may be entirely absent because adenocarcinoma usually arises in the periphery of the gland. Later, obstructive symptoms of hesitancy, frequency, nocturia, and incomplete emptying occur because of disease progression with involvement of the bladder neck and urethra. It should be remembered, however, that obstructive symptoms can occur from benign growth even though a carcinoma exists concomitantly in the periphery of the gland. The frequency of presenting symptoms has not changed appreciably since the report of Barnes in 1940[54] (Table 24-2). Barnes observed that the most common symptoms were dysuria, slow stream, urinary frequency, and complete retention. Back and hip pain were more indicative of metastases. Hematuria is more commonly seen with benign hyperplasia; however, when present in the setting of tumor it is indicative of bladder neck and/or trigone invasion. Other less common symptoms include enlarged supraclavicular nodes, lower bowel complaints, hematospermia, and lower extremity edema or weakness.

Table 24-2
Symptoms in Prostatic Carcinoma

Symptoms	Gross Count	%
Dysuria	283	42
Slow stream	271	40
Urinary frequency	260	39
Complete retention	159	24
Back or hip pain	100	15
Dribbling of urine	98	15
Hematuria	90	13
Pain in bladder	49	7
Constipation	32	4
Rectal or perineal pain	30	4
Not recorded	21	3

Reproduced with permission from Barnes.[54]

Rectal Examination

In 1926 Young and Davis wrote: "The principal resource in the diagnosis of prostatic carcinoma is the rectal examination."[55] This statement continues to be true today as one becomes suspicious of prostate cancer by feeling areas of induration on rectal palpation. Characteristically, carcinoma of the prostate is a discrete hard nodule or area of dense induration within the substance of the gland. With further progression of the disease the margins become obscured and induration is often felt, extending into the region of the seminal vesicles and the bladder neck. With further progression of disease the prostate may actually become contiguous with or fixed to the pelvic side walls. It should be remembered, however, that not all areas of induration will represent carcinoma. Asymmetrical growth and areas of induration occur with focal benign hyperplasia, prostatic infarct, granulomatous prostatitis, prostatic calculi, and because of previous transurethral resections. Digital examination is reported to be 50% to 75% accurate in diagnosing prostate cancer and about 50% of palpable nodules are eventually proven to be carcinomatous in origin.[56]

Biopsy

Once the diagnosis of prostate carcinoma is entertained, confirmation is made by means of biopsy. Methods of obtaining histologic confirmation include open perineal biopsy, transperineal or transrectal needle biopsy, transrectal fine needle aspiration cytology, transurethral resection biopsy, and cytology of expressed prostatic fluid. The most widely used of these technics are the transperineal or transrectal core biopsies and transrectal aspiration cytology. Needle biopsy is 90% accurate in the hands of a skilled operator with a low morbidity and a very low incidence of needle tract seeding. Fine needle aspiration cytology is at least as accurate, with a sensitivity range of 86% to 97% and a specificity range of 96% to 100%.[57] This level of accuracy, however, depends on the level of training, skill, and interest of the cytopathologist. Open biopsy has the advantage of sampling under direct vision, but requires anesthesia and among its morbid complications is a 29% total impotence rate.[58] It is usually used only in conjunction with total perineal prostatectomy. Transurethral resection has limited value because early carcinomas do not involve the periurethral tissue and would likely be missed on biopsy. Cytology of prostatic fluid secretion has likewise been shown to be a poor method for diagnosing prostatic carcinoma.[59]

Intravenous Urography

An intravenous urogram is usually performed to evaluate the upper urinary tracts, bladder function, or degree of obstruction. It may reveal a filling defect in the bladder, bilateral hydroureteronephrosis, nonfunction of one or both kidneys, and the relative amount of postvoid residual urine.

Cystoscopy

The main role of cystoscopy in the diagnosis of prostate cancer is in the determination of whether the tumor involves the periurethral tissue alone and whether or not there is tumor extension to the bladder neck or trigone. These findings directly affect the options employed in management.

Acid Phosphatase Determination

The most important biochemical test in patients with prostate carcinoma is the assay for serum acid phosphatase. A number of different methods are and have been used for determining the prostatic fraction of serum acid phosphatase activity. Most of these methods are based on substrate specificity. Perhaps more sensitive and specific methods are radioimmunoassay, counterimmunoelectrophoresis, or immunoenzyme assays. In patients with benign prostatic hypertrophy and prostatic carcinoma the percentage of patients with elevations in prostatic acid phosphatase was reported by Romas[60] and is shown in Table 24-3. It should be remembered that elevations in serum acid phosphatase can also occur from prostatic massage, prostatic infarct, transurethral resection of the prostate, and from a host of other disease processes including Paget's disease, multiple myeloma, reticuloendothelial diseases, and other carcinomas (breast, stomach, colon, adrenal, kidney) with hepatic or osseous metastases.

In reviewing the data from the three main VACURG studies involving 4128 patients with prostate cancer using serum

Table 24-3
Prostatic Acid Phosphatase Elevations in Patients with BPH and Prostatic Carcinoma

			Elevations (%)		
Stage	No.	Chemical	*CIEP*	*IEA*	*RIA*
BPH	82	9	1	8	17
A	27	7	0	26	30
B	12	33	25	25	33
C	29	55	52	62	72
D	18	91	94	94	100

CIEP = counterimmunoelectrophoresis, IEA = immunoenzyme assay, RIA = radioimmunoassay.

acid phosphatase determinations by the substrate disodium phenylphosphate (King-Armstrong units), several conclusions were reached: (1) 18% of patients with metastases had normal levels of serum acid phosphatase; (2) 39% of those with elevated acid phosphatase levels had metastases on skeletal x-ray film or physical examination; (3) the prognosis for patients with elevated serum acid phosphatase concentrations without metastases is better than that for patients with metastases; and (4) given bony metastases, a normal serum acid phosphatase level is more favorable for survival than an elevated level.[61]

Radioisotope Bone Scan

With the advent of technetium 99 radionuclide bone scans earlier detection of metastatic bone lesions has become possible. Although bone scans detect all metabolically active bone lesions and can be nonspecific, they have been shown to be significantly more sensitive than skeletal survey films in the early detection of metastatic bone disease.[56] The incidence of patients having scans with positive findings and normal skeletal surveys ranges from 12% to 50%. Similarly, 2% of patients with radiographic evidence of metastases have bone scans with negative findings.[62] On the other hand, the problem of a positive bone scan in an area without arthritis and negative findings on skeletal films continues to be a dilemma in deciding on therapy. Whether these areas should be biopsied prior to performing a definitive curative procedure or ignored and the procedure performed is controversial.

Lymphangiography

Bilateral pedal lymphangiography has some application in deciding on therapy ports when a patient is treated by external beam therapy. The technic primarily opacifies nodes in the external iliac, common iliac, and periaortic chains. Whether adequate opacification of the obturator, and hypogastric nodal chains occurs remains an area of controversy. Paulson[63] has reported that "in the best of hands" lymphangiography for prostate carcinoma will have a false-positive rate of 12% to 15% and a false-negative rate of between 22% and 44%. The overall accuracy of this technic is limited because (1) the obturator and hypogastric nodes are not consistently visualized; (2) there is difficulty distinguishing between fatty infiltration and tumor; and (3) microscopic foci of tumor cannot be detected.[56] When a lymphangiogram is performed and is postive, a fine needle aspiration biopsy can be done to prove metastatic disease and determine the type of therapy.

Computed Axial Tomography

Computed axial tomography (CT) of the pelvis does not seem to occupy an important place in the evaluation of prostate cancer because nodes less than 1 cm are difficult to identify and the majority of nodes involved with prostate cancer are rarely larger than 1 cm. Although Levine et al[64] reported that CT scanning did not seem to identify node-positive or node-negative extension with any greater accuracy than lymphangiography, the experience to date does indicate that this technic is capable of identifying a large volume of nodal extension, which may be confirmed by needle aspiration. The false-negative rate with CT scans reported by Olson is 35.5% and the false-positive rate 11.8%.[65]

Staging Pelvic Lymphadenectomy

Staging pelvic lymphadenectomy may be used prior to definitive irradiation or in conjunction with interstitial radiotherapy or radical surgery. The incidence of nodal metastases according to the clinical stage of carcinoma of the prostate from various series is shown in Table 24-4. Because of the false-negative rates, the difficulty in performing and interpreting lymphangio-

Table 24-4
Incidence of Pelvic Nodes According to Clinical Stage for Prostate Carcinoma

	Clinical Stage				
Author(s)	A_1	A_2	B_1	B_2	C
Wilson et al[66]	0/4(0)	0/8(0)	5/36(14)	9/20(45)	10/19(53)
Grossman et al[67]	0/3(0)	25/47(53)	3/18(17)	4/14(29)	5/9(56)
Lieskovsky et al[68]	0/2(0)	1/8(13)	3/16(19)	12/39(31)	11/17(65)
Brendler et al[69]	0/1(0)	3/22(14)	11/58(19)	14/27(52)	10/17(59)
McLaughlin et al[70]	–	–	4/19(21)	5/17(30)	12/24(50)
Golimbu et al[71]	0/4(0)	6/16(38)	–	–	–
Freiha et al[72]	0/0(0)	0/2(0)	2/13(15)	10/44(23)	24/41(58)
Paulson[63]	0/3(0)	8/29(28)	–	16/52(30)	10/26(39)
Whitmore[73]	–	–	0/16(0)	11/36(30)	24/39(62)

grams, and the less than ideal sensitivity of CT, it is not surprising that extraperitoneal pelvic lymph node dissection is recommended for the best assessment of the regional nodes in patients with localized prostate carcinoma. The greatest drawback to the routine use of this procedure is that it requires an operation and in a number of different series a possible morbidity or complication rate of approximately 27% has been found.[74] The most common complications are wound problems, followed by atelectasis, ileus, sepsis, pulmonary embolus, thrombophlebitis, lymphocele, and lower extremity and penile edema. The complication of lymphedema seems to be most closely associated with the extent of the dissection and the extent of the field of postoperative radiation therapy. With the advent of the modified node dissection by Paulson[63] and by Fisher et al[75] the percentage of lymph nodes per stage involved by tumor has not changed and postoperative lymphedema has been less. This more limited dissection is now generally accepted as the current standard.

TREATMENT: OPTIONS AND RESULTS

The management of localized prostatic cancer continues to incite controversy in urologic circles as evidenced by the variety of treatment methods available. Before embarking upon a discussion of the therapeutic options three features of prostatic cancer that confound efforts to define any potentially curative or optimal method of treatment must be pointed out.[76–78] First, the disease occurs in an age group (over 60) wherein the risk of death from a variety of causes other than prostatic carcinoma is high. This is clearly supported by the VACURG data which showed that the probability of dying from cancer of the prostate when a patient had an early-stage neoplasm was less than the probability of dying from other causes, even when the patient was treated conservatively with endocrine therapy. It continues to be generally accepted, however, that the higher the grade and stage of tumor and the younger the patient at presentation, the greater the probability of death from prostatic cancer. It may be assumed then, that aggressive treatment in such patients may not necessarily alter survival rates.

Second, the natural history of prostatic cancer in terms of rate and patterns of progression is unpredictable. Prostatic carcinoma is frequently a slowly progressive tumor, and as such, may remain confined to the prostate for the life of the host, or it may progress despite the treatment employed. In general, the pattern of stage progression is a function of both growth rate and metastatic potential. The theoretical possibilities for the pattern of progression may be expressed schematically for the four clinical stages as follows:

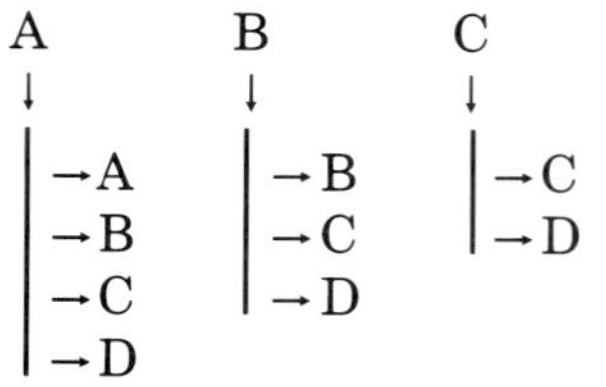

A	B	C
↓	↓	↓
→A	→B	→C
→B	→C	→D
→C	→D	
→D		

There is clinical evidence that each of these possibilities does occur; however, the frequency of occurrence and the factors determining such occurrence are uncertain. Despite growth estimations by tumor grade and thymidine-labeling indices, flow cytometry measurements of DNA content, image analysis determinations of nuclear roundness, and forward light scatter measurements, accurate prediction of growth rate or metastatic potential remains impossible.

Third, the earlier the tumor stage, the greater the number of behavioral patterns of the tumor and the larger the number of treatment options. Available treatment options include follow-up only until a patient becomes symptomatic, radical retropubic or perineal prostatectomy, radiation therapy (external beam megavoltage, interstitial, or both) endocrine therapy, or a combination of methods. Because of improvement in staging modalities over the past 25 years, uncontrolled application of specific treatment regimens at different institutions using different staging criteria, different patient selection criteria, different means of calculating survival results, different means of evaluating the presence of metastatic disease, and the overall similarity of 5-, 10-, and 15-year survival rates with and without disease of patients treated with different regimens, it is impossible to establish unequivocally a more favorable or superior method of treating prostatic carcinoma with respect to survival. Therapy should be judged by its effect on the duration and quality of life, compared with the adverse effects of the basic condition on the duration and quality of life.[76]

Transurethral Resection

Transurethral resection of the prostate is performed commonly to relieve vesical outlet obstruction. Incidental carcinoma of the prostate found under these circumstances depends on patient age but varies between 1.9% and 60%[1,79] (Table 24-5). When three or fewer foci of well-differentiated carcinoma are found on microscopic sectioning the clinical stage is A_1 (T_{1a}). These patients should undergo repeat transurethral resection with simultaneous transrectal or perineal biopsy in order to be certain no residual tumor is present. McMillen and Wettlaufer reported a 26% incidence of residual tumor in 27 patients so rebiopsied.[80] If no further tumor is found the transurethral resection is considered definitive therapy and the patient is followed only on a 6-month basis. If residual tumor is present or the grade of the tumor is less differentiated, consideration should be given to more definitive therapy.

Table 24-5
Incidence of Incidental Carcinoma of Prostate Found at Transurethral Resection (TURP)

Age Decade	Range (%)	Incidence at TURP (av %)
30–39	0.0–4.0	1.9
40–49	4.4–17.0	6.3
50–59	5.3–14.0	10.4
60–69	17.8–23.0	18.5
70–79	21.0–36.0	28.7
80–89	17.6–48.5	37.1
90–99	40.0–80.0	60.0

Adapted from Stamey.[5]

In 1956 Green and Simon[81] reported that the presence of this incidental carcinoma had no adverse effects on patient survival, with the observed 5- and 10-year survival approaching age-adjusted survival rates of patients without prostate cancer. In a further review of four additional series plus 148 patients in the VACURG study with focal stage A disease, only 6.8% of patients demonstrated progressive disease and only five patients (1.9%) out of 262 treated conservatively died of prostate cancer.[82] In 1972 Hanash et al[83] reported on 50 patients with stage A tumors that were treated only by transurethral resection, and determined that the 5-, 10-, and 15-year survival was equal to age-matched expected survivals. Those patients who had poorly differentiated tumors, however, did not survive. The report of Hanash et al[83] re-emphasizes the fact that grading is important and although fewer than three foci of tumor may be found, those patients with less than well-differentiated disease should be treated definitively. With any other stage of disease transurethral resection should be considered palliative and performed only for diagnosis or relief of vesical outlet obstruction.

Radical Surgery

The term radical prostatectomy connotes surgical extirpation of the prostate gland and seminal vesicles (prostatovesiculectomy). It is certainly one treatment option to be considered in patients with localized prostatic cancer that has not extended beyond the capsule and is without evidence of metastases (stages A_2, B, T_1, T_2). The first perineal prostatectomy was performed by Kuchler in 1866 and was later modified and popularized by Young in 1904.[56] Retropubic prostatectomy was described by Millin in 1947[84] and later reported by several others.[85–88] In addition, cystoprostatovesiculectomy and total pelvic exenteration have been used by Coffey,[89] Hinman and Smith,[90] Westerborn,[91] Whitmore and MacKenzie,[92] and McCullough and Leadbetter.[93] Despite extensive experience and long-term follow-up, there is no consensus on the appropriate role of radical surgery in the treatment of this disease.

Perineal prostatectomy has the following advantages over the retropubic prostatectomy: it is less time-consuming in experienced hands; the prostate is readily approachable by the perineal route because of its low-lying position; there is less physiologic disturbance to the patient; fewer blood transfusions are required; and there is better visualization of the vesical neck allowing an easier vesicourethral anastamosis. Its disadvantages are that it does not allow access to the pelvic lymph nodes and most urologists' experience with the perineal approach is limited. Because of the importance of determining pelvic lymph node involvement, two separate procedures with two separate anesthesias three to five days apart are frequently necessary.

The principle arguments in favor of radical retropubic prostatectomy involve technical considerations: surgeons are generally more comfortable with this approach, the pelvic lymphadenectomy can be done at the same time, and if the prostate is high-riding, it may be more readily exposed. The disadvantages of the retropubic approach include greater blood loss, a postoperative period that is more prolonged and difficult for the patient, and the difficulty in anastomosing the vesical neck and bladder to the urethra as compared with the more precise perineal approach.

The operative mortality rates for radical prostatectomy range from less than 1% to 4% regardless of the approach.[94–96] Until the reports of Walsh and associates[97] virtually all of these patients became impotent. If the pelvic nerve plexus is carefully identified and it and the autonomic innervation to the corpora cavernosa are preserved, perhaps a proportion of patients with (B_1 or T_{2a}) lesions undergoing radical surgery will retain their potency. Otherwise, impotence may be partially remedied in most instances by insertion of one of the silastic penile prostheses. Incontinence, either stress or total, may occur in up to 21% of patients initially, but permanent incontinence usually occurs in less than 2% to 10%.[96,98] Other complications include rectal injury with a resultant fistula, bladder neck contracture, urethral stricture, and, much less frequently, hemorrhage, wound infections, or abscesses.

The 10- and 15-year survival statistics for patients undergoing radical prostatectomy are shown in Table 24-6. Many of these results are difficult to compare as some are based on clinical staging and others on pathologic staging. Realizing that a number of tumor-free patients do die of other causes before 15 years are reached, the 15-year survival for disease pathologically confined to the prostate (stage B_1, B_2 or T_2) is reasonable. The proponents of radical surgery will reiterate that to cure carcinoma of the prostate, all tumor must be excised. Certainly, until 15-year follow-up is available with all modes of therapy, radical prostatectomy will continue to be the standard for comparing the efficacy of other forms of treatment. It should be remembered that only 15% to 20% of all prostatic carcinomas are stage B (T_2). Also, as emphasized by Elder et al[107] only about one third of clinical B_2 lesions (T_{2b}) are really pathologically B_2 (T_{2b}) lesions, as 66% of the patients cited in this series had histologic extension behind the capsule or positive lymph nodes.

Radical prostatectomy has been employed for patients with stage A_2 (T_{1b}) carcinoma. The majority of these tumors are less differentiated and have a more virulent biologic potential as manifested by a high incidence of pelvic node involvement. Golimbu et al[108] reported that 68% of tumors were moderately to poorly differentiated and 37.5% were associated with the presence of positive pelvic lymph nodes. Corriere et al[109] reported that 60% of 47 patients with A_2 disease when treated by radical prostatectomy developed recurrent disease. Although it remains a controversial point, radical prostatectomy after extensive transurethral resection may be more difficult technically with a higher rate of complications.

Radical prostatectomy for stage C or D (T_3, T_4) has been performed with 15-year survival rates of up to 20%.[110,111] Interpreting survival times with this procedure is difficult since some of these patients were carefully selected having only small well-differentiated lesions and frequently having received adjuvant endocrine therapy. Most urologists do not favor radical surgery for these lesions and use one of the forms of radiation therapy.

Radiation Therapy

The first use of intraurethral radium in the management of prostate carcinoma was by Pasteau in 1911.[112] Other reports during this period described the use of radium sources with specially positioned applicators located adjacent to the prostate but placed intravesically, intraurethrally,

Table 24-6
Estimated or Actuarial Survival after Radical Prostatectomy

Author	No. Patients	Stage	10 Years	15 Years
Jewett[99]	103	B_1	50%	27%
Walsh and Jewett[100]	57	B_1	–	51%
Jewett[101]	79	B_2	41%	18%
Correa et al[102]	24	B	62%	38%
Berlin et al[103]	116	B	57%	38%
Belt and Schroeder[104]	185	B	55%	31%
Culp and Meyer[105]	162	B	72%	54%
Williams et al[106]	52	B	35%	10%

or transrectally.[113-117] These authors understood the principles of fractionation and tried with the aid of surface applications of external beam supplements, insertion of perineal radium needles, or direct insertion of radium needles into a surgically exposed gland to achieve as homogeneous a radiation dose as possible.

Through the 1920s and 1930s large numbers of patients with prostatic carcinoma were treated using various types of radium applications and external beam therapy.[117-120] The height of this era was probably the report by Barringer,[121] which described a series of 352 consecutive cases of prostate cancer treated with some form of interstitial therapy between 1922 and 1936. Two of these cases at postmortem examination 6 and 7 years posttreatment died without evidence of cancer. At this time endocrine therapy was introduced and except for Flocks et al,[122] who reported on the use of interstitial liquid gold 198, little was done with radiotherapy until the linear accelerator was developed. The use of interstitial gold did not become popular because of the hazards and difficulties of working with the isotope and the inability to control lymph node metastases.

Definitive external beam radiotherapy for prostate cancer utilizing megavoltage x-rays generated by a linear accelerator was initiated at Stanford by Bagshaw in 1956.[123] In 1964 Budhraja and Anderson[124] reported their results on 53 patients with prostate cancer by surgery, stilbestrol, and radiotherapy. Thirty-six of these were treated with megavoltage therapy between 4000 and 5900 rad. These patients tolerated the treatment well with the only complications being transient skin reactions and mild diarrhea. This series showed that radiotherapy was not harmful and was beneficial in patients who relapsed after estrogen treatment. In 1965 Bagshaw et al[125] reported on their results with linear accelerator treatment of patients with apparently operable prostate cancer. Their series is today the standard for comparison with other treatment modalities.

The most recent survival data reported by Bagshaw[126] includes 458 patients with disease limited to the prostate (B or T_2) and 385 patients with extracapsular extension (C or T_3). The 5-, 10-, and 15-year results for the first group are 80%, 59%, and 37%, and for the second group 60%, 36%, and 22% respectively.[126] Prognosis was affected most importantly by the presence of lymph node metastases. In fact, 90% of patients without lymphadenopathy survived 9 years.[123] Other important prognostic factors include extent of anatomical involvement, histologic pattern or grade, and the presence of ureteral obstruction. Local recurrence rates for stage A have been reported by Jazy et al[127] as 7%, stage B, 16%, and stage C, 34%. These recurrence rates may be expected to be even higher as the positive biopsy rates for small B, large B, and for C lesions reported by Bagshaw are 38%, 59%, and 74% respectively.[126] The implication of positive biopsies questions the efficacy of radiation; however, there is little doubt that definitive radiation does cure certain tumors.

Other controversies regarding radiation therapy center around the total radiation dose and the field to be irradiated. Initially only the prostate and periprostatic tissue were irradiated by the Stanford group. After 1971 treatment volumes were extended to include the pelvic lymph nodes below the iliac bifurcation and, in selected patients, the para-aortic nodes. The protocol designed by that group for stages B and C tumors was to treat the whole pelvis with 5000 to 5500 rad with an additional 1500 to 2000 rad to the prostate if on exploration of the lymph nodes or lymphangiogram there was evidence of disease. If no tumor was evident in the nodes, only the prostate was irradiated. If there was extracapsular extension, both the prostate and pelvis were irradiated.[128] Pistenma et al[128] reported in 1977 that patients with localized prostate carcinoma and no documented adenopathy derived no benefit from regional lymphatic irradiation. They also reported that whole pelvic irradiation with proven adenopathy might be of benefit. In 1981, McGowan[129] also reported that no advantage was found with extended field irradiation for localized disease, but with extraprostatic extension whole pelvic irradiation improved disease-free 5-year survival from 35% (localized radiation only) to 63%. There continues to be no absolute proof that whole pelvic irradiation with presence of lymph node metastases improves overall survival. There is likewise no consensus on the adequate radiation dosage level for prostatic cancer control. The dose used by Bagshaw is 7000 to 7600 rad to the center of the gland.[130] Harisiadis et al[131] found that a dose less than 6500 rad in 6.5 weeks was inadequate. Hussey, cited by Harisiadis et al, reported that 6500 rad in 6.5 weeks was sufficient to control 95% of tumors confined to the gland, but anything larger should have a dose of 7000 rad.[132]

The complications of external beam irradiation during therapy include diarrhea, rectal urgency, dysuria, and frequency. Few of these symptoms are lasting or permanent. Impotence occurs in between 13% and 40% of cases, and late complications of therapy include urinary incontinence (7%), chronic cystitis (4% to 8%), and chronic proctitis (1% to 4%).[133] With extended field therapy serious small bowel complications occurred in 67% of patients in the Stanford series. Edema of the genitalia has occurred in up to 55%.[12] Because of these problems extraperitoneal lymphadenectomy has largely been abandoned and the complication rate thereby reduced tremendously.

Overall, external beam therapy probably has the greatest applicability stage for stage. Virtually any patient with localized disease can be treated for a cure. It is more readily available than interstitial technics since special expertise is required for the latter if equivalent results with a minimum of complications are to be attained. There is no doubt that megavoltage teletherapy is effective treatment for certain prostate cancers and is an alternative to radical surgery or interstitial therapy.

Interstitial Irradiation

The modern era of interstitial irradiation began in the 1970s with the introduction of encapsulated radiation sources. Interstitial irradiation, in general, has several advantages when compared to external beam irradiation or radical surgery. The implant dose may be accurately adapted to the size and shape of the tumor; the higher cumulative radiation dose is delivered continuously over the useful life of the isotope; the hypoxic tumor center receives a larger dose than the oxygenated periphery; there is less damage to normal tissues because they receive less irradiation; staging and treatment are combined in a single procedure; and the procedure is applicable to a larger patient population than is radical surgery. The disadvantages of interstitial irradiation are the necessity for a surgical procedure, the possibility that large extracapsular tumors with ill-defined margins may not be adequately treated, and the fact that some prostatic carcinomas may not be radioresponsive.

Three isotopes are used for implantation today: iodine 125, gold 198, and iridium 192. Each has its own radiobiologic characteristics. Iodine 125 is a low energy (27 keV) radionuclide of iodine with a 60-day half-life and a radiation field of 1 cm which delivers between 16,000 and 20,000 rad to the prostate. Because of its low energy emission it has a long shelf life, a protracted period of tumor irradiation (1 year), and is the safest isotope for the personnel handling it, the patient, the patient's family, and the surrounding tissue. Gold 198 has a short half-life (2.7 days), is a high gamma energy emitter (0.41 meV), and has a half-value layer of 2.5 cm in lead and 6 cm in tissue. These properties increase the radiation exposure to operating room personnel, limit the number of implantable seeds to less than a full therapeutic dose because of unacceptable levels of irradiation to normal tissues outside the implanted volume, and lead to a higher rate of bladder and rectal complications. Because supplemental external beam therapy is required to bring the usual 2500-rad dose to a therapeutic level of 6000 to 7000 rad, the treatment period is prolonged, the expense is increased, and a greater morbidity may be anticipated from the combination of surgical procedure and external irradiation.

Iridium 192 is a gamma emitter with an average energy of 340 keV, a half-life of 75 days, and an average tissue spread of 6 cm. The advantages of this isotope and its technic of implantation, as described by Syed et al,[134] include no radiation exposure to operating room personnel because the isotope is afterloaded in the patient's room and the radiation sources cannot be passed later in the feces or urine. In addition, the use of a template gives a more uniform radiation dose distribution, allowing for treatment of large stage C (T_3, T_4) lesions and patients who have had prior transurethral resections for vesical outlet obstruction. The disadvantages, as with ^{198}Au, include the necessity of adjuvant external beam therapy, the prolonged treatment period, and the greater morbidity from the combination of external beam therapy and surgery.

Candidates for prostatic implantation vary depending upon the specific isotope and technic of implantation used. In general, all patients with localized disease can be treated with one of the isotopes or implantation technics. Use of ^{125}I is limited to those patients with B or small C lesions (T_2, T_{3a}) with no significant obstructive symptoms and no periurethral tumor. Larger local tumors and posttransurethral resection patients are poor candidates for ^{125}I as accurate and effective seed placement is difficult and the inadvertant loss of seeds occurs because a small amount of implantable tissue is likely to be present postresection. As a result certain areas of the tumor may not be adequately irradiated. For the most part, ^{198}Au is used under the same circumstances as ^{125}I; however, selected posttransurethral resection patients may be implanted. These patients would include some with A_2 (T_{1b}) and selected C (T_{3a}, T_{3b}) lesions. Iridium 192 usage is more universally applicable, including nearly all localized disease. This is a function of the use of a template and the fact that the implanted irradiation is temporary. The only patients excluded would be those with stage A_2 with minimal prostatic tissue remaining posttransurethral resection (less than 1 cm).

Bilateral pelvic lymphadenectomy and prostatic implantation is a relatively simple, straightforward, well-tolerated procedure with few complications. The complications from the first 300 cases reported from Memorial Hospital have been fully analyzed.[135] The operative mortality was 0.67%, with an intraoperative complication rate of 6% and postoperative complication rate of 23%. Cardiovascular complications including pulmonary emboli, thrombophlebitis, and lower extremity edema occurred in 7%. Other pelvic complications, which occurred in about 10%, included lymphocele formation (4.7%), hematoma, abscess, and pelvic cellulitis. With the use of the modified node dissection since 1978 lower extremity and genital edema has become virtually nonexistent.[136] Some degree of irritative urinary symptoms occur in about 25% of patients, but these are usually mild and last at most only a few weeks. Significant rectal symptoms are likewise uncommon. Occasionally a patient may have a small amount of bleeding secondary to localized radiation proctitis. This problem responds well to conservative therapy and the use of steroids. The devastating complication of rectourethral fistula has been reported[137]; however, this complication has not been seen in the Memorial Hospital experience. Although the exact cause of this problem may not be determinable, underlying factors certainly include technical expertise in seed placement, use of too many seeds with too high energy, inaccurate dosimetry calculations, and the inappropriate use of additional external beam therapy. Finally, sexual potency is preserved in more than 90% of patients treated.[136]

The most recent results of ^{125}I therapy were reported by Herr in 1983 on 586 patients treated at Memorial Hospital.[136] The observed 5-year survival for patients with B_1 lesions was 95% (79% disease-free); for B_2 lesions 81% (53% disease-free); for C lesions (T_3) 71% (45% disease-free); and for large C lesions (T_4) 21% (19% disease-free). The overall survival at 5 years was 84% and at 10 years 68%. The impact of positive pelvic nodes on absolute survival in this group of patients was dramatic with 83% of the patients with negative nodes alive at 9 years compared to 55% of patients with positive nodes. The results of ^{198}Au implantation are similar.[138] The overall 5- and 10-year survival for B_1 patients was 100% and 84%, respectively (71% and 54% disease-free); for B_2 lesions 81% and 52% (59% and 26% disease-free); and for C_1 lesions 86% and 73% (46% and 40% disease-free). The overall survival at 5 years was 90% and at 10 years 68%. As with the ^{125}I data, survival with negative lymph nodes was much better at 5 and 10 years than with positive lymph nodes (74% *v* 32% at 5 years and 53% *v* 18% at 10 years).[139] Since the template technic with ^{192}Ir is relatively new, no 5-year follow-up data are available.

The effectiveness of radiotherapy, be it external beam or interstitial, may be challenged by the findings of persistent tumor on biopsy performed 6 to 36 months post-treatment. Data reported by Scardino[140] following ^{198}Au therapy revealed a 38% overall positive biopsy rate. As the stage of disease increased so did the positive biopsy rate. Those with negative biopsies had only a 4% local recurrence rate and those with positive biopsies had a 37% local recurrence rate. Although it seems that the persistence of tumor after irradiation is a poor prognostic sign, radiation therapy is curative in a number of individuals. It seems that a more important aspect in treating prostate cancer is to try and determine which tumors are radioresponsive and which should be treated by surgery.

Stage D Endocrine Therapy

John Hunter, in 1874, was the first to recognize that removing the testes caused prostatic atrophy in animals.[141] In 1893, White reported that following castration the muscular and glandular elements of the canine prostate atrophy.[142] He therefore advocated castration as the treatment of choice for prostatic obstruction. In 1941, Huggins and associates,[143–145] introduced and firmly established the scientific basis for endocrine therapy for the treatment of prostatic carcinoma. They described eight patients with metastatic prostate cancer and elevated serum acid phosphatase levels who had bilateral orchiectomy with subsequent marked decreased in acid phosphatase and clinical regression of tumor. When they later administered testosterone to some of these patients the serum acid phosphatase activity increased again to an abnormal range. Bruchovsky and Wilson[146] in 1968 demonstrated that the biologic effects of androgens on the prostate depended on conversion within the prostate to dihydrotestosterone by the enzyme 5-α-reductase. After the conversion, dihydrotestosterone combines with a specific steroid receptor protein and is translocated to the nucleus where it binds to nuclear chromatin. This converted androgen then triggers the biochemical events which lead to the synthesis of protein by the prostate cells.[147]

It is well established that between 70% and 80% of patients with advanced prostatic cancer will show a clinical response to hormonal therapy.[148] These responses are highlighted by objective and/or subjective changes such as a decrease in the size of the primary and/or metastatic tumor, a decrease in the serum acid phosphatase level, relief of bone pain, improvement in vesical outlet obstructive symptoms, and increase in weight and RBC count, and improvement in appetite and overall sense of well-being.[149] Although there is an obvious clinical response to this therapy with an improved quality of life, it has not been possible to determine unequivocally that orchiectomy, estrogen therapy, or a combination of both increases overall survival. For this reason controversy continues to exist as to what form of endocrine therapy should be used and when in the course of the patient's disease endocrine therapy should be initiated.

The treatment of prostatic adenocarcinoma is based on the premise that the tumor growth is androgen-dependent. The reduction or inhibition of androgen stimulation may then be accomplished by removing the primary source of androgen production; by removing or suppressing luteinizing hormone–releasing factor and thereby reducing the release of pituitary luteinizing-releasing hormone and the testicular production of testosterone; by the direct inhibition of androgen synthesis at the cellular level; and by blocking androgens or their effects at the cellular level.[150]

Ablation of androgen sources

Orchiectomy The testicles account for 95% of androgen production in men. By removing both testes the normal testosterone level can be reduced from 200 to 1200 ng/100 mL to an average of 43±32 ng/100 mL.[151] In most men the testosterone level will remain uniformly suppressed for up to 2 years postorchiectomy.[152,153] The subsequent appearance of endocrine-unresponsive symptomatic disease after bilateral orchiectomy is not associated with demonstrated increases in androstenedione, dehydroepiandrosterone, or testosterone, showing that there is no detectable increase in testosterone levels from the activation of secondary androgen sources.[154–156] Likewise, estrogen rescue of those who progress despite orchiectomy is not likely.

The advantages of orchiectomy over other forms of therapy include: (1) the easy accomplishment of surgery with the patient awake under local anesthesia, (2) elimination of the problem of patient compliance, (3) the immediateness of the therapeutic response, and (4) the avoidance of the cardiovascular complications of estrogens. The disadvantages include: (1) loss of libido, (2) the psychological trauma of castration, and (3) irreversibility of the operation, whereas estrogens may be discontinued once the desired state of palliation or response is achieved.

Adrenalectomy and hypophysectomy The rationale for adrenalectomy and hypophysectomy in those patients relapsing after orchiectomy or estrogen therapy is to remove the extratesticular androgen sources that may sustain clones of cells at low androgen levels as well as remove prolactin.[56] Bilateral adrenalectomy was first reported by Huggins and Scott in 1945 on four patients; all died from adrenal insufficiency.[157] In 1953 the procedure was revived by Harrison et al who noted some short-lived symptomatic improvement.[158] Bhanalaph et al in 1974 performed adrenalectomy in castrates and could show no further decrease in plasma testosterone levels.[159] Although the adrenal gland may be an insignificant source of testosterone, adrenalectomy has been shown to induce a 20% to 40% subjective response in endocrine-relapse patients.[160] The duration of response, however, is short.

Surgical hypophysectomy has been performed since 1948 for relapse of metastatic prostate cancer to remove the stimulation of ACTH and prolactin. This procedure has been uniformly unsuccessful with any subjective response being of short duration.[161] Recently, selective chemical hypophysectomy has been achieved by administering a new gonadotropin-releasing hormone analogue. It stimulates gonadotropin-releasing hormone and initially increases the release of follicle-stimulating hormone (FSH) and luteinizing hormone (LH) from the pituitary. As usage increases it blocks the release of LH.[161] At present its use is in randomized clinical trials with diethylstilbestrol (DES). The only advantage it may have is a decreased number of side effects when compared to orchiectomy or DES alone.

Estrogen therapy Since Herbst first reported the use of exogenous estrogen in 1942,[162] exogenous estrogens have played an important role in treating prostate cancer. Estrogens suppress the release of LH from the anterior pituitary and thereby eliminate the stimulus for the testicular production of testosterone. Estrogens are also thought to act by increasing circulating testosterone-estrogen–binding globulin, thereby decreasing circulating free testosterone, and possibly by directly inhibiting testosterone production by the testes.[161] Diethylstilbestrol is the most commonly used oral estrogen. Other synthetic agents such as conjugated estrogen, ethynyl estradiol, and chlorotrianisene have been shown to reduce plasma testosterone levels to castrate levels but offer no advantages over DES.[82] The major controversy over the use of DES is the optimal daily dose and when to initiate therapy.

Kent et al,[163] Robinson and Thomas,[164] and Shearer et al[165] have shown that doses of less than 1 mg DES have essentially no effect on reducing serum testosterone levels; however, 1-mg doses can suppress testosterone levels by approximately 50%. The second VACURG study showed that serum testosterone levels need not be reduced to castrate levels to be effective.[166] In this study there was no difference in therapeutic response when 5-mg or 1-mg daily doses were administered.

The results of the first VACURG study revealed the increased risk of cardiovascular complications of a 5-mg daily dose of DES.[167] In that study, patients with low-stage disease (A, B, or T_1, T_2) who received 5 mg DES had poorer survival rates than those patients not receiving estrogen. Upon analyzing the cause of death, it became evident that a number of patients died from cardiovascular complications and not from prostate cancer. These findings suggested that endocrine therapy did not prolong survival and should be withheld because of the cardiovascular side effects until patients become symptomatic. It has subsequently been shown that 3 mg a day of DES consistently suppresses serum testosterone levels and that dosages of up to 30 mg a day do not further suppress testosterone levels.[163,168] Although it is logical to infer that 3 mg DES would be the optimal dose, there is no study equating the efficacy of therapy with the plasma testosterone level and there are no clinical data on the incidence of cardiovascular complications with the use of 3 mg/d.

The proper timing of endocrine therapy also remains controversial. It has been demonstrated in the VACURG trials that patients with stage C tumors who received placebo therapy had a higher rate of progression to stage D than those stage C patients who were treated with endocrine therapy. Likewise, the asymptomatic stage D patients treated by placebo developed symptoms earlier than the stage D patients treated with endocrine therapy. Overall survival from the time of initial diagnosis, however, was not significantly different between the two groups of patients. Therefore, whether endocrine therapy is begun early or late continues to be based upon the personal preference of the treating physician.

Antiandrogens Antiandrogens work by competing with endogenously produced androgens for receptor sites on the target tissue. Primarily they compete with dihydrotestosterone for the cytoplasmic receptor protein that allows dihydrotestosterone to enter the cell nucleus.[169] Cyproterone acetate is a progestational agent that blocks the dihydrotestosterone receptor complex and inhibits the release of pituitary LH. Although it has been used effectively in Europe its only advantage over DES is that it does not cause gynecomastia. Flutamide, a nonsteroidal, nonprogestational antiandrogen, works by blocking the dihydrotestosterone receptor complex. Although it has been shown to decrease pain, relieve obstruction, and decrease prostate size,[170] its only advantage over orchiectomy or DES is that in a number of patients potency is spared.

Inhibitors of androgen synthesis Since testosterone is synthesized from cholesterol in several steps, any drug that effectively blocks the action of any enzyme in this sequence will reduce the serum testosterone level. Aminoglutethimide inhibits the adrenal production of androgens, cortisol and aldosterone by interfering with the conversion of cholesterol to δ-5-pregnenolone. Following orchiectomy, 40% to 50% of patients who relapse have been shown to respond to aminoglutethimide administration.[171,172]

Spironolactone and cyproterone acetate inhibit the 17,20-desmolase enzyme and block the production of androgens. Although it has been found that spironolactone suppresses plasma testosterone from 45 ng/100 mL to 10 ng/100 mL and suppresses plasma levels of androstenedione and dehydroepiandrosterone to 60% and 40% of their control values, there has been only a limited clinical response in those patients treated.[159,173]

Cytotoxic Chemotherapy

Although there has been a substantial amount of investigation of cytotoxic chemotherapeutic agents for advanced prostate cancer, a rational discussion of their efficacy and comparisons between treatment protocols are complicated by many variables. These variables include entry into studies of patients who had been previously untreated, did not respond to hormone therapy, or relapsed on hormone therapy; the fact that some studies have evaluated the response of metastatic disease whereas others have evaluated the response of primary tumor; the wide variety of combinations of agents employed (cytotoxic agents with or without endocrine therapy and/or steroids); the use of nonrandomized trials or comparative trials with no controls; the variations in response criteria used; and the definitions of efficacy including disease-free survival, absolute survival, and duration of an objective or subjective response. Other reasons for delay in the study of chemotherapeutic agents include the previously discussed dramatic response to endocrine therapy, the fact that prostate cancer is a slow-growing tumor and not well suited to chemotherapy, and the advanced age of the patients to be treated, some of whom tolerate the physiologic effects of chemotherapy poorly.[56]

In an attempt to search for effective chemotherapeutic agents and establish strict criteria for evaluation of therapy, the National Prostate Cancer Project (NPCP) embarked on a clinical trials program in 1972. A recent summary of the objective response rates using NPCP response criteria was published by Schmidt and colleagues (Tables 24-7 and 24-8).[174,175] Standard therapy in this trial consisted of continued hormonal therapy, prednisone, analgesics, and palliative radiation. In those patients without prior irradiation, active single agents included methotrexate, cisplatin, 5-fluorouracil, cyclophosphamide, estramustine phosphate, semustine, and decarbazine. Hydroxyurea and procarbazine hydrochloride actually demonstrated inferior response rates and were fairly toxic.[175] In those patients who had prior irradiation, active agents included streptozocin, and estramustine phosphate sodium, alone and in combination with cisplatin.[175] Other conclusions reached through the NPCP trials are: (1) Chemotherapy has an advantage over conventional therapy in relapsing stage D disease; (2) responders to chemotherapy survive significantly longer than nonresponders; (3) objective partial regressions (PR) are seen only with chemotherapy in relapsing stage D disease; (4) active single agents

Table 24-7
Objective Response Rates for Antitumor Agents Evaluated in Trials of Patients with Hormonally Refractory Disease without Prior Pelvic Irradiation* (October 1982)

Drugs	Patients	Objective Response Rates (%)
Methotrexate	58	41
Cisplatin	50	36
5-Fluorouracil	33	36
Cyclophosphamide	119	34
Estramustine	50	34
Semustine	27	30
Decarbazine	55	27
Standard	36	19
Hydroxyurea	28	15
Procarbazine	39	13

*Adapted from Schmidt.[176]

Table 24-8
Objective Response Rates for Antitumor Agents Evaluated in Trials of Patients with Hormonally Refractory Disease without Prior Pelvic Irradiation* (October 1982)

Drugs	Patients	Objective Response Rates (%)
Single Agents		
Streptozocin	38	32
Estramustine	113	25
Cisplatin	42	21
Standard	21	19
Vincristine sulfate	34	15
LEO 1031	62	13
Combinations		
Estramustine + LEO 1031	54	13
Estramustine + vincristine	29	24
Estramustine + cisplatin	42	33

*Adapted from Schmidt.[176]

include cyclophosphamide, fluorouracil, decarbazine, estracyt, methotrexate, cisplatin, and streptozocin; and (5) there is an advantage in adding chemotherapy to estrogens in patients with untreated stage D disease.[175]

It should be emphasized that no "magic bullet" for prostate cancer is available[176]; however, some further answers with regard to chemotherapeutic efficacy will be forthcoming from the NPCP trials. Physicians with patients who meet the criteria for entry into one of these trials are encouraged to do so to make additional meaningful information available to future generations of prostate cancer patients.[176]

REFERENCES

1. Johnson DE: Cancer of the prostate. Overview, in Paulson D (ed): *Genitourinary Surgery.* New York, Grune & Stratton, 1983, pp 1–31.
2. *1984. Cancer Facts and Figures.* New York, American Cancer Society, 1983.
3. Klein LA: Medical progress: Prostatic carcinoma. *N Engl J Med* 1979;300:824–833.
4. Owen WL: Cancer of the prostate: A literature review. *J Chronic Dis* 1976; 29:89–114.
5. Stamey TA: Cancer of the prostate. *Monogr Urol* 1983;4:65–92.
6. Franks LM: Latent carcinoma of the prostate. *J Pathol Bacteriol* 1954;68:603–616.
7. von Eschenbach AC, Johnson DE: Adenocarcinoma of the prostate. *Compr Ther* 1978;4:18–26.
8. Higgins FT: The epidemiology of cancer of the prostate. *J Chronic Dis* 1975;28: 343–348.
9. Wynder EL, Mabuchi K, Whitmore WF: Epidemiology of cancer of the prostate. *Cancer* 1971;28:344–360.
10. Winkelstein W, Jr, Einster VL: Epidemiology and etiology, in Murphy GP (ed): *Prostatic Cancer.* Littleton, Mass, PSG Publishing Co, 1979, pp 1–17.
11. Hutchison GB: Epidemiology of prostate cancer. *Semin Oncol* 1976;13:151–159.
12. von Eschenbach AC: Cancer of the prostate. *Curr Probl Cancer* 1981;5:1–54.
13. Huggins C, Hodges CV: Studies on prostatic cancer. I. The effect of castration, of estrogen and of androgen injection on serum phosphatases in metastatic carcinoma of the prostate. *Cancer Res* 1941; 1:293–297.
14. Moore RA, Twombly GH, Pack GT: *Endocrinology of Neoplastic Disease.* New

York, Oxford University Press, 1947, p 194.
15. Kipling MD, Waterhouse JAH: Cadmium and prostatic carcinoma. *Lancet* 1967;1: 730–731.
16. Winkelstein W Jr, Kantor S: Prostatic cancer. Relation in suspended articulate air pollution. *Am J Public Health* 1969; 59:1134–1138.
17. McMichael AJ, Spirtas R, Kupper LL: An epidemiologic study of mortality within a cohort of rubber workers. *J Occup Med* 1974;16:458–464.
18. Hirayama T: Epidemiology of prostatic cancer with special reference to the role of diet. *Natl Cancer Inst Monogr* 1979;53: 149–155.
19. Phillips RL: Role of life-style and dietary habits in risk of cancer among Seventh Day Adventists. *Cancer Res* 1975;35:3513–3522.
20. Andrews GS: Latent carcinoma of the prostate. *J Clin Pathol* 1949;2:197–208.
21. Armenian HK, Lilienfeld AM, Diamond EL, et al: Relation between benign prostatic hyperplasia and cancer of the prostate. A prospective and retrospective study. *Lancet* 1974;2:115–117.
22. Greenwald P, Kirmiss V, Polan AK, et al: Cancer of the prostate among men with benign prostatic hyperplasia. *J Natl Cancer Inst* 1974;53:335–340.
23. Moore RA: The morphology of small prostatic carcinoma. *J Urol* 1935;33:224–234.
24. Mostofi FK, Price EB: *Tumors of the Male Genital System.* Washington, DC, *Armed Forces Institute of Pathology,* 1973.
25. Tannenbaum M, Lattimer JK: Similar virus-like particles found in cancers of the prostate and breast. *J Urol* 1970;103:471–475.
26. Steele R, Lees REM, Kraus AS, et al: Sexual factors in the epidemiology of cancer of the prostate. *J Chronic Dis* 1971;24: 29–37.
27. Heshmat MY, Kovi J, Herson J, et al: Epidemiologic association between gonorrhea and prostatic carcinoma. *Urology* 1975;6: 457–460.
28. Byar DP, Mostofi FK: Carcinoma of the prostate: Prognostic evaluation of certain pathologic features in 208 radical prostatectomies. Examined by the step-section technique. *Cancer* 1972;30:5–13.
29. Broders AC: Carcinoma: Grading and practical application. *Arch Pathol* 1925;2: 376–381.
30. Gleason DF, Mellinger GT, and the Veterans Administrative Co-operative Urological Research Group: Prediction of prognosis for prostatic adenocarcinoma by combined histological grading and clinical staging. *J Urol* 1974;111:58–64.
31. Mostofi FF: Grading of prostatic carcinoma. *Cancer Chemother Rep* 1975;59: 111–117.
32. Gaeta FJ, Asirwatham JE: Miller G, et al: Histologic grading of primary prostatic cancer: a new approach to an old problem. *J Urol* 1980;123:689–693.
33. Utz DC, Farrow GM: Pathologic differentiation and prognosis and prostatic carcinoma. *JAMA* 1969;209:1701–1703.
34. Kramer AS, Spahr J, Brendler CB, et al: Experience with Gleason's histopathologic grading in prostate cancer. *J Urol* 1980; 124:223–225.
35. Gaeta FJ: Glandular profiles and cellular patterns in prostatic grading. *Urology* 1981;17:33–37.
36. Murphy GP, Whitmore WF Jr: A report of the workshops on the current status of the histologic grading of prostate cancer. *Cancer* 1979;44:1490–1494.
37. Diamond DA, Berry SJ, Jewett HJ, et al: New method to assess metastatic potential of human prostatic cancer. Relative nuclear roundness. *J Urol* 1982;128: 729–734.
38. Tribukait B, Esposti PL, Ronstrom L: Tumor ploidy for characterization of prostatic carcinoma: flow cytofluorometric DNA studies using aspiration biopsy material. *Scand J Urol Nephrol [Suppl]* 1980;55:59–64.
39. Tribukait B, Ronstrom L, Esposti PL: Quantitative and cytologic grade in prostatic carcinoma. *Anal Quant Cytol* 1983;5: 107–111.
40. Ronstrom L, Tribukait B, Esposti PL: DNA pattern and cytological findings in fine-needle aspirates of untreated prostatic tumors. A flow-cytofluorometric study. *Prostate* 1981;2:79–88.
41. Zetterberg A, Esposti PL: Cytophotometric DNA analysis of aspirated cells from prosstatic carcinoma. *Acta Cytol (Baltimore)* 1976;20:46–57.

42. Zetterberg A, Esposti PL: Prognostic significance of nuclear DNA levels in prostatic carcinoma. *Scand J Urol Nephrol [Suppl]* 1980;55:53–58.
43. Frederiksen P, Thommesen P, Kjaer TB, et al: Flow cytometric DNA analysis in fine needle aspiration biopsies from patients with prostatic lesions. Diagnostic value and relations to clinical stages. *Acta Path Microbiol Scand* 1978;86:461–464.
44. Bichel P, Frederiksen P, Kjaer TB, et al: Flow microfluorometry and transrectal fine-needle biopsy in the classification of human prostatic carcinoma. *Cancer* 1977; 40:1206–1211.
45. Lammel A, Roters M, Kastendieck H, et al: Flow cytometric determination of DNA distribution in malignant and benign tumors of the prostate. *Urologe* (Ausg A) 1981;20:400–404.
46. Green LF, Mulcahy JJ, Warren MM, et al: Primary transitional cell carcinoma of the prostate. *J Urol* 1975;110:235–237.
47. Rhamy RK, Buchanan RD, Spalding MJ: Intraductal carcinoma of the prostate gland. *J Urol* 1973;109:457–460.
48. Waisman J, Mott LJM: Pathology of neoplasms of the prostate gland, in Skinner DG, deKernion JB (eds): *Genitourinary Cancer.* Philadelphia, WB Saunders Co, 1978, pp 310–343.
49. American Joint Committee on Cancer: *Manual for Staging of Cancer.* Philadelphia, JB Lippincott Co, 1983, pp 159–164.
50. Whitmore WF Jr: Interstitial radiation therapy for carcinoma of the prostate. *Prostate* 1980;1:157–168.
51. Veterans Administration Co-operative Urological Research Group: Carcinoma of the prostate: A continuing cooperative study. *J Urol* 1964;91:590–594.
52. Del Regato JA: Radiotherapy for carcinoma of the prostate: A report from the Committee for Cooperative Study of Radiotherapy for Carcinoma of the Prostate. Colorado Springs, Penrose Carver Hospital, 1968.
53. Jewett HJ: The present status of radical prostatectomy for state A and B prostatic cancer. *Urol Clin North Am* 1975;2: 105–124.
54. Barnes RW: Carcinoma of the prostate: A comparative study of nodes of treatment. *J Urol* 1940;44:169–176.
55. Young HH, Davis DM: *Young's Practice of Urology.* Philadelphia, WB Saunders Co, 1926, pp 621–634.
56. Catalona WJ, Scott WW: *Carcinoma of the prostate,* in Harrison JH, Gittes RF, Perlmutter AD, et al (eds): *Campbell's Urology.* Philadelphia, WB Saunders Co, 1979; pp 1085–1124.
57. Tannenbaum M: Aspiration biopsy of the prostate: The pathologist's viewpoint. *Semin Urol* 1983;1:172–176.
58. Dahlin CP, Goodwin WE: Sexual potency after perineal biopsy. *J Urol* 1957;77: 660–669.
59. Franks LM: The cytodiagnosis of prostate cancer. *JAMA* 1969;209:1698.
60. Romas NA: Prostatic acid phosphatase: Current concepts. *Semin Urol* 1983;1: 177–185.
61. Byar DP: VACURG studies on prostatic cancer and its treatment, in Byar DP (ed): *Urologic Pathology: The Prostate.* Philadelphia, Lea & Febiger, 1977.
62. Bisson J, Vickers M Jr, Fagan WT Jr: Bone scan. *J Urol* 1974;111:665–669.
63. Paulson DF: Pelvic lymphadenectomy is not essential to staging accuracy in all patients with localized prostate cancer. *Semin Urol* 1983;1:204–211.
64. Levine MS, Arger H, Coleman BG, et al: Detecting lymphatic metastases from prostatic carcinoma. Superiority of CT. *Am J Roentgenol* 1981;137:207–211.
65. Olson CA: *Conference: Prostate Carcinoma Issues and Debate.* Held at Essex House, New York, in press.
66. Wilson CS, Dahl DS, Middler RG: Pelvic lymphadenectomy for the staging of apparently localized prostatic cancer. *J Urol* 1977;117:197–198.
67. Grossman LC, Carpinello V, Greenberg SH, et al: Staging pelvic lymphadenectomy for carcinoma of the prostate: review of 91 cases. *J Urol* 1980;124:632–634.
68. Leiskovsky G, Skinner DG, Weisenburger T: Pelvic lymphadenectomy in the management of carcinoma of the prostate. *J Urol* 1980;124:635–638.
69. Brendler CB, Cleeve LK, Anderson EE, et al: Staging pelvic lymphadenectomy for carcinoma of the prostate: risk versus benefit. *J Urol* 1980;124:849–850.
70. McLaughlin AP, Saltzstein SL, McCullough DL, et al: Prostatic carcinoma: in-

cidence and location of unsuspected lymphatic metastases. *J Urol* 1976;115:89–94.

71. Golimbu M, Morales P, Al-Askari S, et al: Extended pelvic lymphadenectomy for prostatic cancer. *J Urol* 1979;121:617–620.
72. Freiha FS, Pistenma DA, Bagshaw MA: Pelvic lymphadenectomy for staging prostatic cancer: is it always necessary? *J Urol* 1979;122:176–179.
73. Whitmore WF Jr: Interstitial radiation therapy for carcinoma of the prostate. *Prostate* 1980;1:157–168.
74. Paul DB, Loening SA, Narayana AS, Culp DA: Morbidity from pelvic lymphadenectomy in staging carcinoma of the prostate. *J Urol* 1983;129:1141–1144.
75. Fisher H, Herr HW, Sogani P, et al: Modified pelvic lymph node dissection in patients undergoing I-125 implantation for carcinoma of the prostate. Read before American Urological Association, Boston, Mass, May 1981, abstract No. 299.
76. Whitmore WF Jr: Retropubic implantation of I-125 in the treatment of prostatic cancer. New York, Alan R Liss, Inc, 1976, pp 223–233.
77. Herr HW: Interstitial irradiation for localized prostatic cancer. *Semin Urol* 1983;1:222–228.
78. Herr HW: Iodine-125 implantation in the management of localized prostatic carcinoma. *Urol Clin North Am* 1980;7:605–613.
79. Sheldon CA: Incidental carcinoma of the prostate: a review of the literature and critical appraisal of classification. *J Urol* 1980;124:626–631.
80. McMillen SM, Wettlaufer JN: The role of repeat transurethral biopsy in stage A carcinoma of the prostate. *J Urol* 1976;116:759–760.
81. Greene LF, Simon HB: Occult carcinoma of the prostate: clinical and therapeutic study in 83 cases. *JAMA* 1956;158:1494–1498.
82. Byar DP: The Veterans Administration Cooperative Urological Research Group. Survival of patients with incidentally found microscopic cancer of the prostate: Results of a clinical trial of conservative treatment. *J Urol* 1972;108:908–913.
83. Hanash KA, Utz DC, Cook EN, et al: Carcinoma of the prostate. A 15-year follow-up. *J Urol* 1972;107:450–453.
84. Millin T: *Retropubic Urinary Surgery.* Baltimore, Williams & Wilkins Co, 1947.
85. Memmelaar J: Total prostatovesiculectomy-retropubic approach. *J Urol* 1949; 62:340–348.
86. Hand JR, Sullivan AW: Retropubic prostatectomy–analysis of one hundred cases. *JAMA* 1951;145:1313–1321.
87. Flocks RH, Culp D, Porto R: Lymphatic spread from prostatic cancer. *J Urol* 1959;81:194–196.
88. Chute R: Radical retropubic prostatectomy for cancer. *J Urol* 1954;71:347–372.
89. Coffey RC: Cystectomy for carcinoma of the bladder: report of cases. *Am J Surg* 1933;20:254–297.
90. Hinman F, Smith D: Total cystectomy for cancer: critical review. *Surgery* 1939;6: 851–881.
91. Westerborn A: Radical treatment of cancer of the prostate by cystovesiculo-prostatectomy. *Surg Gynecol Obstet* 1950;91: 751–756.
92. Whitmore WF Jr, MacKenzie AR: Experiences with various operative procedures for the total exclusion of prostatic cancer. *Cancer* 1959;12:396–405.
93. McCullough DL, Leadbetter WF: Radical pelvic surgery for locally extensive carcinoma of the prostate. *J Urol* 1972; 108:939–943.
94. Jewett HJ, Bridge RW, Gray GF Jr, et al: The palpable nodule of prostatic cancer: 15 years after radical excision. *JAMA* 1968; 203:403–406.
95. Huson HC, Howland RL Jr: Radical retropubic prostatectomy for cancer of the prostate. *J Urol* 1972;108:944–947.
96. Boxer RJ, Kaufman JJ, Goodwin WE: Radical prostatectomy for carcinoma of the prostate: 1951–1976. A review of 329 patients. *J Urol* 1977;117:208–213.
97. Walsh PC, Donker PJ: Impotence following radical prostatectomy: Insight into etiology and prevention. *J Urol* 1982; 128:492–497.
98. Walsh PC: Radical prostatectomy for the treatment of localized prostatic carcinoma. *Urol Clin North Am* 1980;7:583–591.
99. Jewett HJ: The case for radical perineal prostatectomy. *J Urol* 1970;103:195–199.
100. Walsh PC, Jewett HJ: Radical surgery for prostate cancer. *Cancer* 1980;45: 1906–1911.

101. Jewett HJ: The present status of radical prostatectomy for stages A and B prostatic cancer. *Urol Clin North Am* 1975;2: 105–124.
102. Correa RJ Jr, Gibbons RP, Cummings KB, et al: Total prostatectomy for Stage B carcinoma of the prostate. *J Urol* 1977; 117:328–329.
103. Berlin BB, Cornwell PM, Connelly RR, et al: Radical perineal prostatectomy for carcinoma of the prostate: survival in 143 cases treated from 1935 to 1958. *J Urol* 1968;99:97–101.
104. Belt E, Schroeder FH: Total perineal prostatectomy for carcinoma of the prostate. *J Urol* 1972;107:91–96.
105. Culp OS, Meyer JJ: Radical prostatectomy in the treatment of prostate cancer. *Cancer* 1973;32:1113–1118.
106. Williams J, Marshall VF, Gray GF Jr: Radical perineal prostatectomy with bilateral orchiectomy for carcinoma of the prostate. *J Urol* 1975;113:380–384.
107. Elder JS, Jewett HJ, Walsh PC: Radical perineal prostatectomy for clinical stage B_2 carcinoma of the prostate. *J Urol* 1982; 127:704–706.
108. Golimbu M, Schinella R, Morales P, et al: Differences in pathological characteristics and prognosis of clinical A-2 prostatic cancer from A-1 and B disease. *J Urol* 1978;119:618–622.
109. Corriere JN Jr, Cornog JC, Murphy JJ: Prognosis in patients with carcinoma of the prostate. *Cancer* 1970;25:911–918.
110. Schroeder FH, Belt E: Carcinoma of the prostate: a study of 213 patients with stage C tumors treated by total perineal prostatectomy. *J Urol* 1975;114:257–258.
111. Scott WW, Boyd HL: Combined hormone control therapy and radical prostatectomy in the treatment of selected cases of advanced carcinoma of the prostate – a retrospective study based upon 25 years of experience. *J Urol* 1969;101:86–92.
112. Pasteau O, DeGrais P: Traitement des tumeurs de la prostate par le radium, in Frowde H (ed): *Transactions Seventeenth International Congress of Medicine.* London, Oxford University Press, 1913, p 28.
113. Pasteau O, Degrais P: The radium treatment of cancer of the prostate. *Arch Roentgen Ray Soc* 1914;18:396–410.
114. Young HH: *The Diagnosis and Treatment of Early Malignant Disease of the Prostate.* London, Oxford University Press, 1913.
115. Young HH, Fronz WA: Some new methods in the treatment of carcinoma of the lower genitourinary tract with radium. *J Urol* 1917;1:505–534.
116. Young HH: Technique of radium treatment of cancer of the prostate and seminal vesicles. *Surg Gynecol Obstet* 1922;34: 93–98.
117. Deming CL: Results in one hundred cases of cancer of the prostate and seminal vesicles treated with radium. *Surg Gynecol Obstet* 1922;34:99–118.
118. Barringer BS: Carcinoma of the prostate. *Surg Gynecol Obstet* 1922;34:168–176.
119. Bumpus HC: Roentgen rays and radium in the diagnosis and treatment of carcinoma of the prostate. *AJR* 1922;9:269–287.
120. Smith GG, Perison EL: The value of high voltage x-ray therapy in carcinoma of the prostate. *J Urol* 1930;23:331–342.
121. Barringer BS: Prostatic carcinoma. *J Urol* 1942;47:306–310.
122. Flocks RH, Kerr HD, Elkins HP, et al: Treatment of carcinoma of the prostate by interstitial radiation with radioactive gold (AU-198): preliminary report. *J Urol* 1952; 68:510–522.
123. Liskow A: External radiotherapy for localized prostate cancer. *Semin Urol* 1983; 1:217–221.
124. Budhraja SN, Anderson JC: An assessment of the value of radiotherapy in the management of carcinoma of the prostate. *Br J Urol* 1964;36:535–540.
125. Bagshaw MA, Kaplan HS, Sagermore R: Linear accelerator supervoltage radiotherapy. VII. Carcinoma of the prostate. *Radiology* 1965;85:121–129.
126. Bagshaw MA: Radiotherapy of prostatic carcinoma: long- or short-term efficacy. Conference: Prostate Carcinoma Issues and Debate. Held at Essex House, New York, in press.
127. Jazy FK, Aron B, Dettmar CM, et al: Radiation therapy as definitive treatment for localized carcinoma of the prostate. *Urology* 1972;14:555–560.
128. Pistenma DA, Bagshaw MA, Freiha FS: Extended-field radiation therapy for prostatic adenocarcinoma: status report of a limited perspective trial, in Johnson

DE, Samuels ML (eds): *Cancer of the Genitourinary Tract.* New York, Raven Press, 1979, pp 229–247.
129. McGowan DG: The value of extended field radiation therapy in carcinoma of the prostate. *Int J Radiat Oncol Biol Phys* 1981;7: 1333–1339.
130. Bagshaw MA, Ray GR, Pistenma DA, et al: External beam therapy of primary carcinoma of the prostate. *Cancer* 1975;36: 723–728.
131. Harisiadis LN, Veenema RJ, Senyszyn JJ, et al: Carcinoma of the prostate: Treatment with external radiotherapy. *Cancer* 1978;41:2131–2142.
132. Hussey DH: Experience with limited field irradiation for adenocarcinoma of the prostate in, Johnson DE, Samuels ML (eds): *Cancer of the Genitourinary Tract.* New York, Raven Press, 1979, pp 217–228.
133. van der Werf-Messing B: *Radiation Therapy of Carcinoma of the Prostate.* Baltimore, Williams & Wilkins, 1982, pp 195–216.
134. Syed AMN, Puthawala A, Tonsey LA, et al: Management of prostatic carcinoma: combination of pelvic lymphadenectomy, temporary iridium-192 implantation and external irradiation. *Radiology* 1983;149: 829–833.
135. Fowler JE, Barzell W, Hilaris BS, et al: Complications of iodine-125 implantation and pelvic lymphadenectomy in the treatment of prostatic cancer. *J Urol* 1979; 121:447–451.
136. Herr AW: Interstitial irradiation for localized prostatic cancer. *Semin Urol* 1983;1:222–228.
137. Mouli PC, Sharifi R, Ray P, et al: Prostatorectal fistula associated with iodine-125 seed radiotherapy. *J Urol* 1983;129:387–388.
138. Scardino PT, Guerriero WG, Carlton CE: Surgical staging and combined therapy with radioactive gold grain implantation and external irradiation, in Johnson DE, Boileau MA (eds): *Genitourinary Tumors, Fundamental Principles and Surgical Techniques.* New York, Grune & Stratton, 1982, pp 75–80.
139. Scardino PT: Combined interstitial (gold-198) and external irradiation for localized prostate cancer, in *Prostate Cancer Video Conference,* American Urological Association, 1982, pp 136–142.
140. Scardino PT: Positive prostatic biopsy following radiotherapy: Is it significant?, Conference: *Prostate Carcinoma Issues and Debate.* Held at Essex House, New York, in press.
141. Palmer JF: *The Surgical Works of John Hunter FRCS with Notes.* London, Longman, 1837.
142. White JW: The surgery of the hypertrophied prostate. *Ann Surg* 1893;17: 70–75.
143. Huggins C, Hodges CV: Studies on prostatic cancer. I. The effect of castration, of estrogen and of androgen injection on serum phosphatases in metastatic carcinoma of the prostate. *Cancer Res* 1941;1: 293–297.
144. Huggins C, Scott WW, Hodges CV: Studies on prostatic cancer III. The effects of fever, desoxycorticosterone and of estrogen on clinical patients with metastatic carcinoma of the prostate. *J Urol* 1941;46: 997–1006.
145. Huggins C, Stevens RE, Hodges CV: Studies on prostate cancer II. The effects of castration on advanced carcinoma of the prostate gland. *Arch Surg* 1941;43: 209–223.
146. Bruchovsky N, Wilson JD: The conversion of testosterone to 5-alpha-androstan-17-beta-ol-3-one by rat prostate in vivo and in vitro. *J Biol Chem* 1968;243:2012–2021.
147. Walsh PC: Physiologic basis for hormonal therapy in carcinoma of the prostate. *Urol Clin North Am* 1975;2:125–140.
148. Brendler H: Therapy with orchiectomy of estrogens or both. *JAMA* 1969;210: 1074–1075.
149. Resnick MI, Grayhack JT: Treatment of stage IV carcinoma of the prostate. *Urol Clin North Am* 1975;2:141–161.
150. Paulson DF: The role of endocrine therapy in the management of prostatic cancer, in Skinner DG, deKernian JB (eds): *Genitourinary Cancer.* Philadelphia, WB Saunders Co, 1978, pp 388–396.
151. Coffey DS, Isaacs JT: Control of prostate growth. *Urology* 1981;17(suppl):17–24.
152. Robinson MRG, Thomas BS: Effect of hormonal therapy in plasma testosterone levels in prostatic carcinoma. *Br Med J* 1971;4:391–394.
153. Young HH II, Keat JR: Plasma testoste-

rone levels in patients with prostatic carcinoma before and after treatment. *J Urol* 1968;99:788–792.

154. Vermeulen A, Verdonick L: Studies of the binding of testosterone to human plasma. *Steroids* 1968;11:609–635.
155. Mackler MA, Liberti JP, Smith MJV, et al: The effect of orchiectomy and various doses of stilbestrol on plasma testosterone levels in patients with carcinoma of the prostate. *Invest Urol* 1972;9:423–425.
156. Kent JR, Bischoft AJ, Arduino LJ, et al: Estrogen dosage and suppression of testosterone levels in patients with prostatic carcinoma. *J Urol* 1973;109:858–865.
157. Huggins E, Scott WW: Bilateral adrenalectomy in prostatic cancer. *Ann Surg* 1945;122:1031–1040.
158. Harrison JH, Thorn GW, Jenkins D: Total adrenalectomy for reactivated carcinoma of the prostate. *N Engl J Med* 1953; 248:86–92.
159. Bhanalaph T, Varkarakis MS, Murphy GP: Current status of bilateral adrenalectomy for prostatic carcinoma. *Ann Surg* 1974; 179:17–23.
160. Catalona WJ: Prostate cancer, endocrine therapy. *Urol Times* 1982;10:61–64.
161. Spirnak JP, Resnick MI: Carcinoma of the prostate: early endocrine therapy is best. *Semin Urol* 1983;1:269–279.
162. Herbst WP: Biochemical therapeusis in carcinoma of the prostate gland. *JAMA* 1942;120:1116–1122.
163. Kent JR, Bischoff AJ, Arduino LJ, et al: Estrogen dosage and suppression of testosterone levels in patients with prostatic carcinoma. *J Urol* 1973;109:838–865.
164. Robinson MRG, Thomas BS: Effect of hormone therapy on plasma testosterone levels in prostatic carcinoma. *Br Med J* 1971;4:391–397.
165. Shearer RJ, Hendry WF, Sommerville IF, Fergusson JD: Plasma testosterone: an accurate monitor of hormone treatment in prostatic cancer. *Br J Urol* 1973;45:668–677.
166. Bailar JC, Byar DP: Estrogen treatment for cancer of the prostate: early results with 3 doses of diethylstilbestrol and placebo. *Cancer* 1970;26:257–261.
167. The Veterans Administration Co-operative Urological Research Group: Treatment and survival of patients with cancer of the prostate. *Surg Gynecol Obstet* 1967;124: 1011–1017.
168. Adler A, Burger H, Davis J, et al: Carcinoma of the prostate: response of plasma luteinizing hormone and testosterone to oestrogen therapy. *Br Med J* 1968;1:28–31.
169. Walsh PC, Korenman SG: Mechanism of antiandrogenic action: effect of specific intracellular inhibitors. *J Urol* 1971;105: 850–857.
170. Stoliar B, Albert PJ: SCH 13521 in the treatment of advanced carcinoma of the prostate. *J Urol* 1974;111:803–807.
171. Robinson MRG, Shearer RJ, Fergusson JD: Adrenal suppression in the treatment of carcinoma of the prostate. *Br J Urol* 1974; 46:555–559.
172. Sanford EJ, Drago JR, Rohner TJ, et al: Aminoglutethimide medical adrenalectomy for advanced prostate carcinoma. *J Urol* 1976;115:170–174.
173. Walsh PC, Siteri PK: Suppression of plasma androgens by spironolactone in castrated men with carcinoma of the prostate. *J Urol* 1975;114:254–255.
174. Schmidt JD, Scott WW, Gibbons R, et al: Chemotherapy programs of the National Prostate Cancer Project (NPCP). *Cancer* 1980;45:1937–1946.
175. Schmidt JD: Cytotoxic agents effective in prostate cancer. *Semin Urol* 1983;1:299–310.
176. Olsson CA: Cytotoxic agents in prostate cancer: an enigma. *Semin Urol* 1983;1: 321–322.

CHAPTER 25 Bladder Cancer

Frederick A. Klein

For the year 1982 the American Cancer Society estimated that 37,000 new cases of bladder cancer would be diagnosed in the United States and that more than 10,000 people would die from this disease. Overall, bladder cancer accounts for about 2% of all malignant diseases. Approximately 98% of bladder cancers are epithelial in origin, with 92% transitional cell carcinomas, 6% to 7% squamous cell carcinomas, and 1% to 2% adenocarcinomas. The other nonepithelial tumors include sarcomas, pheochromocytomas, malignant lymphomas, mixed mesodermal tumors, and primary carcinoid tumors; however, the occurrence of the above remains rare.[1]

Bladder cancer continues to represent a spectrum of diseases with different causes. The complexity in understanding the etiology, and treatment lies in the fact that it can assume any one of several forms: a superficial low-grade papillary type, manifested by frequent recurrences, a deeply infiltrating high-grade tumor that may metastasize early, or a noninvasive in situ form that may either remain unchanged for several years or go on to rapidly progress to invasive carcinoma. The interrelationship of these different pathways, however, remains unresolved.

Various treatment modalities have been applied to the different forms of bladder cancer. The success of one specific treatment is more often determined by the natural history of the disease, rather than the efficacy of therapy. The main problems are to determine if, or whether, a superficial tumor will recur or progress to an invasive tumor and predict if or whether these cancer cells will metastasize. At this writing the timing of these events and the course of an individual patient's disease is unknown. With the further development and application of effective combination treatment programs and new and more effective screening methods for making an earlier diagnosis of bladder cancer, the incidence of recurrence and survival rates should improve.

EPIDEMIOLOGY

Bladder cancer is a worldwide problem; however, the incidence varies as much as ten times in different countries and may vary considerably even within the boundaries of a single country. Miller[2] has reported the age-standardized incidence per 100,000 people to range from 2.8 to 28.7 in men, and from 0.2 to 7.0 in women. Higher rates continue to occur in industrialized countries as compared with the more underdeveloped regions of Asia and Africa, and the incidence is higher in urban as compared with rural areas.

With regard to age, the incidence of bladder cancer increases as age increases with the peak incidence in the seventh decade. In the MD Anderson Hospital and Tumor Institute (Dallas) experience, less than 1% of bladder carcinomas occurred in patients under 40 years of age.[3] The actual incidence in the United States increases in men from 6/100,000 at age 40 to 24/100,000 at age 50, 50/100,000 at age 60, and 150/100,000 at age 70. In women the rates increase similarly, but occur two to three times less frequently.[4]

ETIOLOGY

Occupational Considerations

The full implications of industrial carcinogens remains unknown. Rehn[5] in 1895 first suggested that aniline dye workers in Germany were at an increased risk for developing bladder cancer. Further work over the next 60 years identified benzidine, 1-naphthylamine, and 2-naphthylamine as the responsible agents rather than aniline.[6] The average latency time to the development of tumors in these workers lies between 16 and 22 years, but has been seen as early as 2 years following initial exposure.[7]

Although the specific carcinogen has not been identified, certain specific industries and occupations do have a higher risk of bladder cancer. These industries or occupations include dye workers, nurses, tailors, hairdressers, leather industry workers, rubber workers, printing, gas industry, laboratory workers, rodent controllers, fuel workers, tar and pitch workers, and cooks and kitchen workers. The true incidence of bladder cancer attributable to occupational exposure has been estimated in three separate reports at 18%,[8] 23%,[9] and 33%.[10] Case,[11] on the other hand, states that only 1% of bladder cancer deaths among men in England and Wales are due to occupational exposure. Tola et al[12] concluded from their work that occupational exposure was not a major factor in the etiology of bladder cancer in Finland. While occupational exposure is known to cause bladder cancer, the number of cases that can be specifically identified to occur as a result of this exposure remains small.

Although epidemiologic surveys and laboratory investigations have identified high-risk factors and proved many chemicals to be tumorigenic for bladder carcinoma, the actual histogenesis remains unclear. As early as 1941, Berenblum[13] showed that carcinogenesis could frequently be separated into two fundamental stages: (1) initiation, where normal cells become latent or dormant malignant cells, and (2) promotion, where dormant initiated cells are stimulated to divide and grow into recognizable tumor cells. Carcinogenesis is now viewed as a multistaged process characterized by complex interactions of carcinogens and various cofactors. Today people are exposed to a multitude of various bladder carcinogens. The effects of this exposure may be additive, synergistic, or antagonistic; however, it is apparent that any one or all three actions may occur at any one time at different sites of the uroepithelium. Cofactors, on the other hand, may act to enhance the uroepithelial cells' response to a carcinogen, suppress the host cells' immune response, modify DNA or RNA turnover rate, or change the metabolic activation of the carcinogens. Hicks[14] has emphasized the implications of multistage carcinogenesis in the control and treatment of bladder cancer. It is unlikely ever to be able to prevent exposure to low level initiating doses of carcinogens and initiation remains an inevitable event with prolonged exposure. Actual development of tumor, however, requires exposure over a prolonged period of time and may indeed be reversible.

Tobacco

Since Holsti and Armala[15] noted an increase of papillary tumors of the bladder in mice after chronic application of tobacco tar to the oral mucosa, there have been numerous case control studies demonstrating an association between cigarette smoking and bladder cancer. Wynder and Goldsmith[16] reported that about 50% of men and 33% of women with bladder cancer were cigarette smokers. Miller[2] reported similar findings, stating that the risk ratio increased with the frequency of consumption. This risk ratio was 1.0, 3.8, and 5.1 in men who smoked less than 10, between 10 and 20, and more than 20 cigarettes a day. In women, the risk ratio rose from 2.3 to 2.6 when more than 15 cigarettes were smoked. With respect to pipe tobacco, cigars, chewing tobacco, or snuff, no difference in the incidence of bladder cancer could be shown by Wynder and Goldsmith.[16] Miller,[2] on the other hand, reported an increased risk ratio of 2.3 for men who smoked more than 50,000 pipefuls of tobacco in a lifetime. Lockwood[17] also incriminated cigars and cigarillos as increasing the risk of bladder cancer.

The exact mechanism by which tobacco smoking might cause bladder cancer is unknown. Hoffman et al[18] found a small amount of the known carcinogen, β-naphthylamine, in cigarette smoke. Kerr et al[19] found increased amounts of tryptophan metabolites in the urine of cigarette smokers. Although the significance of these findings remains unclear, the strong statistical association that exists between tobacco smoking and bladder cancer implies a definite causal relationship.

Dietary Sweeteners

The ban on sodium cyclamate in the United Kingdom and in the United States was prompted by the work of Price et al[20] who induced bladder cancer in rats with a mixture of cyclamate and sodium saccharin. Friedman et al[21] in 1972 confirmed the carcinogenicity of saccharin in experimental animals. Although the doses used to induce carcinoma far exceeded normal human consumption, the question of how much risk for the development of bladder cancer exists when artificial sweeteners are used over a prolonged period of time remains unanswered.

In 1979 a status report by Newell et al concluded that there was not enough data available to establish an association between the use of saccharin and an increased risk of human bladder cancer.[22] Connelly et al[23] in 1978 reported no relationship in humans between the consumption of artificial sweeteners and bladder cancer. Morrison and Buring[24] in 1980 looked at Sweet-N-Low, Sucaryl, saccharin, and cyclamate and concluded that users have little or no increased risk of cancer of the bladder. Kessler and Clark[25] in 1978 in a study of 519 patients with histologically proven bladder cancer concluded that neither cyclamate nor saccharin were likely to be carcinogenic in man. On the other hand, Hicks et al[26] showed that a single small dose of a known initiating carcinogen, N-methyl-N-nitrosourea, when instilled into female rat bladders and followed by oral saccharin or cyclamate causes a significant number of bladder tumors. Cyclamate or saccharin in this instance was a definite promoter.

Berenblum[13] as well as Cohen et al[27] also showed saccharin to be a promoter in the development of bladder tumors once initiation had occurred.

Coffee Drinking

Coffee drinking has been implicated by several investigators as causing an increased risk for bladder cancer. Cole[28] compared women who drank more than one cup of coffee a day with those who did not drink coffee and found that coffee drinkers had a 2.6 times greater risk of developing bladder cancer. The risk in males was 1.3. Simon et al[29] as well as Fraumeni et al[30] also found a greater risk in coffee drinkers in their studies. Miller[31] and Bross and Tidings[32] found only a slightly increased risk in coffee drinkers. It can be concluded that in the absence of a documented dose/response relationship for either sex, coffee cannot be definitely implicated in causing or promoting bladder cancer.

Additional Factors

Other etiologic factors associated with bladder cancer include phenacetin abuse, dietary ingestion of bracken fern and nitrosamines, and chronic bladder infections secondary to *Schistosoma haematobium* or prolonged catheter drainage as frequently occurs in paraplegics. Fokkens[33] reported a fourfold increased risk of developing bladder cancer in phenacetin abusers whose intake exceeded 2000 g. Bracken fern has been shown to cause bladder carcinomas in most animals to which it has been fed, including rats, cattle, guinea pigs, and sheep.[34] *Schistosoma haematobium* infection is well-known to be endemic to Egypt where carcinoma in bilharzial bladders is a continual problem. These carcinomas are usually squamous cell in type (67% to 77%), are well differentiated (70% to 80%), and usually present at an advanced local stage without lymph node involvement or distant metastases.[1]

HISTOPATHOLOGY

Over the past 30 years there have been many changes in the pathologic classification of bladder tumors as well as a great deal of clinical progress in the classification of stages of the disease. There is no uniformly accepted system of grading, and different pathologists may interpret identical pathologic material differently; however, the three major classifications used today have been reported by Mostofi et al (World Health Organization classification),[35] Friedell et al (National Bladder Cancer Project),[36] and by Koss (Armed Forces Institute of Pathology).[37] The detailed differences in these classifications is beyond the scope of this chapter but the basic classifications are shown in Table 25-1. In the Western Hemisphere the most common bladder tumors are transitional cell carcinomas (90%). The next three most common histologic types are squamous carcinomas, adenocarcinomas, and undifferentiated carcinomas. Although the discussion of treatment in general refers to transitional cell carcinomas, the biologic behavior and/or natural history of mixed tumors or other cell types do not differ appreciably and, as such, the principle methods and results of treatment generally apply for all of the epithelial tumors of the same grade and stage.

At present the most important prognostic features are tumor grade, stage, and multicentricity. However, other features such as age; sex; size; site; number and configuration of tumors (papillary or solid), microscopic features, such as blood and lymphatic invasion; cytogenetic features such as karyotype, RNA and DNA content; immunologic features such as retention or loss of blood group antigens by the tumor cells; and other immunologic assessments of the host will be increasingly incorporated into prognostic predictions and treatment decisions to benefit the individual patient.[38] The concept of tumor grading was first introduced by Broders[39] in 1922 who recognized four grades of tran-

Table 25-1
Classification of Transitional Cell Carcinoma of the Bladder

WHO Classification[35]	Friedell et al[36]	Armed Forces Institute of Pathology[37]
Papilloma	Papilloma	Papilloma
Transitional cell carcinoma, grade I, stage 0	Papillary transitional CIS, grade I	Papillary carcinoma, grade I noninvasive
Transitional cell carcinoma, grade I, stage A–D	Transitional cell carcinoma, grade I, stage A–D	Papillary carcinoma, grade I invasive
Transitional cell CIS, grade II,	Flat transitional cell CIS, grade II	Transitional cell CIS, grade II
Transitional cell carcinoma, grade II, stage 0	Papillary transitional cell CIS, grade II	Papillary carcinoma, grade II noninvasive
Transitional cell carcinoma, grade II, stage A–D	Transitional cell carcinoma, grade II, stage A–D	Papillary carcinoma, grade II invasive
Transitional cell CIS, grade III	Flat transitional cell CIS, grade III	Transitional cell carcinoma, grade II
Transitional cell carcinoma, grade III, stage 0	Papillary transitional cell CIS, grade III	Transitional cell CIS, grade III
		Papillary carcinoma, grade III noninvasive
Transitional cell carcinoma, grade III, stage A–D	Transitional cell carcinoma, grade III, stage A–D	Papillary carcinoma, grade III invasive
		Transitional cell carcinoma, grade III

CIS=carcinoma in situ.

sitional cell growth ranging from grade 1 carcinoma (papilloma) to grade 4 carcinoma. The grade 1 and 2 tumors are generally classified as low-grade lesions and grade 3 or 4 tumors as high-grade lesions. The grade of the neoplasm, as such, provides a visual estimate of the growth potential of the lesion and establishes the probability that bladder wall invasion is proportionately higher with higher-grade lesions. In general, survival decreases as grade increases, despite the mode of therapy. Collan confirmed this datum recently showing survival rates of 132 patients with various histologic grades of tumor (Figure 25-1).[40]

Whether a specific papillary lesion is a benign papilloma or a grade 1 papillary

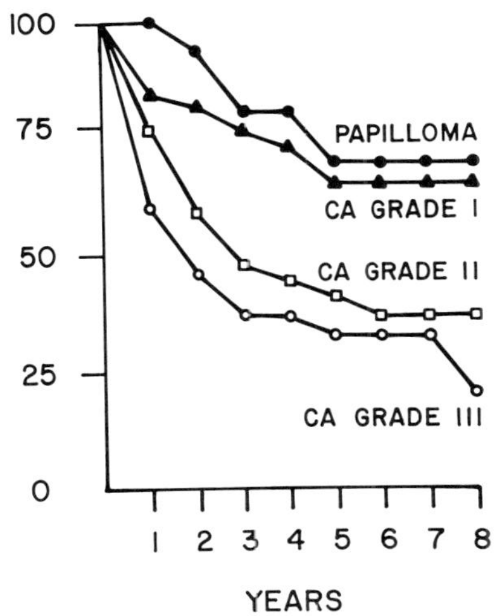

Figure 25-1 Survival rates of 132 patients with various histologic grades of bladder tumor (reproduced with permission from Collan et al[40]).

carcinoma remains a clinicopathologic uncertainty. Clinicians should recognize, however, that whichever term is used, they are identical neoplasms and rarely if ever infiltrate the bladder wall or metastasize. Lerman et al[41] reported on 125 patients with bladder papillomas followed from 11 months to 20 years and reported that only 12 or 9.6% later developed invasive bladder carcinoma. The 5-year survival rate was the same as the age-matched general population. Since as many as 30% of all bladder tumors are such lesions and since local destruction is curative, including these patients in survival reports improves survival data.

Koss suggests that there are indeed two distinct pathways in bladder neoplasia: the papillary and the nonpapillary.[42] The papillary growths with thin stalks are considered relatively harmless as they generally do not invade the muscularis. Nonpapillary lesions such as atypical hyperplasia and carcinoma in situ are looked upon as the common sources of invasive bladder cancer. In fact, diffuse carcinoma in situ, clinically characterized by a history of progressive symptoms of vesical irritability, are in 50% to 80% of cases associated with the development of infiltrating cancers within 4 to 10 years.[43] The problem for the clinician and pathologist alike is recognizing the patient who has concurrent papillary and nonpapillary tumors. In a study by Althausen et al,[44] the incidence of later developing infiltrating cancer in patients with conservatively treated low-stage bladder tumors was correlated with the morphology of the mucous membrane adjacent to the papillary tumors. Three of 41 (7%) patients with normal adjacent mucosa, nine of 25 (36%) patients with atypical mucous membranes, and ten of 12 (83%) patients with carcinoma in situ developed infiltrative lesions in less than 4 years. Automated flow cytometry, electron microscopy, and perhaps microcystoscopy may offer potential means for earlier detection of cancerous change in the near future.

CLINICAL PRESENTATION

The most common presenting symptom of bladder tumors is hematuria. Documented painless microscopic hematuria occurs in 75% to 80% of patients with bladder cancer.[1] This hematuria is usually throughout the entire stream, compared to hematuria which occurs with urethral or prostatitis lesions which is present only at the beginning or the end of the stream. The second most common presenting symptom is bladder irritability, which occurs in about 25% of patients.[45] These symptoms are usually increased urinary frequency, dysuria, and strangury, and usually indicate the presence of carcinoma in situ, a large invasive tumor, or small tumors at the bladder neck. Therefore, the clinical history that should prompt suspicion of bladder cancer includes hematuria (either gross or microscopic), the presence of irritative symptoms, or an occurrence of urinary tract infection in males when prostatitis and urethritis have definitely been ruled out.

Another group of patients presents with complaints attributable to the development of distant metastases or extensive local invasion. Generally about two thirds of all bladder cancers are localized to the bladder at first diagnosis and only about 7% show clinical evidence of distant metastases.[45] In contrast, prostatic and kidney carcinoma have an incidence of metastatic disease of 60% and 40%, respectively, at first diagnosis. Once the diagnosis of bladder cancer is suspected the urologist should proceed to make the diagnosis and determine the clinical extent of the disease as described below without delay.

STAGING OF BLADDER CANCER

Clinical staging may be defined as the clinician's effort to assess the actual extent to which the growth potential of a particular bladder tumor has been expressed at the time of diagnosis. Accurate clinical staging is of importance because it assists the establishment of prognosis for a given lesion at the time of initial diagnosis, the planning of therapy, and the assessment of results as they correlate with a particular stage of disease. The clinical staging of bladder cancer is based primarily upon the depth of penetration found on cystoscopy, bladder biopsy, and bimanual examination. Other data obtained from cytology, history, physical examination, hemogram, blood chemistries, chest films, lung tomography, intravenous pyelography (IVP), radioisotope scans, arteriography, ultrasonography, lymphangiography, and computerized transaxial tomography (CT) are also of importance. The use of these technics will be dealt with in detail below.

The formal clinical staging of bladder tumors began with the work of Jewett and Strong[46] in 1946, when they reported a staging system based on the extent of tumor penetration through the bladder wall. They felt that as long as a tumor was confined to the submucosa, it was potentially curable; but when it penetrated through to perivesical fat, its chance of cure was decreased significantly. In 1952, Jewett[47] made a further distinction between stages B_1 and B_2. In his clinical review, patients with B_1 lesions behaved like those with stage A lesions; and patients with B_2 lesions behaved more like those patients with stage C lesions.

Marshall,[48] in 1952, extended this classification by distinguishing a stage in which no submucosal infiltration had occurred (stage 0, CIS) and a stage in which lymph node involvement was already present (stage D). He likewise confirmed Jewett's observations of the significance between superficial tumors and deep muscle invasion by the tumor.

The principal present alternative to the Jewett-Marshall staging classification is the TNM (tumor-nodes-metastases) system of the Union Internationale Contre le Cancer (UICC)1[49,50] (Table 25-2). The advantages of the UICC system over the Jewett-Marshall system may be summarized as follows:

1. The formal distinction between clinical and pathologic staging (T, P)
2. The inclusion of a specific designation for CIS (Tis, Pis)

Table 25-2
Staging: Comparison of the Original Jewett-Strong Classification with Jewett's and Marshall's Modification and the TNM System

Jewett and Strong[46]	Jewett[47]	Marshall[48]		TNM *Clinical*[49]	TNM *Pathologic*[50]
			No tumor-definitive specimen	T-0	P-0
		0	Carcinoma in situ	Tis	Pis
			Papillary tumor s̄ invasion		
A	A	A	Invasion lamina propria	T_1	P_1
B	B_1	B_1	Superficial	T_2	P_2
			muscle invasion		
	B_2	B_2	Deep	T_{3A}	P_3
C	C	C	Invasion perivesical fat	T_{3B}	
		D_1	Invasion contiguous viscera	T_{4A-B}	P_4
			Pelvic nodes		N_{1-3}
		D_2	Distant metastases		M_1
			Nodes above aortic bifurcation		
		D_2			N_4

Reproduced with permission from Skinner DG, deKernion JB (eds): *Genitourinary Cancer.* Philadelphia, WB Saunders Co, 1978, p 271.

3. The potential for distinction between the local extent of the primary tumor (T, P) and the extent of metastasis (N, M)

With regard to workable treatment planning, it is customary to divide bladder carcinoma into three groups: low stage, O, A, B (Tis, T_1, T_2); high stage, B_2 and C (T_3, T_4); and metastatic, D (N+, M+). The inherent weakness with these systems is the division of B_1 from B_2. It remains controversial regarding therapy whether B_1 lesions may be curable by transurethral resection alone, or whether any muscle invasion requires aggressive therapy by means of radiation and/or radiation and radical cystectomy. Ultimately, the presence or absence of muscle on biopsy and the clinician's impression of completeness of resection determines optimal treatment in this situation.

Clinical Staging Technics

The clinical staging of bladder cancer has been based for the past 35 years primarily upon cystoscopy, biopsy, and bimanual examination. It is important in all patients, however, to synthesize the data obtained from routine history and physical examination, hemogram, blood chemical analysis, chest films and pulmonary tomography, IVP, radioisotope scans, cystography, arteriography, ultrasonography, lymphangiography, and CT to determine or rule out the presence of metastatic disease and to identify other conditions that may ultimately affect treatment decisions. The specific indications for using a majority of the staging examinations mentioned above will be discussed below; however, at the present time logistical and cost effectiveness considerations make their routine use of debatable value.

The mainstay of clinical staging of bladder cancer remains cystoendoscopy under anesthesia (noting the size, location, number, and gross morphology of the tumors), bimanual examination (for clinical evidence of bladder wall infiltration), and systematic transurethral resection and cold-cup lesional and random biopsies of the bladder. Cold-cup and resection biopsies are not only important to determine tumor architecture, cell grade, the depth of tumor penetration and infiltration of the lymphatic and vascular structures, but are important in determining the presence of generalized urothelial instability and thereby influencing patient treatment and prognosis. To specifically evaluate multicentricity, cold-cup biopsy samples should be performed at the margin of the visible tumor, of any endoscopically suspicious areas, and at random sites of normal-appearing areas of the bladder (anterior wall, side walls, posterior wall, and dome) and the prostatic urethra.

Urinary cytology, obtained either by bladder barbotage or voided urine, is also of significance in determining spatial multicentricity. When the cellular grade of the cytologic specimen differs from that of the primary resected carcinoma, it suggests that there is tumor elsewhere in the urinary tract. This finding requires random biopsies looking for carcinoma in situ, and possibly further exploration of the upper tracts and urethra. Bladder barbotage specimens do produce more cellularity and often have less contaminating debris; however, good collection technics and the experience of the cytopathologist are more important factors in determining the reliability of cytology specimens. Overall, the accuracy in cytodiagnosis of high-grade bladder lesions is 80% to 95%; with low-grade lesions it falls between 22% and 30%.[51–53]

The false-negative reading of urinary cytology with low-grade tumors reflects the degree of nuclear anaplasia. False-positive urinary cytology specimens, however, are relatively rare and only occur in the presence of severe bladder infection associated with the presence of bladder calculi.[53] With reliable cytopathology, the presence of positive cytology means that higher-grade transitional cell neoplasms or possibly carcinoma in situ are present.

Intravenous pyelography is routinely performed on patients with bladder carcinoma in order to help detect urothelial tumor multicentricity and anatomical or functional abnormalities in the upper urinary tracts which may influence therapy. The presence of unilateral or bilateral ureteral obstruction, together with a tumor involving one of the ureteral orifices, does imply the presence of more deeply invasive bladder tumors, and helps in clinical staging. Fractional, double-, or triple-contrast cystography, as described by Kafkas[54] has been advocated as a better way to outline bladder tumor characteristics when they project into the bladder or into bladder diverticula. With double-contrast cystography, barium as well as air can be used to outline the tumors. It is felt by Kafkas[54] and others[55-57] that this technic better evaluates bladder wall thickening and possible perivesical tumor spread. Many false-negative and false-positive results have been obtained. For this reason the technic is not widely used in staging.

Several studies have demonstrated the accuracy of staging with pelvic arteriography. Ninety-five percent accuracy has been reported with stage C and D lesions by Lang,[58] and 91% accuracy has been reported by Winterberger et al.[59] In these same series, without arteriography, staging accuracy was only 55%. Although pelvic arteriography does seem to be an accurate way of staging, several reasons why this technic has not been adopted are evident. Whether the lesion is a stage B_2 or C lesion really makes little difference with regard to operative therapy; the technic does not evaluate lymph node involvement, and the uncomfortable and invasive nature of the technic precludes its routine use.

Pedal lymphangiography permits evaluation of internal iliac and external iliac lymph nodes. The primary lymphatic drainage of the bladder, however, is to the hypogastric or obturator nodes followed by iliac and periaortic drainage. This fact alone limits the usefulness of this technic. Interpretation of lymphangiography also remains in question as previous infection and/or surgery can cause lymphatic obstruction, peripheral defects, and enlargement which may be read as a false-negative result. Likewise its sensitivity in picking up microscopic metastatic disease is low. Johnson et al,[60] however, in a study of 49 patients, used lymphangiography to exclude people from unnecessary surgery if frankly positive nodes were present. In this study, no cases were false-positives. They feel that if a positive lymphangiogram and fine needle aspiration of the lymph node proves metastatic disease, that the therapeutic course of the patient will be altered. Most other investigators, however, do not rely heavily on this procedure.

Computerized transaxial tomography of the pelvis and bladder has also received increasing attention as a possible means of evaluating bladder tumor extent as well as the presence of pelvic and retroperitoneal lymph node involvement. Further evaluation with this technic shows that it does not distinguish between superficial and deep muscle–invading tumors; it is unreliable in patients who have had previous surgery and often is difficult to interpret posttransurethral resection or radiation therapy. With specific reference to lymphadenopathy, it only depicts nodes that are approximately 1 cm in size and certainly cannot diagnose microscopic metastatic disease.[31]

Intracavitary ultrasonography studies have recently been advocated to determine invasiveness of a specific bladder tumor.[62-65] Although this technic is promising, it is doubtful that it will alter the necessary therapy for any given lesion. Likewise, special intercavitary probes are required and at the moment they are not readily avialable at most institutions in the United States.

Radioisotopic bone scans and liver scans as well as the whole lung tomography are useful adjunctive procedures that should be performed when specific indications are present. In the face of normal liver function studies, Felix et al[66] in 1976 reported that almost no false-positive liver scans occurred. Likewise, with reference to isotope bone scanning, with no specific symptomatic areas the likelihood of discovering a metastatic lesion is low. With a normal chest radiologic examination the yield from additional whole lung tomography is too low to merit routine use.

The error in clinical staging, estimated by using the routine mentioned above, is illustrated by data from Memorial Sloan-Kettering Cancer Center with the pathologic stage determined by radical cystectomy and pelvic lymphadenectomy (Table 25-3). This experience supports the following clinical staging generalizations:

1. Understaging is far more common than overstaging.
2. The greatest error in staging (33%) occurs in those patients clinically classified as B_1 (T_2).
3. Patients with clinical stage B_2–C (T_3) frequently (37%) show invasion of contiguous organs or metastases in the lymph nodes.
4. Judging clinical staging only on the basis of distinguishing low-stage neoplasms, O, A, B_1 (Tis, T_1, T_2) and/or advanced stages B_2–C, D, (T_3, T_4), 52 of 66 patients (79%) clinically judged to have low-stage tumors did, indeed, have them pathologically, and 65 of 71 patients (91%) of those judged to have advanced neoplasms did, indeed, have advanced neoplasms pathologically.[38]

TREATMENT

In addition to the natural considerations of patient age, mental capacity, physical condition, morbidity, mortality, and the functional inpact of the treatment regimen recommended, the primary considerations with regard to making a therapeutic decision lie with the stage of the tumor, the grade of the tumor, the presence of multicentricity, and, in special circumstances, tumor location. Tumor stage provides an estimate of the extent of the lesion and as such provides a basis for clinical judgment regarding the minimal therapy necessary to control the tumor. Tumor grade provides a rough indication of the inherent aggressiveness of a particular lesion, with higher grade correlating with more aggressive treatment. Tumor multicentricity is factored into the treatment modality decision on the basis of clinical judgment. Polychronotopism (the number of existing tumors in space and the number of tumor occurrences in time), as well as the rate of

Table 25-3
Pathologic Versus Clinical Stage

Clinical Stage (No.)	Pathological Stage						
	IS	*A*	*B_1*	*B_2*	*C*	*D_1*	*D_2*
		Understanding					
IS (7)	7	–	–	–	–	–	–
A (17)	–	15	2	–	–	–	–
B_1 (42)	–	–	28	9	1	3	1
B_2 (39)	–	–	–	16	8	6	9
C_2 (26)	–	–	–	6	11	4	5
D_1 (6)	–	–	–	–	–	3	3
		Overstaging					
Total 137	7	15	30	31	20	16	18

Patients with bladder cancer treated by radical cystectomy with pelvic lymph node dissection who did not receive irradiation (MSKCC experience).

Reproduced with permission from Whitmore.[38]

new tumor occurrences, are the factors to be considered in deciding on more radical treatment. Generally, the greater the number of these tumors, the greater the need for radical treatment. Transurethral surgery is the most effective and most commonly recommended treatment for superficial disease. For deeply invasive tumors, categorical recommendations cannot be made; however, the most convincing data seem to demonstrate the value of combined or integrated radiation therapy and radical surgery.

Methods of Treatment

Local excision or fulguration (transurethral resection or open cystotomy) The rationale of local excision or fulguration in the treatment or superficial disease is that the bladder carcinoma is a focal process and unless the depth of infiltration precludes a safe and sure excision and/or fulguration, the method is a good low-risk means of controlling the lesion.[50] This technic should be limited to the local control of focal and superficial lesions, O, A, B_1, (Tis, T_1, T_2), carcinoma in situ (CIS), *Tis*, and for the palliation of more deeply invasive tumors. The morbidity and mortality of this method of management is extremely low, as there is minimal if any change in urinary and sexual function. Another important advantage to this approach is the ease with which it can be repeated.

A summary of results of transurethral treatment by clinical stage of disease is shown in Table 25-4. Although specific data are lacking with regard to multicentricity–the number of local recurrences and new tumor occurrences–some new lesions most certainly developed within the 5-year follow-up period and must have been successfully controlled by transurethral measures. Likewise, to what extent these failures were due to local recurrence, new tumor formation, or distant metastases cannot be obtained from the data and as such these 5-year survival rates do not necessarily indicate disease-free intervals.

In summary, transurethral resection and/or fulguration of superficial lesions should be considered adequate and final treatment when no muscle invasion is evident on the pathologic specimen and when there is no increase in frequency of tumor recurrence or the development of multiple tumors. Whether or not further treatment is indicated in a patient with surgically staged B_1 disease is wholly a clinical judgment to be made by the operating surgeon. If the lesion is thought to have been completely excised, it is a reasonable approach to bring the patient back in 6 weeks and rebiopsy the same area. If there is no residual disease, then one may consider the lesion controlled. If residual disease does remain, more aggressive surgery is certainly indicated. In a poor-risk elderly patient, transurethral resection or fulguration with careful follow-up examinations

Table 25-4
Five-Year Survival (%) Following Transurethral Treatment by Clinical Stage in Patients with Bladder Cancer

Author	Year	O	A	B_1	B_2	C	D
Flocks[67]	1951		77	--54--		2	
Nichols and Marshall[68]	1956	--81--		-----15-----			
Cox et al[69]	1968	71	47	8	0	0	
Marberger et al[70]	1972	-----43-----			--14---		0
O'Flynn et al[71]	1975		62	59	--20---		
Barnes et al[72]	1977		73	--31---			
Williams et al[73]	1977	--72---					

may even be the treatment of choice.

Local excision and fulguration are usually performed by the transurethral route; however, open suprapubic cystotomy may be used. The specific indications for this approach would be anatomical considerations of inaccessibility transurethrally (stricture), the location of the tumor causing inaccessibility, lack of instruments for the procedure, or lack of technical ability to perform transurethral work.

Although there is limited data available with regard to complications and control by this route, there is no suggestion that this technic produces significantly different results stage for stage than traditional transurethral ablation. The disadvantages of the procedure are that local wound implantation can occur, morbidity and inconvenience are increased over transurethral procedures, and the advantage of repeatability is lacking.[38]

Intravesical chemotherapy Because the concepts of multifocal field change disease and tumor implantation at the time of resection have been implicated as the main etiologies of the high incidence of subsequent bladder tumor formation following initial endoscopic management, the concept of intensive topical chemotherapy was initiated. The institution of postresection adjuvant chemotherapy has been studied hoping to reduce the bladder tumor recurrence rate of 50% to 70% previously reported.[74] The advantages of intravesical therapy mainly reside in the fact that administration is easy, a high dose of the cytotoxic agent is delivered directly to the tumor, the side effects are minimal, and therapy encompasses the whole bladder. Not only have intravesical agents been used in an adjuvant setting to decrease recurrence rate; they have been advocated in an attempt to avert cystectomy or definitive irradiation in patients with multifocal tumors not controlled by endoscopy alone; in patients with medical contraindications to anesthesia; in multifocal carcinoma in situ; and finally for tumors not amenable to resection due to their inaccessibility. These drugs are placed directly into the bladder through a catheter at varying weekly intervals according to specific protocols. The most common and most active drugs presently used are thiotepa, mitomycin, doxorubicin hydrochloride, and BCG vaccine. Each agent, its side effects and efficacy, will be discussed below.

Thiotepa The use of thiotepa to treat bladder tumors was described originally by Jones and Swinney[75] in 1961 and by Veenema et al[76] in 1962. Initially, this alkylating agent was used for patients in whom tumors were so numerous as to be unresectable or recurred so rapidly that repetitive anesthesia was unfeasible. They found that in these patients, approximately 30% to 50% of the bladder tumors were partially or completely destroyed.[76] Subsequent reports have shown that the overall response rate, including both complete and partial regression (greater than 50%) following definitive therapy with thiotepa ranges between 45% and 80%.[76-78] Likewise, thiotepa prophylaxis has been shown to reduce the incidence of subsequent tumor recurrences. Prout et al[79] reported on the long-term fate of the National Bladder Cancer Collaborative Group A thiotepa prophylaxis patients and found a statistically significant difference at 24 months. Fifty-three percent of the prophylaxis group was tumor-free compared to 27% of the controls. At 54 months, however, both recurrence rates equalized. Commonly used dosages range from 30 mg to 60 mg once a week for 4 weeks, followed by monthly instillations for up to a year. Instillation is usually recommended within the first month following definitive transurethral resection or fulguration.

In the studies of the National Bladder Cancer Collaborative Group A, patients receiving thiotepa had a significantly better chance of being tumor-free at 1 year than a control group not receiving the drug: 66% *v* 40%.[78] In the Veterans Administration cooperative group[80] and the EROTC study,[81] the number of tumors per patient month was reduced; however, the overall recurrence rate was not affected.

The major side effect of thiotepa is myelosuppression. Although the incidence of this problem is variable, the major risk seems to occur if the drug is instilled immediately following surgery when mucosal alteration is at its greatest, when there is significant infection, or in the presence of extensive tumor. If the drug is instilled 2 to 4 weeks following the initial resection the chance of significant myelosuppression remains low.

Mitomycin Mitomycin is probably the second most frequently utilized agent for bladder cancer in the United States at the present time. Its use developed largely because it has minimal absorption from the urinary bladder and thus minimal side effects. Instillation is usually 40 mg administered in 50 mL saline weekly for 8 weeks with or without monthly maintenance systemic chemotherapy.

In a dose response study performed by Bracken et al,[82] 43 patients were treated with doses ranging from 20 to 60 mg. All patients had an index lesion to monitor response. The response rate of 70% in this group included 49% complete responses and 30% partial responses.[82] In an earlier study of patients with superficial disease by Mishina et al[83] in Japan, 44% (22/50) patients experienced complete remission and 32% (16/50) partial remission. Soloway and Ford[84] in a study of 36 patients revealed a complete response rate at 12 weeks follow-up of 45% (16/36) while an additional 33% (12/36) had a partial response. Of the six patients in the series with carcinoma in situ, three had a complete response. Drug toxicity in these series was minimal. The overall response of bladder tumors to mitomycin is probably not statistically significantly better than with thiotepa. The major drawback of mitomycin is its expense.

Doxorubicin Doxorubicin is another antitumor drug effective in the intravesical treatment of bladder carcinoma. The majority of experience with doxorubicin has occurred in Europe and the optimal treatment dose and schedule have not been well standardized.

Jakse et al used 40 mg in 20 mL saline biweekly or 80 mg in 40 mL saline monthly in 25 patients with carcinoma in situ.[85,86] At follow-up evaluation ten of 15 patients (66%) had negative cytology and negative cystoscopy. Of these, seven remained disease-free with follow-up of 50 months.

Schulman et al[87] reported on a trial of doxorubicin prophylaxis using 50 mg in 50 mL saline instilled 24 hours following transurethral resection. Intravesical instillation then occurred twice during the first week, weekly for 4 weeks, and monthly for 1 year. Sixty-one percent (50/82) of patients were reported to be tumor-free at 1 year. Twenty-five percent (21/82) of patients, however, had severe irritative symptoms and many were unable to complete the full course of therapy. Abrams et al[88] used 50 mg in 50 mL saline instilled into the bladder 30 minutes following transurethral resection, and compared his patients with a control group not receiving chemotherapy. At 6-month follow-up, 72% of the patients receiving the drug and 39% of the controls had decreased numbers of tumors and were considered to have had a response. There was no statistically significant difference in this group.

Garnick et al[89] reported on 27 patients with polychronotopic superficial disease or carcinoma in situ who were treated prophylactically with 60 mg doxorubicin in 50 mL saline beginning 1 week after surgery with subsequent doses instilled every three weeks for a total of 8 doses. With the response calculated by using each patient as his own control, the 2-year incidence of tumors prior to and after receiving doxorubicin was 75% and 18%, respectively. Niijima,[90] for the definitive therapy of bladder tumors, used two-hour instillations of doses of 20 to 30 mg and 50 to 60 mg three times a week for 2 weeks. The complete plus partial response rates were 56%, 72%, and 74% respectively. Edsmyr et al[91] used doxorubicin 80 mg in 100 mL saline monthly with recystoscopy and biopsy every 4 months as definitive therapy in patients with carcinoma in situ or Tis tumors. The results with a minimum of five instillations revealed that of the eight patients with carcinoma in situ all were endoscopically negative and seven of eight (88%) were cytologically negative at follow-up. Of these 18 patients with Tis lesions, nine (50%) were reported as complete and five (28%) as partial responses.

BCG vaccine Nonspecific immune therapy utilizing BCG 120 mg in 50 mL normal saline instilled into the urinary bladder once a week for 3 to 6 weeks has shown initially excellent results at relatively low cost and low morbidity. Although this therapy still awaits approval by the Food and Drug Administration, it is presently undergoing clinical trials at several institutions. Since the initial report by Morales et al[92] that BCG given intravesically and percutaneously every week for 6 weeks after cystoscopy and fulguration markedly reduced the rate at which new tumors were seen and caused no serious toxicity, subsequent randomized trials have been undertaken. Camacho et al[93] reported on 51 patients randomized between transurethral resection (TUR) alone and TUR plus BCG. The tumor frequency in the TUR alone group was not significantly altered with a prestudy incidence of 2.97 tumors per patient month and a post-TUR incidence of 2.37 tumors per patient month. The BCG group, however, had a prestudy incidence of 3.6 tumors per patient month compared to 0.75 tumors per patient month following BCG administration. The side effects in this study were dysuria, hematuria, urinary frequency, mild low-grade fever, and malaise; however, no patients had to discontinue therapy.

Lamm et al[94] conducted a prospective randomized trial utilizing intravesical plus percutaneous BCG in the same dosage regimen. The recurrence rate in their control group was 46% compared with 22% in the BCG group. Another prophylaxis study was reported by Brosman.[95] He randomized patients to receive regular thiotepa 60 mg in 60 mL saline or BCG, 120 mg in 50 mL saline. Nine of 19 (47%) patients who received thiotepa had a recurrence within 2 years compared with none of 39 patients in the BCG group. In the definitive report on the prospective randomized trial of BCG from Memorial Hospital by Pinsky et al[96] 86 patients were randomized to TUR alone or TUR plus BCG. There was a reduction in the number of tumor recurrences in all of the BCG-treated patients *v* 27 (31%) of the TUR only patients. Significant conversion of cytology from positive to negative, less tumor progression requiring cystectomy, and a prolonged disease-free interval as well as increased time to progression of disease were all significantly greater in the BCG group.

It would appear from these results that the combination of standard therapy and BCG is certainly more effective than standard therapy alone in patients with recurrent superficial bladder tumors. Due to the fact that there is more than one BCG strain available with different viability and conditions of growth, the optimal dose, timing, and route of administration are yet to be determined.

Segmental resection The rationale for segmental resection (partial cystectomy) is that bladder cancer is a focal process and that the existing tumor in the bladder can be completely excised by removing a full thickness portion of the bladder wall. Five-year survival statistics according to clinical stage are shown in Table 25-5. Reasonable results have been obtained in these retrospective studies, primarily with the lower stage lesions. In fact, the specific results with respect to stage O and stage A are not significantly different from those obtained from transurethral resection. With respect to B_1, B_2, and C lesions, segmental cystectomy results are somewhat better. It should be kept in mind that these patients, however, are carefully selected to meet specific preoperative criteria.

The primary indication for segmental cystectomy is the patient with a solitary tumor, deeply infiltrative (stage B_1, B_2 or C), in whom the clinician feels that he can perform a safe and sure local excision and whose tumor size and location permits full thickness excision with a minimal 2-cm margin of normal bladder wall peripheral to the lesion. In addition, previously performed random cold-cup bladder biopsies should show no evidence of dysplasia or concomitant carcinoma in situ. Tumor multicentricity is an absolute contraindication to segmental resection since the risk of recurrent tumor in this setting increases the probability of treatment failure.

The advantages of segmental cystectomy are preservation of urinary and sexual function. These advantages, however, do not represent a viable alternative to other radical surgery in the majority of patients.

The problem of local recurrence and wound seeding is real. There is some evidence that preoperative radiation, in a manner similar to integrated irradiation and cystectomy as reported by Whitmore,[109] has some benefit. Likewise, in 1969 Van der Werf-Messing[110] demonstrated a reduction in the incidence of local wound seeding in T_3 tumors to 0% after open bladder radium seed treatment of the primary lesion. The final advantage of segmental cystectomy is absolute surgical staging of the specimen and extended tumor evaluation obtained by performing pelvic lymphadenectomy prior to partial cystectomy.

Suprapubic radium needle implantation The use of suprapubic radium needle implantation for bladder carcinoma has been reported by van der Werf-Messing.[110] Five-year survival rates for her patients were 75% for clinical stage A or T_1 lesions, 61% for clinical stage B_1 or T_2 lesions, and 25% for stage T_3, or B_2 and C lesions. The selection criteria for these patients were rigid; the patients were considered for this procedure only if there was a solitary tumor that measured less than 5 cm in diameter.

Suprapubic wound recurrence is associated with this technic, occurring in 23% of T_3 patients treated with implantation only. This complication was significantly decreased when implantation was coupled with preoperative radiation. This finding led to the current use of preoperative irradiation prior to segmental cystectomy. The radiation regimen is 1050 rad given in equal fractions, over three days prior to implantation.

Total cystectomy Excision of the entire bladder is mainly indicated when the bladder tumor is of high stage (B_1, B_2, C, or

Table 25-5
Five-Year Survival (%) Following Segmental Resection by Pathologic Stage in Patients with Bladder Cancer

Author	Year	O	A	B_1	B_2	C	D
Marshall et al[97]	1956	-----62-----			--62---		
Riches[98]	1960	--58---		--36---		--0---	
Magri[99]	1962		80	--38---		26	
Jewett et al[100]	1964		58	58	16	16	
Masina[101]	1965	--82---		--50---		38	
Cox et al[69]	1968	43	73	20	33	16	0
Long et al[102]	1972	80	67	43	20	9	
Resnick and O'Connor[103]	1973	75	57	55	16	11	20*
Utz et al[104]	1973		68	47	40	29	0
Evans and Texter[105]	1975		69	43	14	0	
Novick and Stewart[106]	1976	--67---		--53---		17	25
Brannan et al[107]	1978		79	80	45	6	
Cummings et al[108]	1978	100	79	80	45	6	

*Prostatic invasion.

T_2, T_3) or when the size and location of the tumor or multicentricity make a more conservative procedure impractical.

The term radical cystectomy connotes removal of the bladder and prostate, seminal vesicles, perivesical fat, and peritoneum surrounding the bladder in the male; and the bladder, urethra, anterior vaginal wall, and genital organs in the female. Simple cystectomy, on the other hand, means removal of the bladder with the plane of dissection between the muscular bladder wall and the perivesical tissue. A radical cystectomy means the plane of dissection is adjacent to the pelvic side wall and rectum. The inclusion of a pelvic lymph node dissection is separate.

Five-year survival rates following simple cystectomy or radical cystectomy with pelvic lymphadenectomy are shown in Table 25-6. In comparing the 5-year survival statistics between simple cystectomy and radical cystectomy, there is no real significant difference. The most logical reason for radical cystectomy not causing improvement in survival is that most of the failures that occur do so because of distant metastases.

In those patients with B_2, C, or T_3 lesions, the incidence of positive lymph nodes runs between 15% and 25%.[38] The surgical curability in these patients remains low with the best survival statistics reported to be between 13% and 17%.[119-121] These survival statistics primarily reflect those patients with minimal node involvement.

External beam radiation therapy Definitive therapy with external beam radiation remains a useful and important treatment for patients with invasive bladder cancer. Primary therapy usually consists of between 6000 and 7000 rad to the bladder with or without accompanying lymph node treatment. The greatest advantage of irradiation lies in its preservation of renal function. It also avoids the operative morbidity and mortality inherent to such surgical procedures. The risks of radiation therapy alone, however, are not minimal. Its complications can include a poorly predictable incidence of radiation cystitis and proctitis as well as a significant rate of impotence. The bladder may also be affected by radiation cystitis causing bladder contraction and the possibility of significant bladder hemorrhage. In some patients, bleeding and bladder symptoms may even require palliative diversion although tumor is conspicuously absent from the bladder.

Five-year survival results from multiple

Table 25-6
Five-Year Survival (%) in Bladder Cancer Patients Following Simple or Radical Cystectomy

Investigators	Stage B_1	Stage B_2	Stage C
Cystectomy			
Brice et al[111]	25/68(37%)	7/63(11%)	8/88(9%)
Jewett et al[100]	2/4(50%)	2/12(16%)	5/43(12%)
Cox et al[112]	5/11(45%)	2/5(40%)	2/11(18%)
Poole-Wilson and Barrard[113]	8/32(25%)	(combined with stage B_1)	1/8(12%)
Long et al[102]		6/11(55%)	2/20(10%)
Pomerance[114]	3/23(13%)	6/21(29%)	1/41(2%)
Cordonnier[115]	10/19(52%)	4/41(28%)	5/28(18%)
Wajsman et al[116]	14/28(50%)	21/64(32%)	
Radical Cystectomy			
Long et al[102]	3/4(75%)	1/4(25%)	5/10(50%)
Whitmore et al[117]	18/30(60%)	8/31(26%)	2/19(11%)
Pearse et al[118]	9/14(64%)	6/12(50%)	3/15(20%)

series are shown in Table 25-7. All grades and stages of bladder carcinoma have on occasion been controlled by means of external beam irradiation alone. In practice, definitive radiation therapy is considered when localized bladder carcinoma is not amenable to other conservative means of therapy. Primary irradiation is also an option for those patients who refuse cystectomy, with the understanding that some tumors may not be radioresponsive. Likewise, there is no significant evidence to show that definitive irradiation prevents the future formation of bladder tumors. It is thus a frequent finding that new lesions develop during the follow-up period even if the primary lesion is well controlled by radiation therapy. The local failure rate with definitive radiation hovers around 50%.[136]

Although the role of tumor grade, configuration, and size have been correlated with the results of radiotherapy, it remains impossible to consistently predict radiation responsiveness. Whether response to radiation is a function of the primary tumor or of the host's ability to help eradicate the tumor remains uncertain. Ideally, it would be best to determine before radiotherapy which tumors are radioresponsive and which are not. This possibility is the subject of several ongoing research projects. Whether tissue culture studies or perhaps flow cytometry will be helpful may be determined in the near future.[142,143]

Salvage cystectomy Survival rates associated with cystectomy performed after failure of radiation therapy do not differ significantly from those with similar tumor stages treated originally by cystectomy alone. The results from several series are shown in Table 25-8. Because of these results, definitive radiotherapy has remained an alternative to cystectomy alone and to integrated irradiation and cystectomy regimens. Although the risks of salvage cystectomy are higher than cystectomy or integrated irradiation and cystectomy, they do not seem to be insurmountable. Early reports of operative mortality by Higgins et al[147] and Edsmyr et al[148] were between 15% and 33%. Crawford and Skinner[149] in 1980 reported an 8.1% (three patients) mortality in 37 patients; Smith and

Table 25-7
Five-Year Survival (%) Following External Megavoltage Radiotherapy by Clinical Stage in Patients with Bladder Cancer

Author	Year	0	A	B_1	B_2	C	D
Wallace[122]	1959		24	----11----		11	
Dick[123]	1962		73	----46----		0	
Brady and Gislayson[124]	1963		----100--------		-----22-----		0
Collins[125]	1964		33	23	----0------		
Sagerman et al[126]	1965			----33----		25	
Kurohara et al[127]	1965		-----32--------		----13-----		
Crigler et al[128]	1966		-----32--------		----28-----		6
Pointon and Evan[129]	1969		38	19	----27-----		
Frank[130]	1970			57	----31-----		10
Edsmyr et al[131]	1967			34	----25-----		7
Finney[132]	1971		24	----22----		33	
Miller and Johnson[133]	1973		50	26	21	19	9
Combes et al[134]	1974		---23----		----10-----		0
Morrison[135]	1975		---41---		----28-----		6
Goffinet et al[136]	1975				35	20	8
van der Werf Messing[137]	1975		28	28	----10----		10
Fish and Fayos[138]	1976		60,51	25,43	20,25	0,13	0,11
Cummings et al[139]	1976		-----73------		----36-----		
Birkhead et al[140]	1976				----18-----		11
Rider and Evans[141]	1976		56	50	----18-----		28

Table 25-8
Five-Year Survival Rates (%) in Patients with Bladder Cancer After Salvage Cystectomy for Irradiation Failures by Pathologic Stage

Author	Year	0	A	B_1	B_2	C	D
Miller et al[133]	1973	--	7	--	----21----		25
Wallace and Bloom[144]	1976				----52----		
Whitmore et al[117]	1977	55	68	43	33	20	8
Smith and Whitmore[145]	1981	71	63	47	----26----		9
Johnson[146]	1983	--	67	--	----	25	--

Whitmore[145] in 1981 reported a 5% (four patients) operative mortality in 80 patients. At the MD Anderson Hospital and Tumor Institute there have been no postoperative deaths in over 62 patients operated on since 1969.[146] Likewise, hospital stay is prolonged over those treated by integrated irradiation and cystectomy in less than one third of the cases. It should be emphasized, however, that these patients represent a highly selected group; those cured of their bladder cancer by irradiation are excluded as are those who died of local or metastatic disease before they could be considered for salvage cystectomy. It remains certain nevertheless, that salvage cystectomy is worthwhile in some patients.

Integrated irradiation and cystectomy This approach is used at most centers today in patients whose tumors are not amenable to other conservative means of management. The clinical and experimental evidence supporting the use of preoperative irradiation rests on the assumption that radiation destroys any microextension of tumor and reduces the number of viable cells in order to prevent local implantation or distant dissemination of the disease during the surgical procedure. In addition, there is some evidence to show that a small burden in regional lymph nodes may be controlled by radiation therapy given preoperatively. Table 25-9 shows the results of integrated irradiation and cystectomy from several series. The overall survival rates, compared to cystectomy alone, are approximately doubled. In general, several conclusions can be made with regard to the efficacy of integrated irradiation and cystectomy in the management of invasive bladder cancer. In patients with low-stage neoplasms (O–A, B_1–Tis, T_1, T_2), there is no definite improvement in survival from the use of preoperative radiation. In patients with high-stage tumors (B_2, C–T_3), the increase in survival rate over cystectomy alone seems to give an advantage to preoperative irradiation. Whether 2000 rad, 4000 rad, or 4500 rad is used as a preoperative regimen does not seem to make any difference, nor does tumor stage affect survival with respect to grade. As would be expected, however, patients with low-grade and low-stage tumors in general survive better. With high clinical stage lesions, whether the tumor is low grade or high grade, survival is not significantly altered.

The primary effect of radiation and improved survival is seen in those patients in whom tumor regression has occurred as a consequence of irradiation (pathologic stage P less than clinical stage T). In those patients who are not downstaged (P greater than or equal to T), survival rates are similar to those of patients treated by cystectomy alone. Although demonstrable downstaging depends on the preoperative radiation dose and interval to cystectomy, survival for these isolated T_3 lesions, despite dose, is not significantly different.

The primary effect of radiation in this group seems to be a reduced incidence of pelvic recurrence. If the patient's tumor has been significantly downstaged, local control of the neoplasm has been extremely high. The only true studies randomizing

Table 25-9
Results of Integrated Irradiation and Cystectomy for Muscle-Infiltrating Tumors

Author	Year	Dose and Time	T_2	T_{3a}	T_{3b}
Miller and Johnson[133]	1973	5000 rad in 5 wk	--	----53%----	
Prout et al[150]	1973	4500 rad in 4.5 wk	--	----36%----	
van der Werf-Messing[151]	1973	4000 rad in 4 wk	43%	----40%----	
Reid et al[152]	1976	2000 rad in 4 d	--	----34%----	
Wallace and Bloom[153]	1976	4000 rad in 4 wk	--	----33%----	
Whitmore et al[154]	1977	4000 rad in 4 wk	59%	34%	33%
Whitmore[155]	1981	2000 rad in 5 d	41%	----40%----	
Boileau et al[156]	1980	5000 rad in 5 wk	38%	51%	57%

preoperative irradiation with surgery *v* surgery alone was reported by Prout et al[150] and Slack et al.[157] Those studies demonstrated the advantage of integrated therapy over surgery alone in patients with clinical high stage (B_2-C, T_3) lesions. Five-year survival of 36% was obtained with integrated irradiation therapy and surgery compared to a 5-year survival of 22% with surgery alone. Although there has been concern regarding the healing capacity and morbidity and mortality related to preoperative irradiation, with the exception of some minor wound infections and slightly decreased wound healing, no additional risks have been demonstrated.

Treatment Failures

Treatment failure may be divided into five categories. These include new tumor formation in the bladder; new tumor formation in the renal pelvis, ureter, or urethra; iatrogenic implantation or dissemination of tumor; local recurrence because of incomplete primary resection; and regional and distant metastases.[38]

New formation As long as the patient with a history of bladder tumors retains the bladder, there remains a risk for the development of new lesions. In general, multicentricity at initial presentation is the primary predictor of recurrent disease. Grade and stage of disease, A, B, H isoantigen deletion, urinary cytology, random bladder biopsies for the presence of dysplasia and concomitant neoplasia, flow cytometry DNA determinations, karyotyping, tissue culture characteristics, and monoclonal antibody marking have all been suggested as having some predictive value in identifying which bladders are at high risk for developing high-stage recurrent disease. Unfortunately, most of these studies remain experimental and the extent to which any one will demonstrate predictive accuracy remains to be determined.

New tumor formation in the renal pelvis, ureter, or urethra Transitional epithelium lines the entire urinary tract from the tip of the renal calyx to the urethral meatus; this area is at risk for the development of subsequent tumor. Any carcinogenic influence not only bathes the epithelium of the bladder but continually bathes the whole urinary tract epithelium. In general, patients treated for bladder carcinoma have an approximate 5% incidence of developing upper tract tumors and between a 5% and 10% chance of developing tumors in the urethra. The risk in both areas is highest in those with polychronotopic disease.[38] The highest risk of upper tract tumors (25%) occurs in those patients whose course includes a history of both bladder and urethral lesions.[158]

Iatrogenic implantation or dissemination of tumor Iatrogenic local recurrence or dissemination of tumor cells can be the result of wound implantation or lymphatic or vascular dissemination prior to or at the time of treatment. Local tumor implantation in open wounds is a risk of methods employing suprapubic excision, segmental resection, and/or suprapubic implantation of radioactive material. It seems that the risk of implantation is greater with higher-grade tumors when compared with lower-grade tumors. Even during radical cystectomy pelvic recurrence may be due to tumor cell spillage in the wound at the time of transection of the urethra at the prostatic apex in the male, or from incomplete excision of the urethra in the female. Because of this possibility, preoperative irradiation with or without the use of intravesical chemotherapy or formalin during the time of cystectomy has been advocated.[36]

Endoscopic procedures may affect implantation of bladder cancer cells by allowing them to get into the interstices of the bladder wall defect at the time of the resection. Likewise, transsection of lymphatics and blood vessels opens up spaces for potential dispersement or dissemination of the tumor. There is some evidence to show that postoperative intravesical chemotherapy may reduce the incidence of new tumor formation and possibly that of dissemination.

Local recurrence because of incomplete primary excision Local recurrences following endoscopic resection may be due to inaccuracy of clinical staging (understaging), technical limitations in the extent of local excision, and the natural history of the tumor. Jewett and Eversol[159] have demonstrated that local recurrence was more frequent with high-grade lesions than with low-grade lesions. The occurrence of frank carcinoma in situ or severe mucosal dysplasia in other portions of the bladder may also be a potential source of local recurrence. Because of the nature of carcinoma in situ, lesions may not be recognized at the time of resection and thus may be presumed to be an inevitable cause of failure. Although local recurrence with low-stage tumors is frequent, there is no convincing evidence that radical surgery *v* conservative therapy produces a better survival rate. This fact implies that the control of appropriately selected low-stage tumors is excellent and that treatment in this manner does not have a deleterious effect on survival with continued use.

Local recurrence in the bladder after segmental resection connotes poor case selection. As mentioned previously, selected random bladder biopsies should be performed and must not show carcinoma in situ or evidence of severe dysplasia for a patient to be a candidate for segmental resection. Due to these rigid criteria, segmental resection is seldom used. Following cystectomy, local recurrence in the pelvis can be blamed on tumor spillage from the bladder or urethra at the time of surgery, from unrecognized microextensions transsected in the course of resection, or from incompletely resected regional lymph node metastases. Appropriate preoperative irradiation, however, might logically be expected to reduce pelvic recurrence rates. In reviewing data from Memorial Sloan-Kettering Cancer Center, there is no question that preoperative irradiation reduced pelvic recurrence in all patients treated with this regimen.[38] The most common site of primary failure in patients with invasive disease, however, is distant metastases, which for the most part remain independent of pelvic recurrence rates.

Regional metastases The incidence of regional lymph node metastases, according to stage of disease, is shown in Table 25-10.[160] Because pelvic lymph nodes are, or seem to be, the first echelon of metastasis as evidenced by autopsy studies, the inclusion of a systematic bilateral pelvic lymph node dissection prior to radical cystectomy was intended to improve the cure rate in patients with deeply infiltrating tumors. Clinical survival data, however, show that only selected patients (those with microscopic involvement of one lymph node) are helped by this procedure. Even those patients who go on to die of bladder cancer after integrated irradiation and radical cystectomy wtih lymph node dissection generally die of distant metastases to the liver, lung, and bone without ever demonstrating metastases to regional lymph nodes. Jewett and Strong[46] first reported that 36% of the patients who died of distant metastases from bladder cancer died with no evidence of lymph node metastases.

Distant metastases The principal sites of distant metastases are bone, lung, and liver, but any organ may be involved. In a report by Babaian et al[161] at MD Anderson Hospital the major sites of involvement in decreasing order were lymph nodes, liver, lung, bone, adrenals, intestines, heart, brain, kidney, spleen, and pancreas.[161] The higher the stage of primary tumor, the higher the incidence of disseminated disease. How much preoperative staging error has to do with the development or rapid appearance of distant metastases remains uncertain. With improvement in staging, however, a significant number of patients with previously unrecognizable metastatic disease may be selected preoperatively.

Treatment of Disseminated Disease

Surgical palliation When considering surgical palliation of advanced carcinoma, several points should be considered: (1) Will the expectation of palliation justify the procedure? That is, can a surgical procedure be justified to significantly alter the course of the patient in an end-stage situation? (2) Will the procedure increase the length of survival? (3) Will the cost of the procedure be justified inasmuch as the possibility of leaving the hospital remains in question? (4) What do the patient and family want?

Table 25-10
Incidence of Lymph Node and Regional Metastases with Different P Stage Categories

P Category	Lymph Nodes (%)	Regional Metastases (%)
Pis	1	1
P 1	5	10
P 2	10	20–30
P 3	20	40–50
P 4	40	60

Transurethral resection Transurethral resection of bladder tumors or fulguration of bladder tumors to control irritative symptoms and hemorrhage is a plausible means of treating patients with metastases. As much tumor bulk as possible can be removed, often with effective control of local hemorrhage. The advantage of transurethral resection is that it can be repeated at frequent intervals, is cost-effective and well tolerated by the patients.

Cystectomy Palliative cystectomy may be considered in patients with severe pain and/or bleeding that cannot be controlled by any other means. Patients who are considered for palliative cystectomy have usually failed radiotherapy, segmental resection, transurethral resection or fulguration, and the instillation of different intravesical agents. In this situation, palliative cystectomy may be the only choice; however, morbidity or mortality from the procedure remains significant. There are no statistical data regarding palliative cystectomy.

Urinary tract diversion The role of palliative supravesical diversion remains uncertain. It is well known that palliative diversion for ureteral obstruction to prolong survival with obstructed ureters and impending uremic death is not indicated with bladder cancer. The average survival following diversion is approximately 3 months, and a good majority of patients do not leave the hospital. The role of supravesical diversion when lymph nodes are positive remains controversial. Certainly, a good majority of patients who are treated with radiation therapy for bulky tumor have intractable symptoms of frequency, urgency, and often hemorrhage. In these patients, supravesical diversion without cystectomy may be indicated. Patients who may benefit most from palliative supravesical diversion without cystectomy, are those patients presenting with unresectable local lesions or metastatic disease who have significant voiding symptoms and remain untreated for their local primary tumor.

Radiation therapy Although transitional cell carcinoma of the bladder is known to be responsive to radiation therapy, few patients with stage D disease are ever cured by radiation alone. The primary indication for irradiating the bladder with metastatic disease is for treatment of hemorrhage. External beam radiation, however, often makes local irritative symptoms such as spasm, pain, and frequency worse and may lead to palliative diversion. For focal bony metastases, radiotherapy does have a role in decreasing pain. Usually 2000 to 3000 rad over a 2- to 3-week period is significantly palliative.

Other methods of symptomatic treatment for severe hemorrhage may include the use of hydrostatic balloon pressure therapy, introduced by Helmstein,[162] and Holstein et al[163] or the use of intravesical agents such as silver nitrate or intravesical formalin. The uses and complications of each of these procedures have been recently outlined by Klein and Smith[164] but may be summarized as follows. Control of hemorrhage should be obtained by the least invasive method possible. The hydrostatic pressure technic has not been used with much success in the United States. The use of silver nitrate has been successful in a number of patients with minimal side effects. The advantage of silver nitrate is that it may be used on the floor, without anesthesia, whereas intravesical formalin requires anesthesia. Complications of intravesical formalin have been reflux and renal failure as well as bladder perforation. Therefore, the smallest concentration possible to diminish the hemorrhage is indicated as initial therapy. Usually a 0.5% to 1% concentration is used first, followed by 4% formalin. The use of 10% formalin has been associated with the most complications and should be reserved for intractable life-threatening hemorrhage.

Chemotherapy of advanced disease For patients with multiple distant metastases the only hope for survival is systemic chemotherapy. Transitional cell carcinoma is a chemotherapeutically responsive tumor and four efficacious agents are available: cisplatin, methotrexate, doxorubicin, and vinblastine sulfate. Recent data suggest that some combined regimens may produce additional therapeutic benefits over single-agent therapy. These combinations are cisplatin-doxorubicin, cisplatin-doxorubicin-cyclophosphamide, methotrexate-vinblastine, and cisplatin-dichloromethotrexate. In general, response rates (greater than a 50% reduction in the summed products of all tumor measurements for at least 1 month) with single agents ranges from 15% to 40% and with combined regimens from 25% to 50%.[165] Most remissions, however, are partial rather than complete. The combined results of the various agents alone and in combination have been compiled recently by Yagoda[165] and are presented in Table 25-11.

CONCLUSIONS

At the present time successful management of bladder cancer requires clinical judgment based upon an understanding of the natural history of the disease and the efficacy and attendant risks of individual therapeutic options. With improvement in clinical staging and a better understanding of predictive factors, the quality of these judgments will improve treatment applications, end results, and eliminate unnecessary treatment.

Treatment has generally relied on the most conservative methods that will control the existing disease. Superficial lesions are treated with transurethral resection or fulguration and intravesical chemotherapy. Although the risk of recurrence is high (60%), there is no compelling evidence to show that dissemination is influenced by conservative local therapy as long as that lesion is controlled. Likewise, the risk of conservative treatment to survival and quality of life is appreciably less than that of radical treatment. Subsequent radical treatment is recommended for high-grade and multifocal, rapidly recurring, or inac-

Table 25-11
Chemotherapy Results for Bladder Cancer

	No. of Patients	Percent CR + PR
Single Agents		
AMSA	19	11(0–25)
Bisantrene	12	0
Bleomycin sulfate	79	5(0–10)
Cisplatin	320	30(25–35)
Cyclophosphamide	98	31(22–40)
Doxorubicin	223	18(13–23)
5-Fluorouracil	75	35(24–46)
Methotrexate	236	29(23–35)
Mitomycin	42	13(3–23)
PALA	12	0
Vinblastine	38	16(4–28)
Teniposide	108	16(9–23)
Etoposide	29	0
Yoshi 864	11	18(0–41)
Zinostatin	19	5(0–15)
Combined Regimens		
Cisplatin	320	30(25–35)
+ CTX	102	26(17–35)
+ ADM	72	46(34–58)
+ ADM + CTX	202	46(39–53)
+ ADM + 5-FU	44	44(29–59)
Methotrexate	236	29(23–35)
+ VLB	46	34(20–48)
+ CTX + ADM	26	38(19–57)
+ CTX + 5-FU + VCR ± CA + ACT-D	4	50(1–99)
+ ADM + CTX	28	38(20–56)
Doxorubicin	223	18(13–23)
+ CTX	37	18(6–30)
+ CTX + 5-FU	24	21(5–37)
+ 5-FU	103	39(30–48)
+ CTX + BLEO	23	35(15–55)
+ VM-26	24	19(3–35)

CR = complete remissions, PR = partial remissions. Number in parenthesis = 95% confidence limits. AMSA = 4′(9-acridinylamino methanesulfone-m-anisidide), PALA = phosphonoacetyl-l-asparate, CTX = cyclophosphamide, ADM = doxorubicin, 5-FU = 5-fluorouracil, VLB = vinblastine, VCR = vincristine, ACT-D = Actinomycin D, BLEO = bleomycin sulfate, VM-26 = teniposide.

cessible lesions not controllable by conservative means.

For patients with invasive high-grade lesions integrated irradiation and cystectomy seems to currently yield the best overall survival rates with the lowest pelvic recurrence rates. The beneficial effects of preoperative irradiation are largely confined to those patients whose tumors are downstaged to Po by such treatment. The optimal regimen remains to be determined. Definitive irradiation without question cures some patients with invasive disease. For those with recurrent or persistent disease after irradiation, salvage cystectomy is recommended. The role of adjuvant chemotherapy posttreatment for T_3 or T_4 lesions with or without positive nodes is currently under investigation and remains undefined. In those patients with distant metastases, systemic chemotherapy is the treatment of choice. At the moment combined regimens with cisplatin, methotrexate, doxorubicin, and vinblastine seem to be most effective.

Bladder tumors are heterogeneous and therefore respond differently to identical treatment. The goal is to identify prognostic factors relative to specific treatment modalities that will identify and correctly prescribe the treatment that will be best for the individual patient. Multidisciplinary efforts by basic scientists, and groups of clinicians including surgeons, radiotherapists, chemotherapists, pathologists, and immunologists will provide greater insights into these problems, improve survival rates, and rationalize specific treatment plans.

REFERENCES

1. Johnson DE, Boileau MD: Bladder cancer–overview, in Johnson DE, Boileau MA (eds): *Genitourinary Tumors.* New York, Grune & Stratton, 1982, pp 399–447.
2. Miller, AB: Bladder cancer–epidemiology, in Wilkinson PM (ed): *Advances in Medical Oncology, Research and Education.* Elmsford, NY, Pergamon Press, 1979, vol 2: *Clinical Cancer–Principal Sites.* pp 201–206.
3. Johnson DE, Hillis S: Carcinoma of the bladder in patients less than 40 years old. *J Urol* 1978;1201:172–173.
4. Cole P, Monson RR, Haning H, et al: Smoking and cancer in the lower urinary tract. *N Engl J Med* 1971;284:129–134.

5. Rehn L: Blasengeschwülste bei Fuchsin-Arbeitern. *Arch Klin Chir* 1895;50:588–600.
6. Case RAM, Hosker ME, McDonald DB, et al: Tumors of the urinary bladder in workmen engaged in the manufacture and use of certain dye stuff intermediates in the British chemical industry. *Br J Ind Med* 1954;11:95–104.
7. Price JM: Etiology of bladder cancer, in Moltry E Jr (ed): *Benign and Malignant Tumors of the Urinary Bladder.* Flushing, NY, Medical Examination Publishing Co, 1971, pp 189–261.
8. Cole P, Hoover R, Friedell GH: Occupation and cancer of the lower urinary tract. *Cancer* 1972;29:1250–1260.
9. Veys CA: Two epidemiologic inquiries into the incidence of bladder tumors in industrial workers. *J Natl Cancer Inst* 1969;43:219–226.
10. Anthony HM, Thomas GM: Letter to the editor. *J Natl Cancer Inst* 1971;46: 1112–1113.
11. Case RAM: Some environmental carcinogens. *Proc R Soc Med* 1969;62: 1061–1066.
12. Tola S, Tenho M, Korkala ML, et al: Cancer of the urinary bladder in Finland. *Int Arch Occup Environ Health* 1980; 46:43–51.
13. Berenblum I: The mechanism of carcinogenesis. A study of the significance of carcinogenic action and related phenomena. *Cancer Res* 1941;1:807–814.
14. Hicks RM: Multistage carcinogenesis in the urinary bladder. *Br Med Bull* 1980;36: 39–46.
15. Holsti LR, Armala P: Papillary carcinoma of the bladder in mice obtained after per oral administration of tobacco tar. *Cancer* 1955;8:679–682.
16. Wynder EL, Goldsmith R: The epidemiology of bladder cancer—a second look. *Cancer* 1977;40:1246–1268.
17. Lockwood K: On the etiology of bladder tumors in Kobenhaun-Frederiksberg. An inquiry of 369 patients and 350 controls. *Acta Pathol Microbiol Scand* 1961; (suppl):145–165.
18. Hoffman D, Masuda Y, Wynder DL: Alpha-naphthylamine and beta-naphthylamine in cigarette smoke. *Nature* 1969;211: 255–256.
19. Kerr WK, Barkin M, Levers PE, et al: The effect of cigarette smoking on bladder carcinogens in man. *Can Med Assoc J* 1965; 93:1–7.
20. Price JM, Biava CG, Oser BL, et al: Bladder tumors in rats fed cyclohexylamine or high doses of a mixture of cyclamate and saccharin. *Science* 1970;167:1131–1132.
21. Friedman L, Richardson HL, Richardson ME, et al: Toxic response of rats to cyclamate in chow and semi-synthetic dyes. *J Natl Cancer Inst* 1972;49:751–764.
22. Newell GR, Hoover RN, Kolbye AC: Status report on saccharin in humans. *J Natl Cancer Inst* 1978;61:275–276.
23. Connolly JG, Rider WD, Rosenbaum L, et al: Relationship between the use of artificial sweeteners and bladder cancer, letter to the editor. *Can Med Assoc J* 1978;119:408.
24. Morrison AS, Buring JE: Artificial sweeteners and cancer of the lower urinary tract. *N Engl J Med* 1980;302: 537–541.
25. Kessler II, Clark JP: Saccharin, cyclamate and human bladder cancer: no evidence of an association. *JAMA* 1978;240:349–355.
26. Hicks RM, Chowaniee J, Wakefield J St J: Experimental induction of bladder tumors by a two-stage system, in Slaga TJ, Sivak A, Bourwell RK (eds): *Carcinogenesis: Mechanisms of Tumor Promotion and Carcinogenesis.* New York, Raven Press, 1978, vol 2, pp 475–489.
27. Cohen SM, Arai M, Jacobs JB, et al: Promoting effect of saccharin and DL-tryptophan in urinary bladder. *Cancer Res* 1979;39:1207–1217.
28. Cole P: Coffee drinking and cancer of the lower urinary tract. *Lancet* 1971;1: 1335–1337.
29. Simon D, Yen S, Cole P: Coffee drinking and cancer of the lower urinary tract. *J Natl Cancer Inst* 1975;54:587–591.
30. Fraumeni JF Jr, Scotto J, Dunham LJ: Coffee drinking and bladder cancer. *Lancet* 1971;2:1204.
31. Miller AB: The etiology of bladder cancer from the epidemiological viewpoint. *Cancer Res* 1977;37:2939–2942.
32. Bross ID, Tidings J: Another look at coffee drinking and cancer of the urinary

bladder. *Prev Med* 1973;2:445–451.

33. Fokkens W: Phenacetin abuse related to bladder cancer. *Environ Res* 1979;20: 192–198.
34. Price JM: Etiology of bladder cancer, in Maltry E Jr (ed): *Benign and Malignant Tumors of the Urinary Bladder.* Flushing, NY, Medical Examination Publishing Co, 1971, pp 189–261.
35. Mostofi FK, Sobin LH, Torloni H (eds): *Histological Typing of Urinary Bladder Tumors; International Histological Classification of Tumors.* Geneva, World Health Organization, 1973, No. 10.
36. Friedell GH, Bell JR, Burney SW, et al: Histopathology and classification of urinary bladder cancer. *Urol Clin North Am* 1976;3:53–70.
37. Koss LG: Tumors of the urinary bladder, in Koss LG (ed): *Atlas of Tumor Pathology,* fasc 2, series 2, Washington, DC, Armed Forces Institute of Pathology, 1975.
38. Whitmore WF Jr: Management of bladder cancer. *Curr Probl Cancer* 1979;4:1–48.
39. Broders AC: Epithelioma of the genito-urinary organs. *Ann Surg* 1922;75:574–580.
40. Collan Y, Makinen J, Heikkinen A: Histological grading of transitional cell tumors of the bladder–value of histological grading (WHO) in prognosis. *Eur Urol* 1979;5:311–318.
41. Lerman RI, Hutter RVP, Whitmore WF Jr: Papilloma of the urinary bladder. *Cancer* 1970;25:333–353.
42. Koss LG: Mapping of the urinary bladder: its impact on the concepts of bladder cancer. *Hum Pathol* 1979;10:533–548.
43. Tannenbaum M, Romas NA: The pathobiology of early urothelial cancer, in Skinner DG, de Kernion JB (eds): *Genitourinary Cancer.* Philadelphia, WB Saunders Co, 1978, pp 232–255.
44. Althausen AF, Prout GR Jr, Daly JJ: Non-invasive papillary carcinoma of the bladder associated with carcinoma in situ. *J Urol* 1976;116:575.
45. de Kernion JB, Skinner DG: Epidemiology, diagnosis and staging of bladder cancer, in Skinner DG, de Kernion JB (eds): *Genitourinary Cancer.* Philadelphia, WB Saunders, 1978, pp 213–231.
46. Jewett JH, Strong GH: Infiltrating carcinoma of the bladder–relation of depth of penetration of the bladder wall to incidence of local extension and metastases. *J Urol* 1946;55:366–372.
47. Jewett HJ: Carcinoma of the bladder–influence of depth of infiltration on the 5 year results following complete extirpation of the primary growth. *J Urol* 1952; 67:672–680.
48. Marshall VF: The relation of the preoperative estimate to the pathologic demonstration of the extent of vesical neoplasms. *J Urol* 1952;68:714–723.
49. Union Internationale Contre le Cancer: *TNM Classification of Malignant Tumors.* Geneva, Imprimerie G de Buren, 1974.
50. Prout GR: Bladder carcinoma and a TNM system of classification. *J Urol* 1977;117: 583–590.
51. Droller MJ: Bladder cancer. *Monogr Urol* 1982;3:131–154.
52. Esposti PL, Zajicek J: Grading of transitional cell neoplasm of the urinary bladder from smears of bladder washings–a critical review of 326 tumors. *Acta Cytol (Baltimore)* 1972;16:529.
53. Farrow GM: Pathologist's role in bladder cancer. *Semin Oncol* 1979;6:198–206.
54. Kafkas M: Study and diagnosis of bladder tumors by triple contrast cystography. *J Urol* 1973;109:832–834.
55. Connolly JG, Challis TW, Wallace DM, et al: An evaluation of the fractionated cystogram in the assessment of infiltrating tumors of the bladder. *J Urol* 1967;98: 356–360.
56. Sakkas JL, Androulakis JA, Cambouris T, et al: Fractionated cystogram in the diagnosis of tumors of the bladder–modification in technic. *South Med J* 1974;67:10–12.
57. Schmidt JD, Weinstein SH: Pitfalls in clinical staging of bladder tumors. *Urol Clin North Am* 1976;3:107–127.
58. Lang EK: The roentgenographic assessment of bladder tumors. A comparison of the diagnostic accuracy of roentgenographic techniques. *Cancer* 1969;23:717–724.
59. Winterberger AR, Kenny GM, Choi SH, et al: Correlation of selective arteriography in the staging of bladder tumors. *Cancer* 1972;29:332–337.
60. Johnson DE, Kaesler KE, Kaminsky S, et al: Lymphangiography as an aid in stag-

ing bladder carcinoma. *South Med J* 1967a;69:28–30.
61. Seidelmann FE, Cohen WN, Bryan PJ: Computed tomographic staging of bladder neoplasm. *Radiol Clin North Am* 1977; 15:419–440.
62. Schuller J, Walther V, Schmiedt E, et al: Intravesical ultrasound tomography in staging bladder carcinoma. *J Urol* 1982; 128:264–266.
63. Holm HH, Northeved A: A transurethral ultrasonic scanner. *J Urol* 1974;111: 238–241.
64. Gammelgaard J, Holm HH: Transurethral and transrectal ultrasonic scanning in urology. *J Urol* 1980;124:863–868.
65. Nakamura S, Niijima T: Staging of bladder cancer by ultrasonography–a new technique by transurethral intravesical scanning. *J Urol* 1980;124:341–344.
66. Felix EL, Bagley DH, Sindelar WF, et al: The value of the liver scan in preoperative screening of patients with malignancies. *Cancer* 1976;38:1137–1141.
67. Flocks RH: Treatment of patients with carcinoma of the bladder. *JAMA* 1951; 145:295.
68. Nicols JA, Marshall VF: The treatment of bladder carcinoma by local excision and fulguration. *Cancer* 1956;9:559–565.
69. Cox CE, Cass AS, Boyce WH: Bladder cancer–a 26 year review. *Trans Am Assoc Genitourin Surg* 1968;60:22–30.
70. Marberger J, Marberger M Jr, Decristofora A: The current status of transurethral resection in the diagnosis and therapy of carcinoma of the urinary bladder. *Int Urol Nephrol* 1972;4:35.
71. O'Flynn JD, Smith JM, Hanson JS: Transurethral resection for the assessment and treatment of vesical neoplasms. *Eur Urol* 1975;1:38–40.
72. Barnes RW, Dick AL, Hadley HL, et al: Survival following transurethral resection of bladder carcinoma. *Cancer* 1977;37: 2895–2897.
73. Williams JL, Hammonds JC, Saunders N: T2 bladder tumours. *Br J Urol* 1977; 49:663–668.
74. Prout GR Jr: The surgical management of bladder carcinoma. *Urol Clin North Am* 1976;3:149–175.
75. Jones HC, Swinney J: Thiotepa in the treatment of tumors of the bladder. *Lancet* 1961;2:615–618.
76. Veenema RJ, Dean AL Jr, Roberts M: Bladder carcinoma treated by direct instillation of thiotepa. *J Urol* 1962;88: 60–63.
77. Edsmyr F, Boman J: Instillation of thiotepa (Tifosyl) in vesical papillomatosis. *Acta Radiol Therapy Phys Bio* 1970;9: 395–400.
78. Koontz WW Jr, Prout GR Jr, Smith W, et al: The use of intravesical thiotepa in management of non-invasive carcinoma of the bladder. *J Urol* 1981;125:307–312.
79. Prout GR Jr, Koontz WW Jr, Coombs LJ, et al: (National Bladder Cancer Collaborative Group A): Long-term fate of 90 patients with superficial bladder cancer randomly assigned to receive or not to receive thiotepa. *J Urol* 1983;129:677–680.
80. Byar D, Blackard C: Comparisons of placebo, pyridoxine, and topical thiotepa in preventing recurrence of stage 1 bladder cancer. *Urology* 1983;22:556–561.
81. Schulman C, Sylvester R, Robinson M: Adjuvant therapy of T1 bladder carcinoma: Preliminary results of an EROTC randomized study, in Bonadonna G, Mathe G, Salmon SE (eds): *Recent Results in Cancer Research*. Berlin, Springer-Verlag, 1979, vol 68, pp 338–345.
82. Bracken RB, Johnson DE, Von Eschenbach AC, et al: Role of intravesical mitomycin C in management of superficial bladder tumors. *Urology* 1980;16:11–15.
83. Mishina T, Oda K, Murata S, et al: Mitomycin C bladder installation therapy for bladder tumors. *J Urol* 1975;114:217–219.
84. Soloway MS, Ford KS: Subsequent tumor analysis of 36 patients who have received intravesical mitomycin C for superficial bladder cancer. *J Urol* 1983;130:74–78.
85. Jaske G, Hofstadter F, Marberger H: Intracavitary doxorubicin hydrochloride therapy for carcinoma in situ of the bladder. *J Urol* 1981;125:185–190.
86. Jaske G, Hofstadter F, Marberger H: Topical doxorubicin hydrochloride therapy for carcinoma in situ of the bladder–a follow up. *J Urol* 1981;131:41–42.
87. Schulman CC, Denis LJ, Oosterlinck W, et al: Early adjuvant adriamycin in superficial bladder cancer, Read before Annual Meeting of the American Urological Association, Boston, Mass, 1981.

88. Abrams PH, Choa RG, Gaches GC, et al: A control trial of single dose intravesical adriamycin in superficial bladder tumors. *Br J Urol* 1981;53:585–587.
89. Garnick MB, Schade D, Israel M, et al: Clinical pharmacologic evaluation of intravesical adriamycin for recurrent superficial bladder cancer. Read before Annual Meeting of the American Urological Association, Kansas City, Mo, 1982.
90. Niijima T: Intravesical therapy with adriamycin and new trends, in *Diagnostics and Treatment of Superficial Urinary Bladder Tumors.* Stockholm, Montedison Lakemedel, 1979, pp 37–44.
91. Edsmyr F, Berlin T, Boman J, et al: Intravesical therapy with superficial bladder cancer. *Eur Urol* 1980;6:132–136.
92. Morales A, Eidinger D, Bruce AW: Intracavitary bacillus Calmette-Guerin in the treatment of superficial bladder tumors. *J Urol* 1976;116:180–184.
93. Camacho F, Pinsky C, Ker D, et al: Treatment of superficial bladder cancer with intravesical BCG. *Proc Am Soc Clin Oncol* 1976;116:180–184.
94. Lamm DL, Thor DE, Winters WD, et al: BCG immunotherapy of bladder cancer–inhibition of tumor recurrence and associated immune response. *Cancer* 1981;48: 82–88.
95. Brosman SA: Experience with BCG in patients with superficial bladder cancer. *J Urol* 1982;128:27–30.
96. Pinsky CM, Camacho FJ, Kerr D, et al: Intravesical administration of BCG in patients with recurrent superficial carcinoma of the bladder: Report of a prospective, randomized trial. *Cancer Treat Rep* 1985;69(1):47–53.
97. Marshall VF, Holder J, Ma KT: Survival of patients with bladder carcinoma treated by simple segmental resection. *Cancer* 1956;9:568–571.
98. Riches E: Choice of treatment in carcinoma of the bladder. *J Urol* 1960;84: 472–480.
99. Magri J: Partial cystectomy–a review of 104 cases. *Br J Urol* 1962;34:74–87.
100. Jewett HJ, King LR, Shelley WM: A study of 365 cases of infiltrating bladder cancer–relation of certain pathological characteristics to prognosis after extirpation. *J Urol* 1964;92:668–678.
101. Marsina F: Segmental resection for tumors of the urinary bladder–ten year follow-up. *Br J Surg* 1965;52:279–283.
102. Long RT, Grummon RA, Spratt JS, et al: Carcinoma of the urinary bladder (comparison with radical, simple and partial cystectomy and intravesical formalin). *Cancer* 1972;29:98–105.
103. Resnick MI, O'Connor VJ Jr: Segmental resection for carcinoma of the bladder–review of 102 patients. *J Urol* 1973; 109:1007–1010.
104. Utz, DC, Schmitz SE, Fugelso PD, et al: A clinicopathologic evaluation of partial cystectomy for carcinoma of the urinary bladder. *Cancer* 1973;32:1075–1077.
105. Evans RA, Texter JH Jr: Partial cystectomy in the treatment of bladder cancer. *J Urol* 1975;114:391–393.
106. Novick AC, Stewart BH: Partial cystectomy in the treatment of primary and secondary carcinoma of the bladder. *J Urol* 1976;116:570–574.
107. Brannan W, Ochsner MG, Fuselier HA Jr, et al: Partial cystectomy in the treatment of transitional cell carcinoma of the bladder. *J Urol* 1978;119:213–215.
108. Cummings KG, Mason JT, Correa RJ Jr, et al: Segmental resection in the management of bladder carcinoma. *J Urol* 1978;119:56–58.
109. Whitmore WF Jr: Integrated irradiation and cystectomy for bladder cancer. *Br J Urol* 1980;56:1–9.
110. van der Werf-Messing B: Cancer of the bladder treated by suprapubic radium implants–the value of additional external irradiation. *Eur J Cancer Clin Oncol* 1969; 5:277–285.
111. Brice M, Marshall VF, Green JL, et al: Simple total cystectomy for carcinoma of the urinary bladder–one hundred fifty-six consecutive cases five years later. *Cancer* 1956;9:576–584.
112. Cox CE, Cass AS, Boyce WH: Bladder cancer–a 26 year review. *J Urol* 1969; 101:550–558.
113. Poole-Wilson DS, Barrard RJ: Total cystectomy for bladder tumors. *Br J Urol* 1971; 43:16–24.
114. Pomerance A: Pathology and prognosis following total cystectomy for carcinoma of bladder. *Br J Urol* 1972;44:451–458.
115. Cordonnier JJ: Simple cystectomy in the management of bladder carcinoma. *Arch Surg* 1974;108:190–191.

116. Wajsman L, Merin C, Moore R, et al: Current results from treatment of bladder tumors with total cystectomy at Roswell Park Memorial Institute. *J Urol* 1975; 113:806–810.
117. Whitmore WF Jr, Batata MA, Ghoneim MA, et al: Radical cystectomy with or without prior irradiation in the treatment of bladder cancer. *J Urol* 1977;118: 184–187.
118. Pearse HD, Reed RR, Hodges CV: Radical cystectomy for bladder cancer. *J Urol* 1978;119:216–218.
119. Whitmore WF Jr, Marshall VF: Radical total cystectomy for cancer of the bladder–230 consecutive cases five years later. *J Urol* 1962;87:853–868.
120. LaPlante M, Brice M II: The upper limits of hopeful application of radical cystectomy for vesical carcinoma–does nodal metastasis always indicate incurability? *J Urol* 1973;109:261–264.
121. Dretler SP, Ragsdale BD, Leadbetter WF: The value of pelvic lymphadenectomy in the surgical treatment of bladder cancer. *Trans Am Assoc Genitourin Surg* 1972; 64:79–81.
122. Wallace DM: *Tumours of the Bladder.* Edinburgh, E & S Livingstone, Ltd, 1959, pp 312.
123. Dick DAL: Carcinoma of the bladder treated by external irradiation. *Br J Urol* 1962;34:340–350.
124. Brady LW, Gislason GJ: The management of carcinoma of the bladder using supervoltage modalities. *AJR* 1963;89:150–154.
125. Collins CD: Influence of previous surgery on results of megavoltage radiotherapy in carcinoma of bladder. *Lancet* 1964;2: 988–990.
126. Sagerman RH, Bagshaw MA, Kaplan HS: Linear accelerator supervoltage radiation therapy–carcinoma of the bladder. *AJR* 1965;93:122–127.
127. Kurohara SS, Rubin P, Silon N: Analysis in depth of bladder cancer treated by supervoltage therapy. *AJR* 1965;95: 458–467.
128. Crigler CM, Miller LS, Guinn GA, et al: Radiotherapy for carcinoma of the bladder. *J Urol* 1966;96:55–61.
129. Pointon CS, Evan CM: Clinical trials in malignant disease. Part 8: Cancer of the bladder. *Clin Radiol* 1969;20:95–98.
130. Frank HG: Policy and results of treatment by radiotherapy of carcinoma of the bladder in Leeds. *Clin Radiol* 1970;21:425–430.
131. Edsmyr F, Jacobson F, Dahl O, et al: Cobalt 60 teletherapy of carcinoma of the bladder. *Acta Radiol Ther Phys Biol* 1967;6: 81–99.
132. Finney R: The treatment of carcinoma of the bladder by external irradiation. Part 2: A clinical trial. *Clin Radiol* 1971;22: 225–229.
133. Miller LS, Johnson DE: Megavoltage irradiation for bladder cancer–alone, postoperative or preoperative?, in *Proceedings of the Seventh National Cancer Conference.* Philadelphia, JB Lippincott Co, 1973, p 771.
134. Combes PF, Regis H, Daly N: Résultats du traitement des cancer de la vessie par télécobalt (174 caus). *J Radiol Electrol Med Nucl* 1974;55:841–843.
135. Morrison R: The results of treatment of cancer of the bladder–a clinical contribution to radiobiology. *Clin Radiol* 1975; 26:67–75.
136. Goffinet DR, Schneider MJ, Glatstein EJ, et al: Bladder cancer–results of radiation therapy in 384 patients. *Radiology* 1975; 117:149–153.
137. van de Werf-Messing B: *Cancer of the Urinary Bladder Treated at the Rotterdam Radiotherapy Institute from 1950–1974.* Rotterdam, Rotterdam Radiology Institute and Erasmus University, 1975.
138. Fish JC, Fayos JV: Carcinoma of the urinary bladder, *Radiology* 1976;118: 179–182.
139. Cummings KR, Taylor WJ, Correa RJ, et al: Observations on definitive cobalt 60 radiation for cure in bladder carcinoma: 15 year follow-up. *J Urol* 1976;115:152–154.
140. Birkhead BM, Conley JG, Scott RM: Intensive radiotherapy of locally advanced bladder cancer. *Cancer* 1976;37:2746–2748.
141. Rider WD, Evans DH: Radiotherapy in the treatment of recurrent bladder cancer. *Br J Urol* 1976;48:595–601.
142. Pontes JE, Pierce JM, Pokorny M, et al: Biological effects of short course radiation in transitional cell carcinoma of the bladder. *Invest Urol* 1980;17:413–415.
143. Klein FA, Whitmore WF Jr, Wolf RM, et

al: Presumptive downstaging from preoperative irradiation for bladder cancer as determined by flow cytometry–preliminary report. *Int J Radiat Oncol Biol Phys* 1983;9:487–491.

144. Wallace DM, Bloom HJG: The management of deeply infiltrating (T3) bladder carcinoma–controlled trial of radical radiotherapy versus preoperative radiotherapy and radical cystectomy (first report). *Br J Urol* 1976;48:587–594.
145. Smith JA, Whitmore WF Jr: Salvage cystectomy for bladder cancer after failure of definitive irradiation. *J Urol* 1981;125:643–645.
146. Johnson DE: Salvage cystectomy. *Semin Urol* 1983;1:53–59.
147. Higgins DM, Hamilton RW, Hope-Stone HF: The hazards of total cystectomy after supervoltage irradiation of the bladder. *Br J Urol* 1966;38:311–318.
148. Edsmyr F, Moberger G, Wadstrom L: Carcinoma of the bladder–cystectomy after supervoltage therapy. *Scand J Urol Nephrol* 1971;5:215–221.
149. Crawford ED, Skinner DG: Salvage cystectomy after irradiation failure. *J Urol* 1980;123:32–34.
150. Prout GR Jr, Slack NH, Bioss ID: Preoperative irradiation and cystectomy for bladder carcinoma, IV. Results in a selected population, in *Proceedings of the Seventh National Cancer Conference*, Los Angeles, 1972. Philadelphia, JB Lippincott Co, 1973, p 783.
151. van der Werf-Messing B: Carcinoma of the bladder treated by preoperative irradiation followed by cystectomy. *Cancer* 1973;32:1084–1088.
152. Reid EC, Oliver JA, Fishman IJ: Preoperative irradiation and cystectomy in 135 cases of bladder cancer. *Urology* 1976;8:247–250.
153. Wallace DM, Blood HJG: The management of deeply infiltrating (T3) bladder carcinoma–controlled trial of radical radiotherapy versus preoperative radiotherapy and radical cystectomy (first report). *Br J Urol* 1976;48:587.
154. Whitmore WF Jr, Batata MA, Halaris BS, et al: A comparative study of two preoperative radiation regimens with cystectomy for bladder cancer. *Cancer* 1977;40:1077–1086.
155. Whitmore WF Jr: Integrated irradiation and cystectomy for bladder cancer, in Connolly JG (ed): *Carcinoma of the Bladder.* New York, Raven Press, 1981, pp 235–249.
156. Boileau MA, Johnson DE, Chan RC, et al: Bladder carcinoma; results with preoperative radiation therapy and radical cystectomy. *Urology* 1980;16:569–576.
157. Slack NH, Bross ID, Prout GR Jr: Five year follow-up results of a collaborative study of therapies for carcinoma of the bladder. *J Surg Oncol* 1977;9:393–405.
158. Schellhammer PF, Whitmore WF Jr: Transitional cell carcinoma of the urethra in men having cystectomy for bladder cancer. *J Urol* 1976;115:56–60.
159. Jewett HJ, Eversol SL: Carcinoma of the bladder–characteristic modes of local invasion. *J Urol* 1960;83:383–389.
160. Whitmore WF Jr: Management of invasive bladder neoplasms. *Semin Urol* 1983;1:34–41.
161. Babaian RJ, Johnson DE, Llamas L, et al: Metastases from transitional cell carcinoma of the urinary bladder. *Urology* 1980;16:142–144.
162. Helmstein J: Treatment of bladder carcinoma by a hydrostatic pressure technique–report on 43 cases. *Br J Urol* 1972;44:434–450.
163. Holstein P, Jacobson K, Pedersen JF, et al: Intravesical hydrostatic pressure treatment–new method for control of bleeding from the bladder mucosa. *J Urol* 1973;109:234–236.
164. Klein FA, Smith MJV: Urinary complications of cyclophosphamide therapy–etiology, prevention and management. *South Med J* 1983;76:1413.
165. Yagoda A: Chemotherapy for advanced urothelial cancer. *Semin Urol* 1983;1:60–74.

CHAPTER 26 Obstructive Uropathy in the Elderly

Antonia Harford
Domenic A. Sica
Edward T. Zawada, Jr.

Urinary tract obstruction (UTO) is a common cause of renal disease and may result from an obstruction to flow at virtually any level of the urinary tract. The spectrum of obstructive uropathy encompasses a number of clinical manifestations; these include hematuria, pain, infection, and ultimately renal insufficiency. The renal insufficiency that occurs may do so acutely (days), subacutely (weeks), or chronically (months). Of particular importance, especially in the care of the elderly, is the fact that return of renal function can be readily achieved with relief of the obstruction. The presence of obstruction is not always obvious, so that on occasion, uremia is the presenting sign. Thus, it is essential to be aware of the clinical situations in which obstruction occurs and how best to both diagnose and treat this potentially reversible disturbance.

INCIDENCE AND CAUSES

The incidence of hydronephrosis as reported from a series of 32,360 autopsies was 3.8% (3.6% in females and 3.9% in males).[1] In nearly all instances an obstructing lesion was shown to be the cause of the hydronephrosis. This series did not report if clinical symptoms existed with the hydronephrosis, and it is likely that in many instances the observed hydronephrosis was but an incidental autopsy finding.

The observed incidence of hydronephrosis is somewhat lower in children. Campbell noted an incidence of 2% in an autopsy study of 15,919 children. In this study the observed hydronephrosis was most commonly found in those children under the age of 12 months. Clinically recognized obstruction in childhood exhibits a considerably less skewed distribution. In one series only 114 of 512 cases observed were present in those under the age of 12 months.[2]

In the middle years of adulthood, hydronephrosis occurs more commonly in females, a fact attributable to the incidence of pregnancy[3] and carcinoma of the cervix in this age group.[4] Among males in this same age group stone disease is the most common cause of acute ureteral obstruction with an observed frequency of hospitalization of 1/1000 Americans per year (220,000 individuals).[5]

In the older age groups pelvic malignancies[6] continue as a dominant cause of obstruction in females. But, as a result of both benign[7] and malignant prostatic disease,[8] bladder tumors,[9] and urethral strictures,[10] males now outnumber females when a sex incidence of obstructive uropathy is considered in the elderly.

In a recent study, population-based data was accumulated by the Kaiser-Permanente Medical Care Program on the incidence of kidney and urinary tract disease. This group has a membership exceeding 1 million persons and is demographically representative of the general population in the San Francisco Bay area. Discharge diagnoses encoded by the International Classification of Diseases, Adapted (ICDA) were derived from 506,782 hospitalizations by 352,322 subscribers in the 5-year period from 1971 to 1975 as related to a kidney or urinary tract disease. The most common diagnoses were urinary tract infections (ICDA 590.0–590.0, 595.0, 599.0), benign prostatic hypertrophy (ICDA 600), and renal ureteral calculi (ICDA 592). When age-specific rates for these diagnoses and bladder cancer (ICDA 188) are calculated, there is a clear predominance of these illnesses in those over the age of 50 (Figure 26-1).[11] Though these data do not relate directly to the incidence of obstruction in this age group, they do demonstrate that factors prominent in the development of obstruction in the elderly account for the majority of hospitalizations related to kidney and urinary tract disease.

Obstruction to the flow of urine can occur at virtually any level of the urinary tract, from the tubule (uric acid nephropathy) to the urethral meatus (phimosis), and the causes may be secondary to either mechanical or neuromuscular processes (Table 26-1). As previously noted, the age and the sex of the population will frequently suggest both the site and the cause of the obstruction. This observation is especially germane to the elderly, a population group in which obstructive uropathy is frequently attributable to a characteristic group of disorders (Figure 26-2).

Functional disturbances (neuromuscular) are common causes of obstruction in the elderly. These may include adynamic ureteral segments or neurogenic dysfunction of the bladder and/or sphincters.

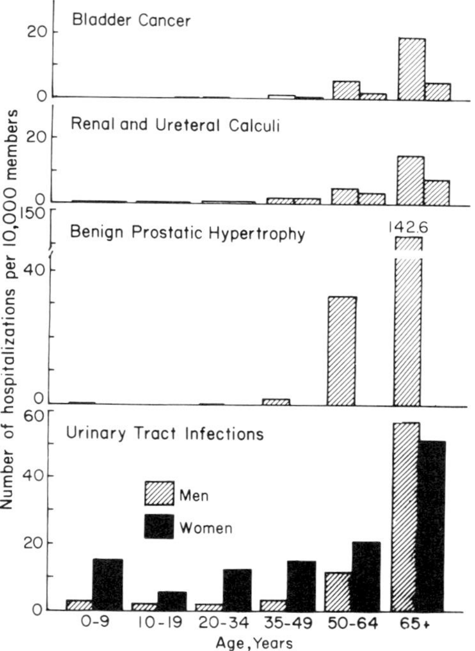

Figure 26-1 Age and sex-specific rates of hospitalization per 10,000 health plan members with four major kidney and urinary tract diseases from 1971 to 1975 (reproduced with permission from Hiatt and Friedman[11]).

Table 26-1
Frequent Etiologies of Urinary Tract Obstruction in the Elderly

Site	Etiology
Intrarenal	Urate nephropathy* Multiple myeloma* Intratubular obstruction* (sulfonamides, methotrexate, furosemide, dextran) Nephrolithiasis* Tumor Blood clot
Renal pelvis	Hydronephrosis* Papillary necrosis* Nephrolithiasis Tumor Blood clot Ureteropelvic stricture (acquired, postinfectious, congenital)
Ureter	Retroperitoneal fibrosis–idiopathic* Secondary (drugs, tumor, metastasis, aortic aneurysm) Retroperitoneal hemorrhage* Retroperitoneal abscess* Ureteral stricture* (infection, tuberculosis, congenital, posttrauma, postradiation Ureteral tumor Nephrolithiasis Tuberculosis
Bladder and posterior urethra	Benign prostatic hypertrophy* Prostatic carcinoma* Bladder carcinoma* Neurogenic bladder* (diabetes, neurologic disorders, narcotics, anticholinergics, antihistamines) Inflammatory disease of prostate* Infectious prostatitis* Blood clot Diverticulum Sarcoma Posterior or median bar of the prostate Contraction of the bladder neck
Urethra	Strictures* (acquired, postinfectious, traumatic) Phimosis* Posterior or anterior valves Meatal stenosis Carcinoma of penis Carcinoma of urethra Paraurethral abscess

*Causes most common to the elderly.

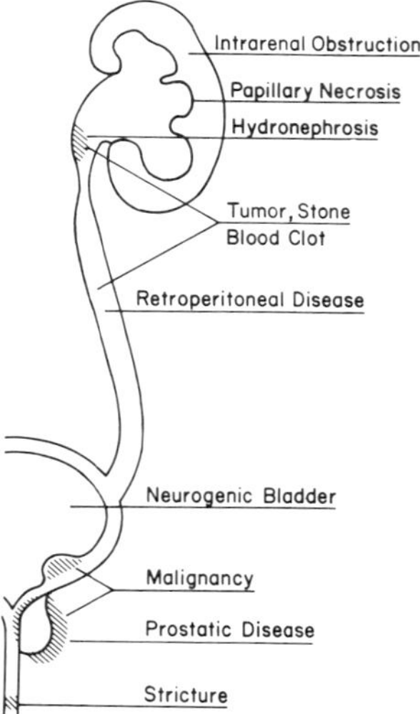

Figure 26-2 Common causes of obstruction in the elderly.

Neurogenic bladder disturbances can occur because of diseases such as diabetes[12] or may be the result of untoward drug effects from the use of anticholinergics, antihistamines, tranquilizers, or α-adrenergics. Ureteral and/or urethral compression (extrinsic or intrinsic) comprise another category of obstructive uropathy. Numerous etiologies exist in this category but those most common in the elderly include pelvic malignancies, prostatic enlargement from carcinoma or benign prostatic hypertrophy, nephrolithiasis, retroperitoneal disease, or development of a stricture within the urethra.

EFFECTS OF OBSTRUCTION ON RENAL FUNCTION

The kidney is inevitably destroyed when complete obstruction of its collecting system has existed for any period of time which generally exceeds 6 to 8 weeks. Less severe obstruction, so-called partial obstruction, will impair a number of renal functions in a predictable fashion. Dependent upon the extent, duration, and level of obstruction, restoration of normal drainage may allow a return toward base- line values for any of these several renal functions that are variably impaired by obstruction.

Renal Damage

Both tubular and glomerular function are lost as the result of obstruction. An impaired ability to concentrate the urine is a characteristic feature of obstructive uropathy occurring in the setting of acute or chronic, unilateral or bilateral, or complete or partial obstruction.[12–16] This contributes to the polyuria and nocturia observed in obstructive uropathy which on occasion presents as a syndrome characterized by passage of large quantities of dilute urine and a resistance to administered vasopressin.[17,18] This phenomenon appears to be directly related to the obstruction since it has been observed in the involved kidney alone in the instance of unilateral obstruction[12] and has disappeared with correction of the obstructing lesion.[19] An additional tubular function lost shortly after the onset of obstruction is the capacity to excrete acid effectively. The ability to attain a minimum urinary pH (< 5.3) is limited and in most instances would suggest the presence of a distal renal tubular acidosis[12,13,15] though in the presence of a postobstructive diuresis proximal bicarbonate wasting has been observed.[19] Subsequent to or at the time of development of tubular dysfunction, reductions occur in both the glomerula filtration rate (GFR) and renal blood flow (RBF).[12,13,20,21] Progressive renal failure will then occur but only if bilateral obstruction exists. Recovery of renal function is fairly complete if obstruction is relieved shortly after its onset; however, if obstruction is prolonged, *irreversible* tubulo-interstitial changes will occur. These are characterized by tubular dilatation, atrophy, and by interstitial fibrosis with a predominent mononuclear cell infiltration.[22]

Postobstructive Diuresis

It has been observed that a period of negative sodium balance follows the release of a lower urinary tract obstruction, this period lasting from hours to days. This has been termed "postobstructive" diuresis, and in reality has come to signify several different functional states. It may describe the transient increase in the flow of dilute urine that occurs shortly after the relief of obstruction, or it may define the occasional excretion of large quantities of sodium that had been retained during the obstructive period or that were administered intravenously (IV) as replacement fluid. Finally, it may be used to designate a state where *inappropriately* large salt and water losses occur.[23]

In most patients following the relief of obstruction the naturiesis is both mild and physiologic reflecting excretion of quantities of salt and water accumulated during the period of obstruction. Persky et al[24] studied six patients following relief of an episode of urinary retention and observed that supplemental fluids or electrolyte solutions were not required in any instance. Similar results were obtained by Eiseman et al[25]; they noted a persistent diuresis (urine volume > water intake by 8 L/d) in only one of 24 patients with correction of urinary retention. Muldowney et al[26] have also demonstrated that an increase in total body exchangeable sodium occurs in association with long-standing obstruction and that not until the exchangeable pool of sodium has returned to normal would urinary sodium excretion match its intake.

There are a very limited number of cases reported in which fluid losses proved inappropriate and volume depletion resulted if there was not full replacement of urinary losses.[25-28] In all instances the obstruction was bilateral and caused by the prostate obstructing the bladder outlet. The pathogenesis of this disorder is not well understood. It had been thought that damage to the tubules caused by obstruction led to the defect in sodium reabsorption. However, postobstructive diuresis has not been observed to occur following relief of *unilateral* obstruction.[13,20,29] Gillenwater et al[13] have observed that following the release of unilateral obstruction, that the fractional excretion of sodium from the previously obstructed kidney was greater than that of the normal kidney. Despite this, a diuresis was absent since the lowered GFR in that kidney and the resultant decrease in filtered sodium more than compensated for any alteration in the fractional excretion rate of sodium.[13] Although the GFR is equally reduced at the time of release of complete bilateral obstruction, a diuresis can occur because there exists a more significant defect in the tubular reabsorption of sodium. Such a diuresis may reflect the effects of accumulated quantities of urea or other natriuretic factors.[27,30] Rarely, the diuresis lasts from weeks to months, far exceeding the time required for elimination of any retained substances.[25,31] In these patients, it is posible that the magnitude of tubular damage exceeds by a considerable degree that having occurred to the GFR; once relief of obstruction has occurred the improved GFR would only act to amplify the now prominent tubular defect.

Information pertaining to the duration and extent of obstruction is frequently lacking in the clinical situation. As such, at least in man, little information is available that might shed light on any of the mechanisms involved in the renal functional changes. Therefore, experimental efforts have been directed toward the use of laboratory animals to better delineate the pathophysiologic events surrounding obstruction.

Renal Function During Unilateral Obstruction

Hydrostatic pressure changes occurring within individual nephrons and the renal pelvis are critical in determining the effects of obstruction on the GFR, RBF, and tubular function. Whether the unilateral obstruction is *acute* or *chronic* will then ultimately determine the extent of alterations in these same renal functional parameters.

When urine flow is impeded, there occurs

an immediate increase in hydrostatic pressure. The subsequent intrapelvic pressure rise is transmitted retrograde with a resultant rise in proximal tubular pressure. Proximal tubular pressure rises until GFR ceases; termed the stop-flow pressure, this proximal tubule pressure is then equal to the difference between glomerular capillary hydraulic pressure and arterial oncotic pressure ($P_{GC} - \pi_A$) and is reached more rapidly if the animal is undergoing active diuresis.[32,33] As the proximal tubular pressure increases it has been demonstrated that a reduction in single nephron GFR occurs within 20 minutes.[34,35] This is due in part to the increase in proximal tubular pressure and secondarily to alterations in the surface area or permeability of the glomerulus.[35] An additional consequence of the rise in proximal tubular pressure is an increased permeability of the tubule wall to small molecular weight substances such as mannitol or sucrose.[36]

Another change seen to occur early after unilateral or bilateral obstruction is that of an increase in RBF.[37,38] The increased RBF does not occur if the renal vessels have been previously dilated as occurs with a prior mannitol diuresis[39] or if intense vasoconstriction exists prior to the obstruction as might result from operative trauma.[40] This vasodilation is transient and generally gives way to vasoconstriction with a decrease in RBF to 50% of control values by 24 hours.[38,41] The mechanism of this initial increase in RBF is not solely explained on a myogenic basis,[42] or by a decrease in local angiotensin concentrations since renal vein renin levels increase shortly after obstruction.[36,40] A more likely explanation for the early rise in RBF is that it is mediated by an increase in local concentrations of vasodilating prostaglandins since it can be attenuated if not abolished by prior treatment with prostaglandin synthetase inhibitors.[43–45] Further evidence supporting prostaglandins as mediators of the increase in blood flow is available from the work of Nishikawa et al[6] and Needleman et al.[47] These investigators have shown that basal production of PGE_2 and of PGI_2 in the isolated perfused rabbit kidney is increased and that there exists increased responsivity of vasodilatory prostaglandins to stimulatory agents such as bradykinin or angiotensin II.[46,47]

As a result of the decrease in GFR and urine flow rate in some cases of partial ureteral obstruction, the absorption of sodium and chloride becomes more complete. Under these circumstances the final urine sodium concentration can be reduced.[34,38] In this way obstructive uropathy on occasion may present a picture mimicking that of prerenal azotemia.

Experimental studies have helped elucidate the effects of prolonged unilateral obstruction. Within about 24 hours the initially elevated intrapelvic pressure has begun to decline, and with an increasing duration of obstruction intrapelvic pressures enter the normal range (Figure 26-3).[49] If complete obstruction is continued, proximal tubular pressure will drop to normal or below the normal range and the kidney surface, if examined, would reveal numerous collapsed tubules.[29,50] Both of these changes suggest that afferent arteriolar vasoconstriction has occurred. This suggestion, that afferent arteriolar resistance has increased, is supported by the observation that RBF drops once ureteral obstruction has been maintained for more than several hours.[51,52]

Several mediators for this vasoconstriction have been proposed. Angiotensin has been suggested as a candidate, but evidence gathered to date has suggested otherwise. Depletion of renin in the kidney[40,53] or the intrarenal arterial administration of saralasin[54] have not prevented the observed decrease in blood flow. Also, renal denervation and adrenergic blockade (α and β) have little effect on the decrement in blood flow.[40] An additional mediator recently proposed for this vasoconstriction is thromboxane A_2. This potent vasoconstrictor is produced in increased quantities by the severely

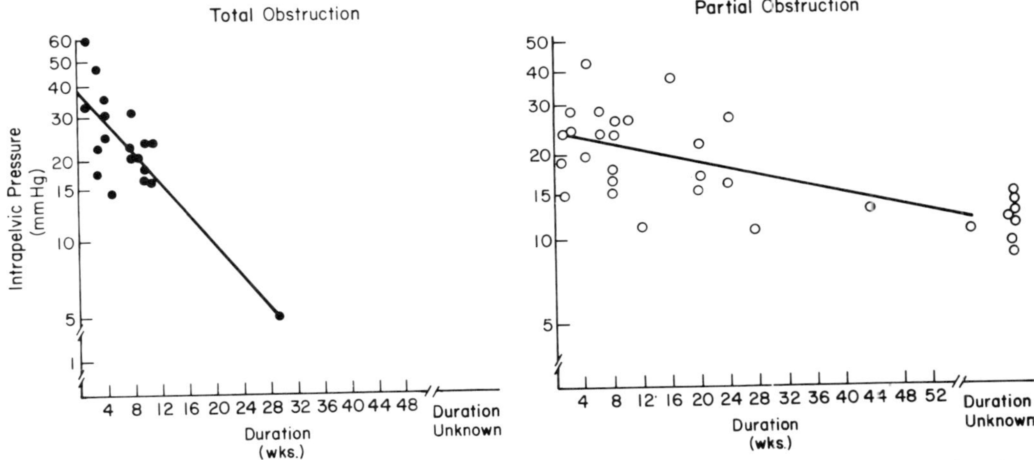

Figure 26-3 Relationship of intrapelvic pressure to the duration of ureteral obstruction in patients with complete (left) and partial (right) obstruction: "Duration Unknown" refers to obstruction present for at least 1 year. (Reproduced with permission from Michaelson [49])

obstructed isolated perfused rabbit kidney.[55] In addition, administration of a selective thromboxane synthetase inhibitor, imidazole, to rats obstructed for 24 hours helped restore GFR and RBF toward preobstruction levels.[56] It must be stated, though, that the activation of thromboxane production requires severe degrees of obstruction (>18 hours in the isolated perfused hydronephrotic rabbit kidney).[57] Also, Ichikawa and Brenner showed that indomethacin (a nonselective prostaglandin synthetase inhibitor and therefore a nonspecific thromboxane synthesis inhibitor) administration to rats with partial ureteral obstruction for 4 weeks was still accompanied by decreased renal blood flow.[58] This observation would then suggest that the identity of the vasoconstrictor substance is still not firmly established and that there may exist a fine balance among the various prostaglandin species in the ultimate maintenance of renal blood flow.[59]

Renal Function During Bilateral Obstruction

The hemodynamic and tubular changes that accompany bilateral obstruction are somewhat different than those observed with unilateral obstruction. Notably, the bilaterally obstructed kidneys do not appear as greatly damaged as kidneys with unilateral obstruction. Unlike unilateral obstruction where with prolongation of the obstruction there is observed a normalization of proximal tubular pressure, with bilateral obstruction proximal tubular pressure remains elevated for a greater period of time and its decline is seldom to levels below normal.[29,60] This alteration in the proximal tubular pressure profile most likely reflects a lesser degree of afferent arteriolar constriction. This postulate is borne out by less significant alterations in both total RBF[45] and in single nephron glomerular blood flow[52] than are observed following unilateral ureteral obstruction.

It is not readily apparent why these models have dissimilar proximal tubular pressure measurements and vascular resistances. Again, it may reflect differences in functional alterations in the prostaglandin cascade,[45] but there do exist more basic differences between unilateral and bilateral obstruction. Whereas, with unilateral obstruction there is at most a 50% reduction in renal function (doubling of serum creatinine), with bilateral obstruction renal function is variably reduced with clearly discernible compositional changes of circulating blood only if the obstruction is fairly complete. In unilateral obstruction greater than bilateral obstruction, potassium, phosphate, and urea values have been noted more commonly to increase,[60-62] and, in addition, substances which are yet to be biochemically defined, but which are known to possess potential vasodilatory properties, may accumulate to a greater degree in unilateral obstruction.

In addition to lowering the GFR, the alteration in proximal tubular pressure may affect tubular function. Acutely, the lowered GFR and tubular fluid flow rate may result in increased sodium and water reabsorption.[34] However, in time the increased tubular pressure impairs tubular function. This results in normal or increased urine output when the urinary tract obstruction is chronic despite the GFR having been reduced.[13,15,34]

Renal Function After Relief of Obstruction

It is commonly thought that once there has been relief of an obstruction that no further functional deterioration will occur and in fact that there will be some return of that function previously lost. This is particularly germane to the elderly since silent prostatism may progress to the point where its presenting symptoms are those of uremia.[63] Regardless of the age group under scrutiny, it is important to know the extent to which tubular and glomerular abnormalities will return towards base-line values following the relief of obstruction. The degree to which the functional integrity of the tubule can be re-established is dependent upon the duration, location (unilateral or bilateral), and completeness of the obstruction. In many instances, relief of bilateral obstruction (most commonly secondary to prostatism) results in improvement in GFR, RBF, maximal reabsorption of Diodrast (Tm_D),[21] acidification ability,[15,18] and concentrating ability.[15,18] In addition, following relief of obstruction there is a time interval during which there exists a poor homeostatic response when limits are placed on the quantity of sodium and water ingested. This may relate to several variables, the most prominent of which being a decreased reabsorptive capacity for sodium in both the proximal and distal tubules.[29,64] There exist a large number of studies that have examined sodium transport in the postobstructive period;[23] the consensus suggests that two factors in combination substantially contribute to the natriuresis: (1) alterations in collecting duct permeability, the result of prior increased intraluminal pressure, may limit sodium reabsorption (2) as of yet unidentified substances that accumulate during obstruction may be capable of inhibiting proximal tubular sodium reabsorption.

A more important question than that of regaining tubular function is that of how long a kidney can be obstructed and still regain glomerular function? There exist published reports describing return of renal function after years of obstruction but most of these are anecdotal. There are, however, four well-described cases documenting return of renal function after periods of complete obstruction lasting 35, 56, 69, and 98 days.[65-68] These cases probably represent the upper limits to be expected for functional recovery. Such recovery is possibly modified by a number of factors, the most important of which is the coexistence of infection. The extent of recovery has been examined experimentally in dogs following release of complete unilateral obstruction after varying intervals of obstruction. After 1 to 2 weeks of complete obstruction GFR was capable of returning to 70% to 100% of base-line values. Further prolongation of the obstruction to 4 weeks resulted in only 20% to 30% return of normal function, and when obstruction exceeded 6 to 8 weeks little functional recovery was seen following relief of the obstruction.[69,70]

An important consideration in the elderly is whether the aged kidney is capable of undergoing compensatory hypertrophy once there has been significant damage to or removal of the contralateral kidney. Valid studies that address this issue in the elderly (>60 years of age) are lacking. Despite this, there is indirect evidence suggesting that age does not limit the ability of the remaining kidney to restore renal function toward prenephrectomy levels. Ekelund and Gothlin[71] measured renal size (product of length and width) at the time of urography pre- and postnephrectomy for tumor. Of the 33 patients studied, 15 were over age 60 and nine over age 70 years, with the mean time interval after nephrectomy being 25 months (3 to 108 months). In their elderly patients postoperative renal enlargement occurred to an extent similar to that in the younger study subjects. A negative correlation between the degree of hypertrophy and age was not observed. Boner et al, in a study of renal size in 22 kidney donors (age range 22 to 63 years), also noted that the magnitude of renal hypertrophy following contralateral nephrectomy was not dependent on age (>40 years in this instance).[72] Dossetor also observed that compensatory renal hypertrophy occurred in ten of the fifteen patients he studied who were over 40 years old.[73] It is clear from these studies that the elderly individual, in general, is capable of increasing renal size following contralateral nephrectomy. However, more critical than the ability of the remaining kidney to undergo hypertrophy, is whether it retains the ability to increase GFR to an extent similar to that seen in young individuals. Unfortunately, detailed long- term prospective studies examining such a question do not exist. Those studies most applicable relate to the compensatory hypertrophy following donor nephrectomy, and in this instance most individuals described to date are younger than age 50 at the time of organ donation. Available studies would suggest that similar degrees of hyperfiltration could be expected between the ages of 30 and 60 years, regardless of the age at which nephrectomy had occurred.[74-77] In addition, if adjustments are made to the expected GFR increment relative to the expected age-related decline in renal function,[78] the degree of hyperfiltration achieved by older individuals after unilateral nephrectomy compares favorable with the increased filtration observed in younger subjects. Finally, of particular concern is whether any hyperfiltration achieved can be maintained for protracted time intervals without eventual deterioration in function and the development of proteinuria, hypertension, and renal insufficiency. Such a possibility has been elegantly detailed in the work of Brenner et al.[79] In one of the longest prospective evaluations available, Vincenti et al[80] addressed this issue. Twenty patients, who underwent donor nephrectomy between 1964 and 1968, and who had a mean follow-up interval of 15.8 ± 3 years (range 14.5 to 18.5 years) were evaluated long-term for the development of hypertension, proteinuria, or a decline in creatinine clearance compared to clearance values obtained 1 week postnephrectomy. These three clinical markers utilized as measures of renal injury, did not deteriorate. The creatinine clearance stayed constant, and though protein excretion was greater than that found in healthy controls the protein being excreted in excess was not albumin and therefore the significance of this observation was uncertain.[80]

CLINICAL MANIFESTATIONS AND EVALUATION

Symptoms

The symptoms that occur with obstruction are dependent upon the site, cause, and the rapidity with which obstruction develops. Pain is often the initial symptom motivating the patient to seek medical attention. Its absence, however, need not eliminate from consideration the possibility of obstruction. Pain usually follows an acute episode of obstruction and results from stretching of the collecting system, the renal capsule and/or renal pelvis, and correlates with the rate of distension rather than the degree of dilation. If the obstruction is more insidious and the rate of distension sufficiently slowed, there may be no pain at all. In certain instances, particularly in the elderly, the absence of bladder sensation may prove to be a problem of sufficient magnitude that progressive renal insufficiency proves to be the initial sign of obstruction.[63,81]

The location of the pain frequently suggests the site of obstruction in the urinary tract. Costovertebral angle pain may be indicative of ureteropelvic junction obstruction whereas ureteral obstruction may cause flank pain with lower quadrant radiation either to the labia or testes. Suprapubic pain generally indicates bladder distention as may be seen with bladder neck obstruction (prostate disease) or stricture disease. It is important to realize that there are certain situations where urine output is inordinately increased, such as with glycosuria and diuretic use, and in such instances pain may be precipitated by the rapid distention of the urinary tract proximal to the site of obstruction. Also, gastrointestinal (GI) symptoms such as nausea, vomiting or paralytic ileus may accompany an episode of obstruction.

Gross or microscopic hematuria occurs with many of the causes of obstruction but seldom affords any diagnostic insight. A number of "urinary" symptoms exist with the causes of obstructive uropathy. If the obstruction has been sufficiently prolonged then impairment in urinary concentrating ability occurs leading to nocturia and/or daytime oliguria/polyuria. A more common grouping of "urinary" symptoms relate to benign prostatic hypertrophy and include frequency, hesitancy, postvoid dribbling, and a decreased caliber of the urinary stream. Sudden interruption of the urinary stream when it occurs may suggest a bladder stone that has occluded the urethral orifice.

In addition to any findings directly referable to obstruction, it is important to search for any underlying disease that may be potentially responsible. Thus, the clinician should question about a history of malignancy; prior abdominal, genitourinary (GU) or pelvic surgery; prior pelvic irradiation or symptoms suggestive of an occult malignancy (weight loss, fatigue, loss of appetite); or any of the disorders associated with papillary necrosis such as diabetes mellitus or urinary tract infection. Drug-related etiologies of obstruction should also be addressed. In the elderly, the agents most commonly implicated in this respect include antihistamines, anticholinergics, or narcotic analgesics.

Laboratory Evaluation

Routine laboratory evaluation is generally nonspecific. The urinalysis may reveal hematuria, pyuria, or bacteriuria. Occasionally the urine may be entirely normal, if complete unilateral obstruction exists, since abnormal urine may then not reach the bladder. If obstruction is prolonged, urine osmolality tends to be isoosmotic and urinary sodium excretion generally exceeds 20 mEq/L.[15,34] A diagnostic clue can sometimes be obtained by an evaluation of the BUN/serum creatinine ratio. Ordinarily 10/1, it may be higher than this with obstruction as the result of increased passive back-diffusion of urea in a low urine flow rate state.[82] Another clue to the presence of obstruction may be the presence of a hyperkalemic metabolic acidosis of uncertain origin. Batlle et al[83] have documented the presence of either a hyperkalemic distal renal tubular acidosis or a state of aldosterone deficiency (type 4 RTA) in patients with moderate renal insufficiency and obstructive uropathy. They state that on occasion the search for obstruction was undertaken purely based on the presence of an undefined hyperkalemic metabolic acidosis.[83]

Etiology

Numerous etiologies exist for obstructive uropathy. It is beyond the scope of this chapter to cover all of these; therefore, emphasis will be placed on those disorders most common to the elderly (Figure 26-2).

Diffuse *intratubular* obstruction can present as an insidious cause of obstructive uropathy in that standard diagnostic tests will seldom reveal hydronephrosis. This entity may occur as the result of intrarenal precipitation of a number of substances including oxalate, uric acid, calcium, or in certain instances drugs and/or their metabolites. Intratubular calcium oxalate deposition may occur after the administration of the anesthetic methoxyflurane[84] and more rarely enflurane.[85] Rarely, intravenous (IV) glycerol, as may be employed in states of high intracerebral pressure, results in renal oxalosis[86] similar to that observed following ingestion of excessive quantities of ethylene glycol.

Deposition of uric acid within the renal collecting system and/or pelvis has been termed *uric acid nephropathy.* Excessive uric acid excretion may result from the initiation of chemotherapy in the case of active tumors such as leukemia, lymphoma, or large solid tumors.[87] The ensuing destruction of large numbers of tumor cells releases large quantities of nucleic acid which are subsequently converted to uric acid and then excreted in the urine. This uric acid can then precipitate in the collecting system, a site where the most marked reduction in its solubility occurs since the urine is most concentrated and acidified in this portion of the kidney.[88] An excess of uric acid excretion may also result from a decrease in its renal reabsorption as follows from the ingestion of high doses of salicylates[89] or the administration of a number of common radiocontrast agents.[90] In fact, this uricosuric property of radiocontrast agents has been suggested to be one of the factors which might lead to contrast-induced acute renal failure.[91]

The diffuse deposition of calcium within renal parenchymal structures, termed *nephrocalcinosis,* commonly results from states with an increased filtered load of calcium such as hypervitaminosis D[92] or milk-alkali syndrome.[93] On occasion, it may also be the result of the hypercalciuria which attends the administration of furosemide.[94] A number of drugs and/or their metabolites are known to cause intratubular obstruction. Methotrexate[95] is one agent capable of this. Other agents used in the elderly that may cause obstruction in a similar manner include dextran,[96] nitrofurantoin,[97] and sulfonamides.[98] Most sulfonamides currently marketed are very soluble and this has diminished what had been a considerable prior incidence of sulfonamide crystalluria.

One of the most common malignancies of the elderly, multiple myeloma, frequently causes a terminal illness whose course may be accelerated as the result of uremia. In 869 cases of multiple myeloma reported by Kyle, only 2% of patients were less than age 40 with the greatest incidence of the disease being in the seventh decade.[99] The renal failure occurring with multiple myeloma has diverse etiologies including cast-deposition of Bence Jones proteins,[100] hypercalcemia, hyperuricosuria, or as the result of diagnostic studies utilizing contrast agents.[101] This disease can be quite insidious with its initial presentation being that of renal failure and the diagnosis obtained only at the time of renal biopsy.[102] Though renal failure with myeloma is frequently secondary to intratubular obstruction, it should be remembered that since it is a disease of the elderly, that other diseases such as prostatism should be considered in the initial differential diagnosis of unexplained renal failure in myeloma.[103]

Renal papillary necrosis results from ischemic necrosis of various segments of the renal medulla. Rather than representing a distinct clinicopathologic syndrome, it represents the confluence of a number of diseases which affect the kidney. In a recent review of the experience at Ben Taub General Hospital, Houston, Texas, 13 of 27 patients with papillary necrosis were over age 60[104] with a mean age for the entire series of 58 years. Though papillary necrosis is frequently bilateral[104–106] and capable of causing an episode of obstructive uropathy, it is seen more commonly as the *result* of an obstructive event further downstream in the urinary tract. Major series in the literature have reported an incidence of from 26% to 39% for obstructive uropathy in the setting of papillary necrosis[106,107] with one series actually having an 85% incidence of obstructive uropathy.[108] Obstruction may in and of itself not be sufficient cause for many of the episodes of papillary necrosis; it may be that the tendency to develop and to have perpetuated urinary tract infection once obstructed may act as a synergistic factor in the subsequent development of papillary necrosis.[109] The finding of papillary necrosis so commonly in the aged may reflect an underlying predilection for vascular insufficiency to the papilla thereby resulting in ischemic necrosis. Such vascular insufficiency would occur with the changes of arteriosclerosis and would not be unexpected in an aged population.[110]

Urinary tract stone formation is a problem principally limited to patients during their middle decades of life.[111] Despite this, hospital admissions for stone disease do not decline until beyond the age of 70 years and when recurrence of stones is considered some reports demonstrate a prevalence rate that is still rising in patients at age 60.[112] The most common stone type in the elderly is a calcium-containing stone[113] which is usually found in the upper urinary tract. Idiopathic hypercalciuria is the most common metabolic disorder in individuals under the age of 60[114] with virtually no data available on its occurrence in the elderly. A common disturbance, particularly in elderly females, leading to the formation of calcium-containing stones, is primary hyperparathyroidism with a reported incidence of stones of 16%.[115] Infection stones (struvite) form in the renal pelvis, calyces, or bladder particularly when the urine is infected with a urea-splitting bacterium, such as a *Proteus* species.[116] These stones are primarily found in women but may be found in any elderly patient who frequently develops urinary tract infection secondary to an indwelling urinary catheter. These stones may form with few, if any symptoms. These stones when present, can prove to be quite refractory to therapy and may consign the patient to an existence marked by difficult-to-eradicate urinary tract infections and a gradual decline in renal function resulting from intrapelvic obstruction due to struvite stone formation and growth.

A number of diseases are capable of leading to ureteral obstruction. Included in this category are disease processes such as tumors, blood clots, and a number of entities which elicit a fibrotic response in the retroperitoneum. In a series of 50 patients with acute renal failure from bilateral ureteral obstruction compiled by Norman et al[117] the mean age of the patients was 60 (range 24 to 86 years). Prostatic and cervical carcinoma were the dominant forms of pelvic malignancy in this series (Table 26-2). Ureteral obstruction can also occur as the result of the treatment employed in the management of malignancies. Gynecologic surgery for malignancy is by far the most common operative situation wherein there exists the possibility of traumatizing the ureters, with a reported incidence ranging from 1.5% to 9.7% depending on the surgical technic employed.[118] Similarly, but less frequently, ureteral obstruction may follow urologic surgery or extensive surgery of the rectosigmoid region. An additional treatment modality capable of causing obstruction is pelvic irradiation. In general, the reported incidence of obstruction after radiotherapy is low (<3%) and posttherapy recurrence of obstruction is most commonly ascribed to recurrence of the original tumor,[119] though some series have reported an incidence of up to 35% for postradiation periureteral fibrosis.[120] The time of onset of urologic problems after irradiation is somewhat variable but if they are to occur they usually do so within 30 months of the completion of radiation therapy.[121] A final consideration in respect to malignant involvement of the ureter is that relating to metastatic spread from a more distant primary tumor. A number of tumors are capable of this by contiguous spread including lung, stomach, prostate, and ovary,[122] while in the case of other tumors, particularly breast cancer, isolated metastases to the ureter may occur.[123]

Retroperitoneal fibrosis can result in obstructive uropathy when the fibrotic process is sufficiently advanced such that involvement of the ureter has transpired. Retroperitoneal fibrosis may occur either as a primary idiopathic disease or as a secondary process resulting from some stimulus that initiates fibrosis in the retroperitoneum. In an extensive retrospective analysis of 430 cases of retroperitoneal fibrosis, 185 (43%) were classified as idiopathic and 245 cases (57%) were due to a secondary disorder.[124] There are several of the secondary etiologies whose occurrence relates to the elderly. These include malignancy,[125] perianeurysmal fibrosis surrounding abdominal aortic aneurysms,[126] aortic bypass surgery,[127] and the ingestion of certain medications such as methysergide,[128] analgesics,[129] or β-blockers such as atenolol[130] or metoprolol.[131]

Table 26-2
Causes of Bilateral Ureteral Obstruction

Disease or Disorder	No. of Patients
Malignant Carcinoma	38
Cervical	11
Prostatic	8
Bladder	5
Colonic	5
Ovarian	5
Undifferentiated	2
Lymphoma	1
Melanoma	1
Benign	12
Retroperitoneal fibrosis	8
Calculi	2
Ligated ureters	2

Adapted from Norman et al.[117]

The bladder may also serve as a focus for obstruction within the urinary tract. This may result from either outlet obstruction as occurs with bladder stones or carcinoma, or from bulky tumor disease capable of internal obstruction at both ureteral orifices. Of additional importance is the fact that the bladder is not a simple conduit but rather is a viscus which empties under a complex coordination of muscular and neurologic events. With failure of the integrated mechanisms operating to allow effective voiding a *neurogenic bladder* results with clinical manifestations of either urinary incontinence or urinary retention. In the elderly, a number of processes are capable of disturbing the normal reciprocal relationship that exists between bladder and sphincter mechanisms.[132] Cerebrovascular diseases[133] or senile dementia may interrupt the coordination of bladder contraction-relaxation resulting in urinary incontinence. The level of neurologic interruption to the bladder can have a predictable effect on lower tract function. Flaccid bladders with a large volume of residual urine may result from lower motor neuron lesions that may ensue from the peripheral neuropathy of tabes dorsalis, alcoholism, or diabetes mellitus. Noteworthy to the elderly is the vesical dysfunction characteristic of diabetes mellitus. It can be insidious in both its onset and progression and may exist in up to 80% of diabetics manifesting peripheral neuropathy.[134] The importance of its discovery is clear since if it remains untreated it may contribute to progressive renal failure.[135,136] Finally, the elderly are often unwitting victims of a polypharmacy management approach. They are potentially exposed to a number of agents such as antihistamines, anticholinergics, and narcotic analgesics, including meperidine or morphine, which are capable of precipitating acute urinary retention.

Diseases of the prostate possess the capacity to cause renal failure in elderly males either by causing chronic partial urethral obstruction or by totally obstructing the flow of urine. The incidence of benign prostatic hypertrophy (BPH), estimated to be present histologically in 50% of males over age 60, has been stated to account for 10% of all cases of renal failure.[137–140] It is not at all uncommon for the elderly male to present with significant renal impairment as his first clinical evidence of prostatism.[141] Once recognized and treated by temporary drainage, 80% of these patients can be expected to regain some measure of renal function.[142] The problem with the determination of the extent and/or progression of the anatomical bladder neck obstruction caused by BPH is difficult. Despite subjective, objective, and urodynamic assessments of BPH, it remains impossible to actually predict those who will progress to urinary retention or obstructive uropathy.[143,144] If anything limits the patient's appraisal of symptoms, such as deficient bladder sensation, the renal consequences of prostatism can only become that much more difficult to detect and are even more likely to present as renal insufficiency.[63,81]

During childhood urethral strictures are commonly congenital in origin. During the adult years strictures will occur after either prolonged catheterization, infections, or following prostatic surgery. Catheter-related strictures appear to be related to the size of the catheter and the duration of catheterization. They occur at sites where the urethra is most narrow including the external sphincter, the penoscrotal junction, and just inside the external meatus.[10] The most common infective cause of inflammatory strictures is gonococcal or nongonococcal urethritis.[145] Other infective agents capable of giving rise to urethral strictures include *Schistosoma haematobium, Chlamydia* organisms, and *Mycobacterium tuberculosis.* A final etiology for strictures that is of particular concern to the elderly is their occurrence following virtually any form of prostatic surgery but in particular after transurethral surgery. The precise incidence of symptomatic posttransurethral resection stricture is difficult to determine, but it is felt to be as high as 29% in those patients whose transurethral prostate resection was performed through an uncalibrated penile urethra.[146] There is a wide range reported for stricture incidence following prostatic surgery and a safe conclusion from these reports might be that whatever its exact incidence, it is *not* a rare complication. In general, the stricture if it is to occur can be expected to be found within 6 months of the original surgery.[147]

COMPLICATIONS

In addition to a number of direct effects on the kidney, obstruction may lead to a variety of other complications. Because of the concentrating defect observed in obstructive uropathy patients may present with hypertonic dehydration and hypernatremia. Landsberg has reported two patients presenting with altered mental status, serum sodium values of 163 and 183 mEq/L, and partial obstruction who both had significant enough thirst defects to be unable to prevent the development of hypernatremia.[148] The majority of renal stones that develop will ordinarily do so in the setting of a normal urinary tract. Alternatively, triple-phosphate (struvite)[149] and bladder stones[150] are commonly associated with varying degrees of antecedent obstruction. The problem of struvite stones in the elderly is of particular note since once the triad of obstruction, infection, and stones has been established, it is difficult to eliminate any individual component unless the entire complex can be eradicated.

Polycythemia is an uncommon complication of hydronephrosis. In a comprehensive review of the literature by Jaworski and Wolan, nine patients were described.[151] In most instances erythropoietin levels had not been obtained, and in the two cases in which erythropoietin was measured none was detectable. The etiology of the increased red cell mass suggested by this series of patients would appear to be indeterminable though in animals in which unilateral hydronephrosis is present elevated plasma levels of erythropoietin can be found to precede the increase in hemoglobin levels.[152]

Once urinary tract infection has been established in an obstructed system it can prove extremely difficult to eradicate. The frequency of urinary tract infection is greater in obstructed individuals as compared to normals. Beeson has stated that the incidence of urinary tract infection is increased 20-fold in obstructed individuals.[153] This appears to be secondary to the bacterial growthfflpromoting effects of urinary stasis as well as to the defects in host defense mechanisms induced by obstruction. For example, obstruction at the level of the urinary bladder interferes with bacterial eradication in several ways: first, an increased residual urine volume increases the number of bacteria remaining within the bladder at the conclusion of voiding; second, bladder wall distention diminishes blood flow to the bladder mucosa and hence delivery of antibacterial mediators and, finally, bladder distention decreases bladder surface area relative to its total volume and may thereby diminish the efficacy of mucosal bactericidal factors.[154] While complete ureteral obstruction markedly increases infection risk it may be less of a problem with partial obstruction. Hasner has demonstrated an infection rate of 8.6% in 221 men without prior instrumentation, who had BPH and a postvoid residual urine exceeding 50 mL.[155] This emphasizes the fact that in the absence of prior instrumentation many patients who are obstructed will remain uninfected. It cannot be overemphasized that the development of urinary tract sepsis in the elderly should precipitate a search for factors which might impair optimal urinary discharge.

Hypertension is occasionally observed following urinary tract obstruction. The mechanism responsible varies, depending both on the type and duration of the obstruction.[156] In dogs, acute unilateral ureteral obstruction results in increased renin release from the ipsilateral kidney and the development of systemic blood pressure elevations.[157] In humans, it has been similarly observed that lateralizing renal vein renin increments occur and that a reduction in blood pressure will follow relief of the acutely developed unilateral obstruction.[156,158,159] Although it has been suggested that renin release is responsible for the hypertension in acute unilateral obstruction, in chronic animal[40] and human studies of a more chronic nature,[156] renin release appears not to be sustained and peripheral renin values are normal. Thus, established hydronephrosis would not appear to be a stimulant for abnormal degrees of renin secretion. Since corrective surgery may normalize the blood pressure, additional abnormalities unrelated to renin may occur with obstruction and account for the hypertension. It has been commonly observed that bilateral hydronephrosis with subsequent sodium retention and volume expansion can result in hypertension with any blood pressure abnormality having developed being readily reversed with relief of the obstruction.[26,156,160] Palmer has demonstrated remission of hypertension with correction of a ureteropelvic junction obstruction in a patient with a solitary kidney. Renal vein renin values were normal, and a 5 kg postoperative diuresis demonstrated the volume-dependent character of the patient's hypertension.[160]

Postobstructive or so-called reflex anuria has been observed following bilateral ureteral catheterization. Though a brief period of anuria may occur secondary to edema at the ureterovesical junction, in certain instances anuria may persist beyond the time of obstruction apparently reflecting unresolved renal vasoconstriction.[161] As previously discussed, progressive renal failure is an inevitable sequel to prolonged bilateral obstruction. The progression of renal failure with bilateral obstruction would appear to be accelerated when urinary tract infection coexists. This is particularly worrisome since eradication of the infection may be limited by an inability of administered antibiotics to reach the site of infection. The combination of obstruction and infection are of major concern to the elderly since limited functional reserve may prevent major degrees of functional recovery once both events have been corrected. A final complication of obstruction, particularly when infection is present, is the development of papillary necrosis, at least in part based on ischemic necrosis resulting from diminished medullary blood flow.[107,108,162] Even the loss of a single papilla in an elderly patient may prove to be sufficient provocation to lead to a change in the level of renal function sufficient to place the renal failure in the symptomatic range.

DIAGNOSIS

The evaluation for obstruction in a patient with renal insufficiency should begin with passage of a bladder catheter. If the obstructing focus is within the urethra or the result of a neurogenic bladder a diuresis should ordinarily be expected. If the bladder is appreciably overdistended it must be carefully decompressed since in cases of rapid decompression bladder hemorrhage or syncope have been described.

If an increased urinary output does not occur after catheterization of the bladder, obstruction, if present, must be at the level of the ureters or above. The plain film of the abdomen is simple to obtain and may suggest obvious causes of obstruction such as ureteral or bladder stones. The remaining diagnostic tests employed in the workup of obstruction rely on the demonstration of hydronephrosis and include excretory urography, ultrasonography, computed tomographic (CT) scanning, radionuclide scanning, or retrograde pyelography.

In most instances of known or suspected obstruction a primary imaging study employed is excretory urography (Figures 26-4 and 26-5). Even in patients whose renal failure is far advanced an infusion IVP with nephrotomography is capable of demonstrating a nephrogram phase and by utilizing delayed films (6 to 24 hours) oftentimes a pyelogram can be observed and the point of obstruction noted.[162,163] In this instance, the nephrogram is due to the presence of contrast material in cortical tubules which then has as a prerequisite some level of glomerular filtration. Since some filtration occurs even in the case of complete obstruction, subsequent water and solute absorption will concentrate the nonreabsorbable contrast material and give rise to a delayed and prolonged nephrogram.[164]

If both kidneys fail to visualize as occurs with severe prolonged obstruction, complete vascular occlusion, or severe intrinsic renal disease, hydronephrosis can still be detected by the use of ultrasound[165,166] or CT scanning.[167] These procedures are performed without contrast material and may be particularly effective *initial* screening measures in patients likely to develop contrast media–induced acute renal failure such as diabetics or those with preexistent renal insufficiency.[168,169] With ultrasound early changes of obstruction will be represented by mild splaying of the usually compact central echo complex and by enlargement of the renal pelvis (Figures 26-6 and 26-7). The enlargement of the renal pelvis presents as a large anechoic central mass compressing renal cortical tissue (Figure 26-8). Computed tomographic scanning can also demonstrate dilated collecting structures (Figure 26-9) and in instances where retroperitoneal masses cause obstruction, this procedure can frequently define both the mass as well as the presence of obstruction.

Retrograde pyelography may be employed in the patient in whom prior studies have proved nondiagnostic or are contraindicated. This study is often diagnostic of

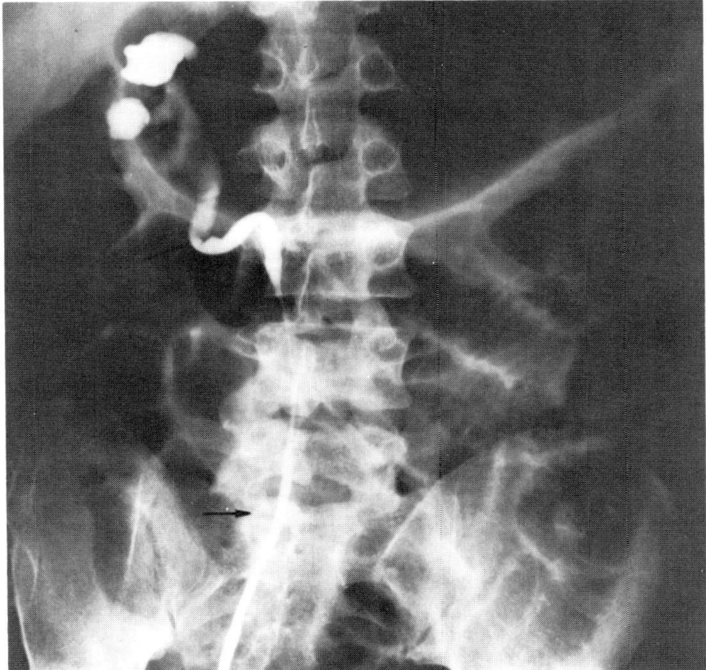

Figure 26-4 Intravenous pyelogram (IVP) of a patient with retroperitoneal fibrosis: Note medial deviation of the ureter (black arrow) as well as dilation of the upper ureter (black arrow) secondary to obstruction by the fibrotic process.

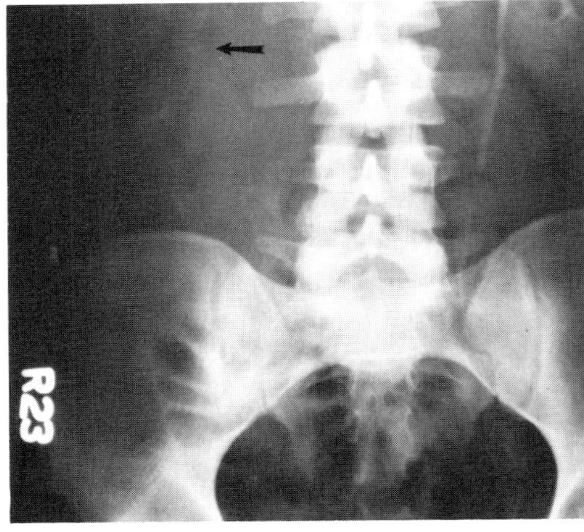

Figure 26-5 IVP of a patient with severe hydronephrosis. The right kidney does not visualize except for a faint opacification around the rim of the kidney (black arrow).

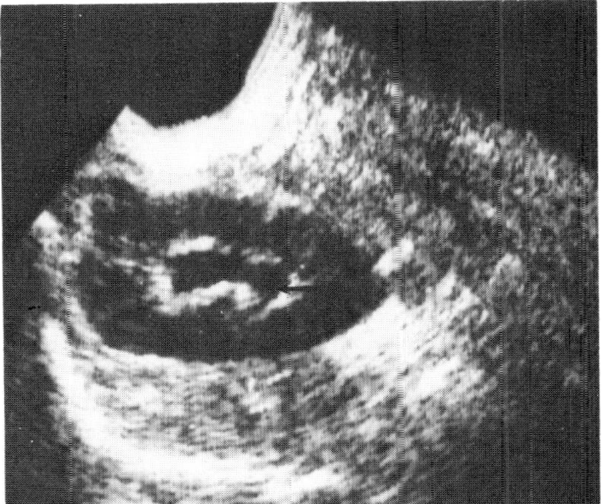

Figure 26-6 Sonographic findings of obstruction as seen in a patient with hydronephrosis in a transplanted kidney. The central echo-free area (black arrow) corresponds to a dilated calyceal system.

the exact site and extent of obstruction and may prove to be therapeutic if the ureteral catheter can be passed beyond the site of obstruction. A final diagnostic test is that of radionuclide imaging (Figure 26-10). It can provide gross anatomical information sufficient to identify the site of obstruction but not the specific cause. Ordinarily the tracer activity can be seen to progress to the site of obstruction while concomitantly demonstrating dilation of the renal pelvis or persistent activity within a ureter.[170]

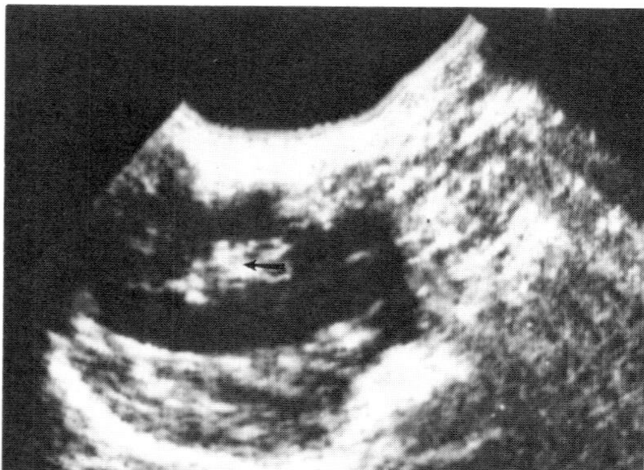

Figure 26-7 Same patient as in Figure 26-6 but following relief of the obstruction. Note the return to a normal central echodense configuration (black arrow).

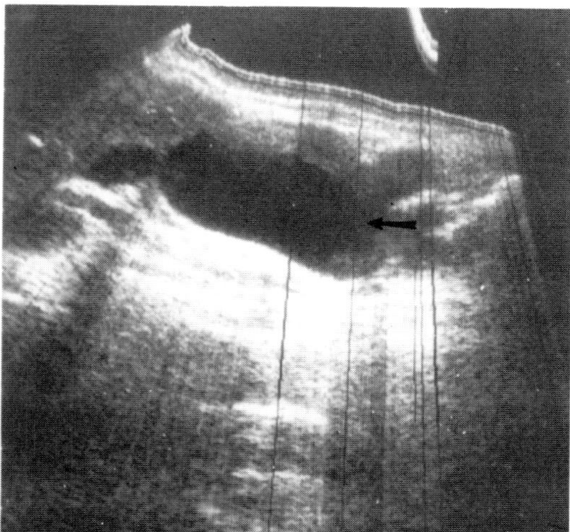

Figure 26-8 Sonogram of the same patient as in Figure 26-5. The large echo-free area (black arrow) represents dilation of the pelvis with destruction of most of the surrounding cortical tissue.

TREATMENT

The obstructed patient whose course is complicated subsequently by infection in the urinary tract has a high mortality rate. Not only is antibiotic coverage necessary but the obstruction should be relieved as promptly as possible. The absence of infection may lessen the urgency of the situation, but nonetheless relief of obstruction should be accomplished quickly in order to minimize the loss of renal function. Other factors exist that may precipitate an aggressive approach to relief of obstruction and include persistent pain, excessive symptoms, recurrent bleeding, or urinary retention.

The remainder of this section is not intended to provide an extensive coverage of what is a burgeoning technical and surgical approach to obstruction. Rather, it will discuss the salient features of both internal and external diversions as well as more permanent forms of urinary diversion onto the skin surface since all of these approaches are ones relevant to an elderly population.

Once the level of obstruction has been determined and a decision has been reached to intervene there are several ways by which it can be accomplished. Whenever possible an *internal* diversion (Figure 26-11) should be attempted to avoid the need for external collection devices. Indwelling ureteral stents have proved quite successful as a long-term means for internal urinary diversion.[171,172] These catheters are made of silicone and therefore can sustain contact with urine for prolonged periods of time without encrustation. Complications, such as infections or extrusions, have not proved to be a detriment to the use of this form of urinary drainage.

External diversion is most readily accomplished by employing some form of tube drainage of the urinary collecting

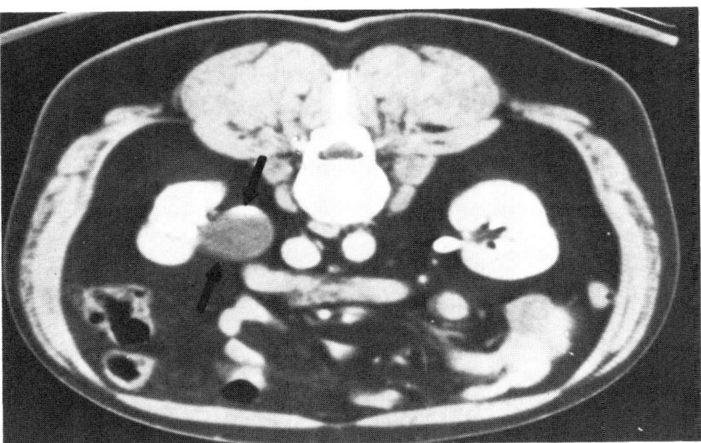

Figure 26-9 CT scan of a patient with a hydronephrotic right kidney secondary to stone disease. Dilation of the calyceal system is demonstrated by the black arrows.

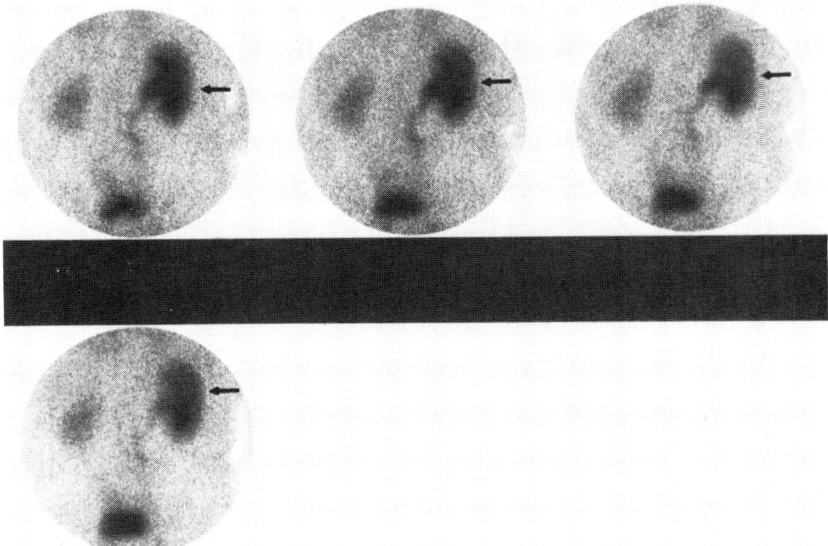

Figure 26-10 Renal scan of a patient with partial obstruction at the area of the right midureter. The administered radionuclide is retained in the enlarged collecting system, renal pelvis, and proximal ureter (black arrows).

system. These so-called nephrostomy procedures have proven quite effective as palliative means of urinary diversion. Nephrostomy placement has previously entailed an open surgical procedure. Now, it is most readily accomplished by a percutaneous procedure (Figure 26-12) under local anesthesia with ultrasonic guidance.[173,174] The complication rate for this procedure is quite acceptable with a low placement failure rate. Complications that may occur include variable incidences of hemorrhage,[175] infection,[176] and dislodgment of the tube.[177]

Prior to use of either of these diversionary modes on a *chronic* basis, strong consideration should be given to two factors particularly as regards their occurrence in the elderly. First, there must be sufficient function in the obstructed kidney to justify a diversionary procedure. This can be determined by careful assessment of the kidney(s) utilizing urography, radionuclide scans, and/or split function testing. Second, if malignancy is the cause of the obstruction any decision to attempt diversion should be tempered by a consideration of the prognosis of individual tumor types and whether or not any future response to tumor therapy can be expected. In this regard the mortality rate in individuals in whom palliative diversions are attempted is high, being 50% and 90% at 3 and 12 months respectively with 64% of survival time being spent in the hospital.[178,179] Patients with prostatic carcinoma or cervical malignancy will fare somewhat better than this and stronger consideration should be

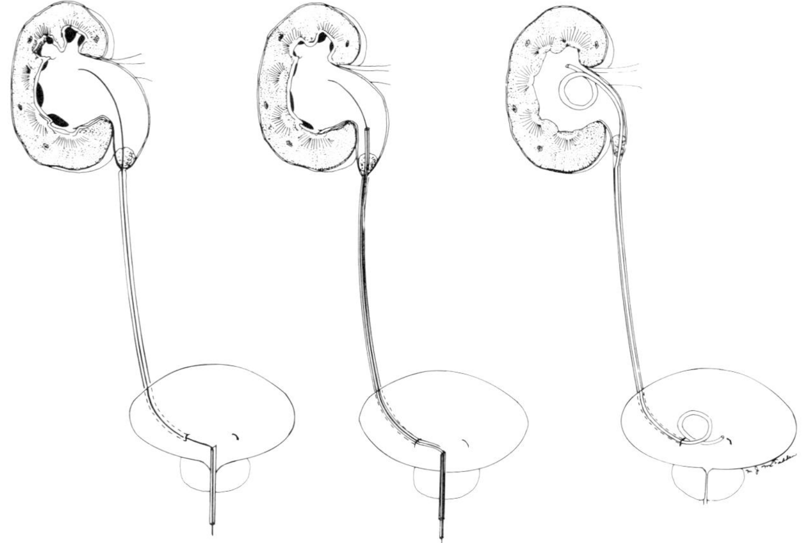

Figure 26-11 Indwelling ureteral stent for long-term internal urinary diversion.

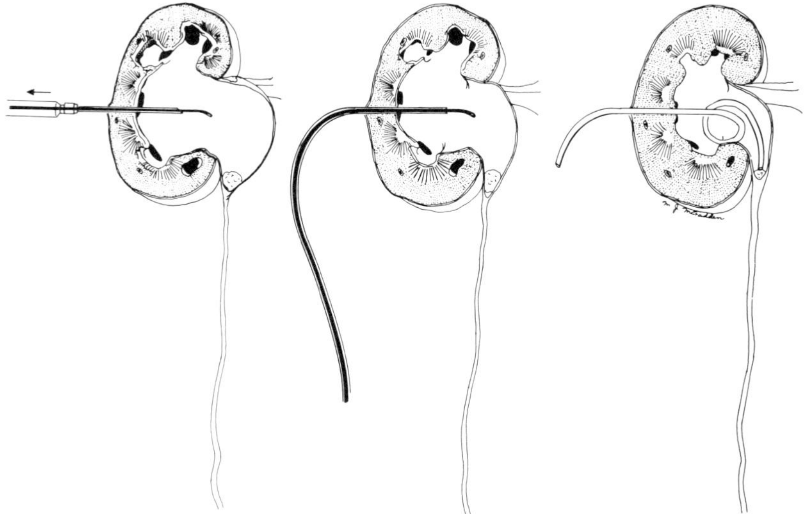

Figure 26-12 External diversion by percutaneous nephrostomy placement.

given to their being diverted.[179–182] Also, if the tumor under treatment is radiosensitive, as is the case in lymphomas[183] or Hodgkin's disease,[184] a diversionary procedure may prove lifesaving until radiotherapy and chemotherapy are sufficiently effective to allow restoration of urinary tract patency.

In patients who require cystectomy for bladder carcinoma, who have the ureterovesical junctions occluded by tumor, or in whom stents have proved unsatisfactory, it may become necessary to construct a more permanent form of urinary diversion. This is usually accomplished by direct drainage of the urinary tract to the exterior by anastomosing a portion of the ureter to an abdominal or flank area termed a stoma. Figures 26-13 through 26-15 demonstrate such anastomoses and represent anterior ureterostomy, lateral loop nephrostomy, and direct flank nephrostomies respectively. Once entry into the stomal area has occurred urine can be gathered in stomal appliances designed to allow free collection of urine with minimal skin irritation. Alternatively, both ureters can be reimplanted into a loop of bowel (ileum or sigmoid colon) whose afferent end is closed and efferent end is open to the skin surface (Figure 26-16).

A final consideration is that of management of bladder outflow obstruction. In this regard, chronic indwelling urethral or suprapubic catheters can be quite effective. Functional bladder obstruction secondary to neurogenic bladder disease can be managed with schedules utilizing frequent or double voiding and/or cholinergic drugs. If possible, any medication which may potentially contribute to impairment in bladder emptying such as muscle relaxants or anticholinergics should be discontinued.

The management of obstructive uropathy in the elderly is not without its rewards. Many elderly patients can adapt quite readily to an imposed life-style change based on alternative methods of urinary drainage. It cannot be overemphasized that current treatment methodology is capable of prolonging the elderly person's life with minimal inconvenience. If the quality of life that will be achieved is meaningful, then both the patient and the physician have several options as to how this may be accomplished. Careful

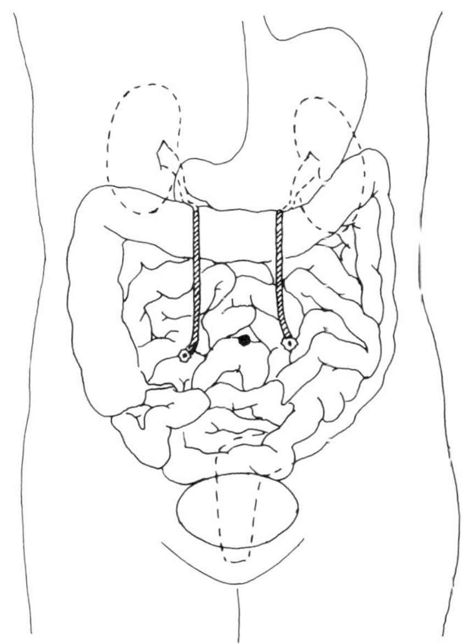

Figure 26-13 Permanent urinary diversion by anterior ureterostomy.

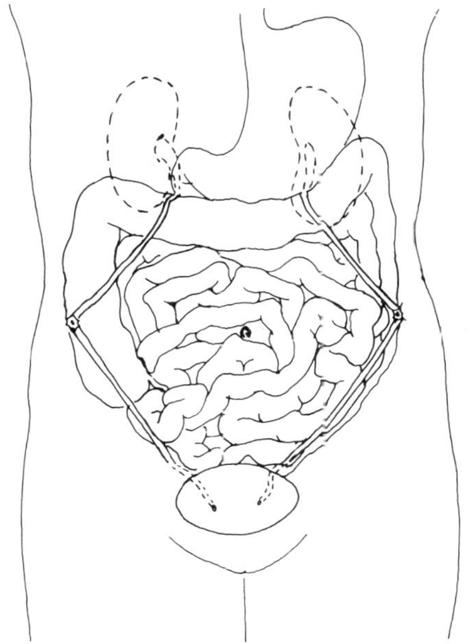

Figure 26-14 Permanent urinary diversion by lateral loop nephrostomy.

selection of the optimal treatment methodology can frequently forestall end-stage renal disease; but even if end-stage renal disease occurs the level of sophistication currently available with dialytic modalities allows for easier management of the elderly patient than in prior years.

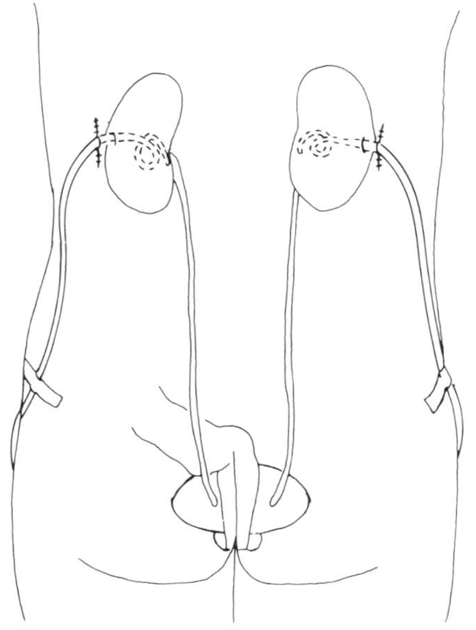

Figure 26-15 Permanent urinary diversion by direct flank nephrostomies.

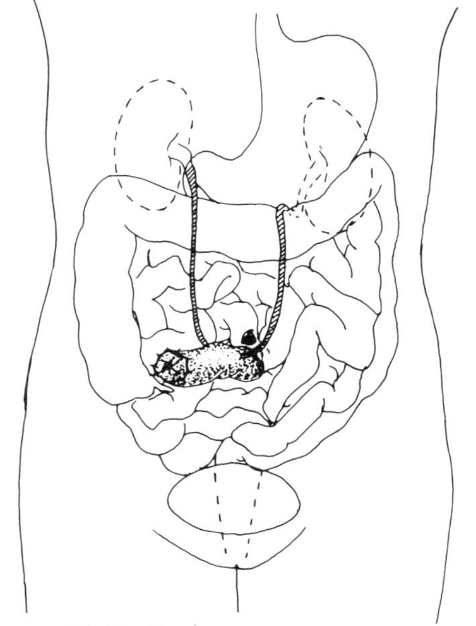

Figure 26-16 Permanent urinary diversion into an ileal bladder; ureteroileostomy.

REFERENCES

1. Bell ET: *Renal Diseases*. Philadelphia, Lea & Febiger, 1946.
2. Campbell MF: Urinary obstruction, in Campbell M, Harrison JH (eds): *Urology*. Philadelphia, WB Saunders Co, 1970, pp 1772–1793.
3. Homans DC, Blake GD, Harrington JT, et al: Acute renal failure caused by ureteral obstruction by a gravid uterus. *JAMA* 1981;246:1230–1231.
4. Alfert HJ, Gillenwater JY: The consequences of ureteral irradiation with special reference to subsequent ureteral injury. *J Urol* 1972;107:369–371.
5. Boyce WH, Garvey FK, Strawviter HE: Incidence of urinary calculi among patients in general hospitals, 1948–52. *JAMA* 1956;161:1437–1442.
6. Taylor PT, Andersen WA: Untreated cervical cancer complicated by obstructive uropathy and oliguric renal failure. *Gynecol Oncol* 1981;11:162–174.
7. Beck AD: Benign prostatic hypertrophy and uraemia. *Br J Surg* 1970;57:561–565.
8. Klein L: Prostatic cancer. *N Engl J Med* 1979;300:824–833.
9. Cole P, Monson RR, Haning H, et al: Smoking and cancer in the lower urinary tract. *N Engl J Med* 1971;284:129–134.
10. Blandy JP: Urethral stricture. *Postgrad Med J* 1980;56:383–418.
11. Hiatt RA, Friedman GD: The frequency of kidney and urinary tract diseases in a defined population. *Kidney Int* 1982;22: 63–68.
12. Zetterstrom R, Ericsson NO, Winberg J: Separate renal function studies in predominantly unilateral hydronephrosis. *Acta Paediatr* 1958;47:540–548.
13. Gillenwater JY, Westervelt FB Jr, Vaughn ED Jr, et al: Renal function one week after release of chronic unilateral hydronephrosis in man. *Kidney Int* 1975; 7:179–186.
14. Better OS, Arieff AI, Massry SG, et al: Studies on renal function after complete unilateral ureteral obstruction of three months duration in man. *Am J Med* 1973; 54:234–240.
15. Berlyne GM: Distal tubular function in chronic hydronephrosis. *Q J Med* 1961; 30:339–355.

16. Berlyne GM, Macken A: On the mechanism of renal inability to produce a concentrated urine in chronic hydronephrosis. *Clin Sci* 1962;22:315–324.
17. Knowlan D, Corrado M, Schreiner GE, et al: Periureteral fibrosis, with a diabetes-insipidus like syndrome occurring with progressive partial obstruction of a ureter unilaterally. *Am J Med* 1960;28:22–31.
18. Wingerg J: Renal function in water-losing syndrome due to lower urinary tract obstruction before and after treatment. *Acta Paediatr* 1959;48:149–163.
19. Falls WF, Stacy WF: Postobstructive diuresis: Studies in a dialyzed patient with a solitary kidney. *Am J Med* 1973;54:404–412.
20. Platts MM, Williams JL: Renal function in patients with unilateral hydronephrosis. *Br Med J* 1963;2:1243–1247.
21. Olbrick O, Woodford WE, Irving RE, et al: Renal function in prostatism. *Lancet* 1957;1:1322–1324.
22. Heptinstall RH: Sundry conditions affecting the renal tubules, in Heptinstall RD (ed): *Pathology of the Kidney.* Boston, Little Brown & Co, 1974, pp 1043–1090.
23. Wright FS, Howards SS: Obstructive Injury, in Brenner B and Rector F (eds): *The Kidney.* Philadelphia, WB Saunders Co, 1981, pp 2008–2044.
24. Persky L, Benson JW, Levey S, et al: Metabolic alterations in surgical patients. X. The benign course of the patient with acute urinary retention *Surgery* 1957;42:290–295.
25. Eiseman B, Vivian C, Vivian J: Fluid and electrolyte changes following the relief of urinary obstruction. *J Urol* 1955;74:222–226.
26. Muldowney FP, Duffy GJ, Kelly DG, et al: Sodium diuresis after relief of obstructive uropathy. *N Engl J Med* 1966;274:1294–1298.
27. Maher JF, Schreiner GE, Waters TJ: Osmotic diuresis due to retained urea after release of obstructive uropathy. *N Engl J Med* 1963;268:1099–1104.
28. Witte MH, Short FA, Hollander W: Massive polyuria and natriuresis following relief of urinary tract obstruction. *Am J Med* 1964;37:320–326.
29. Yarger WE, Aynedjian HS, Bank N: A micropuncture study of post-obstructive diuresis in the rat. *J Clin Invest* 1972;51:625–637.
30. Howards SS: Postobstructive diuresis: A misunderstood phenomenon. *J Urol* 1973;110:537–540.
31. Bricker NS, Shwayri EI, Reardon JB, et al: An abnormality in renal function resulting from urinary tract obstruction. *Am J Med* 1957;23:554–564.
32. Gottschalk CW, Mylle J: Micropuncture study of pressures in proximal tubules and peritubular capillaries of the rat kidney and their relationship to ureteral and renal venous pressure *Am J Physiol* 1956;185:430–439.
33. Yarger WE, Griffith LD: Intrarenal hemodynamics following chronic unilateral obstruction in the dog. *Am J Physiol* 1974;227:816–826.
34. Suki W, Eknoyan G, Rector F Jr, et al: Patterns of nephron perfusion in acute and chronic hydronephrosis. *J Clin Invest* 1966;45:122–131.
35. Blantz RC, Koonen K, Tucker BJ: Glomerular filtration response to elevated ureteral pressure in both the hydropenic and plasma expanded rat. *Circ Res* 1975;37:819–829.
36. Lorentz WB, Lassiter WE, Gottschalk CW: Renal tubular permeability during increased intratubular pressure. *J Clin Invest* 1972;51:484–492
37. Moody TE, Vaughn ED Gillenwater JY: Relationship between renal blood flow and ureteral pressure during 18 hours of total unilateral ureteral occlusion. *Invest Urol* 1975;13:246–251.
38. Moody TE, Vaughn ED Gillenwater JY: Comparison of the renal hemodynamic response to unilateral and bilateral ureteral occlusion. *Invest Urol* 1977;14:455–459.
39. Carlson EL, Sparks HV: Intrarenal distribution of blood flow during elevation of ureteral pressure in dogs. *Circ Res* 1970;26:601–610.
40. Vaughan ED Jr, Shenasky JH, Gillenwater JY: Mechanism of acute hemodynamic response to ureteral occlusion. *Invest Urol* 1971;9:109–118.
41. Hsu CH, Kurtz TW, Rosenzweig J, et al: Intrarenal hemodynamics and ureteral pressure during ureteral obstruction. *Invest Urol* 1978;15:348–351.

42. Kallskog D, Wolgast M: Effect of elevated interstitial pressure on the renal cortical hemodynamics. *Acta Physiol Scand* 1975; 95:364–372.
43. Schramm LP, Carlson DE: Inhibition of renal vasoconstriction by elevated ureteral pressure. *Am J Physiol* 1975;228: 1126–1133.
44. Allen JT, Vaughn ED Jr, Gillenwater JY: The effect of indomethacin on renal blood flow and ureteral pressure in unilateral ureteral obstruction in awake dogs. *Invest Urol* 1978;15:324–327.
45. Gaudio KM, Siegel NJ, Hayslett J, et al: Renal perfusion and intratubular pressure during ureteral occlusion in the rat. *Am J Physiol* 1980;238:F205–F209.
46. Nishikawa K, Morrison AR, Needleman P: Exaggerated prostaglandin biosynthesis and its influence on renal resistance in the isolated hydronephrotic rabbit kidney. *J Clin Invest* 1977;59:1143–1150.
47. Needleman P, Bronson SD, Wyche A, et al: Cardiac and renal prostaglandin I_2 biosynthesis and biological effects in isolated perfused rabbit tissues. *J Clin Invest* 1978;61:839–849.
48. Dibona GF: Effect of mannitol diuresis and ureteral occlusion on distal tubular reabsorption. *Am J Physiol* 1971;221: 511–514.
49. Michaelson G: Percutaneous puncture of the renal pelvis, intrapelvic pressure and the concentrating capacity of the kidney in hydronephrosis. *Acta Med Scand [Suppl]* 1974;559:1–26.
50. Jaenike JR: The renal response to ureteral obstruction: a model for the study of factors which influence glomerular filtration pressure. *J Lab Clin Med* 1970;76: 373–382.
51. Vaughn ED Jr, Sorenson EF, Gillenwater JY: The renal hemodynamic response to chronic unilateral complete ureteral occlusion. *Invest Urol* 1970;8: 78–90.
52. DalCanton A, Corradi A, Stanziale R, et al: Effects of 24 hour unilateral ureteral obstruction on glomerular hemodynamics in rat kidney. *Kidney Int* 1979;15:457–462.
53. Huguenin M, Ott CE, Romero JC, et al: Influence of renin depletion on renal function after release of 24 hours ureteral obstruction. *J Lab Clin Med* 1976;87: 58–64.
54. Moody JE, Vaughan ED Jr, Wyker AT, et al: The role of intrarenal angiotensin II in the hemodynamic response to unilateral obstructive uropathy. *Invest Urol* 1977; 14:390–397.
55. Morrison AR, Nishikawa K, Needleman P: Unmasking of thromboxane A_2 synthesis by ureter obstruction in the rabbit kidney. *Nature* 1977;267:259–260.
56. Yarger WE, Schocker DD, Harris RH: Obstructive uropathy in the rat. Possible roles for the renin-angiotensin system, prostaglandins, and thromboxanes in postobstructive renal function. *J Clin Invest* 1980;65:400–412.
57. Morrison AR, Nishikawa K, Needleman P: Thromboxane A_2 biosynthesis in the ureter obstructed isolated perfused kidney of the rabbit. *J Pharmacol Exp Therap* 1978;205:1–8.
58. Ichikawa I, Brenner BM: Local intrarenal vasoconstrictor-vasodilator interactions in mild partial ureteral obstruction. *Am J Physiol* 1979;236:F131–F140.
59. Morrison AR: Alterations in intrarenal hormones in urinary tract obstruction. *Semin Nephrol* 1982;2:40–45.
60. Jaenike JR: The renal functional defect of postobstructive nephropathy. The effects of bilateral ureteral obstruction in the rat. *J Clin Invest* 1972;51:2999–3006.
61. Buerkert J, Head M, Klahr S: Effects of acute bilateral obstruction on deep nephron and terminal collecting duct function in the young rat. *J Clin Invest* 1977; 59:1055–1065.
62. Beck N: Phosphoturia after release of bilateral ureteral obstruction in rats. *Am J Physiol* 1979;237:F14–F19.
63. Mukamel E, Nissenkorn I, Boner G, et al: Occult progressive renal damage in the elderly male due to benign prostatic hypertrophy. *J Am Geriatr Soc* 1979;27: 403–406.
64. McDougal WS, Wright FS: Defect in proximal and distal sodium transport in postobstructive diruesis. *Kidney Int* 1972; 2:304–317.
65. Lewis HY, Pierce JM: Return of function after relief of complete ureteral obstruction of 69 days duration. *J Urol* 1962;87: 377–378.
66. Graham JB: Recovery of kidney after ureteral obstruction. *JAMA* 1962;181: 993–994.

67. Reisman DD, Kamholz JH, Kantor HI: Early deligation of the ureter. *J Urol* 1957;78:363–375.
68. Roussak NJ, Olecsky S: Water losing nephritis, a syndrome simulating diabetes insipidus. *Q J Med* 1954;23:147–164.
69. Kerr WS Jr: Effect of complete ureteral obstruction for one week on kidney function. *J Appl Physiol* 1954;6:762–772.
70. Kerr WS Jr: Effect of complete ureteral obstruction in dogs on kidney function. *Am J Physiol* 1956;184:521–526.
71. Ekelund L, Gothlin J: Compensatory renal enlargement in older patients. *AJR* 1976;127:713–715.
72. Boner G, Sherry J, Rieselbach RE: Hypertrophy of the normal human kidney following contralateral nephrectomy. *Nephron* 1972;9:364–370.
73. Dossetor RS: Renal compensatory hypertrophy in the adult. *Br J Radiol* 1975;48: 993–995.
74. Edgren J, Laasonen L, Kock B, et al: Kidney function and compensatory growth of the kidney in living kidney donors. *Scand J Urol Nephrol* 1976;10:134–136.
75. Ogden DA: Donor and recipient function 2–4 years after renal homotransplantation: A paired study of 28 cases. *Ann Intern Med* 1967;67:998–1006.
76. Boner J, Shelp WD, Newton M, Rieselbach RE: Factors influencing the increase in glomerular filtration rate in the remaining kidney of transplant donors. *Am J Med* 1973;55:169–174.
77. Donadio JV, Farmer CD, Hunt JC, et al: Renal function in donors and recipients of renal allotransplantation: Radioisotopic measurements. *Ann Intern Med* 1967; 66:105–115.
78. Slack TK, Wilson DM: Normal renal function: C_{IN} and C_{PAH} in healthy donors before and after nephrectomy. *Mayo Clin Proc* 1976;51:296–300.
79. Brenner B, Meyer TW, Hostetter TH: Dietary protein intake and the progressive nature of renal disease: The role of hemodynamically mediated glomerular injury in the pathogenesis of progressive glomerular sclerosis in aging, renal ablation, and intrinsic renal disease. *N Engl J Med* 1982;307:652–659.
80. Vincenti F, Amend WE Jr, Kaysen G, et al: Long-term renal function in kidney donors–sustained compensatory hyperfiltration with no adverse effects. *Transplantation* 1983;36:626–629.
81. Motzkin D: The significance of deficient bladder sensation. *J Urol* 1968;100:445–450.
82. Dossetor JB: Creatinemia versus uremia. *Ann Intern Med* 1966;65:1287–1299.
83. Batlle DC, Arruda JA, Kurtzman NA: Hyperkalemic distal renal tubular acidosis associated with obstructive uropathy. *N Engl J Med* 1981;304:373–380.
84. Frascino J, Vanamec P, Rosen PP: Renal oxalosis and azotemia after methoxyflurane anesthesia. *N Engl J Med* 1970;283: 676–679.
85. Eichhorn JH, Hedley-Whyte J, Steinman TI, et al: Renal failure following enflurane anesthesia. *Anesthesiology* 1976;45:557–560.
86. Krausz T, Sellyei M, Abranyi I: Renocerebral oxalosis after intravenous glycerol infusion. *Lancet* 1977;2:89–90.
87. Kjellstrand CM, Campbell DC, von Hartitzsch B, et al: Hyperuremic acute renal failure. *Arch Intern Med* 1974;133:349–359.
88. Klinenberg JR, Bluestone R, Schlosstein L, et al: Urate deposition disease: how is it regulated and how can it be modified? *Ann Intern Med* 1973;78:99–111.
89. Yü T, Gutman A: Study of the paradoxical effects of salicylate in low, intermediate, and high dosage on the renal mechanisms for excretion of urate in man. *J Clin Invest* 1959;38:1298–1315.
90. Postlethwaite AE, Kelly WN: Uricosuric effect of radiocontrast agents. *Ann Intern Med* 1971;74:845–852.
91. Byrd L, Sherman RL: Radiocontrast-induced acute renal failure: a clinical and pathophysiologic review. *Medicine* 1979; 58:270–279.
92. Howard JE, Meyer RJ: Intoxication with vitamin D. *J Clin Endocrinol Metab* 1948; 8:895–910.
93. Wenger J, Kirsner JB, Palmer WL: The milk-alkali syndrome: hypercalcemia, alkalosis and azotemia following calcium carbonate and milk therapy of peptic ulcer. *Gastroenterology* 1957;33:745–769.
94. Hufnagle KG, Khan SN, Penn D, et al: Renal calcifications: a complication of long-term furosemide therapy in preterm infants. *Pediatrics* 1982;70:360–363.
95. Fox RM: Methotrexate nephrotoxicity.

Clin Exp Pharmacol [Suppl] 1979;5:43–45.
96. Mailloux L, Swartz DC, Copizzi R, et al: Acute renal failure after administration of low-molecular-weight dextran. *N Engl J Med* 1967;277:1113–1118.
97. MacDonald JB, MacDonald ET: Nitrofuratoin crystalluria. *Br Med J* 1976;3: 1044–1045.
98. Dorfman LE, Smith JP: Sulfonamide crystalluria: a forgotten disease. *J Urol* 1970;104:482–483.
99. Kyle RA: Multiple myeloma: review of 869 cases. *Mayo Clin Proc* 1975;50:29–40.
100. DeFronzo RA, Humphrey RL, Wright JR, et al: Acute renal failure in multiple myeloma. *Medicine* 1975;54:209–223.
101. Rees ED, Waugh WH: Factors in the renal failure of multiple myeloma. *Arch Intern Med* 1965;116:400–405.
102. Border WA, Cohen AH: Renal biopsy diagnosis of clinically silent multiple myeloma. *Ann Intern Med* 1980;93:43–46.
103. Martinez-Maldonado M, Jackson Y, Suki WN, et al: Renal complications in multiple myeloma: pathophysiology and some aspects of clinical management. *J Chronic Dis* 1971;24:221–237.
104. Eknoyan G, Qunibi WY, Grisson RT, et al: Renal papillary necrosis: an update. *Medicine* 1982;61:55–72.
105. Harrison JH, Bailey OT: The significance of necrotizing pyelonephritis in diabetes mellitus. *JAMA* 1942;118:15–20.
106. Lauler DP, Schreiner GE, David A: Renal medullary necrosis. *Am J Med* 1960;29: 132–155.
107. Mandel EE: Renal medullary necrosis. *Am J Med* 1952;13:322–327.
108. Simon HB, Bennett WA, Emmett JL: Renal papillary necrosis: a clinicopathologic study of 42 cases. *J Urol* 1957;77: 557–567.
109. Sheehan HL, Davis JC: Experimental hydronephrosis. *Arch Pathol* 1959;68: 185–225.
110. Lagergren C, Ljunqvist A: The intrarenal arterial pattern in renal papillary necrosis. *Am J Path* 1962;41:633–643.
111. Johnson CM, Wilson DM, O'Fallon WM, et al: Renal stone epidemiology: A 25-year study in Rochester, Minnesota. *Kidney Int* 1979;16:624–631.
112. Ljunghall S, Backman V, Danielson BH, et al: Epidemiology of renal stones in Sweden, in Brokis JG, Finlayson B (eds): *Urinary Calculus*. Littleton, Mass, PSG Publishing Co, 1981, pp 13–24.
113. Coe FE, Keck J, Norton ER: The natural history of calcium urolithiasis. *JAMA* 1977;238:1519–1523.
114. Coe FL: Hyperuricosuric calcium oxalate nephrolithiasis. *Kidney Int* 1978;13: 418–426.
115. Tibblin S, Palsson N, Rydberg J: Hyperparathyroidism in the elderly. *Am Surg* 1983;197:135–138.
116. Chute R, Subi HI: Prevalence and importance of urea-splitting bacterial infections of the urinary tract in the formation of calculi. *J Urol* 1943;44:590–595.
117. Norman RW, Mack FG, Awad SA, et al: Acute renal failure secondary to bilateral ureteric obstruction: review of 50 cases. *Can Med Assoc J* 1982;127:601–604.
118. Kontturi M, Kauppila A: Ureteric complications following treatment of gynaecological cancer. *Ann Chir G* 1982;71: 232–238.
119. Dean RJ, Lytton B: Urologic complications of pelvic irradiation. *J Urol* 1978;119: 64–67.
120. Muram D, Oxorn H, Curry RH, et al: Postradiation ureteral obstruction: a reappraisal. *Am J Obstet Gynecol* 1981;139: 289–293.
121. Brady LW, Farber SH: Ureteral injury as a consequence of radiation therapy, in Bergman H (ed): *The Ureter*. New York, Springer-Verlag, 1981, pp 421–426.
122. Ambos MA, Bosniak MA, Megibow AJ: Ureteral involvement by metastatic disease. *Urol Radiol* 1979;1:105–112.
123. Talreja D, Opfell RW: Ureteral metastasis in carcinoma of the breast. *West J Med* 1980;133:252–254.
124. Wagenknecht LV, Hardy JC: Value of various treatments for retroperitoneal fibrosis. *Eur Urol* 1981;7:193–200.
125. Shmookler BM, Laver DH: Retroperitoneal leiomyosarcoma. *Am J Surg Pathol* 1983;7:269–280.
126. Rault R, Kapoor W, Kam W: Perianeurysmal fibrosis and ureteric obstruction: case report and review of literature. *Clin Nephrol* 1982;18:159–162.
127. Rastogi SP, Reid IS: Bilateral ureteral obstruction following aortic bypass surgery. *Clin Nephrol* 1980;14:250–255.

128. Graham JR: Methysergide for prevention of headache: experience in five hundred patients over three years. *N Engl J Med* 1964;270:67–72.
129. Lewis CT, Molland EA, Marshall VR, et al: Analgesic abuse, ureteric obstruction, and retroperitoneal fibrosis. *Br Med J* 1975;2:76–78.
130. Doherty CC, McGeown MG, Donaldson RA: Retroperitoneal fibrosis after treatment with atenolol. *Br Med J* 1978;2: 1786.
131. Thompson J, Julian DG: Retroperitoneal fibrosis associated with metoprolol. *Br Med J* 1982;284:83–84.
132. McGuire E: Urinary dysfunction in the aged: neurological considerations. *Bull N Y Acad Med* 1980;56:275–284.
133. Lorenze EJ, Simon HB, Linden JL: Urologic problems in rehabilitation of hemiplegic patients. *JAMA* 1959;169:1042–1046.
134. Ellenberg M, Weber H: The incipient asymptomatic diabetic bladder. *Diabetes* 1967;16:331–335.
135. Ellenberg M: Diabetic neurogenic vesical dysfunction. *Arch Intern Med* 1966;117: 348–354.
136. Kahan M, Goldberg PD, Mandell EE: Neurogenic vesical dysfunction and diabetes mellitus. *N Y State J Med* 1970;70: 2448–2455.
137. Lytton B, Emery JM, Harvard BM: The incidence of benign prostatic obstruction. *J Urol* 1968;99:639–645.
138. Chisholm GD: Obstructive uropathy–a review of 146 patients with postrenal uraemia. *S Afr Med J* 1967;41:962–964.
139. Keuhnelian JG, Bartone F, Marshall VF: Practical considerations from autopsies on azotemic patients. *J Urol* 1964;91:467–473.
140. Wallach JB, Glass M, Angrist AA: The autopsy incidence of uremia: its clinical implication. *J Urol* 1956;75:356–358.
141. Carter CB, Olichney MJ, Westervelt FB Jr: Renal failure in the elderly. *South Med J* 1970;63:805–808.
142. Roberts JA, Lewis RW: Effect of obstruction on renal function, in Hinman FA Jr (ed): *Benign Prostatic Hypertrophy*. New York, Springer-Verlag, 1983, pp 731–741.
143. Birnhoff JD, Wiederhorn AR, Hamilton ML, et al: Natural history of benign prostatic hypertrophy and acute urinary retention. *Urology* 1976;7:48-52.
144. Abrams P: Prostatism and prostatectomy: The value of urine flow rate measurement in the pre-operative assessment for operation. *Urol* 1977;117:70–71.
145. Singh M, Blandy JP: The pathology of urethral strictures. *J Urol* 1976;115: 673–676.
146. Holtgrewe HL, Valk WL: Factors influencing the morbidity and mortality of transurethral prostatectomy: a study of 2,015 cases. *J Urol* 1962;87:450–459.
147. Lentz HC Jr, Mebust WK, Foret JD, et al: Urethral strictures following transurethral prostatectomy: review of 2223 resections. *J Urol* 1977;117:194–196.
148. Landsberg L: Hypernatremia complicating partial urinary tract obstruction. *New Engl J Med* 1970,283:746–748.
149. Griffith DP: Infection-induced renal calculi. *Kidney Int* 1982;21:422–430.
150. Taylor TA, Bowyer RC: Bladder and prostatic calculi-clinical presentation and composition, in Brockis JG, Finlayson B (eds): *Urinary Calculus*. Littleton, PSG Publishing Co, pp 57–63.
151. Jaworski ZF, Wolan CT: Hydronephrosis and polycythemia, a case of erythrocytosis relieved by decompression of unilateral hydronephrosis and cured by nephrectomy. *Am J Med* 1963;34:523–534.
152. Mitus WG, Toyama K, Brauer MJ: Erythrocytosis, juxtaglomerular apparatus (JGA) and erythropoietin in the course of experimental hydronephrosis in rabbits. *Ann N Y Acad Sci* 1968;149:107–113.
153. Beeson PB: Factors in the pathogenesis of pyelonephritis. *Yale J Biol Med* 1955; 28:81–104.
154. Cotran R, Pennington JE: Urinary tract infection, pyelonephritis and reflux nephropathy, in Brenner B, Rector F Jr (eds): *The Kidney*. Philadelphia, WB Saunders Co, 1981, pp 1571–1632.
155. Hasner E: Prostatic urinary infection. *Acta Chir Scand [Suppl]* 1962;285:7–40.
156. Vaughn EJ Jr, Buhler FR, Laragh JH: Normal renin secretion in hypertensive patients with primarily unilateral chronic hydronephrosis. *J Urol* 1974;112:153–156.
157. Vander AJ, Miller R: Control of renin secretion in the anesthetized dog. *Am J Physiol* 1964;207:537–546.

158. Weidmann P, Beretta-Picoli C, Hirsch D, et al: Curable hypertension with unilateral hydronephrosis. *Ann Intern Med* 1977;87:437–440.
159. Belmon AB, Kropp KA, Simon NM: Renal-pressor hypertension secondary to unilateral hydronephrosis. *N Engl J Med* 1968;278:1133–1136.
160. Palmer JM, Zweiman FG, Assaykeen TA: Renal hypertension due to hydronephrosis with normal plasma renin activity. *N Engl J Med* 1970;283:1032–1034.
161. Shearlock KT, Howards SS: Post obstructive anuria: a documented entity. *J Urol* 1976;115:212–213.
162. Brown CB, Glarcy JJ, Fry IK, et al: High-dose excretion urography in oliguric renal failure. *Lancet* 1970;2: 952–955.
163. Schwatz WB, Hurwit A, Ettinger A: Intravenous urography in the patient with renal insufficiency. *N Engl J Med* 1963; 269:277–284.
164. Sabmom LL, Lanza FL: Glomerular filtration in the rat after ureteral ligation. *Am J Physiol* 1962;202:559–564.
165. Sanders RC: Renal ultrasound. *Radiol Clin North Am* 1975;13:417–434.
166. Ellenbogen P, Scheible F, Talner LB, et al: Sensitivity of gray scale ultrasound in detecting urinary tract obstruction. *AJR* 1978;130:731–733.
167. Sagel SS, Stanley RJ, Levitt RG, Geisse G: Computed tomography of the kidney. *Radiology* 1977;124:359–370.
168. Diaz-Buxo JA, Wagoner RD, Hattery RR, et al: Acute renal failure after excretory urography in diabetic patients. *Ann Intern Med* 1975;83:155–158.
169. Alexander RD, Berkes SL, Abuelo G: Contrast media-induced oliguric renal failure. *Arch Intern Med* 1978;138:381–384.
170. Scharf SC, Blaufox MD: Radionuclides in the evaluation of urinary obstruction. *Semin Nucl Med* 1982;12:254–264.
171. Gibbons RP, Correa RJ, Cummings KB, et al: Experience with indwelling ureteral stent catheters. *J Urol* 1976;115:22–26.
172. Singh B, Kim H, Wax SH: Stent versus nephrostomy: Is there a choice? *J Urol* 1979;121:268–270.
173. Pedersen JF: Percutaneous nephrostomy guided by ultrasound. *J Urol* 1974; 112:157–159.
174. Stables DP, Holt SA, Sheridan HM, et al: Permanent nephrostomy via percutaneous puncture. *J Urol* 1975;114:684– 687.
175. Fowler JE, Meares EM Jr, Goldin AR: Percutaneous nephrostomy: techniques, indications and results. *Urology* 1975;6: 428–434.
176. Perinetti E, Catalona WJ, Manley CB, et al: Percutaneous nephrostomy: indications, complications and clinical usefulness. *J Urol* 1978;120:156–158.
177. Barbaric ZL, Wood BP: Emergency percutaneous nephropyelostomy: Experience with 34 patients and review of the literature. *AJR* 1977;128:453–458.
178. Holden S, McPhee M, Grabstald H: Rationale of urinary diversion in cancer patients. *J Urol* 1979;121:19–21.
179. Brin EN, Schiff M Jr, Weiss RM: Palliative urinary diversion for pelvic malignancy. *J Urol* 1975;113:619–622.
180. Fallon B, Olney L, Culp DA: Nephrostomy in cancer patients: to do or not to do? *Br J Urol* 1980;52:237–242.
181. Khan AU, Utz DC: Clinical management of carcinoma of the prostate with bilateral ureteral obstruction. *J Urol* 1975; 113:816–819.
182. Van Dyke AH, Van Nagell JR Jr: The prognostic significance of ureteral obstruction in patients with recurrent carcinoma of the cervix uteri. *Surg Gynecol Obstet* 1975;141:371–373.
183. Brewer W, Lan WC, Bunts RC: Complete bilateral ureteral obstruction from leukemia and lymphoma. *J Urol* 1967;98:186–190.
184. Loening S, Carson CC III, Faxon DP, et al: Ureteral obstruction from Hodgkin's disease. *J Urol* 1974;111:345–349.

CHAPTER 27 Sexuality in the Elderly

Keith N. Van Arsdalen
Alan J. Wein

The sexual interest and sexual activity of the elderly men and women in our society are determined by a number of physiologic, psychological, and social factors. These influences may accrue gradually over a lifetime or develop suddenly with dramatic effects on both sexual behavior and function. The topic of sexuality in the elderly has recently received a great deal of attention in the press, particularly in various nursing journals, psychiatric/psychological journals, and in publications directed at primary care physicians and geriatricians. Indeed, such interest is warranted since people are now living longer and it has been predicted that by the year 2000, half of the United States population will be over 65 years of age.[1] A review of the literature from the past decade in comparison to that published two and three decades earlier led to a similar conclusion as that reached by Berezin in 1976; ie, recent literature shows little variation in content from that published earlier.[2] In this regard, Kinsey et al appeared to have stimulated a growing public awareness of sexuality with their initial publications.[3,4] Their work included, in part, information on sexuality in the elderly. Masters and Johnson's description of the human sexual response cycle and the associated changes of the body during the various sexual phases was based on laboratory observation[5]; it has provided a classic base of knowledge that most subsequent authors have come to rely on. Their subsequent *Human Sexual Inadequacy* provided complementary information regarding sexual dysfunction as well as a description of the normal physiologic changes that occur with aging.[6] It is essential to read the original description of this as, once again, most subsequent works (including this one) that consider the topic of geriatric sexuality rely heavily on their material. The third major source of information has been the work by Pfeiffer, Verwoerdt and their associates at the Duke Center for the Study of Aging and Human Development.[7–10] They have provided cross-sectional as well as longitudinal data as regards sexuality in the elderly.

Other observations and general precautions are given at this time so that the reader can consider the information reviewed below with a healthy degree of skepticism and inquiry. Foremost in one's mind should be the fact that much of the available information is anecdotal, based solely on case reports and clinical observations. Information is frequently obtained in a nonrandomized fashion by interview technics and then quantified.[11] The resultant statistics may be difficult to interpret or compare and are often, in short, not statistically or scientifically valid.[11] Two themes or basic premises pervade the literature that may introduce bias into many of the studies. The first is that sex in the elderly is desirable if not essential, and hence sexual deprivation results in adverse physical and psychological effects.[12] The second is that most authors are convinced that a negative attitude toward sexuality in the elderly is widespread throughout society. Although this may in fact be true, little proof of this assumption exists and in fact, two studies on sexual attitudes have demonstrated either a lack of negative feelings or even positive feelings toward sex in the elderly.[13,14]

This chapter will review the information that is available concerning normal sexual function in males and females and the normal physiologic changes that occur with aging. Emphasis will be placed on data derived from studies of humans rather than from animal studies. Psychosocial and medical/pathophysiologic parameters that influence sexuality will then be considered; this will culminate in a discussion of the qualitative and quantitative aspects of sexual function as expressed in the elderly.

NORMAL SEXUAL FUNCTION

Anatomy

The physiology of human sexual function involves a complex series of neurologically mediated vascular phenomena that occur with a permissive hormonal and psychological milieu. Masters and Johnson defined the human sexual response cycle and divided it into four phases for descriptive purposes–excitation, plateau, orgasm, and resolution–although the cycle actually progresses as a continuum.[5] Each phase involves genital and extragenital responses that produce dramatic anatomical and physiologic changes. A knowledge of the normal pelvic and genital gross anatomy is helpful in understanding the physiology of the sex act.

The penis, testes, and accessory sex glands are most important in male sexual function. The penis is composed of three cylindrical masses of tissue–two corpora cavernosa and a single ventral corpus spongiosum. Each corporal body is made up of a loose trabecular arrangement of muscular and connective tissue surrounded by a dense fibrous covering called the tunica albuginea. The corporal bodies share a common septum in their pendulous portion such that they function as a single unit.[15] The proximal portions of the corpora cavernosa are anchored to the ventral aspects of the ischial rami and each is covered by the ischiocavernosus muscle. The corpus spongiosum lies in the ventral groove formed by the two larger corporal bodies. The corpus spongiosum contains the urethra and enlarges at its distal end to form the glans penis. Proximally, it is attached to the ventral aspect of the urogenital diaphragm and is covered by the bulbocavernosus muscle.

The blood supply to the penis is derived

from the hypogastric artery as it courses through the deep pelvis and perineum and eventually becomes the internal pudendal artery. Each gives off a perineal, bulbar, and urethral branch before continuing as the penile artery which then divides into the dorsal and profunda arteries. The three major arteries to the penis are paired and are connected by large anastomotic channels.[16] The venous drainage is more complex and has been clearly reviewed elsewhere.[17]

The neural supply of the penis is part of the meshwork which innervates not only the other pelvic organs concerned with sexual function, but the bladder and rectum as well. Three types of fibers (sympathetic, parasympathetic, and somatic) from two areas of the spinal cord (T-10 to L-2 and S-2 to S-4) provide the major innervation. Parasympathetic and sympathetic fibers in the inferior hypogastric or pelvic plexus give rise to the vesical plexus, prostatic plexus, and cavernous plexus. This mixture of fibers of the autonomic nervous system accounts for the present confusion regarding which types of fibers are actually responsible for penile erection.[18]

The testes are normally located in the scrotum and are freely mobile. Each produces testosterone, the major androgenic substance in adult life, and spermatozoa. Testosterone directly enters the blood stream while sperm must traverse the highly elaborate epididymis and vas deferens prior to reaching the urethra for ejaculation.

The periurethral glands of Littre and the bulbourethral or Cowper's glands provide fluid that lubricates the anterior urethra. The latter lie deep within the substance of the transverse perineus muscle of the urogenital diaphragm[19] and fluid is expressed from them by contraction of the surrounding muscle fibers. Their blood supply is from the artery of the bulb and nervous innervation is via the inferior hypogastric plexus.[20] The prostate and the seminal vesicles provide the bulk of the seminal fluid. Each is a muscular structure whose glandular secretion can be actively expressed under neurologic stimulation. The ejaculatory duct results from the fusion of the ampulla of the vas with the ipsilateral duct of the seminal vesicle. This duct, along with the multiple prostatic ducts, opens into the posterior urethra. Blood supply to the duct is from branches of the inferior vesical artery and innervation is by the adjacent subsidiary plexus of the inferior hypogastric plexus.

The relevant female anatomy can be divided into internal and external structures. The latter consist mainly of the labia majora, labia minora, and the clitoris. The labia majora derive embryologically from structures that produce the scrotum in males and these structures are primarily composed of fat pads surrounded by skin. The labia minora vary greatly in shape, size, and pigmentation among individuals. They are usually relatively thin structures that are in apposition in the midline under resting conditions thereby sealing the vaginal vestibule. Unlike the labia majora, they are devoid of fat. Anteriorly, each labium divides to surround the clitoris and form a protective hood or prepuce. The vascular and neural supply to the labia are derived from several sources. The anterior aspects of the labia are supplied by branches of the external pudendal arteries and by the anterior labial nerves that originate in the lumbar plexus as fibers contained in the ilioinguinal and genitofemoral nerves. The posterior labial vessels are branches of the internal pudendal arteries and the posterior labial nerves are branches of the pudendal nerve.

The clitoris is analogous to the glans penis and corporal tissue in the male and contains similar erectile tissue whose anchorage is to the ischiopubic rami. The paired blood supply from both deep and dorsal arteries branching off from the internal pudendal artery is likewise analogous. The major dissimilarity between the clitoris and glans penis lies in the fact that it does not contain the urethra and it is without an obvious nonsexual function. In fact, it appears to have no other function than to be a primary sensory center for sexual stimuli in the female.

The internal genitalia include the vagina, uterus, fallopian tubes and ovaries. The vagina is a thick muscular organ that is flattened in an anteroposterior direction in the resting state with only a potential space existing between its walls. It is lined by stratified squamous epithelium with an extremely rich supporting blood supply that is derived as direct vaginal branches from the hypogastric arteries or as branches of the uterine arteries. No discrete glandular structures have been identified in the vaginal walls. The innervation appears to be by way of the parasympathetic and somatic fibers of the S-2 to S-4 area.

Other than the hormonal contributions of the ovaries, the roles of these structures, the tubes and uterus, are primarily for the purpose of procreation. Their gross anatomy and neuromuscular supply has been well defined elsewhere and will not be considered further at this time.[19]

Physiology

Erection is a neurologically mediated event producing vascular changes which result in engorgement and rigidity of the penis. It is the major genital manifestation of the excitement and plateau phases of Masters and Johnson's male sexual response cycle although scrotal thickening, testicular elevation, and urethral lubrication also occur. The anatomical changes in dimensions and rigidity have been well described and generally include a slight increase in length preceding an increase in circumference, followed by elevation of the penis from the resting position.[17,21] Increases in volume and size do not necessarily parallel changes in rigidity and hence the ability to penetrate the vagina.[21,22]

A vast amount of literature and controversy has accumulated regarding the specific vascular components of erection and the relative importance and role of central and peripheral divisions of the autonomic and somatic nervous systems.[18] Increased arterial perfusion of the corpora cavernosa is the primary event which occurs in the production of an erection, and appears to be secondary to a decrease in arterial and arteriolar resistance.[23-25] Although active regulation of the vascular outlet by either venous compression or constriction does not appear to be absolutely necessary in humans,[26] it is entirely possible that a concomitant change in venous drainage also may occur under normal physiologic conditions. The exact microvascular flow of blood in the flaccid and the erect state is not really known, nor is it understood what role the smooth muscle of the corporal tissue plays in this regulation.

The many theories of the vascular mechanism of erection have usually described shunting of blood through some vessel in the flaccid state and closure of these shunts with diversion of blood into the cavernous spaces during erection. The basic theory that has been taught repeatedly is that of Conti.[27] According to this theory, muscular polsters located in the arteries, arteriovenous (A-V) shunts, and veins control the amount and distribution of blood flow. A more logical synthesis of the recent data generated concerning these structures, as proposed by Benson et al,[28] is that the polsters are simply the earliest manifestation of atherosclerosis in these penile vessels.[28] A shunting mechanism is almost certainly involved in normal erectile activity, but control of these shunts by polsters is not likely.

Any theory of erection must take into account recent elucidated neurophysiologic, neuromorphologic, and neuropharmacologic data. Classically, two types of stimuli have been defined as capable of eliciting erections in a reflex fashion. Those stimuli defined as *psychogenic* include those of an auditory, visual, olfactory, gustatory, tactile, or imaginative nature.[29] *Reflexogenic* stimuli include those of an exteroceptive nature associated with genital manipulation with afferent impulses traveling along fibers of the pudendal nerve. Just as different types of stimuli have been described in eliciting erectile activity, so have different pathways been described in mediating the erection. In general, reflexogenic erections are felt to be mediated by the S-2 to S-4 parasympathetic outflow. From the literature, the thoracolumbar sympathetic outflow would seem to be responsible for the production of erections on a psychogenic basic. In either case, the precise details of postganglionic fiber terminations and their neurotransmitters, and the exact location of the postsynaptic end-organ receptors are really unknown. It is possible that the concept of a purely psychogenic as opposed to a purely reflexogenic erection may be entirely wrong; it can be that if two mechanisms do in fact exist, that they may share a final common pathway with the end result being the same.

The role of the androgenic hormones in regard to male sexual behavior and function is unclear, particularly with regard to the exact amounts of hormone needed for either basal or optimal function. Evidence supporting the physiologic role of androgens in the human is derived primarily from clinical information following surgical or medical castration and from males with hypogonadism. This evidence, along with the fact that it is well known that prepubertal males with very low levels of testosterone are known to have erections, would indicate that a wide range of sexual function exists even in men with very low levels of serum testosterone.[30–32] In most cases, the role of the psyche versus that of lowered testosterone levels has not been fully evaluated, even with the recent use of nocturnal penile tumescence testing.

The information concerning physical changes in the excitement phase of the female sexual response cycle is primarily descriptive and derived from the observations of Masters and Johnson.[5,33] This information is summarized below with great respect for the authors' classic contribution in this field. Lubrication and erection are essentially equivalent and complementary responses and probably have a common physiologic basis, ie, increased arterial inflow. Vasocongestion of the vaginal walls is associated with transudation of fluid producing the characteristic lubrication of the vagina. Glandular secretion is not involved here and the process may be complete within 10 to 30 seconds following exposure to physical or psychogenic stimuli. Other changes of the internal and external genitalia also occur. Vasocongestion of the clitoris and the labia begins with an increase in their size, fullness, and warmth. The proximal portion of the vaginal vault increases in both size and length, in part due to elevation of the uterus and cervix within the pelvis. Breast enlargement, fullness of the areolae, and nipple erection may also begin during this phase.

In men and women, no major event marks the end of the excitement phase and the onset of the plateau phase. The latter is a state of high sexual and neuromuscular tension that follows the build-up period characteristic of the excitement phase. It remains, however, a dynamic, not a static state. Erection and lubrication remain the most obvious of the physiologic changes. Additional fullness of the erection may be noted during the plateau phase, while vaginal transudation and lubrication in the female may actually diminish. The inner end of the vagina may continue to expand while congestion of the outer one third may actually make the canal smaller in this area. Masters and Johnson have termed this constriction the "orgasmic platform." The clitoris may appear to get smaller and hidden due to further increases in the size of the labia minora. Additional breast enlargement occurs with areolar fullness becoming particularly noticeable at this time. The events described are generalizations of the reactions that actually occur. Individual variation is very evident, particularly with regard to the length of time occupied by each phase.

Orgasm in the male is generally associated with the process of emission and ejaculation, and these two phenomena are usually temporally related, occurring at the culmination of a sexually exciting situation. Each has the potential in certain situations, however, to be independent of the other, as well as independent of penile erection.[34,35] Emission refers to the deposition of the glandular secretions from the prostate and seminal vesicles and the contents of the distal vasa into the posterior urethra. The exact nature of the afferent stimuli preceding emission is not clear, but as for erection, exteroceptive stimuli from the genitalia as well as cerebral stimuli are probably involved. Cerebral modification is such that emission may be halted voluntarily up to the sensation of "inevitability," which is due to filling and distention of the posterior urethra. Efferent neural control eminates from the T-10 to L-2 sympathetic outflow.[34]

Ejaculation is a complex phenomenon involving three to seven rhythmic contractions of the pelvic floor musculature compressing the urethra at 0.8-second intervals; this under normal conditions results in expulsion of the semen in an antegrade direction. Although the order is not invariably fixed, the products of the prostate are usually expelled first, followed by those of the vas and finally by the secretions of the seminal vesicles.[34,36] The afferent stimulus for the ejaculatory process appears to be the passage of semen from the posterior urethra to the bulbous urethra. Coordinated sympathetic and somatic nervous outflow must occur. Cerebral localization studies have demonstrated areas associated with emission and ejaculation; these areas are closely associated anatomically to the centers for erection.[35] The factors relating the genital events to the CNS thereby resulting in the intense and profoundly satisfying cerebral sensation and total body appreciation of orgasm are unknown.

Hormonal considerations with regard to emission and ejaculation are similar to those for erection. An important finding, however, is that the absense of testosterone within a short time causes a marked decrease in the volume of the seminal fluid.[34] The relationship of serum androgen levels to orgasm is as of yet not agreed upon. In a recent study, Kraemer et al found that serum testosterone levels increased after an orgasm.[37] Additionally, men with a higher frequency of orgastic release generally had lower levels of testosterone. The suggestion was made that low testosterone levels may serve to stimulate one to sexual activity and orgasm as a means of raising this hormone's level. Fox et al studied one male subject and found plasma testosterone levels to be elevated during and immediately after intercourse compared to levels during resting conditions.[38] Many other authors, however, have been unable to demonstrate any change in testosterone or gonadotrophin levels before, during, and after intercourse and orgasm.[39–41]

Following orgasm, detumescence takes place and a refractory period exists during which time the male is unable to achieve full erection or repeat orgasm. The detumescence phase is generally longer than the initial tumescence phase and occurs with an initial high venous outflow followed by a slower, more gradual emptying. The neurologic regulation of detumescence and the refractory period has not been delineated.

The sensation of orgasm in females likewise represents cerebral interpretation of genital events.[42] Nothing comparable to emission occurs, but rhythmic contraction of the pelvic musculature takes place, also at 0.8-second intervals. Five to 15 contractions may occur involving the pelvic floor and rectal sphincter, the vaginal orgasmic platform, and the uterus. The afferent impulses responsible for orgasm have been a source of great debate.[43] "Vaginal" versus "clitoral" orgasms have been proposed. Neurophysiologic data, however, indicate that the clitoris is richly supplied with nerves and the vagina relatively sparsely supplied. Most experts now agree that there is little evidence to support the idea of a dual orgasm hypothesis based on the particular area of stimulation.[43] The specific neural pathways involved in outflow to the pelvis and in cerebral appreciation of this phenomenon are not clear at the present time.

Following an orgasm, the female may respond to continued stimulation by maintenance of her sexual energy at the plateau phase. She may experience multiple orgasms without the subsequent refractory period which all males experience. The neurophysiologic and vascular basis of this phenomenon is not understood. When the resolution phase is entered, however, the labia minora rapidly shrink, the clitoris "detumesces" and once again becomes easily visible. As in males, a gradual, slow period of resolution follows what were initially rapid changes. Gradual resolution of the marked pelvic vasocongestion takes place over 30 to 60 minutes with return of the vagina to its resting size and return of the uterus to its previous location. Finally, as also noted for males, a clear relationship does not exist regarding hormonal levels, sexual behavior, and orgastic need and/or frequency in women.[39,41,44]

Physiologic Changes with Aging

A variety of physiologic changes occur with aging in both men and women that may then alter sexual function. The naturally occurring alterations are discussed in this section, with pathophysiologic conditions considered below. It should be emphasized, however, that even normally occurring processes may be misinterpreted by a given individual with serious psychological and functional sequelae. Just as one does not spontaneously go from being young to being old, one does not suddenly notice a marked change in sexual interest or activity in the absence of major physical disability or life stresses. In women, however, the menopause and the cessation of menstruation do provide a more obvious signal that biological change has taken place. The elderly female is one who has gone through this period of her life. In men, a concomitant phenomenon or "male climacteric" cannot be marked on a calendar as can the start of irregular menses and/or the individual's last menstrual period. Masters and Johnson used the term "older men" in reference to the 50 to 70-year-old group and "younger man" to describe males in the 20 to 40-year old group.[6] A dividing age must be set for discussion purposes; perhaps 50 years old is a reasonable age for this purpose, but in each sex, however, the transition is really a gradual one as regards anatomical and physiologic changes.

Healthy elderly men go through the same sexual response cycle as younger men with differences of degree noted in each phase. The ability to achieve an erection takes longer in response to both exteroceptive and psychogenic stimuli. More attention may need to be given to direct penile and genital stimulation. This may relate to decreased tactile sensitivity of the penis demonstrated with aging.[45] The resultant erection takes longer to reach maximal fullness and turgidity.[33] The plateau phase is also longer for the aging male and may be exploited by him and his partner for increased mutual satisfaction. Overall, the ejaculatory demand decreases and the need to ejaculate with each coital encounter may not be necessary. Ejaculatory control, therefore, may be noticeably improved. The orgasmic phase generally produces a fairly standard physiologic response and cerebral appreciation in younger men, but may be quite variable in the elderly.[6] The sensation of inevitability may be less well appreciated or may be prolonged due to prostatic spasm during emission of its content to the seminal fluid.[6] Seminal volume is reduced and expelled through the urethra with less of an expulsive force. Although reduced in volume, the semen continues to contain all of its normal components. Sperm production may decrease with age, but fertility can certainly persist.[46] Following ejaculation, penile detumescence may be very rapid and the following refractory period very prolonged.

Other less noticeable changes also may occur including decreased testicular elevation or decreased frequency of rectal sphincter contractions associated with orgasm. Overall, the net effect of aging in the male appears to be one of diminished responsiveness and prolonged phases of the response cycle. The role played by testosterone in this regard is not clear. Several studies have demonstrated decreasing levels of testosterone with increasing age,[47,48] but a recent longitudinal study demonstrated no significant decrement in testosterone levels with increasing age.[49,50] The latter studies also demonstrated only a slight association between serum testosterone level and the degree of sexual activity. Low testosterone levels were found in only a small percentage of men with diminished sexual activity.[50]

In women, the sexual response also tends to decrease with aging compared to that occurring in earlier years, and in addition, major physical changes take place. Most of the changes can be ascribed to the cessation of estrogen production by the ovaries with involution of the steroid-dependent structures of the genital tract.[6,51] Of particular note is the thinning of the vaginal mucosa, resulting in an atrophic, friable, noncorrugated appearance.[6] As a result, lubrication occurs more slowly and with less transudation of fluid during the excitement phase. The vaginal walls are also less elastic and do not expand and lengthen as they had previously. Uterine elevation is less, further reducing the changes in vaginal size.

Fatty tissue is usually lost from the labia majora and mons pubis, and atrophy of the labia minora occurs.[6] The dramatic changes in size and fullness of the labia due to vasocongestion are not as marked in the elderly female. The clitoris does not change in either size or apparently in sensitivity.[6] Sensitivity studies similar to those performed in men have been attempted; unfortunately the vibrometer used to study males proved too erotic with clitoral placement in females, so comparable data with aging are not available.[45] Due to loss of the protective coverings provided by the now atrophic labia minor, the clitoris may be more exposed and more easily irritated, with pain rather than pleasure elicited by direct manipulation.[6]

The orgasmic platform appears to develop normally during the plateau phase and contracts repetitively during orgasm. The number of contractions, however, is usually less. Uterine contractions that occur during orgasm also continue to occur, though less frequently. Of note, these uterine contractions may be associated with similar sensation as in the younger female, or they may present as painful spasms felt in the lower abdomen, vagina, and vulva, particularly in the severely estrogen-deficient female.[6] The ability to experience multiple orgasms is preserved. The resolution phase is shortened, with rapid return of the internal and external genitalia to their resting states.

It can therefore be seen that complementary changes occur in the male and female with aging. Erection and lubrication take longer in the respective partners, making intromission less likely until each is ready. A prolonged plateau phase occurs in each, and orgasm, when achieved, is usually less intense and of shorter duration than earlier in life. The demand for orgastic release, however, is also less intense and not necessarily the object of every sexual encounter. Physical contact, closeness, and touching may be equally satisfying.[52] The resolution phase is shorter in each of the sexes, bringing each more rapidly back to base line. The fertility potential appears to persist for the elderly male, while ending for the female with completion of menopause. Other differences also exist, particularly with regard to the physical changes that occur in the aging female. These are easily attributable to lack of endogenous estrogens and may in part be reversible with estrogen replacement. The debate surrounding this issue will not be considered herein. The role of hormonal changes in males is less clear, as testosterone levels do not demonstrate changes as marked as those noted for estrogen levels in females.

OTHER INFLUENCES ON SEXUAL FUNCTION

Pathophysiology

It is evident from the above discussion that the intensity and level of sexual function may not be the same in the young and the old, but clearly the mechanisms remain intact in healthy people throughout their lifetime. A multitude of factors of an intrinsic and extrinsic nature influence sexual responsiveness and sexual activity in each group. These influences in the elderly range from the physical to the psychological to the social aspects associated with aging.

It has been stated that the psychological complications are much more limiting than the normal physiologic changes with regard to sexual function.[53] This is probably true in healthy men and women and the psychological aspects will be considered below. Clearly, however, physical health is very important for normal sexual function and alterations in health may be particularly important with regard to sexual dysfunction.[54] Erectile dysfunction secondary to a naturally occurring and progressive organic disease usually results in deteriorating sexual ability and a similar pattern of impairment in all sexual and nonsexual situations.[55] Organic dysfunction implies that some abnormality exists in the neurologic, vascular, hormonal, or end-organ mechanisms involved in the process of erection. Diseases, surgical procedures, and drug usage have all been implicated in erectile dysfunction in males of all ages. The commonly occurring processes in the elderly are discussed below. The interested reader is referred elsewhere for a more inclusive discussion of sexual dysfunction.[54]

Neurologic diseases of the central and peripheral nervous system are often accompanied by erectile dysfunction in the elderly male. Common cortical lesions affecting sexual function include cerebrovascular accidents, Parkinson's disease, Alzheimer's disease, posttraumatic encephalopathy, and neurosurgical procedures. Cerebrovascular accidents yield a decrease in sexual activity and libido in one third of patients so affected. Right-sided paralysis leads to impaired libido more often than does a disturbance of the opposite side.[56] Parkinson's disease and Shy-Drager syndrome both involve degeneration in the area of the substantia nigra and can result in erectile dysfunction.[57]

Multiple sclerosis and major trauma are two processes that affect the neurologic function of the spinal cord. There is variability in the degree of sexual dysfunction, which probably relates directly to the degree of neuronal damage and the specificity of the lesions. With multiple sclerosis, the process of ejaculation, as well as erection, is usually impaired. Although libido is often intact, it may be moderately or severely impaired also.[58] With spinal cord injury, the level and completeness of the injury are important in determining the sexual responses that are preserved. Erection is able to occur more commonly in higher lesions than lower lesions; the opposite is true for ejaculation. Incomplete lesions at any level generally allow for better sexual function than complete lesions at comparable levels.[59] It should be realized, however, that even under the best of circumstances, the erectile capacity and coital frequency is markedly reduced compared to the preinjury levels.[60] Other spinal cord lesions such as herniated disks or tumors, amyotrophic lateral sclerosis, and tabes dorsalis may also produce sexual dysfunction.

Thiamine, B_{12}, and nicotinic acid deficiencies have led to impotence which can be persistent if significant neuronal damage has occurred. Central and peripheral neuropathies are probably causally interrelated with general debility; in such situations all aspects of sexual function may be impaired.

Cardiovascular causes of sexual dysfunction may be the most obvious from an etiologic standpoint. Central cardiogenic impotence is basically related to poor output states such as congestive heart failure or anginal syndromes occurring during sexual excitement. Subsequent pain or fear of pain in these circumstances can lead to impotence despite initially adequate endorgan engorgement.[61] Obliterative peripheral vascular disease as classically described by Leriche and Morel can also lead to inadequate end-organ perfusion.[62] Fibrosis, calcification, and luminal obstruction of small vessels of the cavernous tissue have been demonstrated to occur with aging.[63] The earliest manifestation of this process may be intimal smooth muscle hyperplasia at the branch points of the arteries involved. These structures were originally felt to be the physiologic regulators of blood flow (polsters) but in fact they probably represent pathologic entities related to atherosclerosis.[28] The presence of adequate femoral, dorsalis pedis, or posterior tibial pulses is not sufficient evidence to preclude significant vascular disease elsewhere; such disease might affect the pudendal artery and more distal small vessel input into the corpora cavernosa.

The most common endocrine abnormality associated with sexual dysfunction is diabetes mellitus. The incidence of impotence in diabetic males tends to increase with age, beginning much earlier and being much more common than in the general population. Approximately 15% of diabetic men 30 to 34 years old are impotent; this increases to approximately 55% by 60 years of age.[64] The severity of the diabetes, duration of the disease, type of medication, or quality of control is apparently unrelated to the incidence of sexual dysfunction.[65] Although diabetes is primarily an endocrine disturbance, hormonal factors per se do not appear to be directly related to the sexual dysfunction. The etiologic factors for impotence appear to be the neurologic and vascular complications of the disease. The neuropathy of diabetes has long been considered by many to be the major etiologic factor in diabetic impotence.[65,66] Only recently has emphasis been placed on the vascular factor with regard to the microangiopathic changes that appear approximately 15 years earlier in the diabetic than in the nondiabetic.[65,67] Jevtich et al reviewed the vascular and neuropathic changes in a group of impotent diabetics and presented compelling evidence that penile arterial disease is the primary factor responsible for impotence.[67] A number of other less common endocrine disorders has also been associated with sexual dysfunction.[54]

Urologic surgery for prostatic disease has been associated with variable degrees of impotence, depending on the surgical approach employed. Radical prostatectomy by either a transabdominal or perineal route would be expected to produce impotence, as major pelvic neurologic and vascular destruction usually occurs with these operations. Exceptions do occur, however, and potency is perhaps retained in more patients than previously presumed.[68,69] This raises the question of the significance of preoperative suggestion by the surgeon that impotence is inevitable.[70] Finkle and Prian noted a 29% incidence of impotence after simple perineal prostatectomy, 13% after suprapubic prostatectomy, and 5% after transurethral resection of the prostate.[71] However, unless transabdominal or transurethral prostatectomies for benign disease are complicated by serious surgical complications or postoperative infection, there is little to support a direct cause and effect relationship for surgery with subsequent impotence. Objective studies comparing preoperative and postoperative nocturnal penile tumescence monitoring have shown no instance of complete loss of penile erection postoperatively, and generally the postoperative status equaled the preoperative status despite occasional discrepancies as determined by sexual history.[72,73] The level of patient anxiety, preoperative explanation of the surgical procedure and expected outcome, and the patient's general satisfaction with life, may make the difference between postoperative potency and impotence.[74] Retrograde ejaculation does result following prostatectomy and it is therefore suggested that a detailed explanation of this surgical consequence be given to the patient in an effort to prevent misunderstanding and to help maintain the preoperative level of function.

In addition to the various types of prostatectomy, radical cystectomy with urinary diversion, extensive pelvic lymphadenectomy, and total penectomy are urologic cancer procedures that are commonly performed in the elderly and that may be associated with sexual dysfunction. Partial penectomy may be associated with decreased sensation due to removal of the glans penis, but erectile ability may still be satisfactory for vaginal penetration, and ejaculation as well as orgasm may be retained.[70]

Sexual dysfunction after surgery for lower bowel disease appears to be related to the extent of the resection and the age of the patient. Proctocolectomy is generally performed for benign disease, and impotence occurs in from 0% to 20% of patients. Abdominoperineal resection for the treatment of carcinoma requires a much more extensive dissection and is generally performed in older patients. The incidence of impotence is as high as 100% in the reports reviewed by Yeager and Van Heerden[75] with ejaculatory disturbances appearing to occur less frequently than erectile dysfunction. Once again, it is important to evaluate the psychosexual attitudes and sexual function preoperatively before assuming that these have been disturbed postoperatively.

Aortoiliac surgery for vascular disease results in extensive dissection in the retroperitoneum and pelvis with possible neural and/or vascular disruption. The incidence of postoperative impotence until 1978 ranged as high as 80% in a review of the literature.[76] Subsequently, DePalma et al have preserved postoperative function with a nerve-sparing technique.[76] These results were recently confirmed in a large series reported by Flanigan et al who utilized nerve-sparing dissection and particular attention to preservation or improvement of the pelvic blood flow with vascular bypass.[77] Thirty percent of their patients with preoperative impotence regained sexual function, and no patient with normal preoperative potency became impotent postoperatively.

The effects on sexual function in females of the various disorders considered above have not been as extensively studied with regard to the particular phases of the sexual response cycle. For example, the effect of diabetes on vaginal lubrication is not known. Specific gynecologic problems are encountered in the elderly female; these are due to the previously mentioned decrease in estrogenic influence on the generative tissues and the loss of elasticity and support of the pelvic and genital structures.[51] The thin vulvular and vaginal mucosa is susceptible to infectious processes of various etiologies, but particularly those due to the *Candida* species. The inflammatory process may make this area painful, friable, or pruritic. Associated relaxation of the pelvic supporting structures may produce incontinence that may in turn worsen the above problems.

The incidence of vulvar carcinoma peaks during the geriatric years and any suspicious lesions require rapid investigation.[51] Postmenopausal bleeding and any enlargement of the uterus or ovaries may be associated with endometrial or ovarian carcinoma, respectively, in the elderly age group. Any surgical intervention may temporarily or permanently alter female sexual function. Pain, deformity, and/or limited mobility due to osteoporosis may make sexual activity impossible. Arthritis in general may have similar limiting efects on either partner.

Pharmacologic interference with sexual function is a common and often unsuspected side effect of many of the drugs used so commonly in our society. Much of our knowledge in this regard is based on case reports, with well-controlled studies of the sexual side effects of drugs usually lacking. While the information for males is incomplete, it is virtually absent for females. Although the elderly make up only approximately 11% of the United States population at this time, they fill approximately 30% of the prescriptions that are written and use a disproportionately large number of over-the-counter medications for various problems.[78] The disease states and their treatment, as has been noted above, may affect the individual's real or perceived sexual ability. In addition, some of the most commonly prescribed medications, ie, psychotropic drugs and antihypertensive agents, are also the most common offenders with regard to drug-induced sexual dysfunction. Furthermore, the interactions and possible synergism of different drugs in impairing sexual function is certainly possible, but the true incidence of this is largely unknown. Also with aging, drug effects may be more significant, as drug distribution, metabolism, and excretion may be altered due to changes in cardiac, hepatic, and renal function.[78] Theoretical mechanisms of drug-induced sexual dysfunction include production of CNS sedation and/or depression, anticholinergic or antiadrenergic effects, elevation of plasma prolactin levels, direct antiandrogen effects, antiestrogen effects, and other as of yet unknown mechanisms.

The antihypertensive agents are the largest pharmacologic class of drugs associated with sexual dysfunction and essentially every antihypertensive drug currently in use has been at some time associated with impotence or ejaculatory failure in males.[79] These drugs may be categorized into three major classes–diuretics, vasodilators, and sympatholytics. Diuretics are commonly used agents with relatively rare sexual side effects, although some controversy exists in the literature in this regard.[80–83] Problems with libido have been reported as have problems with erectile and ejaculatory function, particularly with their long-term use. Spironolactone has a high incidence of decreased libido and impotence associated with its use. This may be based on its known antiandrogen effects[79,83] which may result in gynecomastia. The vasodilator hydralazine hydrochloride has generally been felt to be free of sexual dysfunction side effects, although two recent reviews have cited case reports of impotence associated with this drug.[81,83] Minoxidil also seems to be relatively free of these side effects.

The sympatholytic agents are some of the most commonly used antihypertensives and the ones most likely to be associated with sexual dysfunction. These agents all alter sympathetic nervous system activity at various sites of action and may therefore be further subcategorized.[82] Centrally acting agents include methyldopa, clonidine hydrochloride, and reserpine. Collected reviews would seem to indicate male erectile failure in one fourth to one third of patients using methyldopa. Ejaculatory problems are less common.[79,82,83] The mechanisms involved appear to be CNS sedation and depression as well as associated increases in serum prolactin.[79] α- and β-Blockers are also useful agents whose antihypertensive action is on a peripheral level. Phenoxybenzamine hydrochloride and phentolamine are both α-adrenergic receptor blocking agents that have been shown to decrease luteinizing hormone (LH) production and to adversely affect ejaculation on a peripheral level. Prazosin hydrochloride is a selective postganglionic α-1-blocker that appears to have relatively rare adverse sexual effects. This drug, however, is also quite new.[82] Propranolol hydrochloride is a β-blocker that has been associated with impaired libido in men and women as well as with impotence in a small percentage of male patients.[81–83] These effects generally occur at the higher dosage range. Adverse effects on sexual function with the newer agent, metoprolol, have not been reported in humans.

Psychotropic drugs are also commonly prescribed for the elderly and may be associated with sexual dysfunction. Major tranquilizers are used primarily as antipsychotic medications and consist of the phenothiazines, butyrophenones, and thioxanthines. All produce markedly disruptive central effects as attested to by acute dystonic reactions, parkinsonian symptoms, and tardive dyskinesias. Decreased libido, impotence, and inhibition of ejaculation have all been reported with these drugs, although orgasm may remain intact.[80]

Antidepressants are made up of two major groups of compounds—tricyclics and monoamine oxidase inhibitors. The tricyclic antidepressants have prominent sedative and anticholinergic properties and can result in decreased libido and impotence. Impaired and/or painful ejaculation has been described for amitriptyline hydrochloride and imipramine hydrochloride.[81] Imipramine has also been associated with delayed orgasm in women.[81] Monoamine oxidase inhibitors interfere with the metabolism of sympathomimetic amines and although less sedating than the tricyclic antidepressants, they may still be associated with sexual dysfunction, probably by adverse effects on central and peripheral mechanisms.

The minor tranquilizers or antianxiety agents, particularly the benzodiazepine compounds, exert a depressive effect on the limbic system, the septal region, and the brain-stem reticular formation. Libido can be reduced and impotence can also occur.[81] Meprobamate, barbiturates, and other sedative-hypnotics exert a central effect similar to that of the benzodiazepines.

Drugs with primarily anticholinergic effects are useful in a variety of clinical settings as antiparkinsonian agents, antinausea, and antivertigo drugs, muscle relaxants, and antiarrhythmics, as well as inhibitors of urinary tract and gastrointestinal (GI) smooth muscle activity. These agents may all interfere with erectile ability, while the libido is generally left intact.[81] These side effects may be accounted for by inhibition of ganglionic transmission and perhaps by direct antimuscarinic action at the level of the end organ.

Sexual dysfunction may also be induced by a number of other drugs prescribed for a variety of disorders. Clofibrate, used in the treatment of hyperlipidemia, may decrease libido and cause impotence. Interference with androgen activity or metabolism has been postulated as a mechanism.[84] Cimetidine is now widely used in the treatment of peptic ulcer disease. It is an antihistaminic agent without anticholinergic properties, but it has been reported to produce decreased libido and impotence. It has a direct antiandrogen effect and may also increase prolactin secretion.[85] Metoclopramide hydrochloride, useful in improving gastric emptying, will also markedly increase serum prolactin levels.[86] Drugs with direct antiandrogen activity may also be important in the elderly male population. The use of estrogens for the treatment of carcinoma of the prostate is relatively common, as this disease is largely found in this group of patients. Ellis and Grayhack studied 82 patients with carcinoma of the prostate who were treated with orchiectomy, estrogens, or both.[31] Persistent sexual function was noted in all three treatment groups. However, in general, an overall decrease in sexual activity and ability was found following medical or surgical castration. It should be remembered that digoxin may also have estrogenlike side effects with the production of gynecomastia, and hence this drug may also affect sexual function in elderly males.

Finally, drugs with abuse potential are often believed to enhance sexual performance and perhaps have aphrodisiac properties. In reality, they may produce problems with sexual function, particularly with their long-term use. Alcohol and narcotic pain medications, as well as barbituates, may be abused by the elderly. Drugs such as alcohol may have a disinhibiting effect that may be translated into increased libido and perceived as a heightened sexual response under some circumstances.[79] Excessive or chronic use, however, results in decreased sexual responsiveness. Decreased sexual arousal, increased ejaculatory latency, and decreased orgastic pleasure have been noted to parallel the blood alcohol content of human males studied under controlled conditions.[87,88] In women, decreased desire and performance has been noted as well as inhibition of orgasm.[89] Narcotics such as codeine and meperidine hydrochloride are usually associated with a diminution of sexual activity and interest, impotence, and delayed ejaculation with chronic use.[90] Nicotine inhaled as cigarette smoke may have a deleterious effect on potency, probably secondary to local vasoconstriction.[91] This may be particularly troublesome when associated with compromised vascular flow due to atherosclerotic peripheral vascular disease.

Psychosexual Aspects

One of the major psychological determinants of sexual functioning in the elderly relates to the interpretation, or misinterpretation, of the normal physiologic changes that occur with aging. Some couples adapt naturally to their slower response times. In others, however, sexual expectations do not change in a manner corresponding to the physiologic changes; the latter are therefore misinterpreted with a worsening of sexual function on a psychological basis. The male may view his slowly developing erection as the onset of sexual impotence that he expected to inevitably occur sooner or later. The female may feel she is not sexually appealing and hence not able to excite her partner. Her slow lubrication response may be similarly misinterpreted by each partner. The extreme of this situation is encountered in what has been termed the widower's and widow's syndrome by Masters and Johnson.[92] In each case, the subject in question has experienced a prolonged period of voluntary or involuntary sexual continence, usually due to failing health or terminal illness of their spouse. When subsequently faced with a sexual opportunity, they often fail to respond with an adequate penile erection or vaginal lubrication. The changes of aging that usually occur gradually are suddenly and dramatically realized. This psychosexual trauma may result in persistent sexual dysfunction. Alternatively, an understanding and knowledgeable partner or psychotherapy may help resolve the problem.[92]

The interplay of factors here is extremely complex relating in part to attitudes toward sex in general, in part to attitudes toward the elderly, and in relationship to attitudes toward sex in the elderly by the elderly themselves as well as by others. Unfortunately, our culture is overly youth-oriented with aging considered a disease rather than a normal process.[93] Oldness is equated with slowness and inflexibility,[94] and the elderly have been described as a minority of invisible people who are not attractively packaged.[95] These feelings are somewhat self-perpetuating as the elderly of today were the youth of yesterday who had similar notions. The general feelings also do not change much with aging, and the majority of elderly males and females do in fact feel unattractive.[96]

The attitude toward sex in general also follows similar cultural dictates. Sex is felt by young and old alike to be the province of the young. It becomes a self-fulfilling prophecy that sexual activity decreases during middle age and may even become nonexistent.[97] Acceptance of these stereotyped views is beneficial to the younger generation in several ways. It helps to insure the young their possible inheritance and makes it easier to manage the elderly.[93] Inhibiting sex in the elderly also removes them from any type of sexual competition that may be threatening to younger people.[93] For some elderly persons an overt decline in sexual interest may be adaptive and defensive for those who choose to accept it and do not want to change their sexual patterns.[10] This is particularly true for the elderly who never had much interest in sexual activity, for those with a sexually incapacitated partner, and for those who have no available partner. This may be true for aging females who on an average live 7 years longer than men. If married, females usually get married 4 years younger, leaving a potential partnerless span of 11 years or more.[10]

On the other side of the coin, however, an early healthy interest in sex with increased sexual activity usually results in increased sexual activity later in life. Continued sexual activity is highly dependent upon past interest and activity as initially demonstrated by Kinsey[3,4] and later confirmed in other major reports.[5,6,10] Past enjoyment, more than past activity, may be especially important for continued sexual activity and interest in women.[10]

In this regard, sexual knowledge and sexual experience correlate positively with sexual interest and activity. This begins as noted above with knowledge and acceptance of the normal physiologic changes that occur with aging. Sexual knowledge may be gained from friends, physicians, the news media, women's or men's groups, and experience. In general, less factual knowledge is associated with more restrictive views towards sexuality, as demonstrated for both males and females.[96] It was noted, however, that it was not known if increased instruction and education would change sexual attitudes during that period of life.[96] Religion also correlated in this regard–the higher the religious devoutness, the less the associated sexual knowledge and sexual activity.[96,98]

Specific attitudes towards sexuality in the elderly parallel the discussion above. As noted earlier, however, it is believed that negative views are widely held toward sex in the elderly although little evidence exists to support this.[13,14] An early study by Golde and Kogan utilized a sentence completion test to demonstrate that a group of college students felt that sex was unimportant and/or negligible for older people.[99] LaTorre and Kear[13] studied the attitudes of 80 undergraduates and 40 nursing home staff toward sexuality in the elderly. They found no negative attitudes, but did demonstrate that coitus was felt to be less credible in the aged than in young people. The nursing home staff overall showed more negative attitudes towards sex in general than did the college students.[13] Kass, in a separate study, found nursing home staff more liberal than the nursing home residents.[100] Wasow and Loeb, however, showed that most elderly persons felt that sex was appropriate for their age group even if they were not personally involved.[96] Brody reported a study in the *New York Times* that demonstrated more liberal views and sexual expression among the geriatric population than previously assumed.[101] It is therefore clear that while geriatric sexuality may not be viewed negatively by the young or the old, it may nonetheless seem less credible. This may result from the persistence of false stereotypes or simply reflect the fact that sexual activity really does decrease with age and is therefore truly less credible when comparing historical vignettes with young and old characters in any particular testing situation.[13]

Other psychosexual attitudes may also influence sexual function. Sexual boredom may be a common detrimental factor in any long-standing relationship.[92] Masters and Johnson suggest variety in sexual activity to overcome this problem just as one varies the menu from day to day.[92] At the opposite extreme, love is an often overlooked factor in many of the studies. West demonstrated that a series of elderly people judged their past experiences as either pleasant or unpleasant in direct proportion to the feelings of love that they had for their partner.[102] This clearly plays a significant role for elderly couples, if not so much for researchers interested in the field.

Demographic and Social Factors

Various demographic and social factors exert an important influence on sexual function in the elderly. The increasing size of the elderly population was mentioned earlier, as was the fact that women generally survive longer than men and hence may outlive their marital partner by a decade or more. In fact, over the age of 65 years, there are four unmarried women for every man.[11] Sex and marital status both significantly affect sexual interest and activity. In all elderly age groups, sexual interest and activity was higher in men than in women.[8] In the Duke University Study,[10] the authors demonstrated that the male partner was most commonly to blame for stopping intercourse. The average age at this point was 68 years for men and 60 years for women. Other authors, however, have demonstrated that female age may be the most important contributing factor for decreasing frequency of intercourse.[103] Generally, a decline in interest and activity has been demonstrated in both sexes. An interesting subgroup of people, however, has been identified who demonstrate both increased sexual activity and interest with aging.[7] In addition, a biologically advantaged group of aged individuals was also studied, and an age-related decline of interest did not occur in this group, further indicating that other factors besides aging must play a role.[9]

Marital status has not been found to markedly affect sexual activity and interest in men but does significantly alter these parameters in women. Christenson and Gagnon showed that 88% of married 50-year-old women and 70% of married 60-year-old women engaged in intercourse, whereas only 37% and 12% of 50- and 60-year-old unmarried women experienced the same.[98] Pfeiffer and Davis found similar values, indicating that the availability of a socially acceptable partner plays a very important role in relation to activity, if not interest.[10] Further consideration must be given to a comparison of the unmarried females in these studies who are either separated, divorced, or widowed versus those who were never married. The former group maintained more contact with eligible males and were able to utilize their adaptive social skills to develop these contacts compared to the women who were never married.[104] Another interesting point raised by these authors is that masturbation, when used as a frequent sexual outlet, also decreased with aging. This decline obviously cannot be attributable to the lack of availability of a coital partner.[104]

The opportunity to meet others in a group or private setting is somewhat restricted for the elderly. Again, most establishments cater to entertainment and activities that involve young people. Even special events for the elderly require adequate economic resources to provide transportation, clothing, and admission prices in most cases.[105] These minor expenditures may become substantial investments for someone whose income is fixed.[105]

Lack of privacy, particularly with reference to living conditions, also becomes a major obstacle for sexual activity in the elderly. This troublesome situation may exist for those living alone in housing projects for the elderly, for those living with family or friends, and for older persons who live in nursing homes. Jealousy and competition may make sexual expression difficult as does the constant supervision and observation in any of these environments.

CONCLUSION

It is readily evident that sexual function in males and females involves a complex series of neurologic and vascular phenomena occurring within a permissive hormonal and psychological milieu. Throughout one's sexual lifetime, various intrinsic and extrinsic factors affect this normally delicately balanced system. With aging, the system shifts gears as does the rest of the body and physiologic changes normally result in a more gradual and diminished sexual response. It is clear, however, that sexual interest and activity do not come to a grinding halt at any time. For the most part, we have intentionally left out statistics that show $x\%$ of men and $y\%$ of women active at specific ages. At any time in life, some people will be active and others will not, and although a gradual decline in activity has been demonstrated in numerous studies, it is important to realize that for a given individual, statistics are meaningless. Many studies have shown marked individual variation in interest, activity, and means of sexual expression. The quality of the sexual experience and the love and intimacy that are involved cannot be measured by statistics.

It becomes increasingly important for physicians and counselors of the elderly to be aware of their continued sexual needs. It is necessary to recognize that the patient with vague nonspecific complaints, often involving the pelvic area, may be seeking information concerning his or her own sexuality. This information should be sought by the physician when medical or surgical therapeutics are instituted that have a significant chance of impairing sexual function. Finally, it is equally important to realize that despite the increasing interest in this subject, the lives of the elderly consist of much more than just sexual activity. As Pfeiffer has stated, there is no need for the clinician to "whip older people into some kind of sexual frenzy or instill new or uncongenial patterns of sexual expression into their aging patients."[106] Rather, as he advocates, "encouraging and assuring continuity of sexual expression for those for whom this has constituted an important part of their lives in the past" should be the direction we follow.[106] There are obviously very sensitive issues involved in sexual counseling of the elderly. But overall, sexual interest and activity may remain a very real and significant aspect of the lives of elderly men and women. Many challenges still exist with regard to furthering our knowledge of the physiologic, psychological, and social factors involved in normal and abnormal sexual function.

REFERENCES

1. Renshaw DC: Sexuality in older women? *J Clin Psychiatry* 1981;42:3–4.
2. Berezin MA: Sex and old age: a further review of the literature. *J Geriatr Psychiatry* 1976;9:189–209.
3. Kinsey AC, Pomeroy WB, Martin CR: *Sexual Behavior in the Human Male.* Philadelphia, WB Saunders Co, 1948.
4. Kinsey AC, Pomeroy WB, Martin CR, et al: *Sexual Behavior in the Human Female.* Philadelphia, WB Saunders Co, 1953.
5. Masters WH, Johnson VE: *Human Sexual Response.* Boston, Little, Brown & Co, 1966.
6. Masters WH, Johnson VE: *Human Sexual Inadequacy.* Boston, Little, Brown & Co, 1970.
7. Pfeiffer E, Verwoerdt A, Wang H-S: Sexual behavior in aged men and women. *Arch Gen Psychiatry* 1968;19:753–758.
8. Verwoerdt A, Pfeiffer E, Wang H-S: Sexual behavior in senescence. *Geriatrics* 1969;24:137–154.
9. Pfeiffer E, Verwoerdt A, Wang H-S: The natural history of sexual behavior in a biologically advantaged group of aged individuals. *J Gerontol* 1969;24:193–198.
10. Pfeiffer E, Davis GC: Determinants of sexual behavior in middle and old age. *J Am Geriatr Soc* 1972;20:151–158.
11. Ludeman K: The sexuality of the older person: review of the literature. *Gerontologist* 1981;21:203–208.
12. Thomas LE: Sexuality and aging: essential vitamin or popcorn? *Gerontologist* 1982;22:240–243.
13. LaTorre RA, Kear K: Attitudes toward sex in the aged. *Arch Sex Behav* 1977;6:203–213.
14. Damrosch SP: Nursing students' attitudes toward sexually active older persons. *Nurs Res* 1982;31:252–255.
15. Wagner G: Erection, anatomy, in Wagner G and Green R (eds): *Impotence.* New York, Plenum Press, 1981, pp 7–24.
16. Deysach LJ: The comparative morphology of the erectile tissue of the penis with especial emphasis on the probable mechanism of erection. *Am J Anat* 1939;64:111–131.
17. Newman HF, Northup JD: Mechanism of human penile erection: an overview. *Urology* 1981;17:399–408.

18. Wein AJ, Van Arsdalen KN, Hanno PH, et al: Physiology of male sexual function, in Rajfer J (ed): *Urologic Endocrinology*. Philadelphia, WB Saunders Co, in press.
19. Hollingshead WH: *Textbook of Anatomy*. New York, Harper & Row, 1967, pp 714–717.
20. Lich R Jr, Howerton LW, Amin M: Anatomy and surgical approach to the urogenital tract in the male, in Harrison JH, Gittes RF, Perlmutter AD, et al (eds): *Campbell's Urology*. Philadelphia, WB Saunders Co, 1979, pp 3–33.
21. Wagner G: Erection, Physiology and Endocrinology, in Wagner G, Green R (eds): *Impotence*. New York, Plenum Press, 1981, pp 25–26.
22. Wein AJ, Fishkin R, Carpiniello VL, et al: Expansion without significant rigidity during nocturnal penile tumescence testing: a potential source of misinterpretation. *J Urol* 1981;126:343–344.
23. Benson GS: Mechanisms of penile erection. *Invest Urol* 1981;19:65–69.
24. Dorr LD, Brody MJ: Hemodynamic mechanism of erection in the canine penis. *Am J Physiol* 1967;213:1526–1531.
25. Shirai M, Ishii N: Hemodynamics of erection in man. *Arch Androl* 1981;6:27–32.
26. Benson GS, Lipschultz LI, McConnell J: Mechanisms of human erection, emission and ejaculation: Current clinical concepts, in von Eschenbach AC and Rodriguez DB (eds): *Sexual Rehabilitation of the Urologic Cancer Patient*. Boston, GK Hall Medical Publishers, 1979, pp 54–68.
27. Conti G: L'érection du pénis humain et ses bases morphologicovasculaires. *Acta Anat (Basel)* 1952;14:217–262.
28. Benson GS, McConnell J, Schmidt WA: Penile polsters: functional structures or atherosclerotic changes? *J Urol* 1981;125: 800–803.
29. Weiss HD: The physiology of human penile erection. *Ann Intern Med* 1972;76:793–799.
30. Bremer J: *Asexualization. A Followup Study of 244 Cases*. New York, Macmillan Co, 1959.
31. Ellis WJ, Grayhack JT: Sexual function in aging males after orchiectomy and estrogen therapy. *J Urol* 1963;89:895–899.
32. Heim N: Sexual behavior of castrated sex offenders. *Arch Sex Behav* 1981;10:11–19.
33. Kolodny RC, Masters WH, Johnson VE: *Textbook of Sexual Medicine*. Boston, Little, Brown & Co, 1979.
34. Newman HF, Reiss H, Northup JD: Physical basis of emission, ejaculation and orgasm in the male. *Urology* 1982;19:341–350.
35. Siroky MB, Krane RJ: Physiology of Male Sexual Function, in Krane RJ and Siroky MB (eds): *Clinical Neuro-Urology*. Boston, Little, Brown & Co, 1979, pp 45–62.
36. Walsh PC, Amelar RD: Embryology, anatomy and physiology of the male reproductive system, in Amelar RD, Dubin L, Walsh PC (eds): *Male Infertility*. Philadelphia, WB Saunders Co, 1977, pp 3–32.
37. Kraemer HC, Becker HB, Brodie HKH, et al: Orgasmic frequency and plasma testosterone levels in normal human males. *Arch Sex Behav* 1976;5:125–132.
38. Fox CA, Ismail AAA, Love DN, et al: Studies on the relationship between plasma testosterone levels and human sexual activity. *J Endocrinol* 1972;52:51–58.
39. Lee PA, Jaffe RB, Midgley AR: Lack of alteration of serum gonadotropins in men and women following sexual intercourse. *Am J Obstet Gynecol* 1974;120:985–987.
40. Raboch J, Starka L: Reported coital activity of men and levels of plasma testosterone. *Arch Sex Behav* 1973;2:309–315.
41. Stearns EL, Winter JSD, Faiman C: Effects of coitus on gonadotropin, prolactin and sex steroid levels in man. *J Clin Endocrinol Metab* 1973;37:687–691.
42. Cohen HD, Rosen RC, Goldstein L: Electroencephalographic laterality changes during human sexual orgasm. *Arch Sex Behav* 1976;5:189–199.
43. Kaplan HS: *The New Sex Therapy*. New York, The New York Times Book Co, 1974.
44. Persky H, Lief HI, O'Brien CT, et al: Reproductive hormone levels and sexual behavior of young couples during the menstrual cycle, in Gemme R, Wheeler CL (eds): *Progress in Sexology*. New York, Plenum Press, 1977, pp 293–310.
45. Edwards AE, Husted JR: Penile sensitivity, age, and sexual behavior. *J Clin Psychiatry* 1976;32:697–700.
46. Schwartz D, Mayaux MJ, Spira A, et al: Study of 484 fertile men, part II: relation between age (20–59) and semen characteristics. *Int J Androl* 1981;4:450–456.
47. Baker HWG, Burger HG, deKretser DM,

et al: Changes in the pituitary-testicular system with age. *Clin Endocrinol* 1976; 34:730–735.
48. Vermeulen A, Rubens R, Verdonck L: Testosterone secretion and metabolism in male senescence. *J Clin Endocrinol Metab* 1976;34:730–735.
49. Harman SM, Isitouras PD: Reproductive hormones in aging men. I. Measurement of sex steroids, basal LH, and response to hCG. *J Clin Endocrinol Metab* 1980; 51:35–40.
50. Tsitouras PD, Martin CE, Harman SM: Relationship of serum testosterone to sexual activity in healthy elderly men. *J Gerontol* 1982;37:288–293.
51. Glowacki G: Postmenopausal gyn problems. *Hosp Pract* 1977;5:107–113.
52. Glover BH: Sex counseling of the elderly. *Hosp Pract* 1977;12:101–113.
53. Shearer MR, Shearer ML: Sexuality and sexual counseling in the elderly. *Clin Obstet Gynecol* 1977;20:197–208.
54. Van Arsdalen KN, Malloy TR, Wein AJ: Male Sexual Dysfunction, in Rajfer J (ed): *Urologic Endocrinology*. Philadelphia, WB Saunders Co, in press.
55. Levine SB: Marital sexual dysfunction: erectile dysfunction. *Ann Intern Med* 1976; 85:342–350.
56. Kalliomake JL, Markkanien TK, Mustonen VA: Sexual behavior after cerebral vascular accident. *Fertil Steril* 1961;12:156–158.
57. Krane RJ, Siroky MB: Neurophysiology of erection. *Urol Clin North Am* 1981;8:91–102.
58. Lilius H, Valtonen E, Wikstrom J: Sexual problems in patients suffering from multiple sclerosis. *J Chronic Dis* 1976;29: 643–647.
59. Bors E, Comarr AE: Neurologic disturbances of sexual function with special reference to 529 patients with spinal cord injury. *Urol Surv* 1960;10:191–221.
60. Amelar RD, Dubin L: Sexual function and fertility in paraplegic males. *Urology* 1982;20:62–65.
61. Gobel AJ: Sexuality and coronary heart disease. *Patient Management* 1974;3:25.
62. Leriche R, Morel A: Syndrome of thrombotic obliteration of aortic bifurcation. *Ann Surg* 1948;127:193–206.
63. Ruzbarsky V, Michal V: Morphologic changes in the arterial bed of the penis with aging. *Invest Urol* 1977;15:194–199.
64. Smith AD: Causes and classification of impotence. *Urol Clin North Am* 1981;8: 79–89.
65. Schiavi RC: Male erectile disorders. *Annu Rev Med* 1981;35:509–520.
66. Ellenberg M: Impotence in diabetes: a neurologic rather than an endocrinologic problem. *Med Aspects Hum Sex* 1973;7: pp 12–28.
67. Jevtich MJ, Edson M, Jarman WD, et al: Vascular factors in erectile failure among diabetics. *Urology* 1982;19:163–168.
68. Finkle AL, Taylor SP: Sexual potency after radical prostatectomy. *J Urol* 1981;125: 350–352.
69. Walsh PC, Donker PJ: Impotence following radical prostatectomy: insight into etiology and prevention. *J Urol* 1982; 128:492–497.
70. Malin JM: Sex after urologic surgery. *Med Aspects Hum Sex* 1973;7: pp 245–264.
71. Finkle A, Prian D: Sexual potency in elderly men before and after prostatectomy. *JAMA* 1966;196:125.
72. Madorsky ML, Ashamalla MG, Schussler I, et al: Post-prostatectomy impotence. *J Urol* 1976;115:401–403.
73. So EP, Ho PC, Bodenstab W, et al: Erectile impotence associated with transurethral prostatectomy. *Urology* 1982; 19:259–262.
74. Zohar J, Meiraz D, Moaz B, et al: Factors influencing sexual activity after prostatectomy: a prospective study. *J Urol* 1976; 116:332–334.
75. Yeager ES, Van Heerden JA: Sexual dysfunction following proctocolectomy and abdominoperineal resection. *Ann Surg* 1980;191:169–170.
76. DePalma RG, Levine SB, Feldman S: Preservation of erectile function after aortoiliac reconstruction. *Arch Surg* 1978; 113:958–962.
77. Flanigan DP, Schuler JJ, Keifer T, et al: Elimination of iatrogenic impotence and improvement of sexual function after aortoiliac revascularization. *Arch Surg* 1982; 117:544–550.
78. Thompson TL, Moran MG, Nies AS: Psychotropic drug use in the elderly. *N Engl Med J* 1983;308:134–138.
79. Horowitz JD, Gobel AJ: Drugs and im-

paired male sexual function. *Drugs* 1979; 18:206–217.

80. Drugs that cause sexual dysfunction. *Med Lett Drugs Ther* 1980;22:108–110.
81. Drugs that cause sexual dysfunction. *Med Lett Drugs Ther* 1983;25:73–76.
82. Reichgott MJ: Problems of sexual function in patients with hypertension. *Cardiovasc Med* 1979;4:149–156.
83. Papadopoulos C: Cardiovascular drugs and sexuality. *Arch Intern Med* 1980;140: 1341–1345.
84. Schneider J, Kaffarnik H: Impotence in patients treated with clofibrate. *Atherosclerosis* 1975;21:455–457.
85. Peden NR, Cargill JM, Browning MCK, et al: Male sexual dysfunction during treatment with cimetidine. *Br Med J* 1979; 1:659.
86. Falaschi P, Frajese G, Sciarra F, et al: Influence of hyperprolactinaemia due to metoclopramide on gonadal function in men. *Clin Endocrinol* (Oxf) 1978;8: 427–433.
87. Malatesta VJ, Pollack RH, Willbanks WA, et al: Alcohol effects on the orgasmic-ejaculatory response in human males. *J Sex Res* 1979;15:101–107.
88. Rubin HB, Henson DE: Effects of drugs on male sexual function. *Advances Behav Pharmacol* 1979;2:65–86.
89. Viamontes JA: Alcohol abuse and sexual dysfunction. *Med Aspects Hum Sex* 1974; 8:185–186.
90. Mirin SM, Meyer RE, Mendelson JH, et al: Opiate use and sexual function. *Am J Psychiatry* 1980;137:909–915.
91. Forsberg L, Gustavii B, Hajerback T, et al: Impotence, smoking and β-blocking drugs. *Fertil Steril* 1979;31:589–591.
92. Masters WH, Johnson VE: Sex and the aging process. *J Am Geriatr Soc* 1981;29: 385–390.
93. Falk G, Falk UA: Sexuality and the aged. *Nurs Outlook* 1980;28:51–55.
94. Renshaw D: Sex and the senior citizen. *Medical Times* 1979;107:27–33.
95. Weinberg J: Sexual expression in late life. *Am J Psychiatry* 1969;126:159–162.
96. Wasow M, Loeb MB: Sexuality in nursing homes. *J Am Geriatr Soc* 1979;27:73–79.
97. Zinberg NE: Social learning and self-image in aging. *J Geriatr Psychiatry* 1976;9:131–150.
98. Christenson CV, Gagnon JH: Sexual behavior in a group of older women. *J Gerontol* 1975;9:351–356.
99. Golde P, Kogan N: A sentence completion procedure for assessing attitudes toward old people. *J Gerontol* 1959;14:355–360.
100. Kaas MJ: Sexual expression of the elderly in nursing homes. *Gerontologist* 1978;18: 372–378.
101. Brody JE: Survey of aged reveals liberal views on sex. *The New York Times* April 22, 1980, C1–C2.
102. West ND: Sex in geriatrics: myth or miracle? *J Am Geriatr Soc* 1975;23:551–552.
103. Udry JR, Deven FR, Coleman SJ: A cross-national comparison of male and female age on frequency of marital intercourse. *J Biosoc Sci* 1982;14:1–6.
104. Christenson CV, Johnson AB: Sexual patterns in a group of older never-married women. *J Geriatr Psychiatry* 1973;6:80–98.
105. Friedeman JS: Factors influencing sexual expression in aging persons: a review of the literature. *J Psychiatr Nursing* 1978; July: 34–47.
106. Pfeiffer E: Sexuality in the aging individual. *J Am Geriatr Soc* 1974;11:481–484.

INDEX